Language Disorders

A Functional Approach to Assessment and Intervention

Robert E. Owens, Jr.
The College of St. Rose, Albany, NY

PEARSON

Boston • Columbus • Indianapolis • New York • San Francisco • Upper Saddle River
Amsterdam • Cape Town • Dubai • London • Madrid • Milan • Munich • Paris • Montréal • Toronto
Delhi • Mexico City • São Paulo • Sydney • Hong Kong • Seoul • Singapore • Taipei • Tokyo

Editor-in-Chief: *Jeffery Johnston*
Executive Editor and Publisher: *Stephen D. Dragin*
Editorial Assistant: *Michelle Hochberg*
Marketing Manager: *Joanna Sabella*
Production Editor: *Cynthia DeRocco*
Editorial Production Service: *Walsh & Associates, Inc.*
Manufacturing Buyer: *Megan Cochran*
Electronic Composition: *Jouve*
Interior Design: *Jouve*
Photo Researcher: Poyee Oster
Cover Designer: *Laura Gardner*
Cover Art: Vladgrin/Fotolia

Credits and acknowledgments borrowed from other sources and reproduced, with permission, in this textbook appear on the appropriate page within text.

Photo credits: Annie Fuller/Pearson: pp. 1, 65, 103, 131, 151, 175, 225, 245, 265, 281, 327, 361; Jim West/Alamy, p. 17.

Library of Congress Cataloging-in-Publication Data

Owens, Robert E.
Language disorders : a functional approach to assessment and intervention / Robert E. Owens Jr. — 6th ed.
p. ; cm.
Includes bibliographical references and index.
ISBN-13: 978-0-13-297872-9
ISBN-10: 0-13-297872-5
I. Title.
[DNLM: 1. Language Disorders. 2. Child. 3. Infant. 4. Language Therapy. WL 340.2]
616.85'5—dc23

2012049057

10

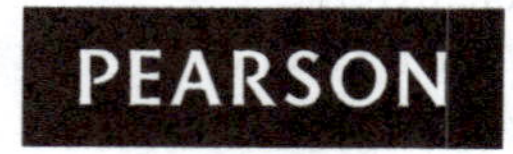

ISBN 10: 0-13-297872-5
ISBN 13: 978-0-13-297872-9

Contents

6 Language Sampling 151

7 Language Sample Analysis 175

8 Narrative Analysis 225

Appendices

Preface

The sixth edition of *Language Disorders: A Functional Approach to Assessment and Intervention* represents an exhaustive compilation of studies conducted by my professional colleagues and of several years of my own clinical work in speech-language pathology with both presymbolic and symbolic children and adults. In this book, I concentrate on children because of the special problems they exhibit in learning language. Adults who are acquiring language, or who have lost language and are attempting to regain it, represent a diverse group that would be difficult to address also in this text.

I call the model of assessment and intervention presented in this text *functional language*. This approach goes by other names, such as environmental or conversational, and includes elements of several other models. Where I have borrowed someone's model, ideas, or techniques, full credit is given to that person. I find assessment and intervention to be an adaptation of a little of this and a little of that within an overall theoretical framework. Readers should approach this text with this in mind. Some ideas presented are very practical and easy to implement, whereas others may not apply to particular intervention settings. Readers should use what they can, keeping in mind the overall model of using the natural environment and natural conversations as the context for training language. I am the first to acknowledge that I do not have a monopoly on assessment and intervention methods, nor do I pretend to have all of the answers.

Within *Language Disorders* I have made some content decisions that should be explained. I group all children with language problems, both delays and disorders, under the general rubric of *language-impaired*. This expedient decision was made recognizing that this text would not be addressing specific disorder populations except in a tangential manner.

Hopefully, you'll be pleased with the sixth edition. Professors who've used the text before will notice some new additions and changes in emphasis. These are based on professional feedback, reviewers' comments, student input, and the changing nature of speech and language services. Here is a partial list of updates and modifications.

- The text is thoroughly updated with the addition of several hundred new sources. This is the result of nearly as many hours of reading or perusing journal articles. In all honesty, I also looked at five other texts on this topic to see how the authors organized and explained language impairment.
- I've added a new chapter on early communication intervention as some reviewers suggested. This is a topic near and dear to my heart, and the model espoused by both the U.S. government and the American Speech-Language-Hearing Association is a functional one.
- I've included a large section on augmentative and alternative communication (AAC). Although strictly speaking, AAC is a mode of communication and not language intervention per se, many of the issues that must be addressed relate to language, and for some children learning language and communication without AAC may be almost impossible.
- New developments, such as inclusion and Response to Intervention or RTI have been added to the classroom intervention chapter in recognition of the effect these are having on what happens in the public schools.
- Since the last edition, the information on Specific Language Impairment and working memory has exploded, so readers will find this section greatly expanded over the previous edition.

- The number of children diagnosed with some variant of autism spectrum disorder (ASD) has continued to explode. I have attempted to expand discussion of this topic and new incidence figures and descriptive criteria.
- Luckily, the number of meta-analyses focusing on the best evidence-based practices has greatly increased since the last edition, although as a profession, speech-language pathologists (SLPs), especially those concerned with language intervention, still lag behind some other medical or medical-related professions. Wherever I have been able to find these professional articles, I have incorporated their results, even when they don't conform to what I might believe. That's how we learn and stay current, isn't it?
- The chapters on language analysis have been strengthened and consolidated into one and the discussion tightened to add more cohesion. In the past, these chapters tended to ramble on about the possibilities for analysis at the expense of the more important how-to.
- As in previous editions, I have included all the relevant information on children from culturally and linguistic diverse backgrounds. I'm in love with the increasingly diverse nature of U.S. society and believe it's essential that we serve those children who need our services to the best of our ability.

No doubt I've forgotten some of the changes. I hope you are pleased with the results.

I hope that you will find this text useful. Those who use the methods found within these pages tell me that they and their clients find them to be useful, effective, adaptable, and fun. Time will tell if you agree.

Acknowledgments

No text is written without the aid of other people. First, I thank the reviewers of this edition; I have tried to heed their sound advice.

No text is undertaken by the author alone, and I have been fortunate to have the support of some wonderful people. First, I must acknowledge my colleagues at my former employer who each nurtured me and encouraged me for so many years. These include Linda House, Ph.D., department chair, and in alphabetic order, Rachel Beck, Irene Belyakov, Linda Deats, Brenda Fredereksen, Beverly Henke-Lofquist, Doug and Cheryl MacKenzie, Dale Metz, Diane Scott, Gail Serventi, and Bob Whitehead. Wow, what a great bunch of folks!

I also owe a big thanks to the faculty and staff at my new home in the Department of Communication Sciences and Disorders at The College of St. Rose in Albany, NY, for believing in me and offering me a spot on their faculty. Their program is exciting and dynamic, and I'm looking forward to my association with them.

I would also like to thank the reviewers for this edition: Joan S. Klecan-Aker, Texas Christian University; Edgarita Long, Northeastern State University; and Gregory C. Robinson, University of Arkansas at Little Rock.

In addition, special thanks and much love to my partner at O and M Education, Moon Byung Choon, for his patience, support, and perseverance. Finally, my deepest gratitude to Dr. James MacDonald, retired from the Department of Speech Pathology and Audiology, The Ohio State University, for introducing me to the potential of the environment in communication intervention.

About the Author

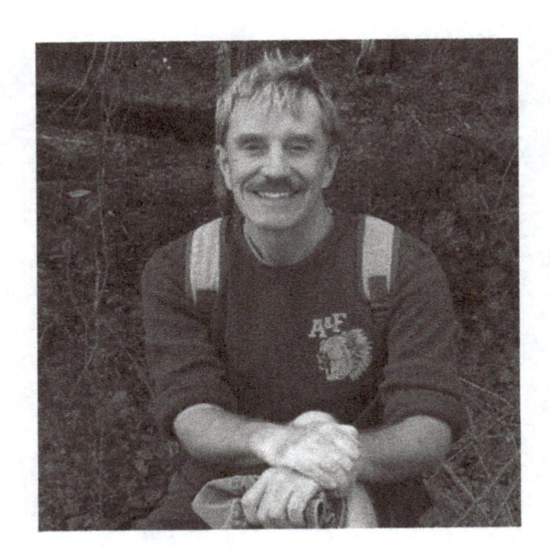

Robert E. Owens, Jr. Ph.D. ("Dr. Bob") is an Associate Professor of Communication Sciences and Disorders at the College of St. Rose in Albany, NY, and a New York State Distinguished Teaching Professor. He teaches courses in language development and language disorders and is the author of

- *Language Development, An Introduction* (8 editions)
- *Language Disorders, A Functional Approach* (6 editions)
- *Program for the Acquisition of Language with the Severely Impaired (PALS)*
- *Help Your Baby Talk, Introducing the New Shared Communication Method*
- *Queer Kids, The Challenge and Promise for Lesbian, Gay and Bisexual Youth*

His *Language Development* text is the most widely used in the world and has been translated into Spanish, Korean, Arabic, and Mandarin. He has also co-authored *Introduction to Communication Disorders, A Life Span Perspective* (4 editions), written a score of book chapters and professional articles, and authored two as-yet unpublished novels that are sure to win a posthumous Pulitzer prize. Currently, he is authoring a text on early intervention. In love with the sound of his own voice, Dr. Bob has presented over 180 professional papers and workshops around the globe. His professional interests are language disorders in infants, toddlers, and preschoolers, who are also some of his best friends. And he's a gran'pa!

Chapter 1

A Functional Language Approach

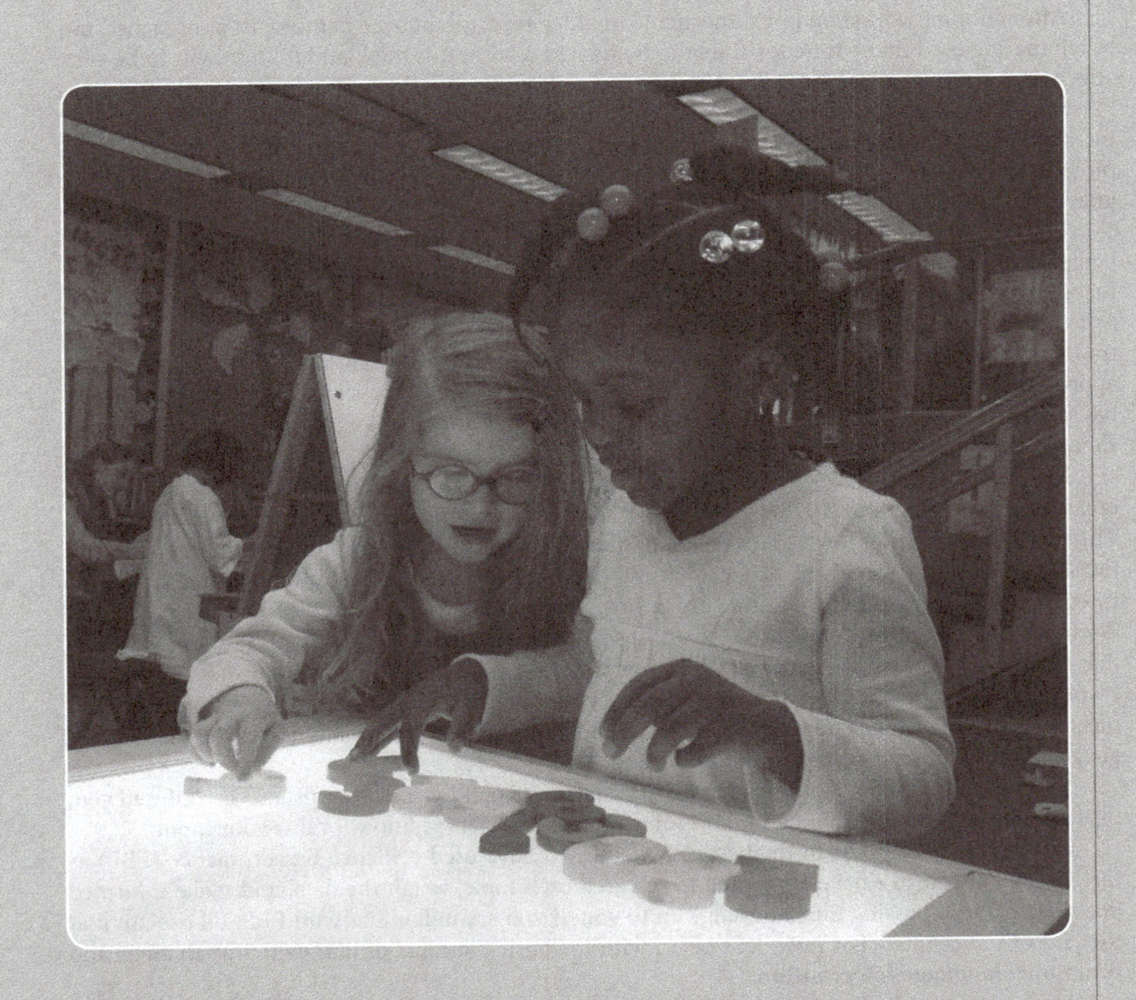

At the risk of sounding like I think I'm something special, which I don't and I'm not, let me begin with two vignettes. A few years ago, I gave a presentation in Buffalo, New York, on a topic other than speech-language pathology and was pleased to see a former student sitting in the rear. Afterward, when I approached her and expressed my surprise at seeing her in attendance, she told me she was there not because of the topic but because she wanted to tell me how much she appreciated the functional intervention methodology I had shared with her in class several years earlier. At the time, according to her, she thought I was describing a standard method of providing intervention and was not aware until she graduated just how different functional intervention is from typical intervention as practiced by her peers. She related to me that, years after graduating, she is still being questioned by colleagues who wondered how she learned to make therapy look so natural and to engage children so well while genuinely seeming to enjoy herself. I can't take credit for that. All I did was provide information. She is a bright, creative speech-language pathologist who was able to implement what she had learned.

After another workshop in Connecticut, an older speech-language pathologist approached me to tell me she used many functional methods she had read in this book and found them to be very effective. Somewhat humbled, I thanked her, but as I moved on, she took my arm firmly and said, "You don't understand. I get it. I get it." As I turned back to her, she explained that functional intervention is not the same as using someone's published language intervention program, it's a philosophy of intervention that influences everything she does with children and adults with language impairment.

Both women get it. In this book, we are going to explore that "it," a functional philosophy of language intervention. I want you to get "it" too. There are many pieces to this model, but luckily, an inability to use some portions, such as working with parents, does not preclude using others, such as teaching through conversation. Nor does use of functional methods negate the need for more traditional methods with some clients and at some times during intervention. But with a functional approach firmly in your mind, you never lose sight of the goal. You never lose sight of intervention based on actual use of the newly trained skill to improve communication. All your clinical decisions should move your clients in that direction.

I've been an SLP and college professor for thirty-five years, but I began my career just as you are, sitting in classes, taking notes, reading texts, and eager but fearful of my first clinical experience. This book is my attempt to give you as much information about language impairment as possible in the shortest space possible. The text is thick and filled with information because this topic is complicated. We'll discuss groups of children as we move through our discussion, children with intellectual disability and others with autism spectrum disorder. Even after we have spent all these words in discussing the topic, we will have only skimmed the surface. You will spend your professional career continually updating your knowledge. And yet, each new child with a language impairment that you meet will challenge your knowledge, your skill, and your creativity. It's what makes the field of language impairment so challenging and rewarding.

So let's proceed together. If you have concerns as we go, if I've made a mistake or confused you, or if I've been insensitive about a topic at some point, please let me know. I value your input.

Throughout this book, to the best of my ability, I have used evidence-based practice (EBP) as the basis for this text. I have attempted to research each topic, weigh the data, and make informed decisions prior to passing the knowledge on to you. If you are unfamiliar with EBP, I'll explain it at the end of the chapter. For now, let's begin with the basic concepts of **language impairment** and **functional language intervention**.

Language is a vehicle for communication and is primarily used in conversations. As such, language is the social tool that we use to accomplish our goals when we communicate. In other words, language can be viewed as a dynamic process. If we take this view, it changes our approach to language intervention. We become interested in the *how* more than in the *what*. It is that aspect of language intervention that I wish for us to explore through this book.

The American Speech-Language-Hearing Association, the professional organization for speech-language pathologists and audiologists, defines *language disorder* as follows:

> A LANGUAGE DISORDER is impaired comprehension and/or use of spoken, written and/or other symbol systems. This disorder may involve (1) the form of language (phonology, morphology, syntax), (2) the content of language (semantics), and/or (3) the function of language in communication (pragmatics) in any combination. (Ad Hoc Committee on Service Delivery in the Schools, 1993, p. 40)

For our purposes, we shall consider the term *language disorder*, which I'll call *language impairment, to apply to a heterogeneous group of developmental disorders, acquired disorders, delays, or any combination of these principally characterized by deficits and/or immaturities in the use of spoken and/or written language for comprehension and/or production purposes that may involve the form, content, or function of language in any combination*. Language impairment may persist across the lifetime of the individual and may vary in symptoms, manifestations, effects, and severity over time and as a consequence of context, content, and learning task. Language differences, found in some individuals who are English Language Learners (ELLs) and those using different dialects, do not in themselves constitute language impairments.

In attempting to clarify the definition of language impairment, we have, no doubt, raised more questions than we have answered. For example, causal factors, such as prematurity, although important, are omitted from the definition because of their diverse nature and the lack of clear causal links in many children with language impairment (LI). In general, causal categories are not directly related to many language behaviors. Likewise, diagnostic categories, such as traumatic brain injury, are not included in my definition for many of the same reasons. The definition also states that language differences are not disorders, even though the general public and some professionals often confuse the two. We'll explore all of these issues in Chapter 2 and the chapters that follow. For now, relax a little and let's discuss functional language intervention.

The professional with primary responsibility for habilitation or rehabilitation of LI is the speech-language pathologist (SLP). The wearer of many hats, the SLP serves as team member, team teacher, teacher and parent trainer, and language facilitator.

These many roles reflect a growing recognition that viewing the child and his or her communication as the sole problem is an outmoded concept, and increasingly, language intervention is becoming family centered or environmentally based, such as in a classroom. Professional concern is shifting from training targets such as individual morphological endings or vocabulary words to a more functional, holistic approach focusing on the child's overall communication effectiveness.

Traditional and Functional Models

A functional language approach to assessment and intervention, as described in this text, targets language used as a vehicle for communication. It's a communication-first approach. The focus is the overall communication of the child with language impairment and of those who communicate with the child. As stated, the goal is better communication that works in the child's natural communicative contexts.

In a functional language approach, conversation between children and their communication partners becomes the *vehicle* for change. By manipulating the linguistic and nonlinguistic contexts within which a child's utterances occur, the partner facilitates the use of certain structures and provides evaluative feedback while maintaining the conversational flow. That last sentence is worth rereading. From the early data collection stages through the intervention process, the SLP and other communication partners are concerned with the enhancement of the child's overall communication.

Functional language approaches have been used in clinical research to increase mean length of utterance and multiword utterance production; the overall quantity of spontaneous communication; pragmatic skills; vocabulary growth; language complexity; receptive labeling; and intelligibility and the use of trained forms in novel utterances in children with intellectual disability, autism spectrum disorder, specific language impairment, language learning disability, developmental delay, emotional and behavioral disorders, and multiple handicaps. Even minimally symbolic children who require a more structured approach benefit from a conversational milieu. In addition, functional interactive approaches improve generalization even when the immediate results differ little from those of more direct instructional methods. Finally, a conversational approach yields more positive behaviors from the child, such as smiling, laughing, and engagement in activities, with significantly more verbal initiation, than does a strictly imitation approach. In contrast, the child learning through an imitation approach is more likely to be quiet and passive.

In the past, the traditional approach to teaching language has been a highly structured, behavioral one emphasizing the teaching of specific language features within a stimulus-response-reinforcement model. Thus, language is not seen as a process but a product or response elicited by a stimulus or produced in anticipation of reinforcement.

Stimulus-response-reinforcement models of intervention have often taken the form of questions by an SLP and answers by a child or directives by an SLP for a child to respond. Typical stimulus utterances by an SLP might include the following:

Which one sounds better . . . or. . . . ?
Did I say that correctly?
Tell me the whole thing.
Say that three times correctly.

In a more traditional model of intervention, the SLP's responses are based on the correctness of production and might include *Good, Good talking, Repeat it again three times, Listen to me again*, and so on. Table 1.1 offers a simplified comparison of the traditional and functional models.

TABLE 1.1 Comparison of Traditional and Functional Intervention Models

Traditional Model	Functional Model
Individual or small group	Individual, small group, large group, or an entire class
Clinical situation	Actual communication situation
Isolated language targets	Relationship of linguistic units stressed as target is used in conversation
Begin with small units of language and build up to conversation	Target conversation as "fixing" the child's language as needed with minimal prompts
Stress on modeling, imitation, practice, and drill	Conversational techniques stressing successful communication
Use in conversations stressed in final stages of intervention	Use is optimized as a vehicle for intervention
Child's behavior and language constrained by adult	Increased opportunity to use the new language feature in a wide variety of contexts
Little real conversation and use	Premised on real conversation and use
Little involvement of significant others	Parents and teachers used as agents of change

Many SLPs prefer a traditional structured approach because they can predict accurately the response of the child with LI to the training stimuli. In addition, structured behavioral approaches increase the probability that the child will make the appropriate, desired response. Language lessons usually are scripted as drills and, therefore, are repetitive and predictable for the SLP.

In a structured behavioral approach the child can become a passive learner as the SLP manipulates stimuli in order to elicit responses and dispense reinforcement. The SLP's overall style is highly directive. In other words, the clinical procedure is unidirectional and trainer-oriented. Unfortunately, used alone, these approaches are inadequate for developing meaningful uses for the newly acquired language feature.

Although structured behavioral approaches that exhibit intensity, consistency, and organization have been successful in teaching some language skills, they exhibit a major problem — generalization of that learning from clinical to more natural contexts. As such, failure of language-training targets to generalize to other uses is one of the major criticisms of intervention with children with autism spectrum disorders.

Lack of generalization can be a function of several factors, including the material selected for training, the learning characteristics of a child, or the design of the training. Stimuli present in the clinical setting that directly or indirectly affect learning may not be found in other settings. Some of these stimuli, such as training cues, have intended effects, whereas others, such as an SLP's presence, may have quite unintended ones. In addition, clinical cues and consequences used for teaching, such as reinforcement, may be very different from those encountered in everyday situations, thus removing the motivation to use the behavior elsewhere.

In contrast, functional approaches give more control to a child and decrease the amount of structure in intervention activities. Measures of improvement are increased successful communication, not just the number of correct responses. Procedures used by an SLP and a child's communication partners more closely resemble those in the language-learning environment of children. In addition, the everyday environment of a child with LI is included in the training.

Naturally, the effectiveness of any language-teaching strategy will vary with the characteristics of the child with LI and the content of training. For example, children with learning disabilities may benefit more from specific language training than do other children with language impairment. Likewise, children with more severe LI initially benefit more from a structured imitative approach.

In this chapter, we'll further define a functional language approach and explore a rationale for it. This rationale is based on the primacy of pragmatics in language and language intervention and on the generalization of language intervention to everyday contexts. Generalization is discussed in terms of the variables that influence it.

Role of Pragmatics in Intervention

As you'll recall, *pragmatics* consists of the intentions or communication goals of each speaker and of the linguistic adjustments made by each speaker for the listener in order to accomplish these goals. Most features of language are affected by pragmatic aspects of the conversational context. For example, a speaker's selection of pronouns involves more than syntactic and semantic considerations. The conversational partners must be aware of the preceding linguistic information and of each other's point of reference.

In an earlier era, interest by SLPs in psycholinguistics led to a therapeutic emphasis on increasing syntactic complexity. With a therapeutic shift in interest to semantics or meaning in the early 1970s came a new recognition of the importance of cognitive or intellectual readiness but little understanding of the importance of the social environment. The influence of sociolinguistics and pragmatics in the late 1970s and 1980s has led to interest in conversational rules and contextual factors. Everyday contexts have provided a backdrop for linguistic performance.

Among those working with special populations, the focus has been shifting to the communication process itself. Previously, for example, children's behaviors were considered either appropriate or inappropriate to the stimulus-reinforcement situation. Echolalia and unusual language patterns considered inappropriate were extinguished or punished. When emphasis shifts to pragmatics and to the processes that underlie behavior, however, the child's language, even echolalia, can be considered on its own terms. For example, does it serve a purpose for the child?

Older approaches have tended to emphasize childrens' deficits with the goal of fixing what's wrong. In contrast, a functional approach stresses what a child needs in order to accomplish his or her communication goals. It follows that intervention should provide contexts for actively engaging children in communication. In shifting the focus from the disorder to supporting a child's communication, the goal becomes increasing support and opportunities for the child to participate in everyday communication situations.

Increasingly, SLPs are recognizing that the structure and content of language are heavily influenced by the conversational constraints of the communication context. This view of language necessitates a very different approach to language intervention. In effect, intervention has moved from an *entity approach*, which targets discrete isolated bits of language, to a *systems or holistic approach*, which targets language within the overall communication process. The major implication is a change in both the targets and the methods of training. If pragmatics is just one of five equal aspects of language, as seen in Figure 1.1, then it offers yet another set of rules to train and the methodology need not change. The training still can emphasize the what with little change in the how, which can continue in a structured behavioral paradigm.

In contrast, an approach in which pragmatics is seen as the overall organizing aspect of language, also seen in Figure 1.1, necessitates a more interactive conversational training approach, one that mirrors the environment in which the language will be used. Therapy becomes bidirectional and child oriented, and conversation is viewed as both the teaching *and* transfer environment.

Dimensions of Communication Context

Language is purposeful and takes place within a dynamic context that affects form and content and may, in turn, be affected by them. *Context* consists of a complex interaction of many factors:

Purpose. Language users begin with a purpose that affects what to say and how to say it. Here's pragmatics again.

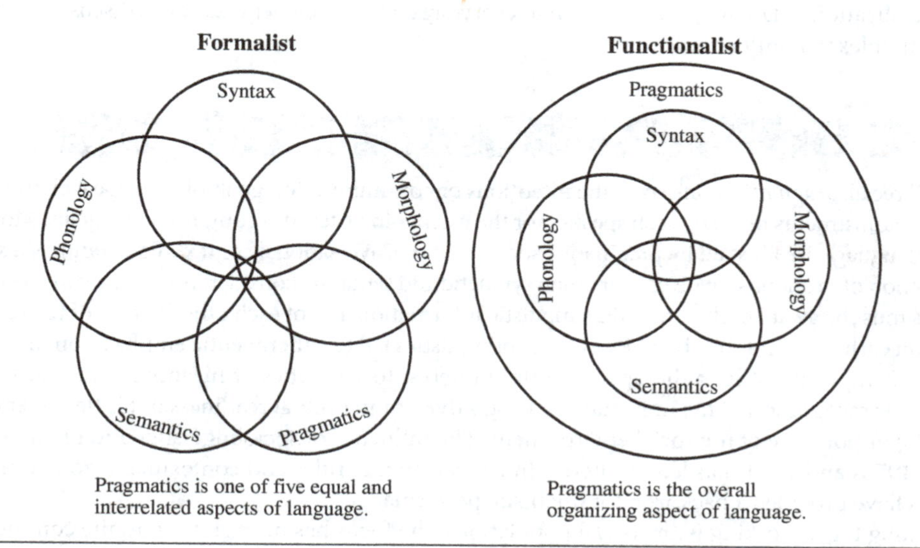

FIGURE 1.1 Relationship of the aspects of language.

Content. Language users communicate about something. This topic affects the form and the style.

Type of discourse. Certain types of discourse, such as a debate or a speech, use a characteristic type of structure related to the purpose.

Participant characteristics. Participant characteristics that affect context are background knowledge, roles, life experiences, moods, willingness to take risks, relative age, status, familiarity, and relationship in time and space. Each participant also belongs to a speech community, which is that group with whom he or she shares certain rules of language.

Setting and Activity. Setting and the activity includes the circumstances in which language users find themselves, which, in turn, affects language, especially the choice of vocabulary.

Mode of discourse. Speech, sign, and written modes require very different types of interaction from the participants.

Within a conversation, participants continually must assess these factors and their changing relationships. Now, it should be easy to see why the pragmatic context is essential to effective intervention.

An SLP must be a master of the conversational context. Unfortunately, it is too easy to rely on overworked verbal cues, such as "Tell me about this picture" or "What do you want?" to elicit certain language structures. As simple a behavior as waiting can be an effective intervention tool when appropriate. Similarly, a seemingly nonclinical utterance, such as "Boy, that's a beautiful red sweater," can easily elicit negative constructions when directed at a child's green socks. If an SLP knows the dimensions of communication context and understands the dimensions, he or she can manipulate them more efficiently.

Summary

In the clinical setting, SLPs need to be aware of the effects of context on communication. How well children with LI regulate their relationships with other people depends on their ability to monitor aspects of the context. Given the dynamic nature of conversational contexts, it is essential that intervention also address generalization to the child's everyday communication contexts.

Role of Generalization in Intervention

One of the most difficult aspects of therapeutic intervention in speech-language pathology is generalization, or carryover, to nontraining situations. Time and again, we SLPs bemoan the fact that although Johnny performed correctly during intervention, he could not transfer this performance to the playground, classroom, or home. When language features taught in one setting are not generalized to other content and contexts, the child's goal of communicative competence is not realized.

For our purposes, let's consider *generalization* to be the ongoing interactive process of clients and their newly acquired language feature with the communication environment (Figure 1.2). For example, if we are trying to teach a child the new word *doggie*, we might repeat the word several times in the presence of the family dog and then cue the child with "Say doggie." If the child repeats the word only in this situation, she has not learned to use the word. If she says the word spontaneously and in the presence of other dogs, however, then we can reasonably assume that the child has learned the word and its use. In other words, the trained content has generalized.

The factors that affect generalization lie within the training content, the learner, and the teaching context but will vary as particular aspects of the teaching situation change. If a response is to occur in a nontraining situation, such as a classroom, then some aspects of that situation should be present in the training situation to signal that the response should occur. In other words, an SLP must consider the effects of the various teaching contexts on generalization to everyday contexts.

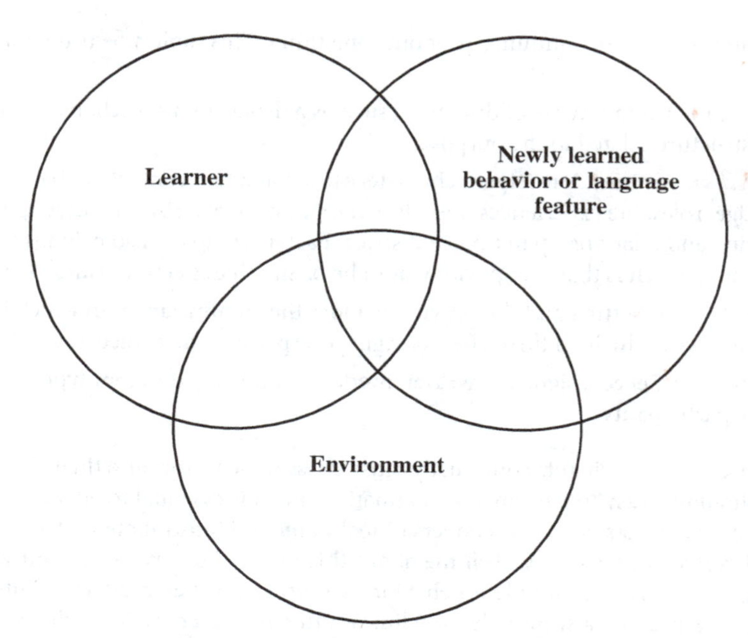

Generalization is the interaction of the individual, the newly trained behavior or language feature, and the environment. All three must be present for generalization to occur.

FIGURE 1.2 Generalization schematic.

Language training may not generalize because it is taught out of context, represents neither a child's communicative functions nor linguistic knowledge or experiences, or presents few communicative opportunities. To some extent, generalization is also a result of the procedures used and of the variables manipulated in language training. Finally, the very targets chosen for remediation may contribute to a lack of carryover.

With each client, an SLP needs to ask: Will this procedure (or target) work in the child's everyday environment? Is there a need within the everyday communication of the client for the feature that is being trained, and do the methods used in its teaching reflect that everyday context? In a recent meeting with a student SLP, the answer to these questions was no. As a result, we decided to forgo auxiliary verb training with a middle-aged adult with intellectual disability in favor of communication features more likely to be used within the client's everyday communication environment, such as ordering at a fast-food restaurant, asking directions, and using the telephone. In other words, we opted for a more functional approach that targeted useful skills in the everyday environment of the client.

Variables That Affect Generalization

Generalization is an essential part of learning. Even the young child using his or her first word must learn to generalize its use to novel content. At first the word *doggie* may be used with other four-legged animals. From feedback—"No, honey, that's a kitty"— the child abstracts those cases in which the word *doggie* is correct and those in which it is not. The child is learning those contexts that obligate the use of *doggie* and those that preclude its use. In other words, the child learns which contexts regulate application of language rules.

Likewise, a young child who can say, "May I have a cookie, please?" has not learned this new utterance until it is used in the appropriate contexts. A child learns the appropriate contextual cues, such as the presence of cookies, that govern use of the utterance.

The contexts in which training takes place influence what a child actually learns. In fact, correctness is not inherent in a child's response itself but is found in the response in context. Saying "May I have a cookie, please?" when none are available is inappropriate. The relationship of context to learning is not a simple one, and the stimuli controlling a response may be multiple.

In a similar way generalization is an integral part of the language intervention process. Thoughts on generalization should not be left until after intervention has occurred. Generalization is not a single-line entry at the end of the lesson plan, nor is it homework.

To facilitate the acquisition of truly functional language—language that works for the child—it is essential that SLPs manipulate the variables related to generalization throughout the therapeutic process. In a functional model, generalization is an essential element at every step. Table 1.2 includes a list of the major generalization variables.

Generalization variables are of two broad types: *content generalization* and *context generalization*. Content is the *what* of training. Content generalization occurs when the child with LI induces a language rule from examples and from actual use. Thus, the new feature (e.g., plural -s) may be used with content not previously trained, such as words not used in the therapy situation. Content generalization is affected by the targets chosen for training, such as the use of negatives, and by the specific choice of *training items*, such as the words and sentences used to train negation.

Overall, the content selected for training reflects an SLP's theoretical concept of language and of strategies for learning and the communication needs of a child. When grammatical units are targeted, different uses or functions for those units are essential if we are to meet a child's communication needs.

If content is the *what*, context is the *how* of training. Context generalization occurs when the client uses the new feature, such as the use of auxiliary verbs in questions, within everyday communication, such as in the classroom, at home, or in play. In each of these contexts there are differences in persons present and in the location, as well as in the linguistic events that precede and follow the newly learned behavior. Generalization can be facilitated when the communication contexts of the training environment and of the natural environment are similar in some way.

Let's briefly look at each variable. We'll come back to them later when we begin to design an intervention approach in Chapter 9.

Training Targets

The very complexity of language makes it impossible for an SLP to teach everything that a child with LI needs to become a competent communicator. Obviously, some language features must be ignored. Target selection, therefore, is a conscious process with far-reaching implications.

Training target selection should be based on the actual needs and interests of each child within his or her communication environments. The focus of instruction should be on increasing the effectiveness of child-initiated communication. Because language is a dynamic process that is influenced heavily by context, language features selected for training should be functional or useful for the child in her or his communication environment.

TABLE 1.2 Variables That Affect Generalization of Language Training

Content generalization	Training targets
	Training items
Context generalization	Method of training
	Language facilitators
	Training cues
	Consequences
	Location of training

Although there is a tendency for beginning SLPs to target specific language deficits, such as plural -s, as an end in themselves, intervention goals should focus on stimulating the language acquisition process beyond the immediate target (Fey, Long, & Finestack, 2003). We can best serve children with LI if we enhance each child's existing resources for learning language more effectively within the intervention context and beyond.

Not all language features occur with equal frequency. It may be necessary, therefore, to create more frequent opportunities for a feature to occur. An SLP must create activities and modify the environment to increase the need for the target.

Generalization is also a function of the scope of the training target and of the child's characteristics and linguistic experience with the target. In general, language rules with broad scope generalize more easily than those with more restricted scope.

The scope of rule application can be a function of the way it is taught. Narrow, restricted teaching reduces training targets to easily identifiable and observable units that may not be found in everyday use environments. Rules interpreted by a child as applying to a limited set of items in a very specific manner will limit generalization.

The child's prior knowledge of language also influences generalization. The failure of training to generalize may reflect training targets that are inappropriate for the knowledge level of a child. For example, it would be inappropriate to train indirect commands (e.g., *can you . . . ?*) prior to the child's understanding and using yes/no questions and direct commands. A child's underlying cognitive abilities are important for target selection.

In conclusion, training targets should be selected on the basis of each child's actual communication needs and abilities. The targets selected for training should be functional or useful in a client's everyday communication environment.

Training Items

The items selected for intervention, such as the specific verbs to be used in training the past tense or the sentences to be used in training negation, and the linguistic complexity of these intervention items also can influence generalization. In general, it is best if these items come from the natural communication environment of the child with LI. Structured observation of this environment can aid intervention programming. For example, an active child may use the verbs *walk*, *jump*, and *hop* frequently. It is more likely that use of the past-tense *-ed* will generalize if these frequently occurring words are used in the training.

Individualization is important because of the many potentially different use environments. A child in a classroom may have very different content to discuss than does a child at home.

Targeted linguistic forms, whether word classes or larger linguistic structures, can be trained across several functions. For example, negatives used with auxiliary verbs can occur in declaratives ("That doesn't fit"), imperatives ("Don't touch that"), interrogatives ("Don't you want to go?") and intentions, such as denying ("I didn't do it") or requesting information ("Why didn't you go?").

For optimum generalization, then, it is necessary to select training items from a child's everyday environment. In addition, these items should be trained across different linguistic forms and/or functions and across both linguistic and nonlinguistic contexts.

Method of Training

The training of discrete bits of language devoid of the communication context actually may delay learning and growth. Such fragmentation allows minute analysis units to eclipse the essential language qualities of intentionality and synergy. In other words, language use is overlooked. Intervention that focuses on these specific, discrete, structural entities fosters drills and didactic training. These, in turn, adversely affect the flow, intentionality, and meaningfulness of language.

If language is viewed holistically, then the training of language involves much more than just training words and structures. Clients learn strategies for comprehending language directed at them and for generating novel utterances within several conversational contexts.

Training should occur in actual use within a conversational context. In a stroke of genius, Carol Prutting (1983) called language intervention into question with the "Bubba" criterion. *Bubba* is Yiddish for "grandmother." If we were to explain our conversational intervention approach to our Jewish grandmother, she would reply: "Oh, I could have told you that. It just makes sense to use conversations to train for conversations. Why didn't you ask me?" In other words, training in the use of context makes sense.

Our intervention methodology should flow logically from our concept of language. If language is a social tool and if the goal is to train for generalized use, then it follows that language should be trained in conditions similar to the ultimate use environment. It is important, therefore, to view context not as a backdrop for but as the ongoing *process* of intervention.

Conversational methods alone will not guarantee success for every child with LI. A successful SLP will blend methods together as required by the child.

Discussion of the method of training leads naturally to consideration of the other contextual variables. For optimum generalization, training should occur within a conversational context with varying numbers of facilitators, cues, consequences, and locations.

Language Facilitators

Good language facilitators increase a child's potential for communication success. Parents, teachers, aides, and unit personnel, in addition to the SLP, can act as language facilitators because of their relationship with and the amount of time each spends with the child. Interactional partners form communication contexts for each other, and it is essential that the client experience newly learned language in a number of these contexts. Because language is contextually variable, it will differ within the context created by a child with each communication partner. Thus, generalization depends on the number of communication partners we can involve in the intervention process.

Programs that involve a child's communication partners, especially parents, produce greater gains for children than do programs that do not. Parents offer a channel for generalizing to the natural environment of the home. With parent or caregiver training, both parents and teachers can function on a continuum from paraprofessionals to general language facilitators. The key in working with families, especially in early intervention with infants and toddlers, is mutual respect and individualization of services based on each family's priorities and concerns (Sandall, McLean, & Smith, 2001).

Some cultural beliefs may be at variance with the use of parents as language facilitators. For example, some Mexican American mothers believe that schools have the main responsibility for educating children and that parents should not be actively involved (Rodriguez & Olswang, 2003). These same mothers are more likely than Anglo American mothers to attribute LI to factors external to the child, such as God's will or a child–school mismatch. Still, these mothers can be enticed into taking an active role in language intervention if an SLP builds positive rapport and collaboration and is respectful of culturally held beliefs.

Intervention need not be limited to just families. When daycare staff are trained to respond to children's initiations, to engage children, to model simplified language, and to encourage peer interactions, it has a significant effect on the language production of preschool children (Girolametto, Weitzman, & Greenberg, 2003).

With the involvement of language facilitators, the traditional role of an SLP changes. In essence, the SLP becomes a programmer of a child's environment, manipulating the variables to ensure successful communication and generalization. To be effective, an SLP needs to recognize that a child's communication partners are also clients, as well as agents of change. The SLP acts as a consultant, helping each child–parent dyad fine-tune its conversational behaviors.

Training Cues

Goals for the child should include both initiating and responding behaviors in the situations in which each is appropriate. Therefore, an SLP considers training language through a great variety of both linguistic and nonlinguistic cues. The adult encourages child utterances by subtle manipulation of the context and responds to the child in a conversational manner. A functional language approach adapts these techniques as naturally as possible to intervention.

Contingencies or Consequences

The nature of the reinforcement used in training is also a strong determiner of generalization. Everyday, natural consequences are best. If the child requests a paintbrush, she should be given one, unless, of course, there is a good reason not to give it. If that is the case, then the child should not have been required to learn that request.

Weaning the child away from edible or tangible reinforcers in favor of social ones is commendable as long as the social reinforcer is found in the natural communication environment. Verbal or social training consequences such as "Good talking," encountered only rarely in the course of everyday conversations, should be discontinued as soon as possible in favor of more natural responses, such as a simple conversational reply.

Verbal responses that combine feedback about correctness/incorrectness with additional information can be both a language-learning opportunity and a communicative turn that maintains the conversational flow. "Good talking" ends social interaction by commenting on the correctness of the child's utterance only and leaving little that the child can say in return.

Not every utterance is reinforced in the natural environment. In the course of everyday conversations, many utterances elicit no positive response. In typical language intervention, however, every utterance by the child may be reinforced. Behaviors continuously reinforced are easy to extinguish. Intermittently reinforced responses are much more resistant and more closely resemble patterns found in the real world.

Location

The location of training involves not only places but also events. For maximum generalization, language should be trained in various locations, such as the home, clinic, school, or unit, and in the activities in which it is used, such as play or household chores. In contrast, where children are removed from familiar contexts, they may not exhibit their most creative language uses.

Language should be trained within the daily activities of the client. Daily routines can provide a familiar framework within which conversation can occur. The familiar situation provides a frame that allows for a degree of automatization important in the acquisition of such skills as language. Often called *incidental teaching*, this approach attempts to ensure that children learn and have ample opportunity to use language within naturally occurring activities. Generalization increases with the similarity of the learning situation to the transfer situation. If the conditions for training and use are the same, the need for contrived generalization strategies is alleviated. In addition, embedding intervention within the everyday routines and activities of the home or classroom focuses on generalization while reducing the stress for families and teachers that accompanies specialized training procedures.

The ideal training situation is one in which a child with LI is engaged in some meaningful activity with a conversational partner who models appropriate language forms and functions. In this way, a child learns language in the conversational context in which it is likely to occur. It is within these everyday events that language is acquired naturally and to these events that the newly trained language is to generalize.

Within these daily events are naturally occurring communication sequences. Daily events, such as phone calls, friendly meetings, dinner preparation, and even dressing, can provide a framework for language and for language training. The frame provides a guide to help the participants organize their language and their language learning. Routines and familiar situations provide support. An SLP can plan conversational roles and language training through the use of such daily events.

Summary

A basic goal of intervention should be to help a child achieve greater flexibility in the learning and use of language in written and oral modalities of comprehension and production. Such language intervention can be a dynamic process of exchange that occurs during natural events in different environments and with different conversational partners. Reinforcement can be the intrinsic conversational success of a child. The variables relative to content and context can, if manipulated carefully, facilitate generalization of newly learned language features and make intervention seem more natural.

Unfortunately, in practice, generalization is too often the final step in planning client training. Instead, generalization should be considered the first, pervasive, and most basic step in intervention.

Evidence-Based Practice

As clinicians, we should be concerned with providing the best, most well-grounded intervention for our clients that is humanly possible. In other words, we should do what works or is effective. Discerning efficacy and providing the most efficacious intervention is a portion of something called **evidence-based practice (EBP)**. In EBP, decision making is informed by a combination of scientific evidence, clinical experience, and client needs. Research is combined with reason when making decisions about treatment approaches.

Evidence-based practice is based on two assumptions (Bernstein Ratner, 2006):

- Clinical skills grow from the current available data, not simply from experience.
- The expert SLP continually seeks new therapeutic information to improve efficacy.

In the field of speech-language pathology, interest in EBP is relatively new, and there are few concrete guidelines on providing services. Although the American Speech-Language-Hearing Association (ASHA) has established the National Center for Evidence-Based Practice in Communication Disorders, it will take years to establish comprehensive assessment and intervention guidelines. In other words, for now, EBP is still a work in progress. That does not relieve SLPs of the responsibility to provide the best, most efficacious assessment and intervention possible. Until such time as guidelines do exist, SLPs need to base decisions on the best available evidence.

Not all clinical evidence is created equal. Professional journals, called peer-reviewed journals, in which each submitted manuscript is critiqued by other experts in the field and accepted or rejected on the basis of the quality of the research, would seem to be the best source of information. Unfortunately, in the field of speech-language pathology, only a small percentage of the articles concern intervention efficacy. Once research has been located, an SLP is left to decide how much information is enough, how to resolve seemingly conflicting results, and how to adapt the information to individual clients.

It is also important for SLPs to recognize that efficacy is never an all-or-nothing proposition (Law, 2004; Rescorla, 2005). We cannot, for example, promise a "cure." As an old-timer, I've had one knee and one shoulder rebuilt, and although these joints now function better than they did prior to surgery and physical therapy, they are not the joints I had when I was 20. I have regained a portion of my former strength and agility, but it is not perfect. Neither is our intervention in speech-language pathology, especially given the variables that can affect intervention outcomes. This fact makes careful understanding and application of recommended intervention techniques critical.

The decision-making process in EBP is systematic and includes the following several steps (Gillam & Gillam, 2006; Perzsolt et al., 2003):

- **Determine the information needed and ask the correct clinical question.** Questions should include information on the client's performance, the environment, the intervention approach, and the desired outcomes.
- **Find studies that address the clinical question.** When searching for information, many SLPs consult the Internet. The ASHA website is a valuable resource for articles published in ASHA journals and hundreds of other affiliated journals. Effective use of the Internet is addressed below.
- **Determine the level of evidence and critically evaluate the studies.** The quality of information differs and should be prioritized by an SLP. First-order information includes research articles in peer-reviewed professional journals. Other information, such as single-subject or small-group reports, archival records, committee reports, conference proceedings, and opinion papers, should be given less weight. In general, the best research compares the efficacy of similar groups to which children have been randomly assigned so as not to bias the results. It is best if data collectors do not know to which group children are assigned and use valid and reliable measures of performance. Finally, statistical evidence should find that, at a probability (p) of .05 or less, the results would not occur by chance. Because the p value may be meaningless at this point, and it's beyond the scope of this text to discuss probability theory, for now just know that authors report the p value in their research. An SLP must also determine that the participants in the study compare well with the specific child in his or her clinical question.
- **Evaluate the information for the specific case in question.** Issues include the associated costs of intervention in time and money, cultural variables of the child and family, student–parent involvement and opinions, client interests, and agency policies and philosophy.
- **Integrate the information and make a decision.**
- **Evaluate treatment outcomes to measure efficacy.** Of special significance is the use of the targeted language features in everyday natural speaking situations.

These steps alone will not guarantee the best outcome, but they do provide a systematic method for decision making.

Because of the potential for misinformation when researching on the Internet, it is important that an SLP use the most appropriate methods for investigating and retrieving information. Search engines such as Google and Bing search the entire open Internet and often provide information from secondary or tertiary sources or information that is not based on peer-reviewed research at all. It's important to know who authored the information and/or sponsors the site, the purpose and nature of the site, and the currency of the information (Nail-Chiwetula & Bernstein Ratner, 2006). For example, a site sponsored by an intervention materials company may try to promote intervention methods using its materials. Even academic (.edu) or government (.gov) sites may present non-peer-reviewed information. For example, educational sites may present student papers submitted for specific courses. Useful professional sites include the following:

The American Speech Language Hearing Association (www.asha.org/topicindex.htm) offers full text of all articles in its journals for ASHA or NSSLHA members.

PubMed (www.ncbi.nlm.nih.gov/entrez/query.fcgi) is a free database offered by the National Library of Medicine. Full-text articles are unavailable.

Many university libraries offer several databases relevant to speech-language pathology, including CINAHL, ERIC, Language and Language Behavior Abstracts (LLBA), MEDLINE, and PsycINFO. Many offer full-text access. Abstracts do not provide sufficient information for evaluating the quality of research reported.

Searches may yield thousands of entries. It is important that an SLP limit the search in order to yield only the most relevant information. For example, a search term such as *autism* will result in too many references to be useful, unless an SLP has years to sort through the data. Additional words, such as *child*, *language*, and *assessment* will further limit the search. Exact phrases can be placed in parentheses, as in (*autism spectrum disorder*), so that results will be limited to those words in that order. Searches can be expanded by using an asterisk after the word, as in *child**. Search engines then treat *child* as a root word and will also search *children* and *childhood*. Journal searches may be limited by year and author as well. SLPs should be careful with common acronyms that may have other references. Even ASHA yields results other than the American Speech-Language-Hearing Association. Specific techniques for limiting or expanding searches are usually included in the search engine's Help section.

As you can imagine, combing journals for clinical results to guide EBP practices can be time-consuming. Half the SLPs polled in one study stated that they didn't have sufficient professional time to devote to the process of EBP (Zipoli & Kennedy, 2005). A first step, of course, is to critically evaluate one's own clinical practices for their efficiency and effectiveness. In centers with more than one SLP or in local professional organizations, SLPs can form EBP research groups that will benefit from the input and the data-keeping and possible research efforts of each member. Together you can explore the best practices to use with children with LI.

Conclusion

A functional approach emphasizes nurturant and naturalistic methods (Duchan & Weitzner-Lin, 1987). The nurturant aspect requires an SLP/facilitator to relinquish control to the child and to respond to the child's communication initiations. The naturalistic aspect emphasizes everyday events and context because language makes sense only when used within a communication context. The SLP becomes a master in the manipulation of that context in order to facilitate communication and generalization. Language is trained while it is actually used in everyday contexts. As a result, the training generalizes.

Learning and generalization are the result of good planning based on a knowledge of the variables that affect generalization and the individual needs of each child. The content selected for training and the context within which this training takes place are both important aspects of the generalization process. The SLP helps the child determine the best response to fulfill his or her initiations within contexts that facilitate his or her intervention targets. Although the role of an SLP within the functional language paradigm changes from primary direct service provider to language facilitator and consultant, the SLP still has primary responsibility for planning and implementing intervention.

Some professionals cast a wary eye on implementation of such conversational and communication-based approaches to language intervention. The fear is that intervention will deteriorate into a "Hey, man, what's happenin'?" approach, too open-ended to be effective in changing client behavior. Although this danger does exist, it is not inherent in functional approaches. As this text progresses, we'll discuss assessment and training procedures that enable SLPs to maintain a teaching momentum within the more natural context of conversation. It's productive, fun, and, where data exist, evidence based.

In the following chapters, we'll explore LIs, assessment, and intervention. After a discussion of children with LIs, we'll discuss the assessment process and the collection and analysis of conversational and narrative data. In the following chapters, an intervention paradigm and various techniques are presented, along with discussion of special applications to the classroom environment and to literacy.

Chapter 2

Language Impairments

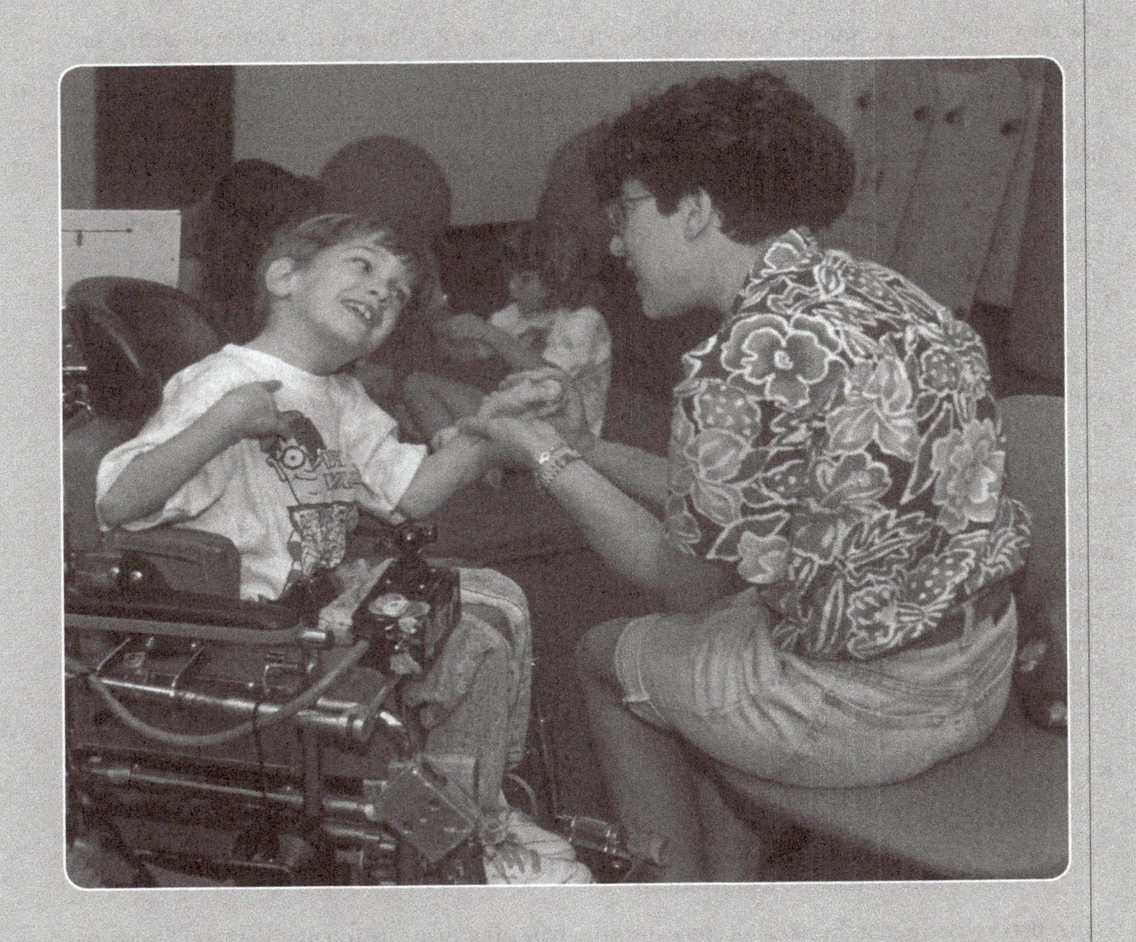

What's wrong, Juan? You seem upset.

Took them things.

Who did, honey? What?

That boy.

Which one? Show me.

Him. (points) *Him took thems.*

Timmy? Timmy took something?

(nods affirmatively) *Thems!*

What? I don't see anything.

Thems, thems things that I build.

Oh, Timmy took your Legos? Timmy took your Legos.

Obviously, we have a communication breakdown. Juan, at age 8, is unable to communicate the simple concept Timmy took my Legos. Juan has a language impairment (LI).

Juan, like many of the children described in this chapter, may have impairments in other areas of development as well. For example, children with intellectual disability are going to experience slower maturity in all developmental areas, not just language. It is reported that some children with LI have nonverbal deficits, as well, in memory and in motor tasks. This and other reported differences may reflect actual deficits or may be confounded by the linguistic aspects of these tasks. We still have much to learn from these children.

In this chapter, we'll discuss the most common diagnostic categories of children with LI. I attempt to personalize this discussion whenever possible, but readers should remember that we are examining groups of children, not individuals. For example, no one child with a language learning disability may exhibit all of the characteristics ascribed to these children in this text. I'll try to explain commonalities and differences across various disorders and to explore the most common language problems seen by SLPs.

At the danger of confusing the issue, let's try to make some general statements about LI, such as how many children have it and how their lives are likely to unfold. In a nationwide survey of 4- to 5-year-old children in Australia, researchers reported that 25.2 percent of parents had concerns about how their child talked and made speech sounds, supported by teachers' reports that 22.3 percent of children were considered to be less competent than others in their expressive language ability (McLeod & Harrison, 2009). Some of these children had speech sound errors. Teachers reported that they considered 16.9 percent of children to be less competent than others in their receptive language ability too. On formal language testing, approximately 15 percent of children were below −1 SD (outside the "normal" range). These figures are closer to the 5–15 percent estimates in the United States.

A second national survey in Australia found that the biggest risk factors for LI include (Harrison & McLeod, 2010)

- being male,
- having ongoing hearing problems, and
- having a more reactive temperament.

I'd bet that you expected the name of some disorder types, but there are too many, as you'll soon see, for any one to dominate. Protective factors found in the same survey are

- having a more persistent and sociable temperament and
- higher levels of maternal well-being.

In general, mothers of preschool children diagnosed with LI are less sensitive and exhibit more depression than mothers of children whose LI has been resolved (La Paro, Justice, Skibbe, & Planta 2004).

Measures of maternal sensitivity include to what degree a mother is a supportive presence and respects her child's autonomy.

It's easy to see that social and environmental factors, especially the child's temperament and the mother's nurturing, play a key role along with biological and psychosocial factors intrinsic to each child. Researchers are now identifying important genetic factors that account for variance in children's conversational language skills (DeThorne, Petrill, Hart, et al., 2008).

If you were one of these children, how would you compensate for a lack of language skill? Young preschool children with LI also gesture more frequently than typically developing or TD children (Iverson & Braddock, 2011). That's one way. Compared to TD peers, children with LI produce a greater proportion of gesture-only communications, often using gestures that add unique information to their co-occurring speech rather than just accompanying it.

It may seem at first glance that these children have difficulty with only one aspect of language, such as syntax, but in reality they often have deficits across the different aspects of language and the processes of communication. For example, many children with pragmatic difficulties also demonstrate poor receptive vocabulary and poor picture-naming abilities. In addition, many of these children also make more semantic errors, nonrelated errors, and omissions and circumlocutions than their TD peers (Ketelaars et al., 2011).

In another example, children with LI have been found to have attention deficits in both visual and auditory modalities, although, as you might expect, the auditory-linguistic deficits are more pronounced (Danahy Ebert & Kohnert, 2011). If a child isn't attending well, this has implications further along in the process. Successful participation in conversational give and take requires active monitoring of one's own comprehension. Think of the effect being distracted has on your own level of comprehension. In narratives, preschool children with LI demonstrate poorer comprehension monitoring, including error detection, evaluation, and correction, than their TD peers (Skarakis-Doyle & Dempsey, 2008).

It's easy to assume from these data that children with LI perform like younger children with similar receptive language skills. That would be incorrect and would overlook the struggles children with LI have with both comprehension and comprehension monitoring, two distinct but related processes.

When we comprehend, we construct meaning, and when we don't, **comprehension monitoring** helps us to detect that a problem has occurred and to attempt to correct it and thus improve the accuracy of our representation fo the meaning. These judgments of communication breakdown and repair are part of a preschooler's emerging metacognitive and metalinguistic abilities. Comprehension monitoring may lie at the intersection of linguistic and cognitive processing. As such, comprehension monitoring calls into play a child's understanding of diverse areas of language, such as pertinent vocabulary, basic grammatical forms, and a rudimentary story representation, as well as skills of detecting errors, evaluation, and regulations of one's own behavior, which are executive functions (Skarakis-Doyle, Dempsey, Campbell, Lee, & Jaques, 2005).

Attention can affect comprehension, which, in turn, can influence and be influenced by the child's social competence, which will be based, in part, on what the child infers from the communication situation. Inference construction within spoken and written narratives and texts is an important social and educational tool for adolescents. Constructing inferences can facilitate the coherent representation necessary for comprehension (Cain, Oakhill, & Bryant, 2001; Virtue, Haberman, Clancy, Parrish, & Beeman, 2006; Virtue & van den Broek, 2004; Virtue, van den Broek, & Linderholm, 2006). Inferencing may occurs in two phases:

- Constructing inferences
- Integrating the inferences into a coherent text base

A complex interplay of comprehension of linguistic input, general world knowledge, and working memory, making inferences in spoken and written discourse has been reported as difficult for individuals with a variety of types of LI (Catts, Adolf, & Ellis Weismer, 2006; Humphries, Cardy, Worling, & Peets, 2004; Moran & Gillon, 2005; Nation, Clarke, Marshall, & Durand, 2004). Unlike their TD peers, the failure of preschool children with LIs to infer speakers' emotions from their speech and facial expressions during conversational discourse leads to less socially competent behavior (Ford & Milosky, 2008). Almost universally, LI affects multiple aspects of language and communication.

The long-term effects of LI for many children are not good, especially without intervention. An Australian longitudinal study of the effects of communication impairment (CI) found that children identified with CI at age 4 to 5 years performed significantly more poorly at age 7 to 9 years than their TD peers on both teacher and parent assessments and on language testing (McCormack, Harrison, McLeod, & McAllister, 2011). Parents and teachers reported slower progression in reading, writing, and overall school achievement. The children with CI reported more bullying, poorer peer relationships, and less enjoyment of school than did their TD peers. These differences were found across age, gender, ethnicity, and socioeconomic status.

Children who are identified as late-talkers at 24 to 31 months still have a weakness in language-related skills in late adolescence (Rescorla, 2009). Although most perform in the average range on all language and reading tasks at 17 years of age, they do significantly more poorly in vocabulary/grammar and verbal memory than SES-matched TD peers. Looking at other aspects of life, a nationwide longitudinal study in the United Kingdom found that when compared to TD peers, children with LI had poorer outcomes in literacy, but also in mental health, and employment even at 34 years of age (Law, Rush, Schoon, & Parsons, 2009). With this background in mind, let's explore different types of LI.

Many categories of disability have language components. In this section, we'll discuss some of these categories in detail, attempting to describe both similarities and differences.

Typical language learning occurs naturally through interaction and conversation with others. This requires that a child be able to

- perceive sequenced acoustic events of short duration.
- attend actively, to be responsive, and to anticipate stimuli.
- use symbols.
- invent syntax from the language of the environment.

In addition, the child must have enough mental energy to do all of the above simultaneously.

Many of the children described in the following section have problems in more than one of these areas. As we discuss each language impairment, try to keep these typical abilities in mind.

There is a danger in describing categories of children and then assigning children to these categories. In general, such categories are helpful for discussion, but there is a danger that the category can become self-fulfilling. Children assigned to the category may then be treated as the category, not as individuals. It is important to remember that the child is not *learning disabled*, but rather is a child *with a learning disability*.

Discussing of LI categories can also cause us to overlook the similarities that exist between children classified within different categories. Many assessment and intervention strategies and techniques can be used across a broad spectrum of children.

Students are often surprised to learn that many children with LI cannot be easily described by any of the categories discussed in this chapter. Such children may have either more than one primary diagnostic category or characteristics that do not fit into any category. Each child represents a unique set of circumstances, so language assessment and intervention should be individualized.

Within each disorder category below, we will limit the discussion to general characteristics, language characteristics, and possible causal factors. Although causal influences vary widely, studies of twins suggest a strong genetic component for many language impairments, especially more severe deficits (DeThorne et al., 2005; Segebart DeThorne et al., 2006). Perception and learning style also are important, as is environmental input. For example, while typically developing (TD) children use one aspect of language to facilitate learning another, such as using semantic knowledge to aid syntactic learning, in a process called *bootstrapping*, children with LI, especially late-talkers, may have different learning styles and use these learning strategies less frequently and/or less effectively (Jones Moyle, Ellis Weismer, Evans, & Lindstrom, 2007).

Unfortunately, we will be unable to discuss all possible language impairments. Some identifiable disorders have been omitted because of the small numbers of children or the paucity of research data. Others—for example, Tourette syndrome, a neurological movement disorder that affects up to 3 percent of children and consists of uncontrolled motor and phonic tics (Jankovic, 2001)—have been omitted because concomitant behaviors place the disorder in a somewhat specialized category and because language impairment is tangential to the primary disorder. In addition, language impairments resulting from low birth weight, prolonged hospitalization, or multiple births are not discussed separately and may be found within other categories described in this chapter (Hemphill, Uccelli, Winner, Chang, & Bellinger, 2002). Some of these causal factors will be addressed in Chapter 3, Early Communication Intervention. Finally, deafness has also been omitted because of the very broad range of issues relative to hearing, speech, and language. Issues of deafness deserve their own text. At the end of the chapter, I'll make a few brief remarks on some of the categories of LI that have been omitted from the more detailed explanations to follow.

Information Processing

Prior to discussing specific disorders, it may be helpful to quickly review the information processing system that serves both thought and language. New research is indicating the importance for both language development and language impairment of this system and of the processing of information.

Each individual processes information in a somewhat different manner. These differences can be explained by structural differences in individual brains and by learned differences, such as the way in which each of us approaches new information or problem solving. These learned differences influence, among other things, decisions about attending, schemes for organization, and rules and strategies for handling information.

Information processing can be divided into four steps: attention, discrimination, organization, and memory or retrieval. These are presented in Figure 2.1. Attention includes automatic activation of the brain, orientation that focuses awareness, and focus. When the brain focuses on a stimulus, a neural or mental "model" is formed in working memory that allows further processing to occur.

We do not attend to all possible stimuli, as can be noted in Stimulus D in Figure 2.1. A child with poor attending skills may not pay attention to important stimuli, with the result that he or she will have poor discrimination.

Discrimination is the ability to identify stimuli from a field of competing stimuli. Decisions are made on the similarity or dissimilarity of stimuli based on the "model" in working memory. In Figure 2.1, Stimuli B and C are perceived to be similar to each other and to information previously stored in Area 2, a fictitious location in the brain.

Incoming linguistic information undergoes two types of synthesis: simultaneous and successive. Simultaneous coding is related to higher thought, and separate elements of the message are synthesized into groups so that all members are retrieved simultaneously. Overall meaning of the message is coded.

In contrast, successive coding occurs in linear fashion, one at a time. Language is processed at the unit level rather than holistically. Both processes are used for decoding and encoding of linguistic and nonlinguistic information.

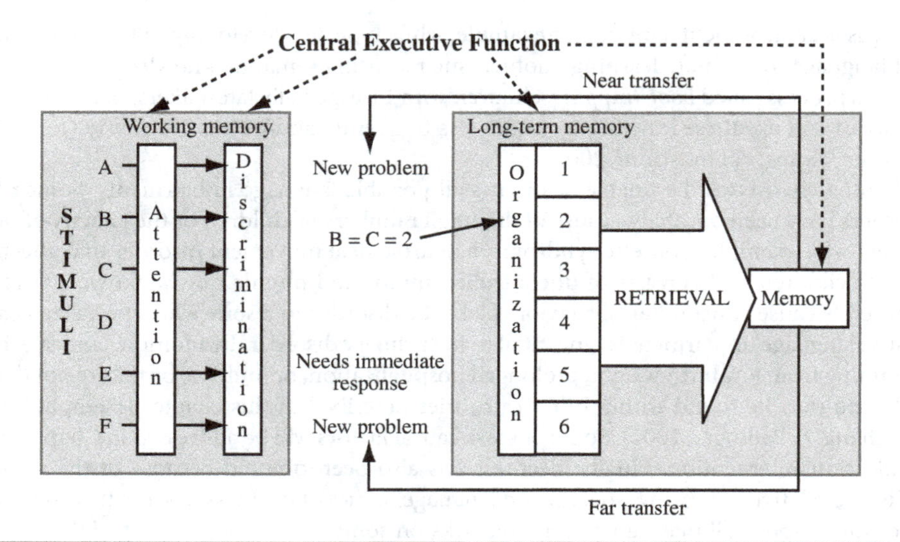

FIGURE 2.1 Schematic representation of information processing.

Organization is the categorization of information for storage and later retrieval. Information that is organized is more easily retrievable. Material that is unorganized or poorly organized will hinder later recall and quickly overload memory capacity. More efficient processing requires increasingly better organization, which, in turn, leaves room for more information to be stored.

Information is stored in networks that relate to all aspects of stored information. The more associations formed, the better memory and retrieval function.

Memory is the retrieval of that information. The capacity for storage and the speed and accuracy of retrieval increases with maturity. Retrieval is limited and dependent on environmental cues, the frequency of previous retrieval, competition from other memory items, and the age of learned information. It is easiest to retrieve information that has been frequently retrieved, has few competing memory items, has distinct environmental cues, and was learned recently and well.

Although not one of the four steps, transfer, or generalization—the application of learned material to previously unlearned information or to new contexts—is important for learning. Transfer exists along a continuum of near to far. Near transfer involves only minimal difference between stored and new information. In contrast, far transfer involves substantial difference. Both types are represented in Figure 2.1. As you might assume, near transfer is easier.

The simplicity of this discussion doesn't do justice to this complex process. Actually, processing occurs on many levels simultaneously (Snyder, Dabasinskas, & O'Connor, 2002). At bottom levels, processing is shallow and involves primarily perceptual analysis. In contrast, top levels of processing are more elaborate and associate the new information with knowledge already stored in the brain. As you might surmise, top processing results in better memory because of the associations formed.

Less complex stimuli are initially processed via perceptual analysis at bottom levels then forwarded to working memory for more elaborate encoding—a process called bottom-up processing—and storage in long-term memory. For more elaborate stimuli, such as language, the brain activates higher, or top-level, processes, such as linguistic and word knowledge. Through these processes, the brain formulates "guesses" of what's coming next, and the low-level processes analyze incoming information perceptually to see how it fits. In other words, language is "heard" in accordance with the guesses that are based on stored linguistic information and the message so far (Samuel, 2001).

The processes may operate either automatically or in a controlled fashion based on the amount and type of information incoming, the demands of the task, and the capacity of the individual.

In contrast to automatic processes, controlled ones are performed consciously and intentionally and make considerable demands on the resources of the brain.

Working memory is the "place" where information is kept active through a system of coding, storage, access, and retrieval (Gillam & Bedore, 2000). Working memory is the place where information, such as an incoming or outgoing sentence, is held while it is processed. While encoding and decoding, working memory must have enough capacity to handle complex information but be flexible to keep up with changing input.

The brain's central executive function (CEF) determines the cognitive resources needed and monitors and evaluates their application while controlling the flow of information. Thus, the CEF is responsible for selective attention and for the coordination and inhibition of stimuli and concepts. Children with LI may exhibit difficulty with CEF in the ways in which they attend to and perceive information and the ways in which concepts are represented (Gillam, Hoffman, Marler, & Wynn-Dancy, 2002).

If a child with LI uses too much energy in bottom-level analyses, he or she may be limiting the amount of language processed. In other words, the child may not have the resources available for automatic top-level analysis. Too much energy expended in bottom-level analysis—because of poor attending, poor working memory, poor discrimination, or poor organization and/or retrieval—limits the child's ability to process language automatically at higher levels of functioning. As we discuss information processing in each disorder, remember the overall process and the effects that each step in the process has on the others.

Diagnostic Categories

One last caution before we begin. The names of some of the disorders we will discuss are in flux. Where this is occurring, I'll warn you. For example, intellectual disability or ID used to be called mental retardation or MR. Although many professionals now use ID, the term, strictly speaking, includes any cognitive disorder that affects intellectual functioning, including traumatic brain injury and Alzheimer's disease. This muddies the picture some. You've been warned; let's go.

Intellectual Disability

The American Association on Intellectual and Developmental Disabilities (AAIDD) defines intellectual disability (ID) as the following:

- Substantial limitations in intellectual functioning;
- Significantly limitations in adaptive behavior consisting of conceptual, social, and practical skills; and
- Originating before age 18 (AAIDD, 2008)

This definition needs some explanation.

Significant limitations means two standard deviations below the mean of 100, a position at the extreme of the human intelligence curve. Approximately 3 percent of the population is below this point, which is at an IQ of 68. The definition is concerned with more than IQ, which is a measure of past learning, and considers *intellectual functioning* plus *adaptive areas*, such as self-help, language, and academic learning. Finally, individuals with ID are considered to be developmental beings, so the definition covers the period during which humans develop into adults. Only individuals who meet all of the criteria are considered to have intellectual disabilities.

The exact number of individuals who have intellectual disability is unknown. Estimates vary from 1 to 3 percent of the population, or approximately 3 to 9 million people in the United States.

Severity varies among individuals and usually changes little over time. Severity typically is associated with IQ, as noted in Table 2.1. Nearly 90 percent of the population with ID is classified as mildly delayed.

Not every child with ID is similar. Differences in severity occur, and other factors, such as amount of home support, living environment, education, type of ID, mode of communication, and age, must be considered. I have worked with very social, very verbal preschoolers and with adolescents and adults who have severe multiple disabilities and very few usable communication behaviors.

Language Characteristics

Language is often one of the most impaired areas for a child with ID and may be the single most important characteristic of the disorder. Even when compared with typically developing (TD) children of the same mental age, children with ID often exhibit poorer language skills.

Although some of this language difference may be attributed to low intellectual functioning, this factor alone does not fully explain the phenomenon. In addition, the cognition–language relationship is an inconsistent one among individuals with ID. For approximately half of the population with ID, both language comprehension and production levels are similar to cognitive levels. In other words, a 6-year-old child with ID might have both a mental age and a language age of 42 months. In 25 percent of the population, both language comprehension and production are below the level of cognition. Finally, in another 25 percent, language comprehension and cognition are at similar levels but language production is below both. Differences between the language of children with ID and those developing typically are presented in Table 2.2.

It cannot be stressed enough that children with ID vary greatly in their communication abilities. Other factors that seem important are prelinguistic communication, chronological age, cognitive skills, and vocabulary comprehension (Vandereet, Maes, Lembrechts, & Zink, 2010). Let's look at two genetic disorders, Down syndrome (DS) and fragile X syndrome (FXS), to get an idea of how children with ID differ.

Children with DS and those with FXS, both explained later, have moderate to severe delays in communication development in speech and in all areas of language (Roberts, Mirrett, & Burchinal, 2001). Some children with FXS also exhibit behaviors associated with autism spectrum disorder (ASD), discussed later in this chapter. These children tend to have more severe language impairment than those without these ASD characteristics (Flenthrope & Brady, 2010; Philofsky, Hepburn, Hayes, Hagerman, & Rogers, 2004). Boys with FXS perform differently in conversation than boys with Down syndrome. Although both groups make more noncontingent, or off-topic, responses than TD boys, those with FXS use more perseverative or overly repetitious speech (Roberts, Martin, et al., 2007). In phonology, boys with FXS make errors similar to those of younger TD youth, while

TABLE 2.1 Severities of Intellectual Disability

Severity	IQ	% of ID Population	Characteristics
Mild	52–68	89	Fewer multiple handicapping conditions
Moderate	36–51	6	↕
Severe	20–35	3.5	
Profound	Below 20	1.5	More multiple handicapping conditions*

*ID most often co-occurs with cerebral palsy and epilepsy.

TABLE 2.2 Language Characteristics of Children with Intellectual Disability

Pragmatics	Gestural and intentional developmental patterns similar to those of children developing normally. Delayed gestural requesting. May take less dominant conversational role. No difference in clarification skills from mental-age-matched peers developing typically. Able to infer communication intent from gestures.
Semantics	More concrete word meanings. Slow vocabulary growth. More limited use of a variety of semantic units. Children with Down syndrome able to learn word meanings from exposure in context as well as mental-age-matched peers developing typically.
Syntax/Morphology	Length-complexity relationship similar to that of preschoolers developing typically. Same sequence of general sentence development as children developing typically. Shorter, less complex sentences with fewer subject elaborations or relative clauses than mental-age-matched peers developing typically. Sentence word order takes precedence over word relationships. Reliance on less mature forms, though capable of more advanced. Same order of morpheme development as preschoolers developing typically.
Phonology	Phonological rules similar to those of preschoolers developing typically but reliance on less mature forms, though capable of more advanced ones.
Comprehension	Poorer receptive language skills, especially children with Down syndrome, than mental-age-matched peers developing typically. Poorer sentence recall than mental-age-matched peers. More reliance on context to extract meaning.

those with Down syndrome have more significant phonological differences than might be expected by delayed development alone (Roberts, Long, et al., 2005).

In general, up through middle elementary school, the overall sequence of communication development of children with ID is similar to that of TD children, but the rate is slower. This pattern can be seen in development of intentions, role taking, presupposition, sentence forms, morphological markers, and phonological processes. **Presupposition** is the speaker's assumption of the listener's perspective, what she or he knows and needs to know.

Even when children are matched for mental age, however, children with ID seem to use more immature language forms than do their TD peers. When we compare the syntax of boys who have FXS with and without ASD to that of boys with DS and TD boys matched for developmental age of 2 to 6 years, we find that although the two FXS groups don't differ in utterance length or syntactic complexity, both the FXS groups and the boys with DS produce shorter, less complex utterances overall with less complex noun phrases, verb phrases, and sentence structures than do TD boys (Price et al., 2008). Overall, both FXS groups produce longer, more complex utterances than the boys with DS.

Although both the oral and written narratives of children with DS are significantly shorter than reading-level matched TD peers, school-age students with DS exhibited many oral and written narrative abilities that were comparable in terms of linguistic complexity, narrative structure, spelling, and punctuation (Kay-Raining Bird, Cleave, White, Pike, & Helmkay, 2008). The use of linguistic devices and cohesive ties are poorer. The predictors of narrative abilities differ with vocabulary comprehension the best predictor of narrative skills for children with DS and age for TD children.

In general, children with DS produce fewer words, fewer different words, and shorter utterances while engaging in more verbal perseveration than mental-age-matched TD peers. **Perseveration** is excessive talking on a topic when it is inappropriate or needless repetition. Males with FXS perseverate more than children with Down syndrome and exhibit more **jargon**, or meaningless unintelligible speech, and more echolalia, or repetition of a partner's speech.

Although children with ID are capable of learning syntactic rules, they tend to rely on less mature word-order rules and a less mature and simpler method of interpretation. Likewise, although capable of requesting clarification when communication breaks down, children with ID are less likely to do so within conversations. Finally, some children with ID, especially those with DS, exhibit poorer receptive language skills than do their mental-age-matched TD peers.

It is possible that the difficulties noted in the language of children with ID reflect problems integrating learning into ongoing events. Possibly these children are using much of their available cognitive energy to monitor and understand the conversation, leaving little for integration of language skills. All of us experience this phenomenon with newly acquired skills until they become more automatic.

Possible Causal Factors

Possible causal factors for ID are many and varied, including, but not limited to, biological and social-environmental causes and information-processing differences related to language comprehension and production (Table 2.3). Any discussion of causality must be tempered with the recognition that for many children the cause of ID is unknown. In addition, more than one causal factor may be at work. In any case, causal factors rarely are related directly to the performance level of the child in question.

Biological Factors. Biological causes are most likely a factor for a majority of children with ID. These include genetic and chromosomal causes, such as Down syndrome (DS); maternal infections, such as rubella or measles; toxins and chemical agents, causing, for example, fetal alcohol syndrome; nutritional and metabolic causes, such as phenylketonuria, or PKU; gestational disorders, primarily in the formation of the brain or skull; complications from pregnancy and delivery; and gross brain diseases, including tumors. In general, a strong correlation exists between biological factors and severity of ID. Remember that although biological causal factors may explain resultant ID in part, they tell us very little about development, specifically language acquisition.

TABLE 2.3 Causes of Intellectual Disability

Type	Examples
Prenatal	
Chromosomal	
Errors in number	Down syndrome
	Klinefelter syndrome
Chromosome deletion	Cri du Chat Syndrome
Chromosomal defects	Fragile X Syndrome
Single Gene Disorders and Genetic Abnormalities	
Metabolic Disorders	Phenylketonuria (PKU)
	Tay-Sachs disease
Neuro-cutaneous Syndromes	Tuberous sclerosis
Brain Malformations	Hydrocephalus
	Microcephalus
	Cerebral malformation
	Craniofacial anomalies

(Continued)

TABLE 2.3 *(Continued)*

Type	Examples
Maternal Infectious Processes	Maternal rubella
	Congenital syphilis
Maternal Toxins and Chemical Agents	Fetal alcohol syndrome
	Drug-exposed fetus
Maternal Nutrition	Severe malnutrition during pregnancy
	Various amino-deficiencies
Trauma	Intracranial hemorrhage in fetus
Perinatal	
Third Trimester Problems	Complications of pregnancy
	Diseases in mother such as heart and kidney
	Disease and diabetes
	Placental dysfunction
Labor and Delivery Problems	Extreme prematurity and/or low birth weight
	Birth asphyxia
	Difficult and/or complicated delivery
	Birth trauma
Neonatal Problems	Severe, prolonged jaundice
Postnatal	
Brain Infections	Encephalitis
	Bacterial meningitis
Head injury	Traumatic brain injury (TBI)
Toxins	Chronic lead exposure
Nutritional Issues	Severe and prolonged malnutrition
Gross brain disease	Tumors
	Huntington disease
Psychosocial Disadvantage	Subnormal intellectual functioning in immediate family and/or impoverished environment
Sensory Deprivation	Maternal deprivation
	Prolonged isolation
Unknown	Perhaps the largest category of causes

Causes are not mutually exclusive and a child may have more than one or mixed causes.

Information taken from: Luckasson, Borthwick-Duffy, Buntinx, Coulter, Craig, Reeve, Schalock, Snell, Spitalnik, Spreat, & Tasse (2002); U.S. National Library of Medicine (2010, December 15); World Health Organization (2010).

Social-Environmental Factors. Social-environmental causal factors of ID are more difficult to identify and may involve many interactive variables. Deprivation, poor housing and diet, poor hygiene, and lack of medical care can affect the development of the child adversely, although the exact effect of each is unknown and varies with each child.

Despite the fact that children with ID display less mature behaviors, there is no evidence that their mothers interact with them less. In general, maternal behavior varies with the child's language level, whether the child has ID or is developing typically. Mothers of children with ID do talk more to their children. By attributing more meaning to their children's less frequent behaviors, these mothers are able to interact more frequently. In short, mothers of children with ID interpret more of their children's behaviors as communicative than do mothers of children developing typically.

Mothers of children with ID match their verbal behavior to their child's language ability while adopting a teaching role. Although they exert more control in play than do mothers of children developing typically, mothers of children with DS are equally or more responsive to their children. Their control behavior includes trying to elicit more responses from their children.

Processing Factors. There may be differences in the cognitive, or information-processing, abilities of the ID population that cannot be attributed to low IQ alone. Children with ID do not seem to process information in the same manner as mental-age-matched TD peers. This difference is especially critical for learning. Cognitive abilities important for learning are attention, discrimination, organization, memory, and transfer.

Attention. In general, individuals with ID can sustain attention as well as mental-age-matched TD peers. Difficulty comes for the individual with ID in the scanning and selection of stimuli to which to attend. Persons with severe or profound ID have more limited attentional capacity and are less efficient at attention allocation.

Discrimination. Individuals with ID have difficulty identifying relevant stimulus cues. This difficulty reflects, in part, the tendency of individuals with ID to attend to fewer dimensions of a task than do TD individuals. If the stimulus dimensions chosen are not the salient or important ones, the individual's ability to discriminate and to compare new information to stored information is limited. Discrimination can be taught, however, and individuals with ID can apply this information to discrimination tasks as well as TD individuals.

In general, discrimination ability and speed are related to severity of ID. The more severe the ID, the slower and less accurate the discrimination.

Organization. Individuals with mild-moderate ID have difficulty developing organizational strategies to aid storage and retrieval. They do not seem to rely on either mediational or associative strategies or to use them as efficiently as individuals developing typically. In **mediational strategies**, a word or a symbol, such as a category name, forms a link between two entities. In associative strategies, one word or symbol aids in recall of another, as in "bacon and ______" or "salt and ______."

Individuals with mild ID exhibit both simultaneous and successive coding; however, these individuals may use these processes differently from TD individuals, especially in complex tasks. Individuals with Down syndrome seem to have greater difficulty with successive processing than do other mental-age-matched individuals with ID. This deficit may be explained in part by the poor verbal auditory working memory abilities of individuals with DS. Although the sequential processing difficulties of children with DS do not affect number sequential recall, the element of meaning present in language may complicate verbal sequential processing for these individuals.

Memory. In general, individuals with ID demonstrate poorer recall than individuals developing typically. The more severe the ID, the poorer the memory skills. Individuals with mild-moderate ID are able to retain information within long-term memory as well as TD individuals, but the retrieval process is slower. No doubt, organizational deficits contribute to difficulty retrieving information.

More obvious differences can be seen in short-term memory. Poor performance by individuals with mild ID may reflect a limited use of associational strategies and organizational/storage deficits. It may be affected also by the rapid rate of forgetting, especially within the first 10 seconds, found in the population with ID.

The working memory deficits of individuals with Down syndrome do not seem to impact the learning of novel words (Mosse & Jarrold, 2011). In fact, novel word learning by children with Down syndrome exceeds what their verbal short-term memory capacity would predict. It's possible that the vocabulary acquisition of children with Down syndrome doesn't rely on verbal short-term memory to the same extent as in typically developing children. In other words, new word learning may rely on another memory process.

Information is retained by rehearsal. It appears that individuals with ID do not spontaneously rehearse and need more time than TD individuals to do so. The need for repeated input and practice retrieval are supported in studies of vocabulary learning among children with Down syndrome (Chapman, Sindberg, Bridge, Gigstead, & Hasketh, 2006).

Memory can also be affected by the type of information. Individuals with ID do more poorly with auditory information than with visual. Within auditory information, nonlinguistic signals, such as a car horn or a doorbell, are much easier for individuals with ID to remember than linguistic information. In general, nonlinguistic signals can be recognized and recalled similarly by individuals with mild ID and without. It is in the recall of linguistic information that differences become evident.

Sentence recall involves reproduction from memory and editing of the recalled text. For individuals with mild ID, difficulty probably is encountered in the second stage.

Auditory memory deficits are exhibited more by individuals with DS than by those with other types of ID. Deficits in auditory short-term memory for words is implicated in the poor performance of children with DS in sentence memory tasks (Miolo, Chapman, & Sindberg, 2005). Phonological short-term recall seems to be especially affected (Seung & Chapman, 2000). This difficulty may be related to poor verbal working memory, a process that enables the hearer to continue to hear a sound after it has ceased. The "echo" may decay more rapidly among individuals with DS than among individuals developing typically. The memory deficit among individuals with DS is specific to verbal information and seems unrelated to receptive vocabulary or auditory or speech difficulties (Jarrold, Baddeley, & Phillips, 2002).

Transfer. Transfer, or generalization, is an area of processing especially difficult for individuals with ID. Although learning may enhance performance, it does not enhance generalization. In general, the more severe a person's ID, the weaker that person's transfer abilities. In addition, persons with ID have difficulty with both near and far transfer, in part because of an inability to detect similarities. Thus, generalization deficits may reflect discrimination and organization problems mentioned previously.

Summary

Generalizations about the language skills of the population with ID are complicated by the many causes of ID and by different severities. Overall, language development follows a path similar to typical development but at a slower pace. Still, differences occur, such as the reliance on less mature forms and the overuse of others. These differences may reflect the information-processing difference found in individuals with ID, especially in the areas of organization and memory.

Problems in information processing help us understand ID and other disorders but do not explain these disorders. Differences may represent the cause, the result, or a concurrent problem. In any case, the differences found in the population with ID suggest certain intervention techniques to be used when working with children with ID. These are represented in Table 2.4.

An SLP must be mindful of individual learning styles as well as those of certain identifiable groups of children. For example, accommodations must be made in intervention for the special learning needs of boys with FXS. In short, with these boys, an SLP can take advantage of their more visual learning style while stressing listening and comprehension. Intervention sessions must also accommodate to these boys' short attention span, difficulty with transitions to new activities or topics, other sensory deficits, and low tolerance of stress (Mirrett, Roberts, & Price, 2003). Some of these children have nonverbal learning disability (NLD), which is characterized by deficits in visual and tactile perception, psychomotor skills, and learning novel information. Although language form is relatively unaffected in children with NLD, subtle pragmatic and semantic impairments exist.

TABLE 2.4 Techniques to Use with Individuals with Intellectual Disability

Attention

1. Aid attending by visually or auditorily highlighting stimulus cues. Likewise, gestures used to highlight important information can enhance the auditory message. Cues should be gradually decreased.
2. Teach child to scan stimuli for relevant cues.

Discrimination

1. Highlight and explain similarities and differences that will aid discrimination. Preschoolers do not understand terms such as same and different. Teachers must demonstrate likenesses and differences, such as hair/no-hair. *Meaningful* sorting tasks with real objects can be helpful. Overall size and shape (not *circle, square,* or *triangle*) and function are relevant characteristics for preschoolers.

Organization

1. "Pre-organize" information for easier processing and storage. No "winging it" here. Visual and spatial cues may be helpful.
2. Train associate strategies. What things go together? Why?
3. Use short-term memory tasks, such as repetition of important information, to aid simultaneous and successive processing. Repetition *and* interpretation are helpful.

Memory

1. Train rehearsal strategies, such as physical imitation. Gradually shift to more symbolic rehearsal tasks.
2. Use overlearning and lots of examples.
3. Train both signal (sounds, smells, tastes, sights) and symbol recall of events. Signals, which are easier to recall, can be gradually reduced.
4. Word associations for new words will improve recall of the words. Likewise sentential and narrative associations will improve recall.
5. Highlight important information to be remembered, thus enhancing selective attending.
6. Use visual memory to enhance auditory memory.

Transfer

1. Training situations should be very similar or identical to the generalization context. Use real items in training, at least initially.
2. Highlight similarities between situations, especially if training and generalization contexts differ. Help child recall similarities.
3. Help child recall previous tasks when approaching new problems.
4. Use people in child's everyday contexts for training.

Learning Disability

The National Joint Committee on Learning Disabilities (1991) has adopted the following definition of learning disabilities:

> Learning disability is a general term that refers to a heterogeneous group of disorders manifested by significant difficulties in the acquisition and use of listening, speaking, reading, writing, reasoning, or mathematical abilities. These disorders are intrinsic to the individual, presumed to be due to central nervous system dysfunction, and may occur across the lifespan. Problems in self-regulatory behaviors, social perception, and social interaction may exist with learning disabilities

> but do not by themselves constitute a learning disability. Although learning disabilities may occur concomitantly with other handicapping conditions . . . or with extrinsic influences . . . , they are not the result of those conditions or influences. (p. 19)

Let's explore this wordy definition a bit. First, as with other disorders, learning disability (LD) is characterized by heterogeneity. It is also important to note that the cause is presumed to be *central nervous system dysfunction,* although other conditions also may be present. Thus, the cause of learning difficulties is not environmental, nor is it these other accompanying conditions. Although not stated, it is assumed that children with LD have normal or near-normal intelligence.

Most children with learning disabilities that I know don't have all of these characteristics. For example, approximately 15 percent of all children with LD have relatively more difficulty with motor learning and coordination. Approximately 85 percent of children with LD have difficulty learning and using symbols. These children are sometimes considered to have a *language learning disability* (LD).

The characteristics of children with LD are many and varied. In general, they divide into six categories: motor, attention, perception, symbol, memory, and emotion. Let's discuss each. Symbol difficulties are discussed under language characteristics later in this section.

Motor difficulties usually involve **hyperactivity**, a condition of overactivity in which children seem to be constantly in motion. Approximately 5 percent of all children have hyperactivity, but the condition is nine times as prevalent in boys as in girls. Not all children with hyperactivity have learning disabilities, nor do all children with LD have hyperactivity.

Children with hyperactivity have difficulty attending and concentrating for more than very short periods of time. Other motor difficulties of LD may include poor sense of body movement, poorly defined handedness, poor hand-eye coordination, and poorly defined concepts of space and time.

Attentional difficulties include a short attention span and inattentiveness. Children with LD seem easily distracted by irrelevant stimuli and easily overstimulated. At present, we are in the middle of an identification frenzy regarding children and adults and their ability to learn and organize their lives.

More and more individuals are being labeled with attention deficit hyperactivity disorder, or **ADHD**, characterized by overactivity and an inability to attend for more than a very short period but without many of the associated difficulties of learning disability. Although ADHD is not a learning disability, children with ADHD often experience problems in social relations that is explained in part by their accompanying pragmatic problems with language use (Leonard, Milich, & Lorch, 2011). Teacher estimates of these children's poor social skills can also be attributed to pragmatic difficulties. ADHD is most likely an impairment in the executive function of the brain that regulates behavior, especially impulsivity.

Some children with learning disabilities may become fixed on a single task or behavior and repeat it. This fixation, mentioned previously, is called perseveration. Several children with whom I have worked would repeat an utterance over and over, seemingly unaware that they were doing it.

Learning disability is not a sensory or reception disorder. It is a perceptual one. Perceptual difficulties are interpretational difficulties. These occur after the stimuli are heard, seen, or received through our senses. As might be assumed then, children with learning disabilities may confuse similar sounds and words and similar printed letters and words. In addition, these children may have difficulty in *figure-ground perception* and in *sensory integration.* **Figure-ground perception** involves being able to isolate a stimulus against a background of competing stimuli. For example, figure-ground discrimination would include being able to listen to the teacher while other things are occurring in the classroom. **Sensory integration**, on the other hand, involves being able to make sense of visual and auditory stimuli occurring at the same time. Each sense may carry part of the message. For example, gestures, facial expression, body language, intonation, and verbal language may be used to convey information. Each alone may be insufficient.

Memory difficulties include short-term and long-term storage and retrieval. Children with LD often have difficulty remembering directions, names, and sequences. Word-finding problems are also common.

Finally, emotional problems also may accompany LD but are not a causal factor. Rather, emotional problems are a reaction or an accompaniment to the frustrating situation in which these children find themselves. Children with LD have been described as aggressive, impulsive, unpredictable, withdrawn, and impatient. Some children may exercise poor judgment, have unusual fears, and/or adjust poorly to change. I worked with a child with learning disabilities who was afraid of shoes, which I think you'll agree is a rather unusual fear. In others, poor adjustment to change, another characteristic, may reflect dependence on routines as a way to compensate for difficulty interpreting language in certain contexts.

Language Characteristics

Usually all aspects of language, spoken and written, are affected to some extent in children with LD. It should be stressed again that although these children may play the TV or radio at a loud volume, or seem to talk too loudly, or squint and rub their eyes when reading, *the problem is not sensory.* Although hearing or vision difficulties may as in all of us, be present, they are not central to the disorder. As mentioned, the difficulties are perceptual.

Children with LD may have difficulty with the give-and-take of conversation and with the form and content of language (Table 2.5). Synthesizing of language rules seems to be particularly difficult, resulting in delays in morphological rule learning and in the development of syntactic complexity. Problems with morphological markers are found both in speaking and writing, with the most common error being omission of bound morphemes (Windsor, Scott, & Street, 2000).

Overall language development for children with LD may be slow. Their language is often like that of younger children, although children with LD may actually use mature structures less frequently. As preschoolers, these children may exhibit little interest in language and may be unable to follow a story or be disinterested in books.

TABLE 2.5 Language Characteristics of Children with Learning Disability

Pragmatics	Little problem with turn taking.
	Difficulty answering questions or requesting clarification.
	Difficulty initiating or maintaining a conversation.
Semantics	Relational term difficulty (comparative, spatial, temporal).
	Figurative language and dual definition problems.
	Word finding and definitional problems.
	Conjuction (*and, but, so, because,* etc.) confusion.
Syntax/Morphology	Difficulty with negative and passive constructions, relative clauses, contractions, and adjectival forms.
	Difficulty with verb tense markers, possession, and pronouns.
	Able to repeat sentences but often in reduced form, indicating difficulty learning different sentence forms.
	Article (*a, an, the*) confusion.
Phonology	Inconsistent sound production, especially as complexity increases.
Comprehension	*Wh-* question confusion.
	Receptive vocabulary similar to that of chronological-age-matched peers developing normally.
	Poor strategies for interacting with printed information.
	Confusion of letters that look similar and words that sound similar.

Word finding is a particular problem, resulting in greater time needed to respond verbally. Retrieval difficulties may result in more communication breakdown, characterized by repetitions, especially of pronouns before words seemingly difficult to retrieve ("*He, he, he* . . . John was . . ."), reformulations, substitutions of indefinite pronouns (*it*), empty words (*one, thing*), delays, and insertions ("He was . . . *oh, I can't remember* . . .").

Word-retrieval difficulties may be complicated by the deficient vocabularies of children with LD. Young children with LD have poor understanding of literal meanings. As these children age, they experience difficulties with multiple and figurative meanings.

The linguistic demands of the classroom are often well above the oral language abilities of these children. The well-documented academic underachievement of children with LD demonstrates the link between language deficits and learning disabilities. Oral language skills are the single best indicator of reading and writing success in school. Difficulty with oral language skills among children with LD is evidenced later in written-language problems, called dyslexia.

Dyslexia is a specific learning disability characterized by difficulties in fluent and/or accurate word recognition and in spelling most often associated with phonological awareness or sensitivity to and awareness of the sound and syllable structure of words (Lyon, Shaywitz, & Shaywitz, 2003). Oral language difficulties are also present (Gallagher, Frith, & Snowling, 2000). It's estimated that possibly as many as 80 percent of children with LD have some form of reading problem and that the incidence of dyslexia in the overall population many range from 5 to 17 percent, depending on how strictly the term is defined (Sawyer, 2006). In either case, a significant portion of the population both with and without LD may exhibit some dyslexic characteristics. The disorder is found among males at twice the rate as females. Although there's no generally agreed-upon definition, when we compare children with dyslexia to their TD peers, some common elements appear (Sawyer, 2006):

- Comparable verbal IQ and/or listening comprehension
- Below average word reading
- Nonsense or non-real word reading (word attack) below real-word reading
- Well below average phonological processing scores

Three distinct types of dyslexia have been described, including

- a language-based disorder that may affect comprehension and/or speech sound discrimination,
- a speech/motor disorder that affects speech sound blending and motor coordination although receptive language is unaffected, and
- a visuospatial disorder that may affect letter-form discrimination although language is relatively unaffected.

The language-based disorder is the most common.

Although reading and writing are different, certain underlying processes influence both. For example, often there is no overall organization to the writing of children with LD. In reading, they also fail to understand the underlying organization, thus treating each sentence as separate and unrelated to the whole.

The behavior of children with LD also demonstrates the interrelatedness of cognition and language. This relationship can be seen in analogical reasoning skills in which known concepts are used to solve novel problems. Children with LD demonstrate difficulty with verbal analogies such as verbal propositions (A is to B as C is to ______), one type of analogical reasoning.

Some of the blame for the problems of children with dyslexia must go to English itself. The rate of dyslexia is twice as high in English-speaking countries as in those with less complex languages. Italian and Spanish, for example, have a more one-to-one relationship between letters, or graphemes, and sounds, or phonemes. In English there are over 1,100 ways to combine the twenty-six graphemes to represent the forty-three or so phonemes.

Possible Causal Factors

Several causal factors may contribute to LD. Central nervous system dysfunction indicates a strong biological basis, but information processing, especially perception, is also important.

Biological Factors. Learning disabilities occur more frequently in families with a history of the disorder and following premature or difficult birth. Children with a parent with dyslexia, especially those with a history of late talking, are at a higher risk for language impairment (Lyytinen, Poikkeus, Laakso, Eklund, & Lyytinen, 2001). These facts strongly indicate a biological link to the disorder. In addition, the use of neurostimulants, such as Ritalin, to enable some children with hyperactivity to concentrate and attend further suggests a biological basis.

It has been suggested that a breakdown occurs along the neural pathways that connect the midbrain with the frontal cortex. This is the area of the brain responsible for attention, regulation, and planning.

Several studies have attempted to find a genetic cause for dyslexia. It is doubtful that there is a single dyslexia gene. More likely is a scenario in which possibly as many as seven chromosomes are involved in various aspects of the disorder (Grigorenko, 2005). Malformations found in the left hemisphere language-processing areas and between these areas and the visual cortex may be related to these genetic changes and to language-processing deficits (summarized in Galaburda, 2005). MRI studies indicate that, when compared to TD children during reading, children with dyslexia exhibited lower activation of the left occipitotemporal region of the brain and heightened activation of Wernicke's area and the frontal lobe areas associated with motor movement, suggesting compensatory use of these areas (Shaywitz & Shaywitz, 2003).

Social-Environmental Factors. Although our definition of learning disability precluded any environmental causality, certain environmental factors are important. The language and, in turn, interactional difficulties of children with LD certainly will influence a child's development.

As mentioned, many of the acting-out behaviors of these children are in response to the very frustrating situations of their lives. Many of the children with whom I have worked had extremely poor self-images. Many were afraid to try anything new; others would do anything for attention and recognition, even if such recognition was negative. The successes or failures that we have as we interact with others have a great influence on our future interactions.

Processing Factors. Children with LD do not appear to function in a manner appropriate for their intellectual level. They seem unable to use certain strategies or to access certain stored information.

Children with LD exercise poor attentional selectivity, concentrating on inappropriate or unimportant stimuli. Appropriate and important information may be screened out along with other information. These children have difficulty deciding on the relevant information to which to attend in both oral and written communication.

In turn, a child with LD has difficulty deciding on the relevant aspects of a stimulus that make it similar or dissimilar to another. Children with LD do more poorly than mental-age-matched TD peers on rule extraction or identification following repeated exposures. Poor discrimination skills may also reflect deficits in working memory (Harris Wright & Newhoff, 2001).

Obviously, information that is poorly attended to and poorly discriminated will be poorly organized. These are children for whom the world often does not make sense, especially linguistically. Their storage categories reflect this confusion. Unlike children with ID, who do not organize spontaneously, children with LD do organize information but too inefficiently for later use.

Memory is related to both storage and retrieval. Growth in word knowledge results in the creation of semantic networks in which words are related and organized. This growth occurs later and more slowly among children with LD. One result is less accurate and slower retrieval by these children.

Effective learners actively process, interpret, and synthesize information by using effective strategies to monitor and organize learning. Children with LD often fail to access or use task-appropriate strategies spontaneously. These problems persist throughout adolescence and into adulthood. Strategies for working with children with LD based on their processing deficits are presented in Table 2.6.

Similar Impairments: Prenatal Drug and Alcohol Exposure

I have decided to place children with fetal alcohol spectrum disorder (FASD) and prenatal drug exposure in the learning disabilities section because of the similarities children with these disorders present in their behavior and in their language. Your professor may have objections to this placement.

When a pregnant woman drinks, the blood alcohol level of her fetus will be the same as her own. Maternal consumption of alcohol during pregnancy can result in **fetal alcohol spectrum disorder** (FASD) for her baby. Disabilities associated with alcohol consumption during pregnancy are approximately 6 in every 1,000 live births (Health Resources and Services Administration [HRSA], 2005). FASD includes but is not limited to

- fetal alcohol syndrome (FAS), which is characterized by developmental disorders, growth deficiencies, and distinct facial characteristics, and
- alcohol-related neurodevelopmental disorder (ARND), which is characterized by significant impairments in several areas of development and distinct facial characteristics.

TABLE 2.6 Techniques to Use with Children with LD

Attention
1. Reduce competing stimuli. Gradually reintroduce these stimuli as child becomes better able to tolerate them. Eventually intervention should move into the classroom with all the competing stimuli.
2. Highlight those aspects of a situation to which the child is to attend.
3. Use visual and physical cues to aid the child in attending to verbal ones.
Perception
1. Train initially with nonspeech environmental sounds, then speech sounds.
2. Use visual and physical cues to aid the child in interpreting verbal ones.
3. Use meaning-based tasks in which a sound change changes the meaning.
4. Visual or hand signals may be used to aid into national interpretation and turn taking.
Organization
1. Help child to see underlying relationships. Use categorizational, associational, and word-class sorting tasks. Use "spreading" model so child realizes many possible associations.
2. Use same/different tasks and match to sample.
3. Be alert that the child's associations may not be the same as adult ones. Try to understand the relationships that may have validity for the child.
Memory and Generalization/Transfer
1. Practice serial recall, first visually (locomotive, touch), then auditorily.
2. Control for infrequent words, linguistic complexity, length, intonation, context, and semantic-logical relationship.
3. Use command following. Control for number of elements and steps.
4. Ask questions about things that happened immediately before. Next, ask questions about slightly distant events. Increase the time lapse. Finally, ask questions concerning what was just said.
5. Teach in the location where you want the feature to be recalled.

Exposure to alcohol *in utero* damages the fetus' central nervous system development, leading to deficits in cognitive, behavioral, and socioemotional functioning (Streissguth & O'Malley, 2001). More specifically, these children will experience difficulties in attention, memory, executive function, learning, behavior control, mental health, and academics across their life spans.

At birth, infants with FASD have a low birth weight and short length often accompanied by central nervous system dysfunction as evidenced in microcephaly or a small head, hyperactivity, motor problems, attention deficits, and cognitive disabilities. IQs range from 30 to 105. In general, these children are concrete learners with poor problem-solving abilities and difficulty generalizing. They are easily distractable, easily overstimulated, impulsive, and perseverative; they have poor memory, interpersonal skills, and judgment; and they exhibit language problems characterized by delayed development, echolalia, and language production that exceeds comprehension. Intervention suggestions are presented in Table 2.7. As infants, children with FASD are irritable and have weak sucking and delayed development. Language deficits include problems with word order and word meaning and difficulties in the give-and-take of conversational discourse (Coggins, Olswang, Carmichael Olson, & Timler, 2003). Most often children with FASD are diagnosed as having a learning disability or ADHD.

The socially competent communicator understands that communicators interact in predictable ways and uses executive function to direct the choice of language and nonverbal behaviors to fit the communication situation. These functions are disrupted in children with FASD who are limited by the amount of linguistic information they can process and have deficits in concept formation, self-regulation, and response inhibition (Jacobson & Jacobson, 2000).

According to parent and teacher behavioral reports, children with FASD performed differently than their TD peers in classroom social communication. In general, children with FASD have significantly more and longer instances of passive/disengaged and irrelevant behavior. Although these children have more occurrences of prosocial/engaged behavior, the proportion and average length of time that they spent being prosocial are smaller and shorter than those of their TD peers (Olswang, Svensson, & Astley, 2010).

Eleven to 35 percent of pregnant women ingest one or more illegal drugs. Although the percentages vary with race, ethnicity, age, socioeconomic status, and geographic location, the use of illegal drugs crosses all these boundaries. The effects on an infant vary with the amount and type of drugs, the method of ingestion, and the age of the fetus. Crack cocaine is especially destructive, with fetal death twice as common as among other noncocaine drug-dependent mothers and sudden infant death syndrome (SIDS) three times as high. Crack cocaine, a rapid-acting cerebrocortical stimulant, easily crosses the placental barrier, decreasing placental blood flow and fetal oxygen supply, reaching significant blood levels in the fetus, and altering the fetus's neurochemical functioning.

TABLE 2.7 Intervention Strategies for Children with Fetal Alcohol Spectrum Disorder

Remove erroneous stimulation.
Provide preferential seating.
Use picture cues to strengthen verbal instructions.
Take care to describe and explain carefully and ask the child to repeat.
Use eye contact or the child's name prior to giving verbal instructions or directions.
"Hook" the child's attention with novel object, topics, and attention getters.
Be patient.
Challenge the child but remember that he or she may be easily frustrated.
Set definite behavioral limits.
Provide a tolerant and patient "buddy" to help the child with social interactions.

Like infants with FASD, those exposed to crack cocaine also exhibit low birth weight and small head circumference; they are jittery and irritable and spend the majority of their time sleeping or crying. An infant may still be unable to reach an alert state by one month of age. Infants exposed to drugs also have hypertonia or poor muscle tone, rapid respiration, and feeding difficulties. Easily overstimulated, these hypersensitive infants actively avoid the human face, which, because of its complexity, may overload them cognitively.

As might be expected, typical mother–child bonding is disrupted, with resultant delays in motor, social, and language development. For her part, an addicted mother's primary commitment is to drugs, and she may fail to attend to her child, and as a consequence, a cycle of infant passivity and parental rejection may be established.

The language characteristics of children exposed to drugs begin with few infant vocalizations, inappropriate use of gestures, and a lack of oral language. By preschool, these children are exhibiting word retrieval problems, short disorganized sentences, poor eye contact, turn-taking difficulties, few novel utterances, and inappropriate or off-topic responses (Mentis & Lundgren, 1995). In kindergarten, the child uses short, simple sentences and has a limited vocabulary, especially for abstract terms, multiple word meanings, and temporal/spatial terms. School-age years are characterized by problems with word retrieval and word order and by pragmatically inappropriate language. Children with drug exposure are usually diagnosed as having a learning disability or ADHD.

Summary

LD is an extremely complex concept. Although it is relatively easy to describe the outward behaviors of children with LD, it is very difficult to explain the underlying processes. In short, biological or neurostructural differences and functional neuroprocessing differences in children with LD affect their ability to attend to, discriminate, and remember linguistic and other stimuli, resulting in language that may be impaired in all aspects and in all modes of transmission and reception.

At this point, before I confuse you any more, it might be helpful for you to stop and jot a few notes contrasting intellectual disability with learning disability. As we proceed, you can add to your list.

Specific Language Impairment

The *ASHA Leader*, a professional publication, describes specific language impairment (SLI) as "characterized by difficulty with language that is not caused by known neurological, sensory, intellectual, or emotional deficit . . . [and may] affect the development of vocabulary, grammar, and discourse skills, with evidence that . . . morphemes may be especially difficult to acquire. . . ." (Ervin, 2001). In other words, this category of language impairment has no obvious cause and seems not to affect or be affected by anatomical, physical, or intellectual problems. One professional has gone so far as to say, SLI "is typically defined in a roundabout way by placing just about everything in the category that is believed to have some connection with language and yet that does not fit any other category well" (Oller, 2003). Although children with SLI exhibit language performance scores significantly lower than their intellectual performance scores on nonverbal tasks, they do not exhibit the perceptual or intellectual difficulties seen in either LD or ID.

SLI is characterized more by the exclusion of other disorders than on some readily identifiable trait or behavior. Clinical identification is difficult and is usually based on the absence of other contributing factors.

Even with a paucity of criteria for characterizing children with SLI, we can make certain definitive statements. Children with SLI may appear to be delayed in one aspect of language, although the language problem is not the result of delay, and children with SLI will not catch up to other children their age without intervention. Even in their apparent delay, children with SLI are unlike children developing typically at any stage of development.

The usual criteria for SLI are a nonverbal or performance IQ above 85 and a low verbal IQ. For most, expressive abilities are significantly below receptive. Although children with SLI have typical nonverbal intelligence, they do exhibit deficits in a variety of nonverbal tasks, suggesting impaired or delayed cognitive functioning, such as manipulating mental images, hypothesis testing, haptic or touch recognition, and conservation, or knowing that quantity remains constant across changes unless quantity is added to or subtracted from (Mainela-Arnold, Evans, & Alibali, 2006). Conservation skills are closely related to language skills and verbal working memory for young school-aged children. These same children have age-appropriate visuospatial short-term and working memory, a right hemisphere function (Archibald & Gathercole, 2006b). An auditory processing disorder in verbal working memory may be evident and will be discussed later (Friel-Patti, 1999; Montgomery, 2002b).

As many as 10 to 15 percent of all children may be "late bloomers" who do not achieve fifty single words and two-word utterances by 24 months of age. Although most of these children seemingly "outgrow" their delay, approximately 20 to 50 percent have language problems that persist into preschool and school age (Paul, 1996). These children form the core of those with SLI.

As many as 7.4 percent of all kindergarten children may have SLI. Although SLI is a changeable condition with maturity, two-thirds of kindergartners with the impairment will still have difficulty with language as adolescents. For example, at age 14, children with SLI still exhibit slower response times in language tasks than do children developing typically (Miller, Leonard, et al., 2006). Even those with more typical language had lingering problems with phonological problems and literacy skills.

In general, children with SLI are perceived more negatively by both teachers and peers (Segebart DeThorne & Watkins, 2001). Young children may have behavior problems; however, these decrease with age (Redmond & Rice, 2002). In elementary school, children with SLI take minor roles in cooperative learning, contribute little, and have fewer high-level negotiating strategies than their language-ability-matched peers developing typically. By late elementary school or middle school, language problems take their toll on self-esteem, and these children perceive themselves negatively in scholastic competence, social acceptance, and behavior conduct (Jerome, Fujiki, Brinton, & James, 2002).

Language Characteristics

As with other language impairments, significant language differences are seen across children with SLI. The language impairment may be primarily, but not exclusively, expressive or receptive, or a combination of the two, and affect different aspects of language, although language form seems to be affected more than other aspects. In addition, the disorder changes within an individual child as he or she matures. Language difficulties of children with SLI extend across early language skills important for reading decoding and comprehension (Boudreau & Hedberg, 1999). Errors seen in speech may also be present in writing.

In general, children with SLI have difficulty (a) learning language rules, (b) registering different contexts for language, and (c) constructing word-referent associations for lexical growth. The result is difficulty in morphological and phonological rule learning and application and in vocabulary development. Morphologic learning is more closely tied to overall language learning than other aspects of language. Pragmatic problems result from inability to use effective forms to accomplish language intentions. Specific language problems are listed in Table 2.8.

Speech disruptions in the sentences of children with SLI, such as inserting pauses or fillers (e.g., *uh* or *well*) or repeating syllables or words, may be a sign of underlying syntactic difficulties, even when the sentences contain no grammatical errors. For example, children with SLI produce significantly more speech disruptions than their same-age peers (Finneran, Leonard, & Miller, in press; Guo, Tomblin, & Samelson, 2008). The rate of pauses is higher at phrase boundaries, possibly indicating lexical and/or syntactic weaknesses in the children with SLI. Speech disruptions may reflect that words or syntactic structures are simply not as well known by or as accessible to these children.

TABLE 2.8 Language Characteristics of Children with Specific Language Impairment

Pragmatics	May act like younger children developing typically. Less flexibility in their language when tailoring the message to the listener or repairing communication breakdowns. Same pragmatic functions as chronological-age-matched peers developing typically, but expressed differently and less effectively. Less effective than chronological-age-matched peers in securing a conversational turn. Those with receptive difficulties most affected. Inappropriate responses to topic. Narratives less complete and more confusing than those of reading-ability-matched peers developing typically.
Semantics	First words and subsequent vocabulary development occurs at a slower rate, with occasional lexical errors seen in younger children developing typically. Poor fast-mapping of novel words. Naming difficulties may reflect less rich and less elaborate semantic storage than actual retrieval difficulties. Long-term memory storage problems are probable.
Syntax/Morphology	Co-occurrence of more mature and less mature forms. Similar developmental order to that seen in children developing typically. Fewer morphemes, especially verb endings, auxiliary verbs, and function words (articles, prepositions) than younger MLU-matched peers. Learning related to grammatical function as in children developing typically. Tend to make pronoun errors, as do younger MLU-matched peers, but tend to overuse one form rather than making random errors.
Phonology	Phonological processes similar to those of younger children developing typically, but in different patterns, i.e., occurring in units of varying word length rather than in one- or two-word utterances. As toddlers, vocalize less and have less varied and less mature syllable structures than age-matched peers developing typically. Poor nonword repetition.
Comprehension	Poor discrimination of units of short duration (bound morphemes). Ineffective sentence comprehension. Reading miscues often unrelated to text graphophonemically, syntactically, semantically, or pragmatically.

Morphological inflections are especially difficult. Morphemes are small units of language that receive little stress in speech. Verb endings and auxiliary verbs pose a particular problem, as does use of pronouns. The two problems are related because pronoun selection (*he* versus *they*) determines some verb endings (*walks* versus *walk*).

Verb morphology is a particular difficulty for young children with SLI. Auxiliary verbs, infinitives, verb endings, and irregular verbs offer persistent problems for both preschool and school-age children (Goffman & Leonard, 2000; Redmond & Rice, 2001). Although most tense markers are mastered at age 4 for children developing typically, children with SLI take an additional three years to achieve the same level of competence. Morpheme use is not a simple case of all or none. Children with SLI use the regular past tense *-ed* less when temporal adverbs, such as *tomorrow* and *already*, are present in the sentence, suggesting that other sentence elements also play a part in use of the tense marker (Krantz & Leonard, 2007). The relatively late appearance of tense markers, such as part tense *–ed,* may be an early indication of SLI (Hadley & Short, 2005). Morphological problems found in English have also been reported for children with SLI learning Spanish and modern Hebrew as a native language (Bedore & Leonard, 2001). Even as adolescents, children with SLI continue to struggle with morphological markers and exhibit an ongoing maturational lag compared to TD age-matched and language-matched peers (Rice, Hoffman, & Wexler, 2009).

Both semantic and phonological deficits contribute to word-learning difficulties in children with SLI (Gray, 2005). For example, compared to their TD peers, children with SLI recognize fewer semantic aspects of objects and actions, such as physical features (color, shape, size), thematic elements (throw, hit, catch within a game), and/or causation (who caused an action, who or what received) (Alt, Plante, & Creusere, 2004). Although word retrieval problems are usually defined as difficulties in accessing words that are already known by a child, children with SLI's drawings, definitions, and recognition responses are also relatively poor indicating that the children's limited semantic knowledge contributes to their frequent naming errors (McGregor, Newman, Reilly, & Capone, 2002).

The sparse underlying lexical–semantic representations in children with SLI cannot fully be explained by difficulty with auditory perception or phonological working memory. Rather, **lexical competition** is a significant factor in these children's poorer word definitions (Mainela-Arnold, Evans, & Coady, 2010).

Lexical competition happens all throughout verbal communication. When we begin to hear a word, our brains activate our best prediction of what that word will be based on the initial phonological information. Hearing the word spoken confirms or does not confirm our prediction. Choices are limited by the phonemes heard and by semantic sensemaking. For example, you're in a fast food restaurant with a friend and she says, "I'll have a "/bI/. . .". You predict she'll say "Big Mac" not *Big Bird, bib*, or *bitter*. The competing words are cancelled automatically. Research suggests that children with SLI experience difficulty inhibiting activations of nontarget competitor words (Mainela-Arnold, Evans, & Coady, 2008).

Although the naming abilities of children with SLI are slower than those of TD age-matched children, they're similar to other children at the same vocabulary level (Sheng & McGregor, 2010). The naming errors of children with SLI suggest immaturities in their semantic representations. A significant subgroup of children with SLI demonstrate deficits in lexical–semantic organization (Sheng & McGregor, 2010). On word association tasks, compared with both TD age-matched and vocabulary-matched peers, children with SLI produce fewer semantic responses (e.g., *cat–pet*), more phonologically based responses (e.g., *cow–now*), and more errors.

That said, for both children with SLI and TD children, fast mapping of new words appears to occur in a similar fashion (Gray & Brinkley, 2011). The phonotactic probability or predictability of the new word and previous lexical knowledge affect word learning in similar ways for both groups of children.

Language comprehension and processing are active processes in which the listener infers the meaning from the auditory message, contextual information, and stored world and word knowledge. Children with SLI do not appear to employ actively all of this available information. In general, they have difficulty constructing an integrated representation of a series of events, whether the series is presented verbally or nonverbally. Thus, vocabulary growth—which occurs typically as the result of inferring meaning from repeated exposure and without direct reference or prompting from adults—will be very difficult for the child with SLI using limited active processing strategies.

Not surprisingly, given their other deficits, children with SLI do less expressive elaboration of oral narratives than their TD age-matched peers, producing narratives that resembled those of younger children (Ukrainetz & Gillam, 2009). The stories of both 6-year-old TD children and 8-year-olds with SLI have fewer appendages such as a preceding abstract, orientations such as a descrition of a character, and evaluations. Children with SLI and younger TD children show poorer performance with simple narrative elements such as character names.

Preschool children with SLI demonstrate a reduced ability to resist distracting input and to inhibit it (Spaulding, 2010). In conversation, many things are occurring at once that require both abilities in order to focus on language.

The conversational behaviors of children with SLI compared with those of mental-age-matched peers TD are marked by both qualitative and quantitative differences. Qualitative differences, such as difficulty initiating interaction and inappropriate responses, lead to increased interruptions by other children and other quantitative changes. The child with SLI is less likely to interact with other children over time as the child experiences repeated failure. As a result, children with SLI often are ignored by other children in the classroom and experience reduced interactional opportunities. Thus, children with SLI have poorer social skills and fewer peer relationships and report less satisfaction with these relationships than age-matched classmates. In short, children with SLI have deficits in their ability to recognize the impact of and to express emotions when compared to typically developing age-matched peers (Brinton, Spackman, Fujiki, & Ricks, 2007).

Compared to TD school-age children, those with SLI, especially those with expressive language deficits, are less successful at initiating play interactions and engage in more individual play and onlooking behaviors (Liiva & Cleave, 2005). Teachers of children with SLI rate their students as exhibiting more reticence and solitary-passive withdrawal (Hart, Fujiki, Brinton, & Hart, 2004). Reticence is characterized by staring at other children but not reacting, doing nothing even when there are many opportunities, and demonstrating fear of approaching other children. Children exhibiting solitary-passive withdrawal seem to enjoy solitude. Although they play with toys and engage in constructive activity, they do so alone. Reticence and extreme aloneness may lead to rejection by others in middle and high school (Rubin, Burgess, & Coplan, 2002). Children with SLI who have poor social skills are three times as likely to be victimized as their TD peers (Conti-Ramsden & Botting, 2004). In short, poor pragmatic skills are related to poor social outcomes. As a result, by the time they get to junior high, many adolescents with SLI perceive themselves negatively in scholastic competence, social acceptance, and behavioral conduct, characterized by choosing to act in the accepted manner (Jerome et al., 2002). For example, although adolescents with SLI engage in both oral and text-based uses of cell phones, they exchange text messages less often than their TD peers (Conti-Ramsden, Durkin, & Simkin, 2010). This suggests that social difficulties may be restricting use, which, in turn, curtails opportunities to develop social networks and to make arrangements for peer social interaction.

Language and literacy play an increasingly larger role in adolescent independent functioning in both TD adolescents and teens with SLI. As a result, adolescents with SLI are less independent than their TD peers. Further, this level of independence is associated with poor early language and poor later literacy skills (Conti-Ramsden & Durkin, 2008). Although they express a desire to interact socially, older adolescents with SLI are at risk of lower global self-esteem and of experiencing shyness (Wadman, Durkin, & Conti-Ramsden, 2008). As teens transition into adulthood, parents of children with SLI are concerned about their child's level of independence, quality of peer relations, his or her social behavior, and the presence of behavioral issues (Conti-Ramsden, Botting, & Durkin, 2008).

Possible Causal Factors

Causes of SLI are difficult to determine and may be as diverse as the children who have the impairment. With such a diverse population, it is not surprising that several possible causal factors have been identified.

Biological Factors. The language and learning problems of children with SLI suggest a neurological disorder. Possible neurological factors include brain asymmetry, in which language functions are located in different areas from those found in the majority of individuals, and delayed myelination, the progressive process of nerve sheathing that results in more rapid transmission of impulses. The reported adeptness of children with SLI in analyzing visual, spatial patterns is considered by some to be evidence of greater reliance on the right hemisphere of the brain. Language processing, at least linear or sequential processing, is concentrated in the left temporal lobe.

Magnetic resonance imaging (MRI) suggests that, compared to TD children, those with SLI exhibit different patterns of brain region activation and coordination that suggest reliance on a less functionally efficient pattern (Ellis Weismer, Plante, Jones, & Tomblin, 2005). These patterns are presented in Figure 2.2. The arrows in this schematic are sized to represent the amount of coordination between brain areas. Note the differences. In addition, those with SLI show reduced activation in the brain areas critical for communication processing (Hugdahl et al., 2004).

Recent studies suggest that many children with SLI have a deficit in the neural circuitry responsible for procedural memory (Ullman & Pierpoint, 2005). Procedural memory is involved in the learning and execution of sequential cognitive information such as language. The problem is not limited to language expression and influences comprehension as well (Tomblin, Mainela-Arnold, & Zhang, 2007).

There is a predominance of males among children with SLI. In addition, there is increased likelihood of a child having SLI if there is a sibling or parent with the disorder (Whitehouse, 2010).

A biological cause is also suggested by this strong familial pattern (Choudhury & Benasich, 2003). Sixty percent of children with SLI have an affected family member, 38 percent an affected parent. The relationship is particularly strong for children with SLI who exhibit expressive language problems. When LI occurs in families with a history of SLI, it is often accompanied by reading impairments (Flax et al., 2003). Further evidence of a biological factor can be found in preterm births. A sizable minority of infants born at 32 weeks or less are at considerable risk for SLI.

Social-Environmental Factors. Although no one has suggested environmental causes, some differences do exist in the interactions of parents with children with SLI and those developing typically. Studies have reported conflicting data on the frequency of recast sentences by parents of children with SLI. Sentence recasts, such as expansions, are adult remixes or modifications in a child's utterance that maintain the focus of the original utterance and can be an effective language teaching technique. For example, an adult could expand "Puppy bite" to "Yes, some puppies bite" or recast as "No, that puppy won't bite."

When parents of children with SLI recast a child's utterance, they are most likely to recast the noun phrase, in contrast to parents of non-SLI children, who are most likely to recast the verb phrase. This is unfortunate because children with SLI have particular difficulty with the verb phrase.

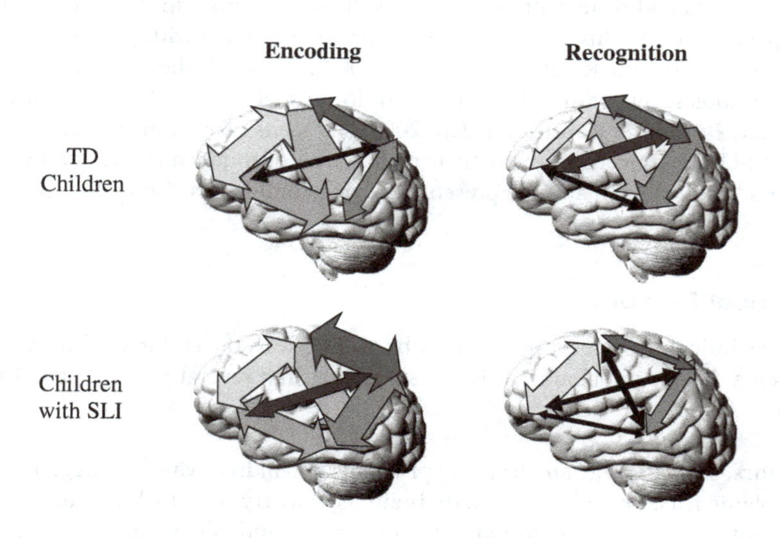

FIGURE 2.2 Neurological processing of TD children and those with SLI.

Size of arrows reflects correlational values.

Source: Ellis Weismer, Plante, Jones, & Tomblin (2005).

Processing Factors. Although children with SLI demonstrate typical nonverbal intelligence, they may also demonstrate cognitive impairments not exhibited on standard intelligence measures. As mentioned previously, these children do not seem to employ active processing strategies that use contextual information and stored knowledge. Information-processing problems of children with SLI occur with incoming information, in memory, and in problem solving. In addition, children with SLI demonstrate slower linguistic and nonlinguistic processing on both expressive and receptive tasks than age-matched children developing typically.

These characteristics suggest limitations in cognitive processing capacity in which tradeoffs exist between accuracy and speed of responding (Ellis Weismer & Evans, 2002). In the rapid give-and-take of conversation this tradeoff results in reduced processing and storage of phonological information, inefficient fast mapping and novel word learning, slow word recognition, and ineffective sentence comprehension (Ellis Weismer, Tomblin, et al., 2000; C. A. Miller, Kail, Leonard, & Tomblin, 2001; Montgomery 2000a).

Specific difficulty with grammatical markers, such as *-ed* and plural *-s*, suggests that the brevity of these morphemes in speech may be a factor. Children with SLI perform considerably below age-matched typically developing children in sensitivity to sound contours and sound duration (Corriveau, Posquine, & Goswami, 2007). In addition, these children demonstrate difficulty in nonword or nonsense word repetition. Taken together, these characteristics may indicate underlying language-processing deficits in phonological working memory, where words are held while processed. More specifically, these difficulties may be in the simultaneous processing of analyzing the phonological structure of nonwords and encoding them for production (Marton & Schwartz, 2002).

Although children with specific language impairment (SLI) demonstrate significant language impairments despite normal-range hearing and nonverbal IQ and an absence of developmental disability, many but not all of these children do show marked deficits in working memory (WM) abilities (Archibald & Joanisse, 2009). Children with SLI differ with respect both to the linguistic deficits they exhibit and to their limitations in WM.

As you may recall from your language development course, several aspects of memory are important for language learning and use, including (Hood & Rankin, 2005)

- short-term memory (STM).
- long-term memory (LTM; including semantic and episodic memory).
- working memory (WM).

STM involves the temporary storage of information, such as immediately recalling items on a shopping list or numbers in a recently heard telephone number or steps in following directions (Alloway, Gathercole, Kirkwood, & Elliott, 2009; Minear & Shah, 2006). **Working memory** is an active process that allows limited information to be held in a temporary accessible state while cognitive processing occurs (Cowan, Nugent, Elliott, Ponomarev, & Saults, 2005). Information in WM is in an active and/or accessible state and temporarily maintained while a mental operation is completed.

Think of WM as a multidimensional system with three separable interactive mechanisms (Bayliss, Jarrold, Baddeley, Gunn, & Leigh, 2005; Gavens & Barrouillet, 2004).

- A central executive responsible for coordinating and controlling the different activities within WM, especially the allocation of mental energy to updating the changing the contents of WM, sustaining attention, and inhibition or the blocking of irrelevant stimuli (Lehto, Juujarvi, Kooistra, & Pulkkinen, 2003).
- A storage device devoted to the temporary retention of verbal material, containing two subcomponents:
  - An articulatory rehearsal process in which phonological information is maintained in memory through a process of silent rehearsal, and

   - A short-term phonological store or phonological short-term memory (PSTM) that is responsible for the temporary storage and processing of phonological representations, which quickly decay unless some covert effort is undertaken to maintain the information.
- A storage device devoted to the temporary retention of visuospatial input.

There may also be a fourth mechanism, the episodic buffer that integrates input into a coherent representation important in the processing and retention of large chunks of connected speech (Baddeley, 2000, 2003). Figure 2.3 presents a diagram of WM.

Tasks that are particularly demanding from either a storage and/or a processing perspective result in fewer resources available for other aspects of the task. The attentional resource allocation mechanism of the central executive governs both the amount of mental energy available to complete a task and the flexibility with which an individual allocates available resources between the simultaneous demands of storage and processing (Montgomery, Polunenko, & Marinellie, 2009).

Individuals vary in their level of resource capacity. Limitations in resources are attributed to the amount of effort and cognitive ability available at a given time. Difficulties arise when tasks place a demand on the system that is greater than the resources available.

Phonological STM is an important word-learning device involving matching sound to meaning (Gathercole, 2006). In morphological and syntactic learning, PSTM may serve as a mediating or moderating mechanism for this analytic process, helping children identify distributional properties or regularities of the input.

WM is also essential to the acquisition of complex academic skills and knowledge across a variety of language-based literacy areas, such as reading, writing, and mathematics (Bull & Scerif, 2001; Cain, Oakhill, & Bryant, 2004; Seigneuric, Ehrlich, Oakhill, & Yuill, 2000). Children with WM deficits, such as those with SLI, exhibit learning difficulties (Swanson & Beebe-Frankenberger, 2004).

Unfortunately, data on the association between WM and language limitations in SLI are sparse. For an in-depth discussion of recent relevant research, I recommend reading two excellent reviews by Montgomery, Magimairaj, and Finney (2010) and Boudreau and Costanza-Smith (2011) from which much of this discussion has been taken.

Relative to age-matched peers, many children with SLI show several significant limitations in WM mechanisms and in processing speed. First, many children with SLI show limitations in PSTM capacity. In addition to lagging behind that of TD children developmentally, the PSTM capacity of children with SLI may level off by about 11 years, three to four years before it does in TD children (Conti-Ramsden & Durkin, 2007; Gathercole, Lamont, & Alloway, 2004). Even comprehension of simple sentences requires significantly more PSTM resources for children with SLI than for their TD peers (Montgomery & Evans, 2009). In general, children with LI and SLI in particular perform more poorly than TD peers on PSTM tasks, especially those involving non-word recognition (NWR) (Ellis Weismer et al., 2000; Leonard et al., 2007). Twin studies suggest that difficulties in PSTM are highly heritable (Bishop, North, & Donlan, 1995).

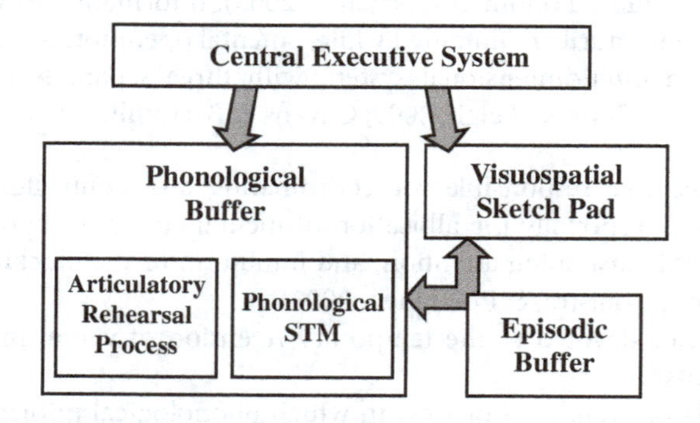

FIGURE 2.3 Schematic diagram of working memory.

Second, many children with SLI show reduced performance relative to age peers in attentional capacity, the limited mental energy available in perform a given task, especially as task complexity increases (Alloway & Archibald, 2008; Archibald & Gathercole, 2006c, 2007; Mainela-Arnold & Evans, 2005; Montgomery, 2000a; Windsor, Kohnert, Loxtercamp, & Kan, 2008).

Although children with SLI have reduced attentional capacity and poor inhibitory control, according to some researchers, they do not seem to exhibit poor resource allocation. Inhibition is preventing irrelevant stimuli from entering WM or becoming the focus of attention. Resource allocation is the ability to devote attention to two different tasks or two different levels of a task. In contrast, other researchers point to poor resource allocation is a significant factor in these children's complex sentence comprehension difficulties. For children with SLI, comprehension of both complex and simple grammar is a mentally demanding activity (Montgomery & Evans, 2009).

Processing capacity limitations and difficulty in executive function inhibition control may explain why children with SLI consistently perform more poorly than their TD peers on tasks that tap into the storage and processing components of WM (Brocki, Randall, Bohlin, & Kerns, 2008; Isaki, Spaulding, & Plante, 2008; Marton, Kelmenson, & Pinkhasova, 2007; Riccio, Cash, & Cohen, 2007).

Third, children with SLI have trouble updating the contents of WM. Updating is maintaining focus at a given level of a task while adding new content.

Fourth, many children with SLI have trouble sustaining attention, the ability to maintain attention over time in order to identify a target in the midst of nontargets, especially in the auditory modality when the amount to which the child is to attend increases (Finneran, Francis, & Leonard, 2009; Montgomery, 2008; Montgomery, Evans, & Gillam, 2009; Spaulding, Plante, & Vance, 2008). Using functional magnetic resonance imaging in combination with behavioral tasks, we can substantiate that adolescents with SLI exhibit (Ellis Weismer et al., 2005):

- Hypoactivation in regions of the brain associated with attentional control, as well as memory, and language encoding and retrieval.
- Differences in patterns of coordination activation among brain regions.

These data provide support for physiological differences related to WM in children with SLI.

This sustained attentinal performance may not be limited to auditory information. For example, children with SLI are significantly less accurate in responding to visual stimuli but not significantly slower than their TD peers in visual sustained attention tasks (Finneran et al., 2009). Although these data support the notion of attention difficulties in children with SLI, they suggest there may be separate attentional capacities for different stimulus modalities.

Finally, processing speed refers to the amount of cognitive work that can be completed in a given unit of time. If information is not processed with a sufficient speed, it is vulnerable to decay and/or interference. Although many children with SLI are slower processors than TD age peers, they do show some developmental improvement in both linguistic and nonlinguistic processing speed between ages 7 and 11 (Montgomery, 2005).

In conclusion, we can say that relative to age-matched peers, the limited WM capacity of children with SLI is due to a combination of deficits in executive-attention mechanisms and verbal-specific storage and slower general processing (Archibald & Gathercole, 2007). These limitations in processing capacity have implications for both comprehension and production and restrict the amount and timeliness of information that can be processed whether on input or output (Hoffman & Gillam, 2004; Leonard, Ellis Weismer, et al., 2007; Montgomery, 2000a).

Although some professionals doubt the existence of distinct receptive and expressive SLI, others report differences in short-term memory (STM) between children whose language difficulties are primarily receptive or expressive. In short, children with receptive SLI seem to have STM deficits with both visual and verbal information, while those with primarily expressive SLI have STM deficits with primarily verbal information (Nickisch & von Kries, 2009).

Deficits in WM and processing speed in children with SLI can have a negative impact on language learning and functioning as we've seen. This may include partial processing of words, grammatical forms, and syntactic structures. Poor ability to process input could mean that children need more exposures to language before they can begin to sense regularities. In the give-and-take of conversation, a child's efficiency with storage, access, retrieval, and coordination of stored representations may be strongly tested. Let's look at the language deficits of children with SLI from the perspective of WM.

In general, children with SLI show slower vocabulary growth and smaller lexicons or personal dictionaries than their age-related TD peers. It should be noted that for some children with SLI, this area of development is a relative strength. That said, a combination of WM deficits, including those in PSTM, may place these children at risk for lexical difficulties (Gathercole, 2006).

Morpheme learning may involve

- perceiving an inflected word (*boys*) and comparing it with the uninflected component (*boy*).
- hypothesizing the grammatical function of the morphological marker.
- placing the marker in a morphological paradigm or model.

Moreover, these operations must be completed in a timely manner to ensure correct morphological analysis, thus emphasizing the speed of processing. This learning process relies on WM because a child must be able to store the novel inflected word, retrieve from long-term memory its uninflected component, and simultaneously perform a comparative morphological analysis before the marker decays from memory. The production of newly learned grammatical morphemes may stretch the WM and processing speed of children with SLI. The need to access a newly learned morphological inflection and then append it to a word while simultaneously formulating and producing an utterance in a timely fashion may exceed the overall processing capacity of children with SLI. The implication of poor processing is that many children with SLI are at risk for constructing incomplete or inaccurate morphological representations.

In general, children with SLI also exhibit poorer sentence comprehension than age-matched TD peers. Comprehension may well represent general cognitive processing limitations in WM and processing speed (Bishop, 2006; Montgomery & Evans, 2009). Performance varies with the types of sentence form measured. For example, immediate processing of simple SVO forms does not entail significant WM, even for children with SLI (Montgomery, 2000a). More complex sentences place additional processing demands on WM. This data should not be interpreted to mean that such processing is automatic for children with SLI because such processing involves significant mental effort for these children but not for their age-matched TD peers (Montgomery, Evans, & Gillam, 2009). Children with SLI show

- poorer sustained attention.
- poorer sentence processing and slower word recognition reaction time to target words.
- poorer sentence comprehension.

This suggests a correlation between attention and comprehension.

As we might expect, children with SLI and WM deficits are likely to have academic difficulties. Most likely deficits in WM interact with other factors, such as past knowledge, the nature of the task and the strategy used by the child, to influence the outcomes in tasks with significant WM demands (Minear & Shah, 2006).

Imagine that you have limited working memory, but communication is occurring at a rapid rate. As the input increases, you are easily overwhelmed, slowing the entire process. Your limited memory makes it increasingly difficult to hold information as more comes in, slowing the process even more. You begin to lose information as more comes in. It's increasingly difficult to relate new information to partially processed old information. Maybe you've experienced this when you've tried to communicate in another language. Now you get some inkling of one aspect of language processing for children with SLI.

Summary

Much discussion has taken place concerning the viability of SLI as a separate category of language impairment. It has been suggested that SLI is not a distinct disorder category but merely represents children with limited language abilities as the result of genetic and/or environmental factors.

One recent study of over a thousand preschool children failed to find a qualitatively distinct group corresponding to children with SLI (Dollaghan, 2004). Some educators have suggested that SLI may not even be a useful concept, especially because clinical tools are unable to diagnose it easily and accurately.

For now, the best diagnostic techniques appear to be rote memory tasks, such as counting or sequential digit recall, nonsense word repetition, rule induction (see description of dynamic assessment of children from diverse backgrounds in Chapter 5), story recall, grammatical completion, especially verb markers, number of different words in a speech sample, and memory plus interpretation tasks while listening or reading. Memory and awareness tasks for intervention are presented in Table 2.9.

TABLE 2.9 Intervention for Memory and Awareness with Children with SLI

Naming letters and objects	Repeating novel and nonsense ("funny") words
Recalling spoken sentences	Rhyming games
Using melody as a memory aid	Recalling of words that begin with specific phonemes
Listening to stories and nursery rhymes	Guessing games based on cumulative cues
Repeating nursery rhymes	Rehearsing verbally
Acting out pictures	Categorizing words and objects
Acting out rhymes	
Using gestures to aid recall	

Pervasive Developmental Disorder/Autism Spectrum Disorder

The fourth, revised edition of the American Psychiatric Association's *Diagnostic and Statistical Manual on Mental Disorders* (DSM-IV) (2000) lists autism along a continuum labeled pervasive developmental disorder (PDD). Autism spectrum disorder (ASD) is at the more severe extreme, while a milder form of the disorder is called pervasive developmental disorder–not otherwise specified (PDD-NOS) (Bauer, 1995a, 1995b). In actual practice, children are labeled as ASD when the severe form of the disorder exists and as simply PDD or another disorder when the milder form exists. Some children with PDD may be labeled with Asperger's syndrome or are mislabeled as learning disabled or ADHD. If this is not confusing enough, other children with PDD may be labeled hyperlexic and may exhibit some characteristics of ASD while others with this label appear more like children with learning disabilities. These labels are not assigned arbitrarily but are based on characteristics exhibited by the child. Don't be too confused by all these labels. We shall try to sort out these differences in the following discussion.

The American Psychiatric Association (2000) defines ASD as an impairment in reciprocal social interaction with a severely limited behavior, interest, and activity repertoire. The *DSM IV* lists several behaviors that characterize ASD. These include

- Social relatedness
  - Nonverbal behavior
  - Failure to develop peer relationships
  - Lack of seeking to share
  - Lack of social/emotional reciprocity
- Communication
  - Delay/lack of speech
  - Impaired conversational ability
  - Stereotyped/repetitive/idiosyncratic language
  - Lack of make-believe/imaginative play
- Restricted/repetitive/stereotyped patterns
  - Stereotyped/restricted pattern of interest
  - Nonfunctional routine or ritual
  - Stereotyped or repetitive motor mannerisms
  - Preoccupation with parts of objects

Not every child with ASD will exhibit all of these characteristics, and several characteristics, especially in children who have ASD but are high functioning, overlap with other disorders such as ADHD and various anxiety disorders. One study found that the characteristics that best distinguish ASD from other disorders and specify ASD are as follows (Hartley & Sikora, 2009):

- Failure to develop peer relationships
- Lack of social/emotional reciprocity
- Nonfunctional routines or rituals
- Nonverbal behavior
- Stereotyped or repetitive motor mannerisms

ASD is found in males four times more frequently than in females and affects 1 in 500 children.

ASD is much more common than previously believed, and the incidence figures have been changing rapidly, most likely because of better diagnosis. In 2012, after a national survey, the U.S. Centers for Disease Control and Prevention (CDC) announced that

- the incidence of ASD among children was 1 in 88.
- boys are more likely to display ASD characteristics by 5-to-1.
- most children with ASD have IQs above 70 (above the cutoff of ID).

Approximately 25 percent of these children exhibit intellectual disability (Chakrabarti & Fombonne, 2001; Fombonne, 2003b).

We must take this with so many grains of salt, given that the discussion that followed the announcement indicated that children with several varieties of PDD were included in the ASD category. We might be on safer ground to assume that ASD occurs in one in 150 births. Still, there is no denying that ASD and related disorders are becoming more common. The changes represent an approximately 500 percent increase in the last fifteen years (U.S. Government Accountability Office, 2005). The CDC attributed this increase to better diagnosis.

In general, the age of detection of ASD varies with severity and developmental delays, especially in communication and social interaction. The more intense the symptoms, the poorer language and overall development (Pry, Petersen, & Baghdadli, 2005). Although it is rare that the disorder is identified prior to 18 months of age, infants with ASD have been described as either lethargic, preferring solitude and making few demands, or highly irritable, with sleeping problems and screaming and crying. Usually, between 18 and 36 months, the signs become more pronounced, including more frequent tantruming, repetitive movements and ritualistic play, extreme reactions to certain stimuli, lack of pretend and social play, and joint attention and communication difficulties including a lack of gestures.

In approximately 20 percent of the cases, parents report typical development until 24 months, especially among girls. Early identification is often difficult because of the lack of obvious medical problems and the early typical development of motor abilities. Infrequently, onset occurs in later childhood. Recent data suggests that young children with PDD exhibit clusters of impairment in joint or mutual attending, symbolic play, and social affective communication.

Development often proceeds in spurts and plateaus, rather than smoothly. Most areas of development are affected by delay and disorder, although occasionally one area, such as mechanical or mathematical abilities, is typical or above. I have worked with children well above average in mathematics but unable to dress themselves or to participate in meaningful conversations. Motor behaviors may include toe walking, rocking, spinning, and, in extreme cases, self-injurious behaviors, such as biting, hitting, and head banging. One adolescent with whom I worked was covered with scars and scabs from self-inflicted scratches and bites. Another child pounded his head with his fist an average of more than 7,000 times in a five-hour school day.

Although it is beyond the scope of this text to discuss intervention for self-injurious behaviors, we should note that they often represent ineffectual ways of communication or stress associated with this lack of communication and can be reduced in some children by providing new more effective ways of communicating (Buschbacher & Fox, 2003).

Children with ASD exhibit sensory modulation dysfunction (SMD). Sensory modulation occurs within the central nervous system (CNS) as it attempts to balance excitation and inhibition inputs arising within one's sensory mechanism with those occurring external to the body. Modulation within the CNS occurs when the electrical properties of neurons change as a result of neurotransmitters or hormones. Typically, sensations are detected and responded to in a routine manner that is appropriate and adaptive (Lane, 2002). SMD is a mismatch between the external demands and a person's internal system characteristics, resulting in behavior that is underresponsive or overresponsive (Hanft, Miller, & Lane, 2000). For children with ASD, stimuli must be within the limits of a child's tolerance and expectation. Children with ASD fluctuate between the two extremes, exhibiting overresponsiveness until overload occurs and results in shutdown of the process and a defensive or withdrawal response.

Over- and underresponsiveness to stimuli may be found in the same child. For example, loud noises may get no response from a child, while whispering results in a catastrophic response. In general, children with ASD tend to prefer shiny objects, especially those that spin; things that can be twirled; and noises they produce themselves, such as teeth grinding. Children with ASD seem to prefer routines and may become extremely upset with change. Individual children may have very definite preferences in taste, touch, and smell. I worked with one child whose only food preference was dill pickles. Self-stimulatory behaviors may include rocking, spinning, and hand flapping.

Relational disorders may be the most distressful aspect of ASD, especially for parents. In particular, children with ASD often avert their gaze or stare emptily and lack a social smile, responsiveness to sound, and anticipation of the approach of others. Parents often are treated as "things" or, at best, no different from other people. The effect on parents can be imagined.

As mentioned, children with a milder form of the disorder are labeled with pervasive developmental disorder–not otherwise specified, PDD-NOS, or simply PDD. Children with **PDD-NOS** exhibit many of the characteristics of ASD but to a lesser degree. For example, they may have difficulty with social behavior and exhibit poor eye contact and poor use of gestures and facial expressions. Their grammar may be disordered, and they may use echolalia. Compared to children with either ASD or Asperger's syndrome, children with PDD-NOS have levels of functioning performance (communication, daily living and social skills, IQ, and age of acquisition of language) between the two (Walker et al., 2004). One subgroup of PDD-NOS has significant impairments in social communication but fewer repetitive behaviors than seen in children with ASD.

Asperger's syndrome (AS), a neurodevelopmental disorder less severe than ASD in which cognitive, language, and self-help skills are supposedly not disordered (American Psychiatric Association, 2000), although there may be subtle language impairments with little delay, along with social interaction difficulties, restricted interests, and repetitive behaviors. In general, compared to children with high-functioning autism (HFA), children with AS have high verbal IQ and low non-verbal or performance IQ, while in most children with HFA the pattern is reversed; however, there is considerable overlap between HFA and AS (Ghaziuddin & Mountain-Kimchi, 2004). In general, adolescents with either HFA or Aspergers rate the quality of their communication life positively but lower than do their TD peers (Burgess & Turkstra, 2010). Communication similarities and differences are presented in Figure 2.4. The heterogeneity of both populations increases the need for thorough evaluation and individualized intervention (Tsatsanis, Foley, & Donehower, 2004).

Language difficulties with AS include verbosity, a pedantic speaking style, inability to understand the rules of social behavior, including conversation, and an intense interest in a limited range of one or two topics. Children with AS may be poorly organized but perfectionist in their demands, with ability to concentrate deeply and difficulty transitioning between activities or topics.

Still other children may be said to have **hyperlexia**, a disorder affecting boys and girls at a ratio of 7:1 and characterized by a spontaneous early ability to read—often at age 2½ or 3—but with little comprehension. Children with hyperlexia have an intense preoccupation with letters and words and extensive word recognition by age 5 but exhibit language and cognitive disorders in reasoning and in perceiving relationships. In addition to delayed language, these children experience difficulty with connected language in all modalities, especially integrating it with context in order to derive meaning.

As with all the disorders discussed, there is a range of severity. Some children with mild forms may be mislabeled as learning disabled depending on the characteristics present. This is not a science but a fine art. Although outcomes for children with ASD represent a broad continuum, only a small percentage achieve full independence and employment as adults (Howlin, Goode, Hutton, & Rutter, 2004).

Language Characteristics

Communication problems are often one of the first indicators of possible ASD. These may include a failure or delay in developing gestures or speech, a seeming noninterest in other people, or a lack of verbal responding. Lack of communication skills is one of the most significant stress factors for families of children with ASD and one of the earliest indicators of the disorder.

All children with ASD are not alike in development of communication skills. In general, children who say and imitate more words, have better pretend-play skills with objects, and use gestures

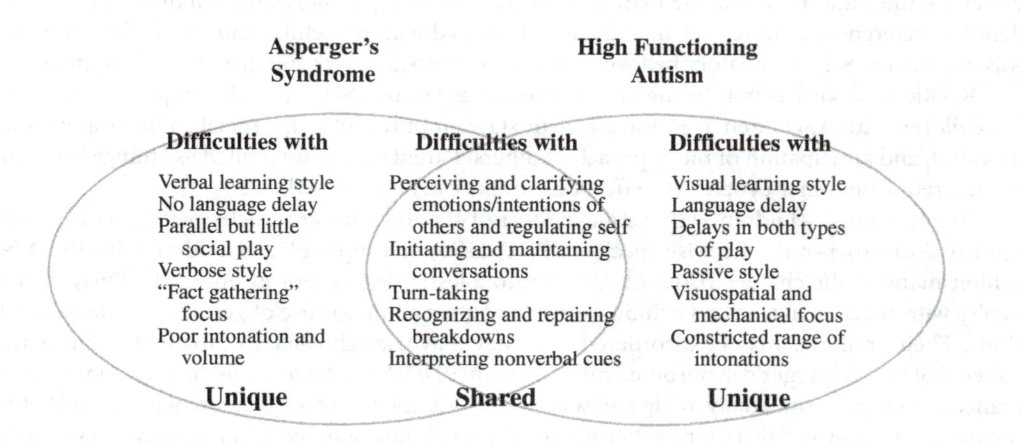

FIGURE 2.4 Similarities and differences in the communication of children with Asperger's syndrome and high-functioning autism.

These characteristics are generalities, and individual children will vary greatly.

Source: Adapted from Rubin & Lennon (2004).

more often to initiate joint attending, such as pointing at entities to direct attention, have the most rapid expressive vocabulary growth (Smith, Mirenda, & Zaidman-Zait, 2007). Calling attention to entities through gestures and sounds seems to be important for comprehension of new vocabulary words (McDuffie, Yoder, & Stone, 2005). The importance of these factors is similar to that found in typical development (Watt, Wetherby, & Shumway, 2006).

Poor social interaction and poor language and communication skills are extremely characteristic of children with ASD. Speech does not seem to be difficult for those who speak, although speech is often wooden and robotlike, lacking a musical quality. Although children with HFA are able to perceive affective stress (sad, happy) and lexical stress (*HOTdog* vs. *hot DOG*) as well as TD peers, they had reduced ability to produce natural prosody in their own speech (Grossman, Bemis, Plesa Skwerer, & Tager-Flusberg, 2010).

While as many as 25 percent of children with ASD may have typical language (Kjelgaard & Tager-Flusberg, 2001), between 25 and 60 percent of the population with ASD remains mute or nonspeaking. Until recently, this lack of speech also has meant that they remained noncommunicating. This situation is changing for some, but not all, children using augmentative and alternative communication (AAC).

Those children using speech and language may demonstrate immediate or delayed **echolalia**, a whole or partial repetition of previous utterances, often with the same intonation. In fact, most children with ASD who learn to talk go through a period of using echolalia. Immediate echolalia is variable and increases in highly directive situations, with unknown words, following an inability to comprehend, in the presence of an adult, in unfamiliar situations, in face-to-face communication with eye contact, and with longer, more complex utterances. Immediate echolalia also has been found to signal agreement in some children. No such data are available for delayed echolalia. One child with whom I worked would repeat many of the utterances directed to him during the day as he lay in bed prior to sleep.

Although communicative dysfunction is one of the central characteristics of PDD, its characteristics vary widely across children. At one extreme are children whose language structure is within normal limits, while at the other are children with ASD who remain essentially nonverbal (Landa, 2000). As a group, children with ASD demonstrate significant delays in language and communicative, especially in pragmatics (Tager-Flusberg, Paul, & Lord, 2005). Even when language structure seems intact, difficulties with the appropriate social use of language or pragmatics persist (Adams, 2002; Landa, 2000; Tager-Flusberg, 2004; Young, Diehl, Morris, Hyman, & Bennetto, 2005).

Children with ASD have difficulties in initiating a conversation and in responding to initiations of others. Once the conversation has begun, they have difficulty with the give-and-take of conversation and with taking turns appropriately (Botting & Conti-Ramsden, 2003). Speakers with ASD may fail to contribute new, relevant information to the topic and may repeat previously mentioned topics or previous utterances or fail to link their utterance to prior ones, resulting in sudden and inexplicable topic changes (Volden, 2002).

The range of intentions is very limited. In addition, intentions may be expressed in an individualistic or idiosyncratic manner, such as saying "Sesame Street is a production of the Children's Television Workshop" for "Goodbye."

The conversations of children with ASD often contain inappropriate, irrelevant, bizarre, or stereotypical utterances (Adams, 2002; Gilchrist et al., 2001; Volden, 2004). For example, a child might say, "Did you know that the Volt is a type of electric car" in the middle of a conversation about what he or she had for breakfast.

Semantics may also be affected. Definitions tend to be very concrete and may not generalize to similar words. Figurative language is also difficult for many children with ASD who tend to interpret phrases such as "Hit the roof" in an overly literal manner to questions.

Children with ASD also seem to have difficulty matching the content and form of language to the context. Occasionally, children will incorporate rote utterances, such as the child who says "Attention, K-Mart shoppers" to get attention. Even those individuals who have acquired language often have peculiarities and irregularities in their communication. Specific language characteristics are listed in Table 2.10.

Language structure is often not disordered. Oral language structure or form is a relative strength for children with ASD. Language form errors that do occur seem to represent a lack of underlying semantic relationships.

Although many children with ASD fail to develop verbal communication skills, verbal children are similar in syntax and phonology to other children matched for mental age. In addition, verbal students with ASD appear to develop language form and speech in a typical developmental sequence (Watson & Ozonoff, 2000).

To help us determine which behaviors are important for development, predictive studies offer some guidance. For example, young children with ASD who were rated as highly inattentive are more likely to have lower rates of change in vocabulary production and language comprehension over the next two years. Those who are highly unresponsive socially tend to have lower rates of change in vocabulary comprehension and production and in language comprehension over next two years. Other behaviors, such as insistence on sameness, repetitive stereotypic motor behaviors, and acting-out, did not seem to predict later language development (Bopp, Mirenda, & Zumbo, 2009).

As you might expect, 18- to 24-month-old children with ASD communicate via gestures, vocalizations, and verbalizations at a lower rate than either TD children or those with developmental

TABLE 2.10 Language Characteristics of Children with ASD

Pragmatics	Deficits in joint attending.
	Difficulty initiating and maintaining a conversation, resulting in much shorter conversational episodes.
	Limited range of communication functions.
	Difficulty matching form and content to context. May perseverate or introduce inappropriate topics.
	Immediate and delayed echolalia and routinized utterances.
	Few gestures used; misinterpretation of complex gestures.
	Overuse of questions, frequent repetition.
	Frequent asocial monologues.
	Difficulty with stylistic variations and speaker-listener roles.
	Gaze aversion, seeming use of peripheral vision.
Semantics	Word-retrieval difficulties, especially for visual referents.
	Underlying meaning not used as a memory aid.
	More inappropriate answers to questions than age-matched peers.
Syntax/Morphology	Morphological difficulties, especially with pronouns and verb endings.
	Construction of sentences with superficial form, often disregarding underlying meaning.
	Less complex sentences than mental-age-matched peers developing typically.
	Overreliance on word order.
Phonology	Phonology variable within individual child, often disordered.
	Developmental order similar to children developing typically.
	Least affected aspect of language.
Comprehension	Impaired comprehension, especially in connected discourse such as conversations.

disabilities, such as ID. In addition, children with ASD use a significantly lower proportion of communication acts for joint attention and have a significantly lower percentage of deictic gestures, instead relying on more primitive gestures than both the other groups of children. Those children with ASD who communicate for joint attention are as likely as other children to coordinate vocalizations, eye gaze, and gestures. Thus, the rate of both communicative acts and joint attention are very stronge predictors of verbal outcome at age 3 (Shumway & Wetherby, 2009).

Possible Causal Factors

In the past, children with ASD have been classified as having an emotional-, physical-, environmental-, or health-related impairment. The cause may be any and all of these, although the primary causal factors are probably biological. Even within this population, neuroanatomical and neurochemical features may differ.

Biological Factors. Approximately 65 percent of all individuals with ASD have abnormal brain patterns. The incidence of autism accompanying prenatal complications, fragile X syndrome, and Ritt syndrome, a degenerative neurological condition, and among those with a family history of autism is higher. In addition, ASD is often accompanied by ID and seizures. All of these suggest a biological basis but do not explain the actual disorder. Other studies have found unusually high levels of serotonin, a neurotransmitter and natural opiate; abnormal development of the cerebellum, the section of the brain that regulates incoming sensations; multifocal disorders of the brain; and impairment of the neural subcortical structures with accompanying impairment in cortical development.

Recent studies have suggested a genetic link in ASD, although is seems doubtful that a solitary autism gene exists (Wentzel, 2000). It is more likely that several genes are involved and may be shared with other disorders.

Social-Environmental Factors. Early studies blamed parents for their child's ASD. No basis has been found for this conclusion. In general, parents interact with their children at the appropriate language level.

Processing Factors. Children with ASD have difficulty analyzing and integrating information. When attending, they tend to fixate on one aspect of a complex stimulus, often some irrelevant, minor detail. In other words, responding is very overselective. This fixation, in turn, makes discrimination difficult.

Aberrant sensory processing may affect the rate of acquisition of language, social, and communication skills in children with ASD and other DDs. More specifically, hypo-responsiveness and sensory seeking behavior, such as self-stimulatory behaviors, are negatively associated with language skills and social adaptive skills.

Overall processing by these children has been characterized as a "gestalt" in which unanalyzed wholes are stored and later reproduced in identical fashion, as in echolalia. In this relatively inflexible system, input is examined in its entirety rather than analyzed into its component parts. Information usually is reproduced in a context that is in some way similar to the initial context. This reliance on unanalyzed wholes could account for the tendency of children with ASD to repeat an agrammatical sentence, rather than to correct it as language-matched children with ID will do. It is possible that children with ASD depend more heavily on simultaneous language processing than on successive language processing.

The behavior of children with ASD suggests that very little of the world makes sense to them. They seem to overload quickly. Information "swallowed" whole could quickly "fill" the system.

Storage of unanalyzed wholes also might hinder memory. Children with autism reportedly are less able to use environmental cues, such as a word or gesture, to aid memory, possibly because those cues do not exist as separate entities in the child's memory. It is also difficult for these children to organize information on the basis of relationships between stimuli.

In addition, children with ASD have difficulty transferring or generalizing learned information from one context to another. This difficulty reflects the inability of these children to identify the relevant contextual information.

Summary

As with other disorders that have been discussed, PDD demonstrates heterogeneity. Great differences are found in severity, especially in communication abilities. In general, these differences affect the pragmatic and semantic aspects of language and may reflect processing difficulties such as stimulus overselectivity and storage of unanalyzed wholes.

Early intervention (EI) is critical to maximizing outcomes for children with ASD, but early identification is often difficult. Although SLPs alone do not make evaluations of children for ASD, they are a vital part of the evaluative team (Prelock, Beatson, Bitner, Broder, & Ducker, 2003). The American Academy of Neurology and Child Neurology Society has suggested that failure to meet the following milestones indicated need for further evaluation (Filipek et al., 1999):

- No babbling by 12 months
- No gesturing by 12 months
- No single words by 16 months
- No two-word spontaneous speech by 24 months
- Loss of language or social skills at any age

In addition, children with ASD also demonstrate deficits in joint attention and symbolic communication (Wetherby, Prizant, & Schuler, 2000). Given the limitations of current research, it may not be possible at this time to make a definitive diagnosis prior to 24 months of age (Woods & Wetherby, 2003).

Although there is no definitive cure for ASD, up to 70 percent of children with ASD are prescribed psychoactive medications to ameliorate disruptive behaviors associated with ASD. These include hyperactivity, inattention, impulsivity, aggression, irritability, self-injury, obsessive compulsiveness, anxiety, and mood disorders. The entire healthcare team, including SLPs, should be involved in monitoring the behavior of children with ASD for medication efficacy, tolerability, and potential side effects. Self, Hale, and Crumrine (2010) offer an excellent tutorial on medications prescribed to treat behaviors associated with ASD, including potential side effects.

Brain Injury

Children with brain injury differ greatly as a result of the site and extent of lesion, the age at onset, and the age of the injury. In general, the smaller the damaged area, the better the **prognosis**, or chance of recovery. Brain injury in children may result from trauma, cerebrovascular accident (CVA) or stroke, congenital malformation of the neural blood vessels, convulsive disorders, or encephalopathy, such as infection or tumors. Each has different characteristics; however, some similarities in language occur. Only the most prevalent types of injury are discussed here.

Traumatic Brain Injury (TBI)

Approximately 1 million children and adolescents in the United States have traumatic brain injury, or TBI, diffuse brain damage as the result of external physical force, such as a blow to the head received in an auto accident. Individuals may range from nearly full recovery to a vegetative state in some very severe cases. Although the chances of survival have improved greatly in recent years, long-term disability is a continuing public health problem.

Deficits may be cognitive, physical, behavioral, academic, and linguistic. *Cognitive deficits* include perception, memory, reasoning, and problem-solving difficulties and may be permanent or temporary and may partially or totally affect functioning ability. Psychological maladjustment or acting-out behaviors, called **social disinhibition**, may also occur. For example, I once evaluated a young man with TBI who kept insisting on kissing my hand. Other characteristics include lack of initiative, distractibility, inability to adapt quickly, perseveration, low frustration levels, passive-aggressiveness, anxiety, depression, fear of failure, and misperception.

Severity may range from a *mild concussion,* defined as a loss of consciousness for less than 30 seconds, through *moderate TBI,* a loss of consciousness or posttraumatic amnesia for 30 minutes to 24 hours, with or without skull fracture, to *severe TBI,* consisting of a coma for 6 hours or longer. Severity of symptoms is not directly related to the deficits mentioned above.

Variables that affect recovery are extremely independent and are complicated by some of the characteristics of the population at risk for TBI. As a group, this population has a lower IQ, higher social disadvantage, poorer schooling, and more behavioral and physical difficulties prior to injury than the general population. Other variables include degree and length of unconsciousness, duration of posttraumatic amnesia, age at injury, age of injury, and posttraumatic ability. In general, shorter, less severe unconsciousness, shorter amnesia, and better posttraumatic abilities indicate better recovery.

Age at the time of injury is a less definitive factor because the child is developing when the injury occurs. Younger children may exhibit more severe and more long-lasting problems. Although younger children have less to recover, they also do not have the benefit of as much past learning as older children.

Age of the injury also can be an inaccurate predictor. In general, the older the injury, the less chance of change, but this aspect is complicated by the delayed onset of some deficits. Neural recovery over time is often unpredictable and irregular.

Language Characteristics. Language problems are usually evident even after mild injuries. Individuals with severe TBI and resultant deficits in executive function demonstrate problems with pragmatics (Douglas, 2010). More specifically, these individuals had difficulty regulating the amount and manner or conversational participation as well as the relevance of their contributions. This can be noted in the narratives and in conversation of these children. Utterances are often lengthy, inappropriate, and off-topic, and fluency is disturbed. Language comprehension and higher functions such as figurative language and dual meanings also may be affected. A child may lose his or her train of thought in conversations, while in narratives the same child may not retain the central focus of the story, thus deleting important information.

By comparison, language form is relatively unaffected. The majority of children with TBI regain the ability to manipulate language form and content. Surface structure may seem relatively unimpaired. A child's language may be relatively effective in school until the third or fourth grade, when students are required to use higher language abilities to analyze and synthesize. Semantics, especially concrete vocabulary, is also relatively undisturbed, although word retrieval, naming, and object description difficulties may be present. Other characteristics are listed in Table 2.11.

Some deficits will remain long after the injury even when overall improvement is good. Although there is considerable variability among children with TBI, many subtle deficits remain, especially in pragmatics.

Possible Causal Factors. Obvious biological and physical factors are involved in TBI. More important is the manner in which informational processing is affected. As mentioned, children with TBI are often inattentive and easily distractible. Attention fluctuates, and they have difficulty focusing on a task.

All aspects of organization—categorizing, sequencing, abstracting, and generalization—are affected. Children with TBI seem stimulus-bound—unable to see relationships, make inferences, and solve problems. They evidence difficulty formulating goals, planning, and achieving. This deficiency often is masked by intact vocabulary and general knowledge.

Finally, children with TBI exhibit memory deficits in both storage and retrieval. Long-term memory prior to the trauma is usually intact. Techniques presented in Table 2.6 might be helpful with these children.

TABLE 2.11 Language Characteristics of Children with Traumatic Brain Injury (TBI)

Pragmatics	Difficulty with organization and expression of complex ideas. Off-topic comments. Ineffectual, inappropriate comments. Frequency of eye gaze is appropriate during conversation. Less complex narratives, containing fewer words and shorter, less sentences complexity, and fewer episodic elements. Short narratives include story grammar and cohesion, as do those of typically developing peers.
Semantics	Word retrieval, naming, and object description difficulties, although vocabulary relatively intact. Automatized, overlearned language relatively unaffected.
Syntax/Morphology	Sentences may be lengthy and fragmented.
Phonology	Few phonological difficulties, but there may be some dysarthria or apraxia due to injury.
Comprehension	Some problems due to inattention and speed of processing. Poor auditory and reading comprehension. Difficulty with sentence comprehension due to difficulty assigning meaning to syntactic structure. Most routinized, everyday comprehension unaffected. Vocabulary comprehension usually unaffected, except for abstract terms.

Cerebrovascular Accident (CVA)

Cerebrovascular accidents occur when a portion of the brain is denied oxygen, usually because of a blockage or rupture in a blood vessel serving the brain. Most frequently, damage is specific and localized. Patterns of recovery suggest that adjoining portions of the cortex, the surface of the cerebrum, augment the functioning of the damaged portion.

CVAs usually are found in children with congenital heart problems or arteriovenous (blood vessel) malformations in the brain. Prognosis is generally good. Naturally, the variability will be great, depending on the site and extent of the lesion. Language problems often accompany left hemisphere damage, although any brain damage has the potential to disturb language functioning.

Language Characteristics. Long-term subtle pragmatic difficulties are common. Language form usually returns quickly, although performance may deteriorate when demands increase. Word retrieval may be extremely difficult at first, with deficits in both speed and accuracy. Language comprehension also is affected initially. Children usually recover, although higher level academic and reading difficulties may persist.

Summary

The underlying relationship between cognition and language varies with age and with the aspect of language studied. At many points in development, we are not able to describe the exact relationship. It is not surprising that we cannot fully explain the mechanisms at work when the brain is injured. Still, we can predict that vocabulary and structural rules will return more easily than higher order functions, such as conversational skills that require complex synthesis of language form, content, and use. Even those children who seem to recover may continue to exhibit long-term subtle pragmatic difficulties.

Maltreatment: Neglect and Abuse

Each year in the United States, approximately 1.2 percent of children, or 900,000 children, are maltreated sufficiently for this information to be reported to the authorities (U.S. Department of Health and Human Services [DHHS], 2007). A study of over 50,000 typically developing children found that 9 percent had been maltreated (Sullivan & Knutson, 2000). The percentage is higher for young children and for those with disabilities. In the same study, 31 percent of children with disabilities and 35 percent of children with speech/language impairment had been maltreated.

Although maltreatment occurs across the income spectrum, children from families earning less than $15,000 per year are over twenty times more likely to be abused than those from families earning at least twice that amount (Kapp, McDonald, & Diamond, 2001). It is believed that the increased economic, social, and health problems and lower levels of education and employment of the poor increase the risk of maltreatment.

Table 2.12 presents the types of neglect and abuse that have been identified. Of the 900,000 maltreated annually, approximately 63 percent are neglected, 17 percent physically abused, 9 percent sexually abused, and 7 percent psychologically abused (U.S. DHHS, 2005). Until recently, these children were not identified as having distinct language problems. The effect of each type of abuse varies with each child.

Neglect and abuse are extreme examples of a dysfunctional family and are a sign of the type of social environment in which the child learned language. Although neglect and abuse are rarely the direct cause of the communication problem, the context in which they occur directly influences a child's development.

Complex trauma, or exposure both to domestic violence or maltreatment and to physical, sexual, and psycho-emotional abuse, rarely occurs in isolation and is often associated with substance abuse, mostly alcohol abuse, by parents. Adults who abuse alcohol are prone to violence, and their children are at risk (Willis & Silovsky, 1998). Whether these causal factors occur alone or together, they can lead to developmental difficulties across the lifespan (Timler, Olswang, & Coggins, 2005).

Children exposed to both prenatal alcohol and postnatal abuse and neglect have lower intelligence scores and more severe neurodevelopmental deficits than traumatized children who are not prenatally exposed to alcohol (Henry, Sloane, & Black-Pond, 2007). Developmental deficits occur in language, attention, memory, visual processing, and motor skills.

Children who have been traumatized experience biological brain changes as a result (Atchison, 2007). Characterized as *hyperarousal,* these changes are associated with acceleration in nervous system areas responsible for perception and processing of potentially threatening sensations. The accompanying release of certain stress hormones, influence thoughts, feelings, and actions. In a state of fear-related activation, the child responds to perceived threats with primitive, reflexive, and

TABLE 2.12 Types of Neglect and Abuse

Physical neglect	Abandonment with no arrangement for care, including inadequate supervision, nutrition, clothing, and/or personal hygiene, and/or failure to seek needed or recommended medical care.
Emotional neglect	Failure to provide a normal living experience, including attention and affection, and/or refusal of treatment or services recommended by professional personnel.
Physical abuse	Bodily injury, such as neurological damage, or death from shaking, beating, and/or burning.
Sexual abuse	Both nonphysical abuse, such as indecent exposure or verbal attack, and physical abuse, such as genital-oral stimulation, fondling, and/or sexual intercourse.
Emotional abuse	Excessive yelling, belittling, teasing/verbal attack, and/or overt rejection.

aggressive reactions. Over time, the hypervigilant state of the child leads to apprehension, fear, attention difficulties, and restlessness (Lane, 2002). Persistent activation of this response can result in a maladaptive, persistent state of fear.

Language Characteristics

Maltreated children have less complex language than nonmaltreated children (Eigsti & Cicchetti, 2004). All aspects of language are affected; however, it is in language use that children who are neglected and abused exhibit the greatest difficulties (see Table 2.13). In general, children who are neglected and abused are less talkative and have fewer conversational skills than their peers. Utterances and conversations are shorter than those of their peers. They are less likely to volunteer information or to discuss emotions or feelings.

In school, these children have depressed verbal language performance. A high correlation is found between deficient verbal and reading ability and neglect and abuse.

Possible Causal Factors

Certainly, negative social-environment factors are important in the development of language by children who are neglected and abused, but biological factors should not be overlooked. Medical and health problems among the poor also can contribute. Direct effect is difficult to determine because of the multiplicity of overlapping factors, especially among the poor.

Biological Factors. Neglect and abuse are not limited to poor families, but in these families or in cases of extreme neglect, biological factors also may contribute. Poor maternal health, substance abuse, poor or nonexistent pediatric services, and poor nutrition can all affect brain development and maturation. Physical abuse also may cause lasting physical or neurological damage. We do not know the long-term effects on the brain of lack of environmental stimulation.

Social-Environmental Factors. As in all children, the early language experiences of a child with a history of maltreatment influence the underlying social cognitive behavior of the infant or toddler (Lohmann & Tomasello, 2003). When children are repeatedly exposed to violence and stress, they compensate through behaviors that ensure their survival. These strategies can interfere with critical brain development in areas of socioemotional learning. As a result, these children have limited ability to predict and interpret the beliefs and intentions of others and to self-regulate their own language

TABLE 2.13 Language Characteristics of Children Who Are Neglected and Abused

Pragmatics	Poor conversational skills. Inability to discuss feelings. Shorter conversations. Fewer descriptive utterances. Language used to get things done with little social exchange or affect.
Semantics	Limited expressive vocabulary. Fewer decontextualized utterances, more talk about the here and now.
Syntax/Morphology	Shorter, less complex utterances.
Phonology	Similar to peers.
Comprehension	Receptive vocabulary similar to peers. Auditory and reading comprehension problems.

use. Some maltreated children exhibit *alexithymia,* difficulty in the identification, regulation, and understanding of feelings in others and, in extreme cases, in themselves. It is hypothesized that traumatic experiences result in a disassociation between right-hemisphere emotions and left-hemisphere expression (Schore, 2001). As a result, children with alexithymia may have behavioral problems or outbursts of aggressive behavior.

Either or both parents may be neglectful or abusing, but it is a mother's or primary caregiver's everyday responsiveness to a child that has the most effect on language development. The quality of the child–mother attachment is a more significant factor in language development than is maltreatment and can moderate or exacerbate the effects of neglect or abuse.

Several factors, including childhood loss of a parent, death of a previous child, pregnancy complications, birth complications, current marital or financial problems, substance abuse, maternal age, and/or illness, can disturb maternal attachment. In turn, mothers may adopt two general patterns of interaction. Most abusive mothers are *controlling,* imposing their will on the child. As controllers, they tend to ignore a child's initiations, thus decreasing the amount of verbal stimulation received by that child. *Neglecting* mothers, however, are unresponsive to their infant's behaviors because they have low expectations of deriving satisfaction from the infant. Either situation includes a lack of support for the development of meaningful communication skills and little active interaction, such as playing games, hugging, patting, or nuzzling, and little nurturing maternal speech toward a baby.

The result is insecure attachment on the part of a child. The child may be apprehensive in the presence of the parent and may avoid interaction to lessen the chance of hostile responses. Early stimulus–response bonds—an infant's notion that her or his behavior results in an adult reinforcing response—may be nonexistent, further depressing the child's behavior. Obviously, this is not an ideal language learning environment.

Summary

Only now are we beginning to understand the effect of caregiver behavior on an infant. Although it seems intuitive that neglect and abuse would cause language and communication problems, especially in language use, the data are only correlational, not cause and effect.

Although no practice that harms children can be condoned, professionals must be either mindful of different cultural practices or risk offending or alienating parents (Westby, 2007). By focusing on the welfare of the child, however, it should be easy to recognize when a family has crossed into maltreatment. It may be helpful to think of cultural childrearing practices as falling on a continuum from beneficial to harmful (Koramoa, Lynch, & Kinnair, 2002). Responses by professionals can vary according to where a practice falls on the continuum. Less-than-harmful corporeal punishment, for example, might best be handled by parental education. Culturally sensitive ways of approaching a family about childrearing and punishment might include the following (Fontes, 2002):

- Explaining the laws regarding such practices
- Exploring the family's goals and suggesting alternative methods
- Explaining the effects of harsh or corporeal punishment
- Gaining the aid of professionals from the same culture

Other Language Impairments

Although we've touched on some of the more prevalent language impairments, we have by no means exhausted the discussion. I've omitted several forms of LI or related conditions for the sake of brevity. Let me at least familiarize you with some category names and brief descriptions. In order, we'll explore *nonspecific language impairment* (NLI), late talkers, childhood schizophrenia, selective mutism (SM), otitis media, and children who have received cochlear implants. Disorders specifically related to literacy have been left for discussion in the chapter on literacy impairments. No doubt, your professor will have others to add to the list.

Nonspecific Language Impairment (NLI)

Children with nonspecific language impairment (NLI) have a general delay in language development, a nonverbal IQ of 86 or lower, and, as in SLI, no obvious sensory or perceptual deficits. Beyond this characterization, the population is poorly described in the disorder literature. Compared to children with SLI, these children perform more poorly on some language tasks and take longer to generalize rule learning (Rice, Tomblin, Hoffman, Richman, & Marquis, 2004).

Late Talkers

Although a significant number of late-talking children, possibly 40 to 50 percent, have persistent language problems throughout the preschool years, it is difficult to predict the effect of early delay on later development (Dale, Price, Bishop, & Plomin, 2003). Nor is the severity of early delay a good prognostic indicator. By age 4, late talkers without persistent LI do not differ from TD children in morphological development (Rescorla & Roberts, 2002); however, more subtle deficits may be present.

Although child health is an important factor in early delay, most early language delay is environmental in origin. Environmental factors persist for children whose parents do not seek professional help such as SLP services (Bishop, Price, Dale, & Plomin, 2003). One environmental factor can be poverty and/or homelessness. Many children in homeless shelters exhibit language delays, but there is no common pattern. In fact, although the majority of both mothers and children in homeless shelters have some type of LI, the lack of a pattern of LI means that they do not form a distinct diagnostic category (O'Neil-Pizozzi, 2003). We'll discuss extreme poverty more under considerations for children from culturally and linguistically diverse backgrounds in Chapter 5.

Childhood Schizophrenia

Childhood schizophrenia, a serious psychiatric illness that causes strange thinking, odd feelings, and unusual behavior, is uncommon, occurring in approximately 1 of every 14,000 children below age 13 (APA, 2000). The disorder is difficult to recognize in its early phases, and the cause is unknown; it may result from a combination of brain changes and biochemical, genetic, and environmental factors.

Although schizophrenia can be controlled by medical treatment, it is a lifelong disease that cannot be cured at the present time. Symptoms may include seeing and hearing things that are not real, called hallucinating; confusing reality and fantasy; exhibiting odd and eccentric behavior; confused thinking and extreme moodiness; and severe anxiety and fearfulness. Behaviors may change slowly over time.

Although there are slightly more males than females with the disorder, it is observed only rarely in children below age 5. In general, the earlier the symptoms appear, the poorer the prognosis. Among preschool children, approximately 30 percent who will develop schizophrenia have behaviors similar to those associated with pervasive developmental disorder (PDD) discussed earlier, such as rocking and arm flapping. It is not until early school age or later that children begin to display symptoms of hallucinations, delusions, and disordered thinking.

Approximately 55 percent of children and adolescents with schizophrenia have language abnormalities, including language delay (Mental Health Research Association, 2007). Although there are few studies of the language of children with schizophrenia, data from adults suggest difficulty with pragmatics, especially in content relevancy (Nicolson et al., 2000). More specifically, adults have problems with appropriateness of topics and intentions, turn-taking, vocabulary, and nonverbal behaviors (Meilijson, Kasher, & Elizur, 2004).

Selective Mutism

Selective mutism (SM) is a relatively rare disorder in which a child does not speak in some situations, such as in school, although she or he may speak normally in others. From 0.2 to 0.7 percent of all children may have SM at some time, with girls nearly twice as likely as boys to be affected (Bergman, Piacentini, & McCracken, 2002; Kristensen, 2000). Related factors include social anxiety, extreme shyness, and LI or second language learning. Although 30 to 50 percent of children with SM are reported to have LI, the nature and extent of this impairment remains undetermined.

Otitis Media

Many young children suffer from chronic otitis media. In general, the cumulative effect of recurrent hearing loss can be a significant factor in delayed language development (Feldman et al., 2003). While otitis media is a factor in LI, children with otitis media do not constitute a separate category. Otitis media may co-occur with categories discussed previously, such as SLI or NLI.

Deafness

Although limited space precludes discussion of the language of children with deafness, it is important to note the effect of two things, early intervention and cochlear implants. Children born with deafness who receive both speech and sign training in infancy can often become proficient, if not perfect, speakers or develop language through sign, or both. Interestingly, children exposed to sign will express their first word in sign at about 8 months, while hearing children often don't speak their first word until four months later.

Those who receive cochlear implants develop language in a manner similar to that of typically developing children. In general, those implanted as infants show more rapid growth in language than those implanted later; however, the relationship is not simple (Tomblin, Barker, Spencer, Zhang, & Gantz, 2005). Although those implanted later have an initial advantage of maturity that enhances language growth, this advantage seems to disappear later as children who received implants at an earlier age begin to develop spoken language at an ever-increasing rate (Ertmer, Strong, & Sadagopan, 2003; Nicholas & Geers, 2007).

Implications

Language impairments are not outgrown. Even with intervention, they are rarely "cured." Typically, language impairments change and become more subtle. Children with preschool LI may continue to have trouble with linguistic and academic tasks. Language impairments in kindergarten are likely to persist well into elementary school (Tomblin, Zhang, Buckwalter, & O'Brien, 2003). Reading performance may be affected. As adults, children with LI may continue to do poorly in speech and language although nonlinguistic skills seem unaffected. With or without intervention, certain ramifications of having an LI affect academic performance and social acceptance.

Poor oral language usually results in poor reading and writing ability. Poor reading often reflects the child's lack of language awareness skills, called *metalinguistic abilities*. This awareness is crucial for reading.

Within the classroom, children with LI form a separate subgroup that interacts increasingly less with their peers developing typically. One's relative communication skills influence participation. Because children with LI are poor communicators overall, they are increasingly ignored. As a result, children with LI are more likely to be overidentified as having a socioemotional disorder (Redmond, 2002). In general, children with LI exhibit more behavior problems and poorer social skills than do their TD peers (Qi & Kaiser, 2004). The poor ability of these children to infer emotional reactions in social situation may contribute to the social difficulties they encounter (Ford & Milosky,

2003). Teachers rate children with LI significantly below their peers in impulse control, likability, and social behaviors such as helping others, offering comfort, and sharing. Increasing reticence to talk leads to withdrawal, especially among prepubescent and adolescent boys (Fujiki, Brinton, Isaacson, & Summers, 2001).

In general, a child's popularity is associated with her or his conversational skills. Children with LI initiate little verbal interaction, are less responsive, use more short and nonverbal responses, and are less able to maintain a conversation. The result is fewer interactions with others.

Children with LI often continue to have poor vocabularies and poor higher level semantic skills. These include difficulties with abstract meanings, figurative language, dual meanings, ambiguity, and humor.

Their syntax and morphology are usually characterized by the continued use of less mature forms. Word formation processes, consisting of a free morpheme plus one or more bound morphemes, are less mature. Similarly, phonological patterns usually reflect those of younger children.

Finally, language comprehension difficulties, especially at higher levels such as detection of ambiguity, may persist. These difficulties reflect the underlying language difficulties evidenced in expressive language. It seems appropriate at this point to note that some professionals and organizations (American Psychiatric Association, 2000; World Health Organization, 2005) label expressive language disorder as a distinct category, principally limited to deficits in language output. Evidence suggests, however, that expressive language deficits are usually accompanied either by limitations in language knowledge or by difficulties in processing of language input (Leonard, 2009).

SLPs are responsible for intervening to correct some language difficulties, to modify others, and to teach compensation skills for still others. In the chapters that follow, we'll explore a model that proposes to do this in the most natural way possible. It's called a functional approach.

Conclusion

At this point, most likely, you are in need of a one-sentence summary that once and for all distinguishes each language impairment from the others. Unfortunately, I do not have one forthcoming. Still, we need to make some sense from the wealth of information presented. At the risk of generalizing too much, let's try. At the beginning of the chapter, I cited six abilities needed for typical language development. It might be helpful to consider these in conceptualizing the language impairments discussed (see Table 2.14).

Perceptual difficulties are reported for some of the disorders mentioned, but not all. Nor are they similar in type and severity. For children with SLI, perceptual difficulties seem to be limited to rapid, sequenced auditory stimuli, but perceptual difficulties are the essence of LD and ASD. Even here the difference seems to be one of perception and sensory integration in LD and responsiveness levels in ASD.

Attentional difficulties also accompany several of the language impairments discussed. Again the variability is great. Children with ASD are either seemingly inattentive or fixated on one, often irrelevant, aspect of a stimulus. In contrast, children with TBI experience attentional fluctuations and seem to attend for only brief periods.

Although all children with language impairment have difficulty using symbols, this difficulty varies. Children with ID and ASD have great difficulty with symbol referent relationships, while those who are neglected and abused have little difficulty with language form and content.

Language is rarely taught formally. Instead, children acquire language by hypothesizing the rules from the give-and-take of conversational speech. This can be a difficult task if the child is inattentive or has difficulty perceiving language, as are children with LD, ASD, and TBI.

The requirement of having enough mental energy is a tricky one. We shall broaden the concept somewhat. Children with ID may lack the mental abilities for some tasks, while those with

TABLE 2.14 Language Learning Requirements and the Difficulties of Children with Language Impairment*

	Language Impairment					
Requirements	ID	LD	SLI	ASD	TBI	Neglect/ Abuse
Ability to perceive sequenced acoustic events of short duration		X*	X	X	X	
Ability to attend actively, to be responsive, and to anticipate stimuli		X		X	X	
Ability to use symbols	X	X	X	X	X	X
Ability to invent syntax from the language in the environment	X	X	X	X		
Ability to interact and communicate with others				X		X
Enough mental energy to do all the above simultaneously	X		X		X	X

*Xs represent problem areas in language learning and use.

SLI and TBI may use vital mental energy on lower level tasks, leaving little for language analysis and synthesis. The frequently reported depression of children with TBI and children who are neglected and abused also limits the cognitive energy available for language learning.

Finally, the ability to interact and communicate with others probably is affected in each of the disorders discussed. The difficulty is in determining whether an inability to interact and communicate reflects a cause of the impairment, a result, both, or just an accompanying feature. Among at least two groups of children—those with ASD and those who are neglected and abused—inability to interact seems directly related to the language impairment exhibited.

Each impairment presents a somewhat different image. In a clinical sense, however, the important features to which an SLP attends are the individual characteristics of each child, not the diagnostic category. Naming and describing a language impairment does not necessarily explain it nor determine clinical intervention.

Chapter

3

Early Communication Intervention

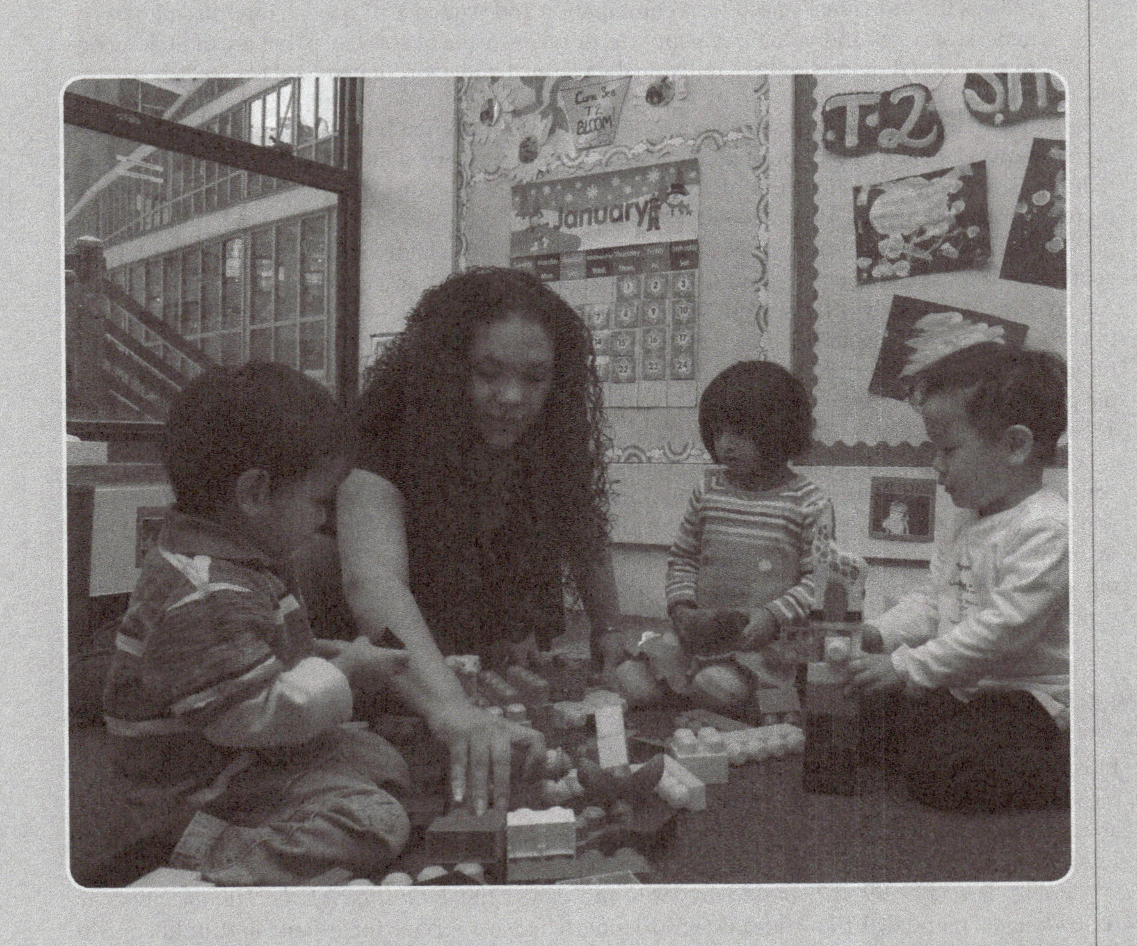

In the United States, approximately 17 percent of children, including one of my grandsons, have a **developmental disability** (DD) (Centers for Disease Control and Prevention [CDC], 2007). The U.S. government, in PL 106-402 (2000), *The Developmental Disabilities Assistance and Bill of Rights Act*, defined developmental disability as a severe, chronic disability that

- is attributable to mental or physical impairment or a combination of impairments.
- is manifested before the age of 22 years.
- is likely to continue indefinitely.
- results in substantial functional limitations in three or more areas of life activity, such as self care, receptive and expressive language, learning, mobility, self-direction, capacity for independent learning, and economic self-sufficiency.
- reflects the individual's need for a combination and sequence of special, interdisciplinary, or generic services, individualized supports, or other forms of assistance that are of lifelong or of extended duration and are individually planned and coordinated (ASHA, 2005c).

Despite the heterogeneity of the population, many of these children have communication and feeding/swallowing problems. Communication deficits among very young children can range from reduced or atypical babbling through limited use of communicative gestures to slow growth of or regression in vocabulary (ASHA, 2008b).

This and other legislation translates into more than 300,000 children being eligible for early intervention services as mandated by Part C of the Individuals with Disabilities Education Improvement Act (IDEA, 2004). **Early intervention** (EI) is an educational approach for young children, ages birth to three years, who have or are at risk for developmental disability. EI's purpose is to provide both remediation and prevention of future difficulties. The focus is on both the child and family. When the primary focus of intervention is speech, language, and/or feeding, we refer to the child's program as **early communication intervention** (ECI).

The model for ECI is a functional one, focusing on the child and family members within the context of everyday communication. This model of intervention may seem different from what you may have seen in the public schools with older children. Working with young children and family members, and also with other professional care providers, may take some adjustment. Let's start our exploration with the legal basis for EI and then we'll explore a model for assessment and intervention, and end with a discussion of augmentative and alternative communication (AAC).

Legal Basis for Early Intervention

EI isn't just a good idea. In the United States and other developed countries, it's mandated by law.

The impetus for EI came from the World Health Organization's focus on healthcare for vulnerable groups, such as mothers and children (WHO, 1981). Several laws outline the requirements for EI in the United States.

Public law (PL) 99-457, passed in 1986 and called the *Education of the Handicapped Act Amendments*, mandated that states establish comprehensive service for infants and toddlers with DD and for their families. The law required that qualified professionals complete an assessment of the child and that both assessment and intervention be provided by a multidisciplinary team. The purpose of the assessment is to confirm the presence and extent of disability and to identify

- a child's unique needs, accomplishments, and strengths.
- a family's strengths and needs as they relate to the child's development.
- the nature and extent of early intervention services appropriate to the child and family.

Eligibility for services varies by state. Determiners include birth weight, gestational age at birth, and medical diagnosis.

Four years later, the U.S. Congress passed the *Individuals with Disabilities Education Act* of 1990 (IDEA). The IDEA requires free, appropriate public education (for children with disabilities. Part C specifies programs for infants and toddlers as provided an Individualized Family Service Plan (IFSP). More on IFSPs later.

The Individuals with Disabilities Education Act was reauthorized in 1997 in PL 105-17. Part C of PL 105-17 strengthens the requirement that services be provided within the context of family. Family members are part of the interdisciplinary team and primary decision makers in the collaborative effort.

In 2004, IDEA was again reauthorized as the *Individuals with Disabilities Education Improvement Act* (IDEIA). The IDEIA requires that these individualized programs be offered in the natural environment or the least restrictive environment (LRE).

Several principles of intervention outlined in the legislation are important in designing EI programs (ASHA, 2008a, b, c, d). Services should be

- comprehensive, coordinated, team-based, and transdisciplinary in nature to optimize the participation of children and their families and integrated to meet the needs of children and their families.
- family-centered and responsive to families' priorities as well as the culture and values of the family, including each families unique situation, culture, language(s), preferences, resource, and priorities.
- individualized for the child and family.
- developmentally supportive and promote children's participation in their natural environment.
- developmentally appropriate for children's age, cognitive level, strengths, and family concerns and preferences.
- provided in the least restrictive and most natural environment for the child and family.
- based on the highest quality and most recent research evidence on intervention effectiveness merged with professional expertise and family preferences.

These elements are also supported by the EI guiding principles of the American Speech-Language-Hearing Association (ASHA, 2008b). Let's explore some of these further.

In 2001, the World Health Organization (WHO) endorsed a new model of disability that considers health and disability in relation to each other and to participation in daily life activities (World Health Assembly, 2001). In other words, the degree of disability is considered in terms of a person's functioning in his or her natural environment. Like the functional model discussed throughout this text, concern is for how and with whom the individual communicates on a daily basis.

Daily activities and routines offer learning opportunities that restricted participation can limit. By enabling or enhancing participation, we help a young child acquire new skills. Participation requires communication.

The Early Intervention Model

Now that we have an idea of the overall EI approach, let's take it apart and briefly look at the individual pieces. These include multidisciplinary teams, the importance of family and culture, the role of caregivers/parents, individualized services and the IFSP, and use of the natural environment.

Team Approach

A team is responsible for selecting the most appropriate service delivery model based on the individualized needs of a child and family. One professional on the team, often the SLP, may be designated as the primary service provider (PSP). This model may help in avoiding fragmenting of services and the PSP may provide services across disciplines while other professionals act in a consultative manner.

Although IDEA 2004 uses the term "multidisciplinary" teams, other team models may be applied depending on the needs of the child and family. Interdisciplinary and transdisciplinary are two other commonly used team models. These three team models frequently differ in the amount of communication and coordination that exists among team members (Paul-Brown & Caperton, 2001).

Multidisciplinary team members, such as an SLP, evaluate a child and determine his or her needs independently. Although separate findings are pulled together, there is little coordination. Families are often not treated as full members of the intervention team, and there is the potential for them to feel overwhelmed by the number of individual professionals consulting with them and making recommendations. There is the potential for gaps or overlaps in services.

An **interdisciplinary team** has established lines of communication among professionals, resulting in a greater degree of cooperation. The family is considered part of the team. Although a child is assessed by different disciplines independently, the team presents the family with a cohesive report. Disciplines may still provide services separately, but they plan cooperatively and coordinate intervention services.

In a **transdisciplinary team** approach parents and facilitators from multiple disciplines share responsibility for planning and implementing, while at the same time contributing their own unique expertise. In this way, transdisciplinary teams fully integrate the family and different disciplines. All members of the team participate in the assessment using a format called arena assessment in which team members observe the child interacting with a family and/or team member(s). At the conclusion, the team develops an integrated service plan through consensus or collaboration with the family.

Importance of Families

Effective early intervention is family centered. Family involvement produces positive effects for children's physical, cognitive, social, and language skills; fosters a parent's sense of personal control and self-efficacy; and increases a parent's overall satisfaction with intervention services (Applequist & Bailey, 2000). In family centered intervention, parents are partners with professionals.

Successful early intervention depends on quality relationships between all parties, children, parents, and intervention facilitators. These relationships have a direct impact on the parent–child relationship.

The children and families who require or request EI services vary tremendously in the characteristics of individual family members. In addition to the individual characteristics of each child, there are varying family histories, current circumstances, and the family's reasons for seeking services.

The results of a meta-analysis of eighteen studies of parent-implemented language interventions with preschool children found such approaches to be an effective approach to early language intervention for young children with language impairments (Roberts & Kaiser, 2011). Young children whose parents participate in intervention activities make more language gains than children whose parents are not involved in intervention (Chao, Bryan, Burstein, & Cevriye, 2006). Working collaboratively, SLPs and families can identify goals and typical daily routines within which these goals might be addressed.

Cultural Concerns

According to PL 99-457, early intervention must by its nature reflect respect for individuality and for racial, ethnic, cultural, and other differences found across diverse family backgrounds and be responsive to each family's needs. At the least, materials distributed to caregivers should be in the native language, procedures should be nondiscriminatory and in the language to which the infant has been most exposed, and multiple methods of assessment should be employed.

Like all children, a child with developmental disability is part of an ecology that includes parents, siblings, extended family members, friends, neighbors, and community agencies. The family is embedded within broader cultural contexts. Ethnic and cultural groups can vary significantly in their beliefs about disability, the nature of family and community supports, medical practices, and use of professional services. To improve ECI participation, collaboration, and service delivery with families from diverse backgrounds, SLPs must understand and respect culturally specific beliefs and values (Garcia, Mendez-Perez, & Ortiz, 2000; Rodriguez & Olswang, 2003; Salas-Provance, Erickson, & Reed, 2002).

Child and Parents/Caregivers

The parent–child or caregiver–child interaction dyad is an especially powerful context for ECI, providing an opportunity to support and extend the experiences of both members. It's essential that we pay attention to interactions between a parent and child because this is the filter through which all intervention will pass regardless of whether we choose to recognize its importance.

At the very least, SLPs should explore with parents their beliefs and knowledge about (Kummerer, Lopez-Reyna, & Hughes, 2007)

- their children's speech and/or language disabilities.
- the difference between and importance of both receptive and expressive language.
- why intervention is recommended.
- the role of speech-language therapy and the speech-language pathologist.
- why it is important for parents to participate in ECI.
- how clinicians will interact with children and the family.
- how the clinician and family can work collaboratively.
- the amount of time and effort needed to remediate children's difficulties.
- how the family can generalize strategies to the home setting.

These topics are important because uninformed or discouraged parents may be less effective as agents of change.

The SLP's role is to support caregivers in becoming competent and confident in their ability to help their children develop communication. To do this, SLPs must integrate their knowledge of and skill in child-focused intervention with adult education principles needed to guide caregivers to implement intervention.

Individualized for Each Child

As with any good intervention, SLP services in ECI must be tailored to the individual child. This requires thorough and ongoing assessment and monitoring of a child's communication behavior and accurate record keeping. Flexibility is the key as a young child develops and new opportunities to intervene become available. As a group, children who begin receiving intervention services at a younger age require fewer intervention visits than those who begin later, regardless of the type of disorder (Jacoby, Lee, & Kummer, 2002).

Individualized Family Service Plan (IFSP)

Part H of the Education of the Handicapped Act Amendments of 1986 and Part C of the reauthorizations of IDEA move EI focus from the child with disabilities to the child as part of a family unit. The primary example of that change is the move to an **individualized family service plan** (IFSP). Based on the individualized educational plan (IEP) for school-aged children, the IFSP addresses both child and family needs that impact a child's development.

At the very least an IFSP should include

- the child and family's current status.
- the recommended services and expected outcomes.
- a projection of the duration of service delivery.

It's essential that the family understands the contents and feels some ownership of the plan through participation in the process. The plan should be reviewed periodically and updated as needed to accommodate the child and family's changing needs.

The IFSP is a collaborative document. Family members should participate in the assessment of the child's strengths and needs, and the IFSP should reflect this collaboration between families and providers in its description of a child's levels of functioning. Families should be included in the planning of the evaluation and encouraged to discuss their concerns and priorities and their resources for promoting the development of their child.

Both child and family outcomes should reflect the family's concerns, priorities, and resources and be written in language the family understands. IFSP outcome statements are very different from the goal and objective statements you will use for a school-age child's IEP. The difference reflects the service plan rather than treatment plan format of the IFSP. Not only is an IFSP more flexible than an IEP, but it can address issues beyond those related only to the child. Once the IFSP has identified services needed to achieve the outcomes identified by the family and other team members, all parties collaboratively plan services toward goals and objectives.

To succeed, family-centered and caregiver-implemented intervention must be based on the caregiver decision making regarding the outcomes, activities, and routines to be used for intervention and on when, where, and how interventions strategies will be embedded. When caregivers are encouraged to participate in decision making, they expand their capacity to generalize intervention strategies to other activities and routines and settings (Kashinath, Woods, & Goldstein, 2006; Wetherby & Woods, 2006).

Natural Environment

The Individuals with Disabilities Education Improvement Act, Part C (IDEIA)(2004) used the term *natural environments* to refer to settings that are typical for infants and toddlers. This contrasts with more traditional intervention settings, such as clinics or medical-based sites. Natural environments include family homes, early care and educational settings, and other community settings where families spend the majority of their time with their children. The most frequent natural environment for intervention services is the family home.

IDEIA requires that individualized programs developed in IFSPs and subsequent IEPs be offered in a child's natural environment or in the least restrictive environment (LRE). When EI services are provided in a non-natural environment, the IFSP must include a justification. As a child reaches the age of eligibility for preschool services, the IDEIA similarly requires these services to be provided in the LRE, which may be a preschool setting.

One goal of IDEIA is to prevent families from having to receive intervention in multiple locations in a non-transdisciplinary manner. Intervention may occur both in individual or groups sessions as long as services are individualized. Hybrid models are common. For example, groups can provide an adjunct to individual intervention services.

Although center-based EI has the potential, if not handled sensitively, to be threatening to some parents, it also offers an opportunity for children and parents to interact with other children and parents. When carefully guided, these interactions can be an enjoyable way for parents to observe other parent–child interactions and to enhance parent interactional skills as an adjunct to home-based services.

Home-based intervention involves more than just location. The context of a family's daily routines and activities offers an opportunity for children to learn and develop within events occurring naturally within the home environment. Parents can use daily routines and activities as opportunities for teaching. Children's activities, such as eating and being bathed, are an integral part of everyday life and a familiar part of a family's day. These activities have a profound impact on the cognitive and communicative functions children develop and offer meaningful and functional opportunities for learning communication. SLPs, working in partnership with families, can coach parents on the ECI methods for including individualized communication activities throughout the day.

Young children learn best when participating in an activity while a caregiver mediates the environment and interactions (Hancock & Kaiser, 2006; Wetherby & Woods, 2006). The SLP can help caregivers understand how young children learn to communicate, enabling the caregivers to make decisions about the best times and ways to interact with their child throughout the day. The probability that caregivers will act as effective communication facilitators is increased when they are involved in problem-solving and planning.

Role of the SLP

This may all sound very different from what you assumed to be the role of an SLP. Within the EI model, the SLP assumes multiple roles relative to infants and toddlers and their families. These include (Woods, Wilcox, Friedman, & Murch, 2011)

- team member, possibly the Primary Service Provider (PSP).
- clinician.
- communication facilitator.
- coach.
- consultant.

While some of these roles are familiar ones, others, such as collaborating with caregivers to embed communication goals into their daily routines and helping caregivers learn to use communication intervention strategies, are not.

In coaching caregivers to learn to embed communication strategies into their daily routines, the SLP acts as both a teacher and a learner. Caregivers are not likely to have the expertise or experience they need to support their child's communication learning. For their part, caregivers inform the SLP about the child's strengths, the nature of the child's daily routines and interests, and which strategies are good fits with the family's culture and values and might or might not work. In other words, both the SLP and caregiver contribute and gain knowledge and skills as partners to support the child's development (Dunst & Trivette, 2009a). This bidirectional teaching and learning relationship is the basis for a truly individualized family-centered approach (Woods et al., 2011).

Children Served in ECI Programs

The more limited a child's communication behavior, the more difficult it is for a child to learn the link between communication behavior and results. Within the first few months of life, typically developing (TD) children learn that their behavior can affect other people in their environment. Making this connection is a vital first link in developing communication intent. In addition, communication impairment impacts other aspects of a child's development. For example, toddlers with language delays appear to show more social withdrawal relative to TD toddlers (Horwitz et al., 2003; Irwin, Carter, & Briggs-Gowan, 2002; Rescorla, Ross, & McClure, 2007). There is also a relationship between the presence of communication impairment and behavioral problems. Language problems in preschool are related to later behavioral/emotional disorders.

TABLE 3.1 Established Risks

Categories
Chromosomal and genetic disorders
Neurological disorders
Congenital malformations
Inborn metabolic errors
Sensory disorders
A typical developmental disorders
Chronic medical illness
Severe infectious disease

Conceptual framework based on Rossetti (2001)

Several factors can contribute to communication impairments. For example, low birth weight and premature birth are both significant predictors of *late language emergence* (LLE), a hallmark characteristic of children with language impairments. Other significant factors in LLE include a family history of LLE, male gender, and early neurobiological growth. Factors such as parental educational levels, socioeconomic resources, parental mental health, parenting practices, and family functioning are less significant. Predictors among 24-month-olds of later language impairment included problems in gross and fine motor development, poor adaptive and psychosocial development, and negative temperament or mood quality.

As outlined in PL 99-457, two broad categories of children are served by early intervention programs, those in **established risk** categories, such as those with Down syndrome, or those in at-risk categories, such as preterm or low birth weight infants. In established risk, there is a strong relationship between the condition and developmental difficulties. Table 3.1 presents examples of established risks. Established risk categories include chromosomal and genetic disorders, neurological disorders, congenital malformations, inborn metabolic errors, sensory disorders, atypical developmental disorders, chronic medical illness, and severe infectious disease (Rossetti, 2001).

Although a child has an established risk, he or she is not precluded from experiencing **at-risk** factors as well. At-risk factors include anything with the potential to interfere with a child's ability to interact in a typical way with the environment and to develop typically. At-risk factors may also be both biological and environmental in nature. At-risk factors may include, but are not limited to the following:

- Preterm birth
- Low birth weight
- Physical abuse
- Severe, chronic caregiver or child illness
- Lack of or limited prenatal care
- Chronic or acute caregiver mental illness or DD
- Caregiver alcohol or substance dependence

Let's look at each type of risk briefly.

Established Risk

As a group, established risks are easier to identify and have a strong link with developmental difficulties. Many of these have been described in the previous chapter and will only be mentioned briefly. Examples of established risk include intellectual disabilities (ID), autism spectrum disorder (ASD), cerebral palsy (CP), and deafness and deaf-blindness.

Intellectual Disability (ID)

Although almost every child is able to learn, develop, and become a participating member of the community, the cognitive limitations of individuals with ID will result in a child's learning and developing more slowly than a typical child. More severe types of ID and accompanying multiple handicapping conditions may be obvious at birth, but administering definitive testing is extremely difficult with young children. My grandson has ID, accompanied by cerebral palsy and blindness; the latter condition not definitively established until he was 5 years old.

Autism Spectrum Disorder (ASD)

Children with moderate-to-severe ASD are almost always delayed in speech and language acquisition and in communication in general (Tager-Flusberg et al., 2005). Early language ability and social competence are related to positive long-term outcomes and verbal skills are the strongest predictors of later functioning (Howlin, Mawhood, & Rutter, 2000; Liss et al., 2001; Lord, Risi, & Pickles, 2004; Mawhood, Howlin, & Rutter, 2000; Stone & Yoder, 2001).

Multiple factors seem to contribute to the development of language skills in young children with ASD. Of importance are (Bono, Daley, & Sigman, 2004; Charman, Baron-Cohen, et al., 2003; Stone & Yoder, 2001; Woods & Wetherby, 2003)

- functional and symbolic use of objects.
- the number and type of gestures.
- ability to initiate joint attention.
- presence of verbal imitation skills.
- number of words produced.
- number of words comprehended.

Several studies of young children with ASD report an association between attention, imitation skills, and language (Bono & Sigman, 2004; Siller & Sigman, 2002; Stone & Yoder, 2001).

Cerebral Palsy

Cerebral palsy (CP) is a group of chronic brain disorders that affect movement, muscle tone, and muscle coordination in approximately half a million people in the United States. Approximately 8,000 babies and infants are diagnosed with CP annually with another 1,500 identified during the preschool years. Damage to one or more motor areas of the brain disrupts the brain's ability to control movement and posture because of the faulty signals sent to the muscles. The degree of severity depends on where and to what extent the brain is damaged. CP is associated with difficulty in swallowing and problems with both speech and language.

Cerebral palsy is not a disease, and it doesn't worsen with time. The majority of newborn brain injury cases, approximately 70 percent, are attributed to events occurring before labor begins. Estimates of the incidence of CP are two per 1000 live births. Risk factors for CP are low birth weight, preterm birth, placental disorders, rubella or other infections of the mother during pregnancy, Rh or other blood incompatability factors, prolonged loss of oxygen, and stroke or bleeding in the infant's brain.

The three main types of CP are spastic, athetoid, and ataxic. These are rarely seen in their pure form and many individuals have mixed CP. In addition, many young children initially exhibit what is termed flaccid or hypotonic CP characterized by poor muscle tone and a floppy posture. The majority of these children manifest one of the other forms of CP as they mature. Characteristics of the types and causes of cerebral palsy are presented in Table 3.2.

An early sign of CP is often failure to develop motor skills similar to other children. My grandson at age 2 moved about by either rolling or "combat crawling" — pulling himself along — on his stomach, and although he could get to his knees, he seemed incapable of crawling independently.

TABLE 3.2 Characteristics and Causes of Cerebral Palsy

Type of Cerebral Palsy	Characteristics	Area of Brain Affected
Spastic	Spasticity, increased muscle tone in opposing muscle groups Rigidity and exaggerated stretch reflex Jerky, labored, and slow movements Infantile reflex patterns	Motor cortex Pyramidal tract
Athetoid	Slow, involuntary writhing Disorganized and uncoordinated volitional movement Movements occur accompanying volitional movement	Extrapyramidal tract, basal ganglia
Ataxic	Uncoordinated movement Poor balance Movements lack direction, force, and control	Cerebellum

Deafness and Deaf-Blindness

Hearing impairment occurs when there is a full or partial decrease in the ability to detect or understand sounds. The degree of impairment can be viewed as a continuum from typical hearing to profound hearing loss or **deafness**. Severity is measured by the degree of loudness or the *intensity level,* measured in decibels, that a sound must attain before being detectible to an individual. A profound hearing loss is a 90 dB threshold or greater. This means that sounds that are quieter than 90 dB or the level of very loud music is not detectable auditorily.

While the above definition of deafness is technically correct, it may be more appropriate to think of deafness in more practical terms. For example, ability to benefit from auditory information is situationally dependent on the type of sound, interfering noise, and the context.

The age at which the hearing impairment develops is crucial to spoken language acquisition. Development of hearing loss either prenatally or during infancy can interfere with both social development and the development of spoken language, because a child is unable to access audible/spoken communication from the outset. In general, among children receiving EI services, those whose hearing loss is identified by 6 months of age demonstrated significantly better language than children identified later. For this reason, nearly all infants in the United States are screened as neonates for hearing loss.

The prevalence of profound hearing loss (90 dB or greater) in newborns in the United States is approximately 1–2 per 1,000 live births. Another 6–8 per 1,000 have severe loss of 70–90 dB (Cunningham & Cox, 2003; Kemper & Downs, 2000). Most children with hearing loss have hearing impairment at birth and are potentially identifiable by neonatal hearing screening, although some types of degenerative hearing loss may not become evident until later.

Young children with major impairments in both auditory and visual abilities have unique communicative, developmental, emotional, and educational needs. Sensory deficits can lead to communication impairment and frequently lead to behavioral challenges.

Total blindness is the complete lack of form and visual light perception. A child described as having only "light perception" can distinguish light from dark but no more. Governments variously define something called **legal blindness**. In the United States, Canada, and most of Europe, legal blindness is defined by a visual acuity with the best possible correction of 20/200 or less in the better eye as compared to 20/20 for typical vision. The 20/200 value means that a person standing 20 feet from an object would see it with the same degree of clarity as a typically sighted person at 200 feet. Approximately 10 percent of those deemed legally blind have no usable vision. In addition to visual acuity, many jurisdictions also consider visual field in the definition of legal blindness. The typical person can see 180 degrees of field. Those with legal blindness may have a visual field of less than 20 degrees.

Having a child with a dual sensory impairment or with other multiple impairments, such as a child with deafness, visual impairment, and cerebral palsy, can create emotional and financial stress on a family. If we consider the family as a unit, then having a child with deaf-blindness or other multiple handicapping conditions is likely to alter most areas of family functioning, in part because of the chronic stress associated with raising such a child.

At-risk Children

Unlike children in established risk categories in which there is a strong link between their condition and developmental disability, those in at-risk categories may or may not experience developmental difficulties, although the possibility exists. In the following section we'll discuss some of the more common at-risk categories, including international adoption, low socioeconomic status, maltreatment/neglect and fetal alcohol spectrum disorder, and premature birth and low birth weight.

International Adoptions

At present, in the United States approximately 19,000 children are adopted from non-English-speaking countries annually (U.S. Department of State, 2007). Nearly two-thirds of these children come from China, Russia, and Guatamala. Infants and toddlers adopted from countries with a different language and culture undergo a unique language learning experience and may be predisposed to LI. Development in the birth language is arrested and replaced by development of the adopted language, because adoptive families usually are unable to maintain the birth language (Glennen & Masters, 2002). If you want to pursue this unique language acquisition process further, I recommend the excellent review by Glennen (2002).

Complicating language acquisition is the fact that 88 percent of all these children are initially raised in institutional orphanages (Johnson, 2000). In addition, many of the countries from which they come have low personal income, poor nutrition, and limited access to healthcare. These risk factors create a less-than-optimal environment for health and early development.

Delays in growth and development are strongly related to orphanage care. It is estimated that children raised in orphanages lose one month of linear growth for every three to five months in an orphanage (Johnson, 2000; Miller & Hendric, 2000). Although specific figures vary, at the time of adoption, a significant percentage of children (18 to 51 percent) are below two standard deviations, meaning that they are in the lowest 2.5 percent, for height, weight, and head circumference. Given the importance of early development, this lack of growth is a concern.

The heightened incidence of several conditions and diseases, such as fetal alcohol spectrum disorder (FASD), iodine insufficiency, hepatitis B and C, tuberculosis, and intestinal parasites, among international adoptees may also adversely affect development of young international adoptees (Johnson, 2000; Miller & Hendric, 2000). Other factors include poor maternal healthcare, high-risk pregnancy or delivery, and premature birth.

Low Socioeconomic Status

The risk of communication impairment is associated with socioeconomic factors such as economic deprivation. Many children with LI come from homes lacking in stable and continuous childcare, adequate nutrition, and even rudimentary medical care.

Beginning at conception, poverty significantly heightens a child's risk for (Halpern, 2000)

- birth complications such as fetal alcohol syndrome.
- physical health problems such as asthma and malnutrition.
- mental health problems.
- inattentive or erratic parental care.
- neglect and abuse.
- removal from the home and placement in foster care.
- deficits in cognitive development and achievement.

Not only are there more risks, but the consequences of these risk factors can be more severe for children in poor families because of exposure to multiple risks. An accumulation of risk factors can increase the negative effects of poverty and increase the risk for developmental disability (Stanton-Chapman, Chapman, Kaiser, & Hancock, 2004).

Maltreatment/Neglect and Fetal Alcohol Spectrum Disorder

As noted in the previous chapter, there is a clear interaction between LI and the factors of caregiver maltreatment/neglect or fetal alcohol spectrum disorder (FASD) (Hernandez, 2004; Hooper, Roberts, Zeisel, & Poe, 2003). Although the United States spends more money fighting child abuse than any other country, it has the highest rate of child abuse in the industrialized world (Lindsey, 2003). Children in immigrant families are more than twice as likely as those from native-born families to experience multiple risk factors critical to their development, including exposure to violence and neglect (Jaycox, Zoellner, & Foa, 2002). Maltreatment and neglect may stem from poverty, stress, and cultural differences. For SLPs working with immigrant families, it is important to remember that these families will have varying views regarding childrearing practices and punishment.

There is a direct relationship between the amount of language input a child receives and the amount of language a child produces. Very socially depriving circumstances will affect language development. In addition, some children who experience extreme deprivation show behaviors, such as rocking, self-injury, and atypical sensory interests, that are more characteristic of ASD although the underlying causes are distinctly dissimilar (Beckett et al., 2002; Fombonne, 2003b; Rutter, Kreppner, & O'Connor, 2001).

For some children maltreatment begins in utero when they are exposed to the negative impact of maternal alcohol use, resulting in **fetal alcohol spectrum disorder** (FASD). Each year, approximately 40,000 infants are born with FASD, costing the United States approximately $6 billion (U.S. Department of Health and Human Services, 2008). At least 2,000 of these children experience severe medical concerns (Braillion & DuBois, 2005).

Preterm and Low Birth Weight Infants

Preterm birth is a major challenge in early healthcare. Most neonatal or newborn deaths occur in preterm infants, and preterm birth is an important risk factor for neurological impairment and disability (Tucker & McGuire, 2004). The rate of preterm births in the United States is a growing public health problem that has significant consequences for families, and costs U.S. society at least $26 billion a year (Preterm Birth, 2006).

Although treatment of preterm infants in a neonatal intensive care units (NICUs) or special care nurseries (SCNs) can greatly improved their survival, these infants remain vulnerable to many complications, including possible death. Long-term problems may include cerebral palsy, intellectual disabilities, visual and hearing impairments, and behavior and social-emotional problems, learning difficulties, and poor health and growth.

Most pregnancies last 37 to 42 weeks and babies born during this window are called full term. **Preterm** labor refers to contractions that begin to open the cervix before week 37. No one knows exactly what causes preterm labor. Eighty-four percent of preterm infants are born between 32 and

37 weeks of gestation. About 10 percent are born between 28 and 31 weeks and are labeled very preterm, while only 6 percent, called extremely premature, are born prior to 28 weeks of gestation (Martin et al., 2006).

Most mortality and morbidity affects very preterm and extremely preterm infants. **Morbidity** is illness or disability. Although survival is possible for babies born as early as 22 to 27 weeks, most likely these children will face a lifetime of health problems. The age of viability or the age at which a fetus can survive outside the womb varies internationally and changes with medical advances but is at present somewhere around 21–22 weeks in the United States.

Although birth weight and gestational age are positively related, they are not interchangeable. The categories for low birth weight (LBW) are:

- Low birth weight: Below 2500 gms or 5.5 lbs
- Very low birth weight: Below 1500 gms or 3.3 lbs
- Extremely low birth weight: Below 500 gms or 1.1 lbs

According to a World Health Organization 1996 report, 6 to 8 percent of all live births are of children with some type of LBW.

Only around two-thirds of low birth weight infants are preterm. Full-term infants may be of low birth weight because they are "small for gestational age," usually defined as below the 10th percentile or in the lowest 10 percent of birth weight babies. Infants may be small for gestational age as a result of *intrauterine growth restriction* (IUGR). Fetal growth restriction is the second leading cause of perinatal morbidity and mortality with prematurity being the first. The incidence of IUGR is estimated to be approximately 5 percent in infants.

Over the past twenty to thirty years the incidence of preterm birth in most developed countries has been about 5 to 7 percent of live births (Tucker & McGuire, 2004). The incidence in the United States, however, is about 12 percent. Several factors have contributed to the overall rise in the incidence of preterm birth in the United States. These include increasing rates of multiple births, greater use of assisted reproduction techniques, such as *in vitro* fertilization, and more obstetric intervention, such as the increased use of caesarian section (Tucker & McGuire, 2004). In the United States, the highest rates for preterm births are among African American women, and the lowest are among Asian or Pacific Islanders (Preterm Birth, 2006). These disparities cannot be fully explained by differences in socioeconomic conditions.

Premature infants tend to need the most care right after birth, with the most preterm generally requiring the greatest attention. Many families find the experience to be an emotional roller coaster that can be extremely difficult for parents. Initially, the infant is kept in the NICU/SCN on an open warmer, a bed that keeps the baby warm by heating the surrounding air. Once the infant's breathing rate is stabilized, the infant is usually placed in an isolette, an enclosed plastic incubator with controlled air temperature. When it is easier for an infant to maintain its own temperature and the infant weighs about 4 pounds and if there are no serious complicating factors, the infant is placed in an open crib.

Most preterm births, approximately 70 percent, are a result of spontaneous labor, either by itself or following spontaneous premature rupture of the membranes (PROM) of the sac inside the uterus that holds the fetus (Goldenberg, Culhane, Iams, & Romero, 2008). PROM may be triggered by the body's natural response to certain infections of the amniotic fluid and fetal membranes. The most important predictors of spontaneous preterm delivery are a history of preterm birth and poor socioeconomic status. Medical and health conditions during pregnancy, such as intrauterine infections and maternal high blood pressure or diabetes, also may increase preterm labor and delivery (March of Dimes, 2007).

The remaining 30 percent of preterm births result from early induction of labor or cesarean delivery due to pregnancy complications or health problems in the mother or the fetus (Iams, 2003). In most of these cases, early delivery is probably the safest approach for mother and baby.

Complications from preterm birth or low birth weight may be (Bromberger & Permanente, 2004; March of Dimes, 2007) any of the following.

- Respiratory. Approximately 70 percent of babies born before 34 weeks of gestation have some type of respiratory difficulty.
- Circulatory. Circulatory problems may be related to immaturity of the heart, internal bleeding, and anemia.
- Immunological. Neonatal immunological problems can lead to many forms of infection because of immature immune systems and may include pneumonia or lung infection, blood infection or sepsis, and meningitis, an infection of the membranes surrounding the brain and spinal cord.
- Feeding and digestive. Preterm or small infants are not able to suck and swallow until they reach approximately 32 weeks of gestational age and may experience serious digestive problems, such as *necrotizing enterocolitis* in which the child experiences temporary or permanent *necrosis* or death of intestinal tissue.

These complications can range from mild to severe.

The increasing survival rates of children who are born very preterm are accompanied by greater risk of neurological disabilities and cognitive dysfunction. Although approximately 80 percent of infants born at 26 weeks and 90 percent of those at 27 weeks survive to one year, about a quarter of these infants will develop serious lasting disabilities, and up to half may have milder problems, such as learning and behavioral difficulties (American College of Obstetricians and Gynecologists, 2002).

At age 5 years, 49 percent of children born at 24–28 weeks of gestation or extremely preterm have some disability (Larroque, Ancel, Marrett, et al., 2008). Cerebral palsy is present in 9 percent of all children born very preterm and 32 percent are intellectually disabled. In the very preterm group, 5 percent have severe disability, 9 percent moderate, and 25 percent mild disability. Special health-care/education resources are used by 42 percent of children born at 24–28 weeks and 31 percent born at 28–32 weeks, compared to only 16 percent of those born full term.

ECI Assessment

Assessment of young children is not like any other type of communication evaluation in speech-language pathology for the simple reason that very young children are very independent when it comes to cooperating or not. Add to this the unreliable responding of these children to standardized testing and the often multiple handicapping nature of their disorders and you sometimes get the feeling that "We're not in Kansas any more, Toto!" By the same token, for those of you who are creative, curious about the world, and think you might like the challenge, early communication assessment and the intervention that follows may be just the right fit for you.

Currently recommended practices within EI focus on comparing a child's skills across and within different developmental domains to provide a clearer picture of the child's overall development and to identify the child's relative strengths and challenges (Crais & Roberts, 2004). In addition to being required by law, this type of developmental "profiling" is thought to provide the best overall portrait of the child and help families and professionals make the most informed decisions.

A child's linguistic skills are built on a foundation of prelinguistic skills that not only serve as an indicator of the child's current skill level but are a strong predictor of the child's potential for language competence later. For very young children, especially those who are not talking, it is important to identify the key components of prelinguistic communication, such as vocalizations, vocabulary comprehension, symbolic play, gesture use, initiating and responding to joint attention, parental interactions, and familial history of language and/or learning impairments (Hadley & Holt, 2006; Mundy, Block, Delgado, Pomaes, Van Hecke, & Parlade, 2007).

Our charges — the infants and toddlers we serve — are small, often sick or with multiple handicaps, and their caregivers may be confused and overwhelmed by their child's needs. We must tailor our assessment to these realities.

An assessment is the child and family's introduction to the early intervention process. The manner in which we as professionals interact with the family and the child can mean all the difference between a satisfying and fruitful experience that can lead to future collaboration if needed and a situation that leaves a family confused, frustrated, and possibly hostile.

Typically, the assessment process for communication is a two-step affair but the lines between them are blurry. First, the team is interested in a more global or overall evaluation. This may be followed by assessment of skills in different areas, such as communication.

In part, professional involvement is influenced by the way in which SLPs and other team members define assessment. Part H of the IDEA specifies that an **evaluation** must be conducted to determine a child's eligibility for services. This requires identifying a child's level of developmental functioning in a manner that is comprehensive, nondiscriminatory, and conducted by qualified personnel. Traditionally, evaluations are more structured and formal and rely on the use of standardized instruments. In contrast, **assessment** is the ongoing process of identifying a child's unique needs; the family's priorities, concerns, and resources; and the nature and extent of the EI services needed by both. As such, assessment activities are usually less formal and rely on the use of multiple tools and methods with the close cooperation of families and professionals. Typically, assessments focus not on what is *wrong* with a child but on identifying what can be done to help. In this way an assessment is truly a first step in intervention.

Transdisciplinary Model of Assessment

Many young children need to be assessed by more than one professional and may have disorders in several developmental areas. In most cases, the SLP will be a central figure in these evaluations and in subsequent intervention decisions.

As mentioned, a transdisciplinary team approach is one in which there is a conscious effort to pool expertise and freely exchange insights and ideas. This is best accomplished if parents and professionals observe the entire evaluation and simultaneously assess the child, a method dubbed **arena assessment**. Instead of the child's being separately assessed by each discipline, a common sample of the child's behavior is collected and recorded as all observe the process.

The format is often play-based. When compared to more formal, structured, discipline-specific methods, play-based assessment is more

- naturalistic.
- ecologically sound.
- context-based.
- child-centered.

It is all too easy to assume that the word *play* implies an open-ended free-for-all in which data are collected haphazardly. Nothing could be further from the truth. A good evaluation requires planning, training, and considerable expertise. In structured play the partner attempts through manipulation of the context to elicit specific behavior from the child. For example, while playing, an adult, either a professional or parent, may role a ball under or behind another object to see if the child will search for it or may play an imitation "game" to see if the child will follow suit. Throughout, the process of interaction takes precedence over the product or result.

As mentioned, EI should be family-centered. In order for families to be empowered, they must be full participants and real decision makers in the EI process (Dunst, 2002). If assessment and intervention recommendations are to be "owned" by families, these proposals must match the family's notions of appropriateness and importance. Parental collaboration is a vital part of ECI.

Assessment serves as an introduction for the family to the ECI process. Our behavior at that time determines whether a family becomes vested in their child's communication development program. As an ECI service provider, I want the family's full engagement in the assessment process and in the possible intervention to follow.

Family Concerns, Priorities, and Resources

IDEA 2004 requires that programs provide an opportunity for a family to identify their concerns, priorities, and resources related to enhancement of their child's development. Six key objectives may guide the gathering of family information (ASHA, 2008b; Bailey, 2004):

- To identify the family's concerns and what they hope to accomplish through their participation.
- To determine how the family perceives the child's strengths and needs relative to their family values, structure, and routines.
- To identify the family's priorities and how service providers may assist with these priorities.
- To identify the family's resources related to their priorities.
- To identify the family's preferred role in the service delivery and decision-making processes.
- To establish a supportive, informed, and collaborative relationship.

Each of these outcomes should be addressed in an assessment and throughout the intervention process.

Informal Communication Assessment

Students approaching the topic of ECI often assume there's little to assess in young children because they may not be talking yet. Actually, the opposite is true. The difficulty comes in trying to winnow down all the possible behaviors and to note only the most important ones. At the present time, researchers are attempting to identify the most significant early communication developments. One of the values of evidence-based practice is that we are beginning to recognize those child behaviors that seem to have the greatest impact on later communication intervention. Let's explore the information that we hope to gain from an evaluation of both the child and caregivers.

Description of Communication

The SLP and other team members attempt to describe as well as possible the present communication system of the child and caregiver. Of importance are the forms/means of communication and communication success.

Successful communication depends on more than just the child. Success requires a responsive partner. We'll discuss caregivers in more detail in the following section. Let's discuss forms/means and success briefly.

Forms/means of Communication. Communication forms are intentional or unintentional behaviors performed by a child in the presence of a caregiver. The means may be physical, vocal, or both. Physical or nonvocal signals may include eye contact, facial expression, communication distance, body movements or contact, gestures, and even aggression to self or others. Vocal signals can range from soft sounds to screaming and crying.

A relationship exists between the early use of various means of communication, such as eye gaze, gestures, and vocalizations, and later language skills in children with communication delays and those with ASD (McCathren, Yoder, & Warren, 2000; Zwaigenbaum, Bryson, Rogers, Brian, & Szatmari, 2005). It is important, therefore, that all forms of communication be identified in an assessment.

Communication Success. Stated simply, communication success occurs when a communicator's goal is attained. The success of a child's communication depends as much on the communication partners and the environment as on the child.

Efficiency improves with the advent of intentional or goal-oriented behavior, demonstrating that the child understands that objects and persons can be used to obtain something desirable. When compared to unintentional behaviors, intentional nonsymbolic communication, such as gesturing, is less ambiguous, more efficient, and more successful. Our task as SLPs is to describe communicative or potentially communicative behaviors as best we can and to attempt to determine how they are used by the child and/or interpreted by caregivers as communication.

Caregiver–child Interactions

In addition to a caregiver's role in an assessment, parents' and other caregivers' behaviors are also evaluated within the context of interacting with the child. It is within this interaction that most of the work of intervention will occur, so the quality of that interaction will be an important factor in a child's learning to communicate better.

Part of any evaluation is determining the sensitivity, responsiveness, and interpretation of intent by caregivers in response to the behavior of the child, especially attempts to communicate. Sensitivity includes noticing the sometimes subtle behavior of the child as he or she displays interest or attempts to interact with an object or a person or to communicate in some way.

A child can learn the impact of certain behaviors through the responsiveness of others. This requires caregivers to be more than just sensitive. Caregiver responses provide consequences that encourage or discourage behaviors. Responsiveness includes

- contingency or the relatedness of the response to the behavior of the child.
- consistency of the adult response.
- timeliness or the quickness with which the adult responds.

A **contingent caregiver response** is one based on the perceived intent of the child.

Presymbolic Behaviors

During the presymbolic period, a typically developing child learns to initiate communication for a variety of purposes and to attend jointly with a partner. Communication becomes purposeful and increasingly symbolic. Of most importance in predicting later language skills in TD children and children with DDs are the following presymbolic behaviors:

- Joint attention and attention-following of gazing and pointing.
- The variety and complexity in symbolic play (Lyytinen et al., 2001).
- Intentional communication and the use of gestures and vocalizations (McCathren et al., 2000). The use of gestures correlates with later receptive language abilities (Watt et al., 2006). Gestures may, in fact, serve as a bridge from understanding language to actively producing language.
- Complexity of presymbolic vocalizations including the variety of consonants and syllable structures.
- Receptive language or the number of words and phrases understood by a child. Numerous studies have demonstrated that receptive language is a significant predictor of later expressive language skills (Lyytinen et al., 2001).

For children with delays in several areas, problems in communication and language often persist.

Communicative intent is particularly difficult to determine. For intent to be present, three observable things should occur.

- The child performs a signal or behavior.
- The signal is directed toward another person.
- The signal appears to indicate some communication function.

That last one can be particularly difficult to judge, because of its sometimes subtle nature. Changes in either the rate or magnitude of behavior can signal intentionality, especially in children with neuromuscular deficits.

In addition to the behaviors mentioned, there are other presymbolic behaviors that may be important for later communication training. Chief among these are

- functional use of objects as a way of learning concepts, such a *spoon-ness*.
- motor imitation.

While neither behavior is sufficient for communication growth, each provides a method for enhancing teaching and learning.

Symbolic Assessment

Once a child is using symbols, whether as words, signs, or some other form of augmentative and alternative communication (AAC), the focus of an early communication assessment changes somewhat. In addition to some of the previously mentioned areas of concern, we now focus on symbols and the ways in which a child uses them to communicate. The areas of a communication assessment that are particularly relevant for a young child using symbols are gestures in combination with speech, symbolic play, receptive language or comprehension, and form and pragmatic functions of expressive language.

For speech or another means to qualify as communicative, it should be produced for the purpose of conveying a message to a partner. For speech to be functional, it also should be frequent, flexible, and purposeful. In other words, perseverative speech or saying the same word repeatedly, imitation of the speech of others, or echolalia is not functional in most cases.

Through several means, the SLP will attempt to collect data on the child's

- phonotactic abilities or range of production of sounds, sound combinations and syllable structures.
- ability to imitate words.
- expressive vocabulary.
- multiword combinations.
- word combination patterns.
- pragmatic functions or intentions.

Single symbols or symbol combinations reflect the intentions previously expressed through gestures. We are on firm ground when we say that words are acquired to fulfill those intentions previously expressed through these gestures. Possible early intentions of speech are presented in Table 3.3.

A child's multi-word combinations will be used to plan the direction of intervention, including new combinations and longer ones. The more traditional way of describing early word combinations is with the early semantic rules, such as *agent + action* and *negative + X*, first described in detail by Roger Brown and others in the early 1970s. The advantage of using the semantic analysis method is that the categories are easy for adults to conceptualize and teach. The second and newer approach comes from constructionist linguistic theory. According to Michael Tomasello and other linguists, young children use at least three different methods of combining words (Tomasello, 2003). These are word combinations, pivot schemes, and item-based constructions. Examples of each are presented in Table 3.4. Constructionist categories suggest a hierarchy for intervention. I suggest you check your language development text for a fuller explanation than we have space to discuss here.

TABLE 3.3 Early Intentions

Primitives Speech Acts	Early Verbal Intentions	Examples
(Gestural and vocal) (Dore, 1974)	(Owens, 1978; Wells, 1985)	
Requesting action	Wanting demands	*Cookie* (Reach)
	Direct request/Commanding	*Help* (Hand object or struggle)
Protesting	Protesting	*No* (Push away, shaking head, or being uncooperative)
Requesting answer	Content questioning questioning	*Wassat?* (Point)
	Hypothesis testing	Doggie?
Labeling	Naming/labeling	*Doggie* (Point)
	Statement/declaring	*Eat* (Commenting on dog barking)
Answering	Answering question	*Horsie* (in response to question)
	Reply	*Eat* (in response to "The doggie's hungry.")
	Exclaiming	Squeal when picked up
Vocal accompaniment	Verbal accompaniment	*Uh-oh* (With spill)
	Expressing state or	*Tired*
Greetings	Greeting	*Hi, Bye-bye*
Repeating/Practice	Repeating	*Cookie, cookie, cookie*
	Practice	*Cookie* (in response to "Want cookie?")
Calling	Calling	*Mommy!*

Adapted from Owens (2012)

TABLE 3.4 Semantic Rules and Constructionist Multiword Utterance Patterns

Semantic Rules	Constructionist Patterns
Demonstrative + Entity: *This doggie, That kitty* **X + Locative**: *Daddy car, Mommy bed, Cookie up* **Negative + X**: *Allgone juice, No cracker*	**Word combinations**: Equivalent words that encode an experience, sometimes as two successive one-word utterances. Examples: *Water hot, Wave bye, Drink cup.*
X + Dative: *Give daddy, Flower mommy* **Modifier + Head** **Attribution + Head**: *Big horsie, Little duckie* **Possessor + Possessed**: *My cup, Doggie bed* **Recurrent + X**: *More juice, 'Nuther cookie*	**Pivot schemes**: One word or phrase structures the utterance by determining intent. Examples: *Throw ball, Throw block, Throw airplane; More juice, More cookie, More bottle*. Several words may fill the "slot," as in "Want + 'things I want'." Examples: *Want blanket, Want up, Want out*.
Agent + Action: *Boy eat, Mommy throw* **Action + Object**: *Eat apple, Kick ball*	**Item-based constructions**: Seem to follow word-order constructions for specific rules. May contain morphological markers. Examples: *Daddy driving,*
Agent + Object (Rare in English): *Daddy cookie, Mommy ball*	*Drive car, Drive to gran'ma's; Baby eat, Hug baby, Baby's bed*

Formal Assessment of Infants and Toddlers

Formal normative tests of language development are inappropriate for measuring language comprehension and production in children below age 3, especially those with ASD (Mirenda, Smith, Fawcett, & Johnston, 2003). Standardized tests, for example, adhere to inflexible performance criteria that are often difficult for young children. On the other hand, alternative parent-completed vocabulary checklists, such as those in the *MacArthur–Bates Communicative Development Inventory (MCDI*; Fenson et al., 2006), have proven to be both valid and cost-effective for assessing vocabulary size and development (Dale et al., 2003).

There are a number of commercially available assessment tools and tests as well as some that have appeared in professional journals. The list of tests is presented in Table 3.5.

By its very nature, nonsymbolic communication lacks convention. Each child–caregiver dyad is in the ongoing process of negotiating the individualistic interactional behaviors that work for them. By definition, nonsymbolic interactions are often extremely individualistic and multi-modality, i.e., vocal and gestural. SLPs attempt to describe these communicative behaviors as thoroughly as possible.

TABLE 3.5 Tests for Young Children

Assessment Tool	Author(s)	Publisher or Journal
Ages and Stages Questionnaires (ASQ): A Parent-Completed Child-Monitoring System, Second Edition (2003)	Bricker, D.D., Squires, Baltimore, MD: Paul J., Mounts, L., Potter, L. Brookes Nickel, R., Trombley, E. & Farrell, J.	Baltimore, MD: Paul Brookes
**Assessment, Evaluation, and Programming System: AEPS Measurement for Birth to Three Years (Volume 1), Second Edition* (2002)	Bricker, D.D. (Ed.)	Baltimore, MD: Paul Brookes
**Bayley Scales of Infant Development, Second Edition (BSID-2)*(1993)	Bayley, N.	San Antonio, TX: The Psychological Corporation
Carolina Curriculum for Infants and Toddlers with Special Needs, Third Edition(2004)	Johnson-Martin, N.M., Attermeier, S.M., & Hacker, B.J.	Baltimore, MD: Paul Brookes
**Carpenter Play Scale* (1987)	Carpenter, R. L.	In L.B. Olswang, C. Stoel-Gammon, T.E. Coggins, & R.L. Carpenter, *Assessing prelinguistic and early linguistic behaviors in developmentally young children.* Seattle: University of Washington Press.
**Casby Scale* (2003)	Casby, M.	*Communication Disorders Quarterly, 24,* 175–183.
**Communication and Symbolic Behavior Scales* (1993)	Wetherby, A., & Prizant, B.	Chicago: Riverside
**Infant-Preschool Play Assessment Scale* (I-PAS) (1996)	Flager, S.	Chapel Hill Teaching-Outreach Project
**Infant-Toddler Language Scale* (1990)	Rossetti, L.	East Moline, IL: LinguiSystem

(*Continued*)

TABLE 3.5 *(Continued)*

Assessment Tool	Author(s)	Publisher or Journal
Language Development Survey (1989)	Rescorla, L.	*Journal of Speech and Hearing Disorders, 54,* 587–599
MacArthur-Bates Communication Development Inventories (2006)	Fenson, L., Dale, P., Reznick, S., Thal, D., Bates, E., Hartung, J., Pethick, S., & Reilly, J.	San Diego, CA: Singular Publishing
Maternal Behavior Rating Scale (MBRS)(1986)	Mahoney, G., A., & Finger, I.	*Topics in Early Childhood Special Education, 6,* 44
A Manual for the Dynamic Assessment of Nonsymbolic Communication (2002)	Snell, M.E., & Loncke, F.T.	Unpublished manuscript University of Virginia at Charlottesville. Available http://people.virginia.edu/~mes5l/manual9-02.pdf
**McCune Play Scale* (1995)	McCune, L.	*Developmental Psychology, 31,* 200–211
Observation of Communicative Interaction (OCI)(1987)	Klein, M., & Briggs, M.	*Journal of Childhood Communication Disorders, 4, 91*
Preschool Language Scale, Fourth Edition (PLS -4)(2002)	Zimmerman, I.L., Steiner V.G., & Pond, R.E.	San Antonio, TX: The Psychological Corporation
Receptive-Expressive Emergent Language Test, Third Edition (REEL-3)(2003).	Bzoch, K.R., League, R., & Brown, V.L.	Austin, TX: Pro-Ed
Sequenced Inventory of Communication Development–Revised (SICD-R)(1984)	Hedrick, D.L., Prather, E.M., & Tobin, A.R.	Los Angeles: Western Psychological Services
Speech and Language Assessment Scale (1993)	Hadley, P.A. & Rice, M.L.	*Seminars in Speech and Language, 14,* 278–288
**Symbolic Play Test* (1988)	Lowe, M., & Costello, A.	Austin, TX: Pro-Ed
**Transdisciplinary Play-Based Assessment: A functional approach to working with young children (TPBA)*(1990)	Linder, T.	Baltimore: Paul H. Brookes

*Use or can be adapted for a structured play format or a combination of formats. In addition, the ***The MacArthur–Bates Communicative Development Inventories*** contain a list of play behaviors that parents can check off.

Assessment Steps

Now that we have most of the pieces for an assessment of a nonsymbolic or minimally symbolic child, we need to organize our assessment in a logical manner to give us the information that we need to describe how an individual child communicates with those in her or his environment. SLPs are primarily responsible for selection and development of age-appropriate screening and assessment procedures (ASHA, 2008b).

Communication Screening

In the United States, children in the established risk category are eligible for services under IDEA 2004 Part C. This is not true for children in the at-risk category, and states have varying criteria for eligibility. It is the responsibility of SLPs to integrate knowledge of at-risk factors with the results of screening tests and, if needed, with more thorough results from communication assessment (ASHA, 2008b).

Screening is a process for determining whether a child is likely to show deficits in communication and/or feeding and swallowing development. More specifically, screening helps SLPs identify young children at risk so that evaluation can be used to establish eligibility and determine the appropriate in-depth assessment. Because screening is the first step in possible receipt of services, it is vitally important that the measures used be valid, reliable, sensitive, specific, and representative whether they are standardized or criterion-referenced (ASHA, 2008b).

Screening measures include direct assessment of the child and/or parental report on a standardized instrument, either of which alone or in combination is appropriate. Of course, the validity of the screening process increases with a combination of measures. Increasingly, the process for initial identification is an interview, often based on a questionnaire focusing on the child's interests and behavior and on caregivers' priorities (Wilcox & Woods, 2011). The interview process provides the SLP with an opportunity to explain the concept of daily activity- and routine-based intervention and participation-based outcomes. This lays the groundwork for a collaborative team process.

Results of the screening should be shared with the family who, in turn, should be encouraged to ask questions. If a child passes the screening, the SLP should make sure the family understands that (ASHA, 2008b)

- screening is only a general estimate of the child's performance at a point in time.
- continued monitoring of the child's progress over time is important.
- the family should return for further screening or a full evaluation if their concerns persist or new concerns arise.

When a child fails a screening, an evaluation is typically conducted to determine if he or she meets legibility for services criteria under IDEA and state guidelines.

Communication Assessment

Typical ECI assessment encompasses in-depth observations and information gathering. Ideally, the assessment is completed within a transdisciplinary context that assesses a child across all developmental domains. Planning and organization are important. Within a transdisciplinary context, team members work collaboratively, pooling members' knowledge and skills across discipline boundaries and including the family's concerns and expertise.

One way to build consensus and a collaborative relationship is to share assessment information in an ongoing way throughout the assessment. Before each task, professionals can explain its purpose to parents, and as each is completed, families and professionals can share their impressions and discuss their findings. Collaboratively, they can begin to generate ideas to enhance assessment and to plan intervention.

Good assessments include several sources of information and multiple methods of collection and will most likely not be obtained in a single sitting. Assessment tools and procedures should be individualized for the child and family, age-appropriate, and culturally sensitive. Because our goal is to obtain the best description possible of a child's functional communication abilities, we are interested in the observations of both professionals and caregivers.

The SLP is interested in the entire communication dynamic of the child, the caregiver(s), and their shared communication environment. Our overall assessment goals are

- to describe the child's communication abilities.
- to relate those abilities to partners in familiar environments/contexts.
- to describe the communication behaviors of the child's partners.
- to identify the child's responses to various facilitative prompts.
- to discover promising intervention techniques.

Ideally, the parents or caregivers will be our primary change agents during intervention.

At the very least, the assessment process should include the following steps. These are presented schematically in Figure 3.1.

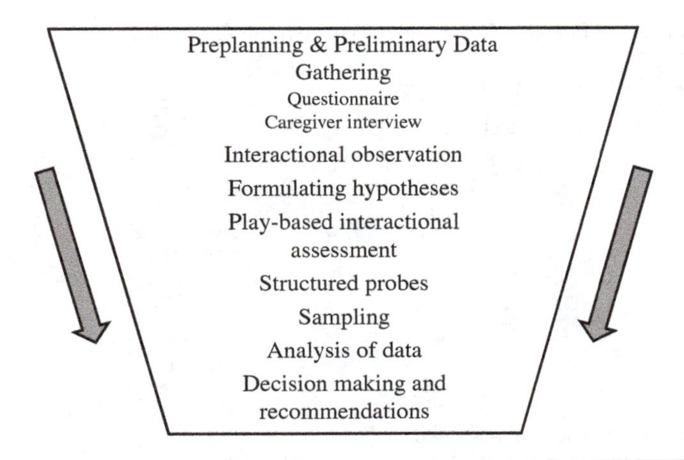

FIGURE 3.1 Schematic of the assessment process.
Each step logically flows from the previous one as we refine and sharpen our description of the child.

- *Preplanning and preliminary data gathering.* In pre-assessment collaborative planning, the process by which families and professionals set the parameters of the upcoming individualized assessment, professionals actively listen to family members' concerns and appreciate the family members' knowledge of the child.
  - *Questionnaire.* Ideally, questionnaires consist of open-ended questions that allow caregivers to elaborate and describe behaviors within everyday routines and contexts, reinforcing the notion that communication is part of each family's day and that intervention can occur in the context of everyday events. Sample questions are presented in Table 3.6.
  - *Caregiver interview.* Through open-ended interview questions, parents are asked to identify (1) ways their child communicates basic needs; (2) the communicative forms and functions or uses that the child routinely exhibits; (3) problem or challenging behavior and its possible communication function; (4) the family's attitudes, concerns, and desires; and (5) successful and unsuccessful ways to motivate communication in the child.
- *Interactional observation.* Through observation of the primary caregiver's communicative interactions with the child, the SLP and team (1) identify situations in which a child communicates most, (2) document the frequency of communication opportunities and the responsiveness of the child's communication partners, and (3) record the forms and functions of the child's intentional communication. A key component of this process is gaining understanding of contextual factors and how they may enhance or constrain participation (Wilcox & Woods, 2011).
- *Formulating hypotheses.* Collaboratively, team members, including the family, begin to formulate hypotheses about (1) the communication observed and (2) the quality of the parent–child interaction and its potential as a vehicle for change while setting parameters for the play-based assessment to follow.
- *Play-based interactional assessment.* Within a play mode, the SLP and parent(s) use "communication temptations," such as eating a treat in front of the child, to entice a child to initiate communication and manipulate the context, such as pausing in the middle of a fun activity, to attempt to elicit communication from the child.
- *Structured probes and testing.* After the more unstructured, child-initiated play portion, the SLP can conduct structured probes, such as dynamic assessment, strategically embedded in natural routines and play. **Dynamic assessment**, discussed in more detail in Chapter 5, is an adult mediated strategy that attempts to probe "teachability" of a behavior and may take

TABLE 3.6 A Sample of Possible Open-Ended Assessment Questions

What are things your child is really good at doing?
How does your child let you know he/she is... Angry? Confused? Happy? Hungry or thirsty? Sad? Surprised? Tired? Uncomfortable?
How does your child let you know he/she needs... Assistance? Toileting?
How does your child show you that she intends to communicate?
How would you feel about your child using other means of communication either as a replacement for or an addition to speech?
What do you and your child mostly communicate about?
What are the biggest obstacles to others understanding your child?
What are the biggest obstacles to others communicating with your child?

a *test-teach-test* form. After observing how the child responds without assistance (test), the SLP provides limited assistance over several trials until the child's behavior changes (teach), and then withdraws the assistance and returns to the original situation to see if learning has occurred (test). The SLP introduces and withdraws prompts as needed by the child to be successful. Even small changes in a child's behavior are considered significant.

- *Sampling.* For children using vocal and/or verbal communication, spontaneous language samples can be useful as a quantitative method for assessing language problems, developing a sound inventory and a babbling analysis, establishing semantic and pragmatic inventories, categorizing sound errors and/or patterns, and making judgments about intelligibility.
- *Analysis of data.* After obtaining information, the team attempts to determine (1) the caregiver's priority activities and routines, (2) ways to enhance the child's communication and participation, (3) possible use of augmentative or alternative communication or other forms of assistive technology to enhance the child's participation, (4) activities and routines that can provide a context for embedding learning opportunities for more complex communication skills, and (5) skills needed for children to successfully participate (Wilcox & Woods, 2011).
- *Decision making and recommendations.* The team members, including the family, review the results and discuss different intervention options while continuing to build consensus between families and professionals.

The order reflects an efficient way to accomplish the evaluative task. Like any good detective, the assessment team discovers more and more as they advance. Each step informs the next as they hone their description of the child and caregiver behaviors and interactional style.

Families who were more actively involved in all aspects of assessment are more likely to contribute to intervention planning and decision making. When families and professionals work collaboratively during the assessment, they set the tone for future collaborative interactions.

Intervention

Language skills emerge out of multiple shared social experiences in which a child's and a partner's attention are jointly focused on events or objects. As the child matures and intentionally communicates with parents, the form of that communication moves from nonsymbolic to symbolic, from gestural and vocal to verbal. It seems, logical, therefore, that intervention should also focus on mapping symbolic forms of communication onto existing prelinguistic functions or intentions. If we target these intentions, intervention becomes functional, fulfilling the child's need for communication while at the same time building on communication uses already in place.

In this context, functional communication is the use of symbols or actions to express basic wants and needs and to obtain desired outcomes. The transactional nature of communication and language development suggests a model for intervention. If ECI targets both child nonsymbolic communication behaviors and parental responses to these behaviors within everyday events, then we can facilitate a child's language development. Within these daily routines, parents can be trained in the use of language-facilitating responses to these child communication behaviors. Caregiver-identified child interests and activities are associated with the greatest gains by children (Dunst, Hamby, Trivette, Raab, & Bruder, 2000; Raab & Dunst, 2007).

A family's daily routines and activities are unique, creating specific interactions that shape a child's development. Routines, such as feeding and bathing, are an important part of everyday family life and an ongoing natural learning environment. Embedding intervention within home-based daily routines is also consistent with current educational practices and legal requirements that services to be provided in the least restrictive environments (LREs).

Once a routine is identified as a good teaching milieu, parents describe the steps in the routine. Next, they determine what props may be needed to support language teaching opportunities. Finally, with help from the SLP, parents identify ways of creating opportunities for their child to use the targeted behavior and give their response options. The family and SLP will discuss the plan, followed by an SLP model of appropriate techniques, role-playing by the parents, and a critique. This provides a great opportunity for brainstorming other techniques that might work. This may, in turn, lead to a revision of the plan by the parents and SLP.

Intervention Strategies

Specific intervention strategies with promising evidence fall into one of three groups: responsive interaction, directive interaction, and blended (ASHA, 2008b). Responsive interaction approaches typically include models of the target communication behavior without an obligation for the child to respond and include

- following a child's attentional or conversational lead with a response.
- responding to a child's initiations, both verbal and nonverbal, with natural consequences.
- extending a child's topic in a reply.
- self-talk and parallel talk describing an action.
- providing meaningful feedback.
- expanding the child's utterances with models slightly in advance of the child's current ability within typical and developmentally appropriate routines and activities.

For example, expansion of the child's utterance to a slightly more mature utterance is a powerful strategy because the adult response immediately connects the child's communication to more mature communication that serves the same purpose.

Incidental teaching is a naturalistic child-directed intervention strategy used during unstructured activities. Usually incidental teaching occurs when a child has shown an interest in something and the adult follows through by interacting around that interest. Such naturalistic interventions result in improved communication skills for young children in the early stages of communication development.

Directive interaction strategies include several teaching strategies possibly best represented by behavioral principles. Behavioral teaching strategies manipulate antecedents and consequences that surround a desired behavior. Another way of saying this is that adults will alter cues and prompts (*Say "Cookie."*) that precede the behavior in a systematic way to elicit the behavior (*Cookie!*) and also manipulate what follows the behavior to give corrective feedback (*I like the way you said "cookie." Here it is.*) while strengthening the desired response and weakening others, such as tantrumming.

Finally, blended approaches have evolved because behavioral strategies frequently fail to generalize to more functional and interactive environments. These are the approaches we've been discussing in this chapter and include teaching in natural environments using strategies for modeling language and responding to children's communication that derive from typical mother–child interactions.

Natural Settings and Partners

Optimal ECI services are provided in natural environments, which offer realistic, authentic, and ecologically valid learning experiences and promote successful communication with caregivers (ASHA, 2008b). Authentic learning has the potential to maximize children's acquisition of functional communication and promote generalization to natural, everyday contexts (Roper & Dunst, 2003). Naturally occurring activities offer opportunities to promote a child's participation and learning throughout the day using familiar activities, materials, and people (Bernheimer & Weismer, 2007; Dunst et al., 2000).

Parents or caregivers are in a unique position in ECI. They are team members and the primary agents of change at the same time that they are clients, patients, consumers, or whatever term is preferred by the servicing agency. The SLP is concerned with changing adult behaviors concurrent with changing the child's. Not only are parents capable of learning and implementing multiple teaching strategies, but positive outcomes for young children are reported (Bibby, Eikeseth, Martin, Mudford, & Reeves, 2001). Parent-implemented intervention with young children has been linked to (Kaiser, Hancock, & Neitfield, 2000)

- increases in verbalizations.
- more spontaneous speech.
- increased use of target utterances.
- longer intervals of engagement.
- more responsiveness in target tasks.
- decreases in disruptive and noncompliant behaviors.

In general, inclusion of parents as language facilitators maximizes the chance that intervention is consistent and frequent and takes place in functional contexts (Goldstein, Walker, & Fey, 2005). The quantity of intervention is increased, ensuring sufficient intensity.

The teaching techniques that parents use with their child do not need to be elaborate or formal. Simplicity is best. Daily activities provide the best time for language learning because the child knows the routine, making participation easier, and has experienced the same actions and words repeatedly within each routine.

A parent might be taught to expand on these behaviors and to encourage the child to imitate in turn. Nonsymbolic behavior can also be interpreted verbally by the parent, adding meaning to the child's behavior. At a symbolic level, expanding a child's utterance into a longer utterance can stimulate a child's development, while replying in kind can be reinforcing and can keep a child participating.

In our rush to intervene, it's easy for SLPs to overwhelm caregivers with too many intervention tasks. Adult learners actually do better with one thing at a time. Feedback should be specific and address the current situation. Parent training should include the following steps (Roberts, Kaiser, & Wright, 2010):

- Teach a specific strategy rather than several strategies, provide a rationale, examples, and a time for practice.
- Demonstrate, practice, coach, and critique, including asking how parent feels about the training and the strategy being taught.
- Plan together for everyday use of the strategy and stress the importance of home routines in intervention.
- Monitor progress of both the child and the adult through easy to use measures of behavior.
- Solicit feedback from the parent by inviting parent questions and comments.

SLPs should be mindful of the need to build parental confidence and avoid feelings of inadequacy or failure. Principles need to be presented multiple times and applied to multiple situations in order to help caregivers learn. Information should be meaningful and individualized.

Although the SLP is responsible for familiarizing families with communication services and supports (ASHA, 2004a), she or he may need to rely on the help of others when working with families from culturally linguistically diverse backgrounds. Some EI programs use cultural–linguistic mediators to aid with effective and mutually satisfying communication between professionals and families (Lynch & Hanson, 2004; Moore & Perez-Mendez, 2006). A cultural–linguistic mediator, knowledgeable about the family's culture and/or linguistic community, facilitates communication between families and EI agencies and providers. Alternative strategies include (Wing et al., 2007)

- involving more acculturated siblings or others.
- using more structured tasks or group settings for language treatment.
- using direct training techniques that are consistent with the family's culture.

Many children with special needs also participate in special care nurseries, childcare settings, or preschools. Longitudinal studies have demonstrated children's gains in both receptive and expressive language skills as a result of participation in daycare programs offering developmentally facilitative activities, high levels of staff training, and optimal levels of social and linguistic responsiveness to children's communication attempts. These settings offer yet another location within which the SLP can attempt to intervene.

A Hybrid Model

Models for inclusion of parents in ECI range from individual to small group. For a number of reasons, a hybrid model has evolved as the most efficacious means of providing ECI services. In this model, the SLP sees the child two or three times per week at home or in a childcare, EI, or preschool program. During these visits, the SLP works with the child and also instructs caregivers in the best methods of training the mutually agreed upon targets behaviors. Parents and teachers are further trained in group or individual meetings where targets are selected, objectives modified, and training continued.

If working with groups of parents and children, six to eight parent–child dyads may be optimal. Larger groups make it difficult for an SLP or other facilitators to attend easily to each individual parent–child dyad and for each parent to participate in discussions and demonstrations. Although parents and children need not be homogeneous in their characteristics, it's best to focus on a narrow range of functional age or abilities. This will facilitate the use of materials and activities that will promote engagement for children in the group.

Intervention sessions with individual caregiver-child dyads may consist of the following format:

- SLP and parent review data kept by the parent on child responsiveness to the intervention.
- Parent models techniques used.

- SLP critiques the parent's teaching.
- SLP and parent decide on targets and methods for the intervening days.
- SLP models methods for the new or revised targets.
- Parent attempts the methods for the new or revised targets.
- SLP critiques the parent's teaching and revisions are made as needed.
- SLP and parent agree on what data will be kept in the intervening days.
- SLP and parent brainstorm new ways to create even more opportunities for communication.
- SLP models new ways to talk with or stimulate the child.
- Parents attempts these new methods.
- SLP critiques.

As you can see, there's plenty to accomplish in a short amount of time.

Group sessions with parents will vary in format, sometimes including the child while at other times only parents or other family members. Wilcox, Bacon, and Greer (2005) offer a wonderful online resource for structuring of these meetings when the intervention target is single word production. Their site, listed in their bibliography, offers handouts, self-assessments, and other materials for parents. Table 3.7 presents a possible format for successive parent meetings. If it is not feasible for parents to meet in groups, the material presented in the following section can also be covered in individual sessions.

As mentioned, it's best to introduce intervention techniques slowly, no more than a few at a time over the course of intervention. At each meeting, no more than two or three techniques can be presented for talking to children, cueing their communication behavior, teaching, and responding to their behavior.

SLPs are also expected to participate in consultation with and education of team members, including families and other professionals; service coordination; transition planning; advocacy; and awareness and advancement of the knowledge base in early intervention. In ECI, SLPs work

TABLE 3.7 Play Group and Parent Class Training Agenda

Sensitivity: Tuning in to Opportunities for Language Learning
Session 1 Group meeting: *Overview and Introduction: Teaching Your Child*
Session 2 Group meeting: *Creating Opportunities for Teaching*
Session 3 Group meeting: *Using Daily Activities to Teach Language*
Session 4 Individual meetings in your home
Session 5 Group meeting: *Encouraging Communication*
Session 6 Group meeting: *Encouraging Communication during Play*
Contingency: Responding to Children's Communications
Session 7 Group meeting: Talking to Young Children
Session 8 Individual meetings in your home
Session 9 Group meeting: Imitating, Interpreting, and Expanding
Session 10 Group meeting: Responding to Your Child's Communications
Session 11 Group meeting: Options for Responding
Session 12 Individual meetings in your home
Consistency: Self-Monitoring Skills and Encouraging More Complex Language
Session 13 Group meeting: *Strategies to Further Enhance Children's Language*
Session 14 Group meeting: *Identifying More Complex Communication and Language*
Session 15 Individual meetings: *Reviewing Progress and Planning Future Goals*

Information from the model presented in Wilcox, Bacon, & Greer (2005).

in collaborative partnerships with families and caregivers and in consultative relationships, sharing essential information and support with team members, including the family and other caregivers, and other agencies and professionals (Buysse & Wesley, 2006).

Augmentative and Alternative Communication

We would be remiss if we didn't consider augmentative and alternative communication (AAC) in any discussion of nonsymbolic children. Some children, my grandson included, need extra assistance to be able to communicate more effectively, to play, eat, or to move more freely. **Assistive technology** (AT) is an essential part of early intervention, consisting of adaptations and devices for children and families that enable children to function more independently. **Augmentative and alternative communication** (AAC) is a form of AT and an intervention approach that uses other-than-speech means to complement or supplement an individual's communication abilities and may include a combination of existing speech or vocalizations, gestures, manual signs, communication boards and speech-output communication devices. You can see from this description that AAC is a multimodality ECI strategy that enables a child to use every mode possible to communicate. Early access to multiple forms of AAC is essential for early communication development in young children at risk for expressive communication impairments. An **AAC system** consists of an integrated group of components used by an individual to enhance communication.

The use of AAC does not mean that speech is ignored. Speech will be a component of most multimodal AAC systems. In this way, a child makes optimum use of vocal and speech skills for communication as part of a multimodal AAC system.

The breadth of communication behaviors involved in AAC has the potential to enhance communication skill overall. AAC can promote communication development in infants and toddlers by (ASHA, 2008b)

- enhancing both input and output.
- augmenting existing vocalizations and speech.
- replacing socially unacceptable behaviors with a more conventional means of communication (Beukelman & Mirenda, 2005).
- serving as a language-teaching tool (Romski & Sevcik, 2005).
- facilitating a young child's ability to more fully participate in daily activities and routines.

Typically, AAC serves as an output mode for communication. The other uses may be equally important for the very young child beginning to develop communication skills (Romski & Sevcik, 2005).

Results of one survey indicated that approximately 12 percent of preschoolers receiving special education services require AAC (Binger & Light, 2006). Given these findings there is a critical need for all SLPs to be prepared to provide AAC services for children who require either some alternative or addition to speech (Cress & Marvin, 2003).

Types of AAC

AAC systems are typically divided into unaided and aided based on the non-use and use of external devices respectively.

- **Unaided AAC** does not require any equipment and relies on the user's body to relay messages.
- **Aided AAC** incorporates the use of communication devices in addition to the user's body.

Unaided AAC systems use the body's own devices to communicate and include signs and gestures but also vocalizations and possibly verbalizations even if unintelligible. Possible sign systems include

- American Sign Language (ASL), the sign language used within the Deaf Community.
- Seeing Essential English (SEE_1) and Signing Exact English (SEE_2), artificially created English-based sign systems.
- Signed English, developed at Gaullaudet University with young children in mind.
- American Indian Hand Talk (Amer-Ind), a form of gestural communication consisting of 250 conceptual signals.

Other sign systems, fingerspelling, and Cued Speech are used infrequently, if at all, with infants and toddlers.

Aided AAC can range from low technology to high technology. Low-tech devices may be electronic or non-electronic, consisting of a static or non-changing display or a single switch single message. In contrast, high-tech devices offer dynamic or changing displays, are usually computer-based, and usually require more training to learn to use. Aided devices consist of

- non-electronic **communication boards** with visual-graphic symbols, such as photographs, line drawings, symbols, or even printed words, are portable, readily accessible, and very adaptable and usually contain pictures which are selected by pointing.
- electronic devices, which are extremely varied and can consist of commercially available AAC devices, individually designed AAC equipment, or adaptations to existing computers. Devices differ primarily by
  - Input mode, varying from simple pressure switches operated by a touch with virtually any body part through touchscreen devices accessed by direct selection or scanning and on to position switches such as a computer mouse.
  - Control electronics.
  - Output or display, ranging from single-message voice output devices, printed messages, and speech-generating devices (SGDS). Voice output can effectively gain the attention of others, and partners also find voice output easy to interpret and understand (Hustad, Morehouse, & Gutmann, 2002).

In **scanning** the message elements are presented in sequence to a child who then makes his or her choice as each element is presented (Beukelman & Mirenda, 2005). Scanning can take many forms.

Possible organizational designs for symbols on aided devices include a taxonomic grid, schematic grid, schematic scene, and iconic organization. In the taxonomic grid condition, vocabulary items are typically organized on different vocabulary pages or screens usually by part of speech, such as nouns and verbs. Schematic grid vocabulary items are organized by different events or contexts, such as food or clothing.

In contrast, schematic scene organization uses integrated scenes with items represented within the scene. For example, selecting a representation of a house may yield vocabulary used at home or a photo of the mother and child playing may house the words *mommy, play, me,* and toy items. Scene displays offer several possible advantages for nonsymbolic young children, including the use of familiar events and acrivities and the use of context (Light & Drager, 2007).

Finally, in iconic displays icons or line drawings are used in combination to retrieve a single word. For example, *people* (category) + *boy* (item) are used in combination to represent "boy."

Evidence-Based Practice

It must be admitted from the outset that our empirical or experimental data on AAC use is thin, especially with very young children, making evidence-based practice a challenge. A review of research articles in peer-review journals since 1980 finds that most studies are single-subject, making comparisons to diverse clinical populations difficult (Campbell, Milbourne, Dugan, & Wilcox, 2006). Although there is some evidence on the efficacy of AAC intervention for infants, toddlers, and preschoolers with a variety of severe disabilities, more studies are desperately needed (Cress, 2003; Romski, Sevcik, & Forrest, 2001; Rowland & Schweigert, 2000).

A meta-analysis of fifty studies across various age groups and populations — not just children — found that although there may be an initial learning advantage for unaided AAC over aided, there is little difference between the two in generalized communication over time (Schlosser & Lee, 2000). A second meta-analysis of twenty-four studies found no evidence to suggest that either signing or aided techniques are more likely to lead to natural speech development (Millar, Light, & Schlosser, 2000).

Even with this less than complete guidance, we can make some definitive statements. For example, AAC can play many roles in early communication development and should be introduced before communication failure occurs (e.g., Cress & Marvin, 2003; Reichle, Beukelman, & Light, 2002). Early access to AAC has been shown to be a means for (Brady, 2000) acquiring some necessary prelinguistic and cognitive skills essential for language development and establishing symbolic communication. In other words, AAC is appropriate for a young child just developing both communication and language skills in order to prevent failure in these areas of development. Although there are not many empirical studies, the ones we have demonstrate improvement in speech skills after AAC intervention (Beukelman & Mirenda, 2005; Cress & Marvin, 2003). For very young children, the use of AAC appears to enhance the development of spoken communication, although reported gains admittedly are often slight (Cress, 2003; Millar, Light, & Schlosser, 2006). Use of AAC not only helps a child communicate but also has a positive impact on parental perception of the child's language development (Romski, Sevcik, Adamson, Smith, Cheslock, & Bakeman, 2001).

A systematic review of the professional literature for over thirty years of AAC research reported that none of the studies demonstrated decreases in speech production as a result of AAC intervention (Millar et al., 2006). Research data clearly suggest that the introduction of AAC will neither cause a child to abandon speech he or she may be using nor prevent acquisition of new spoken words.

Assessment

All individuals communicate along a continuum from prelinguistic through symbolic to fully linguistic. Although one focus of an AAC assessment is to determine the need for AAC, it's more important to explore this continuum and to determine the devices and services that can help a child fully participate in their environment (Romski, Sevcik, Cheslock & Hyatt, 2002).

Standardized tests may be of little help in clearly indicating what the nonsymbolic child knows. Of importance is identifying what facilitates and what inhibits communication at each step in the process. Sadly, it's often easier to identify what a child cannot do, although from a practical standpoint, we can only build on positives. The negatives may provide future targets for intervention.

In addition to a communication assessment similar to that mentioned previously for nonsymbolic children, an SLP should determine a child's

- communication methods.
- physical abilities.
- barriers that affect the child's participation.

This can be accomplished through family/caregiver interviews and informal observation of the child interacting with family, friends, and caregivers during natural daily routines and in typical settings. Team members then engage in a problem-solving process to determine the most appropriate devices, adaptations, services, and/or strategies that will reduce or eliminate these barriers and enhance participation. Problem solving may include trial-and-error usage of a variety of devices and strategies.

There are no prerequisites per se to AAC use. Although some basic cognitive skills are essential in all children for language to develop, the exact relationship is unclear.

Cognition and language interact in a reciprocal manner, and denying a child the means of expression may put her or him at a distinct developmental disadvantage. In fact, the development of language skills through use of AAC may be critically important to cognitive growth for many AAC users. Receptive AAC use can begin at any time in much the same way that parents talk to their infants before the child comprehends speech.

Children ages 12 to 42 months of age with severe expressive impairments have better receptive language scores than expected for either their cognitive or overall developmental status (Ross & Cress, 2006). Receptive language measures may provide a better estimate of a child's mental age than cognitive test scores that can be limited by motor disabilities.

Some of the elements of a communication assessment mentioned previously take on new relevance in an assessment for AAC. Keeping in mind that AAC is or should be a multimodal communication system, the SLP is particularly interested in speech and sound making and current modes of communication. Relevant areas for AAC use include motor skills, visual perception, and sign and symbol recognition. Research data indicate that given the choice, children will use the method of communicating that they find most efficient, and this may vary even by individual symbol (Richman, Wacker, & Winborn, 2001; Sigafoos & Drasgow, 2001). These data suggest that SLPs should not impose artificial restrictions on AAC use.

Within reason, SLPs should give the child and certainly the family a choice of their preferred methods of communication. If the family is not comfortable with an AAC device, they may not use it at home. Several studies have demonstrated that positive results with AAC are critically tied to a family's participation in both assessment and intervention (Angelo, 2000; Goldbart & Marshall, 2004). One of the best ways to know if an AAC system is a good fit is to try it. If possible, a device on loan may help families adjust to this new technology. The choice of an AAC system should be determined by the extent to which that system enhances a child's interaction with people in the child's environment.

To be optimally effective, an AAC system needs to be (Light & Drager, 2005)

- versatile.
- appealing.
- easy to learn.
- dynamic.

Versatile systems meet a child's communication needs in a variety of situations and contexts and provide the potential for growth. SLPs should not overlook the use of multiple modes of communication. A dynamic systems approach is capable of changing and growing as a child learns new skills and matures.

With aided AAC there are several specific issues to be addressed. These include the symbol system, the method and rate of symbol selection, and the organization of symbols. Navigating a system or moving about a device to find a target symbol can pose a particular challenge for young children. Organization and layout of symbols can either facilitate or impede the accuracy and efficiency of a child's ability to locate, select, and functionally use those symbols.

Potentially important factors that may influence learning and use include grouping and arrangement of symbols, color, background, borders, shape, pattern, texture, size, position, and movement/animation (Beukelman & Mirenda, 2005; Scally, 2001). For example, if young children organize concepts by events and context, it would make sense to organize symbols on an aided device in that manner (Shane, 2006).

Three-year-old TD children perform significantly better with a contextual scene format in which foods and utensils are presented in a kitchen scene than a grid format based on separate semantic categories such as foods, utensils, and actions (Drager, Light, Carlson, et al., 2004). In contrast, 2½-year-old children have great difficulty regardless of the format of the display, although contextual embedding is easier (Drager, Light, Curran Speltz, Fallon, & Jeffries, 2003).

Scenes are most helpful when they are displayed initially so that a child may select a scene and then locate the desired symbol (Drager, Light, et al., 2004). For example, in a playground scene the child can touch the *swing* or the *slide* to indicate these items. Actions can be selected by touching children performing these actions.

Color can be used to highlight pictures or items in pictures. SLPs should consider incorporating color in the foreground of line drawings in visual displays. Older TD preschool children are able to locate line drawings featuring foreground color faster than drawings featuring only background color (Thistle & Wilkinson, 2009).

AAC Intervention

In designing an expressive AAC system, it is important to provide a mode or modes that can grow with a child. Each child needs a language system that can facilitate crucial transitions from one level of linguistic complexity to another. If these transitions are not inherent in an AAC system, a child cannot expand his or her communication abilities.

Speakers typically rely on multiple modes of communication to meet their needs (Blackstone & Hunt Berg, 2003). Young children using AAC need the same (Binger & Light, 2006; Light & Drager, 2005). The choice of modes should relate to a child's skills, communication contexts, partners, tasks, and intent (Blackstone & Hunt Berg, 2003).

AAC systems can be made more appealing by (Light, Drager, & Nemser, 2004; Light, Page, Curran, & Pitkin, 2008)

- including motivating, interactive activities.
- incorporating popular movie, book, or television characters and favorite activities.
- incorporating sound effects, such as laughter, music, and songs.
- using bright colors and decorations.
- allowing a child choices.
- making use fun.

Let's face it, we all like doing something that we enjoy and that reflects our desires.

Ease of learning is fostered by reducing the learning demands. In aided AAC, a child must learn

- to operate the equipment, which may be a sophisticated computer-based device.
- to recognize and use the symbol system, such as pictures or drawings.
- to use the technology in communicative interactions.

Typically, an AAC device is just one part of a child's AAC system. It is not uncommon for children to also use signs, gestures, vocalizations, and speech approximations with different in different situations with different communication partners (Beukelman & Mirenda, 2005).

One factor that effects learning and use is response efficiency. Any of the four components of response efficiency — response effort, rate of reinforcement, immediacy of reinforcement, and quality of reinforcement — may have an effect on a child's use of AAC (Johnston, Reichle, & Evans, 2004). Response effort includes both the physical effort required to produce a communicative act and the cognitive effort required to recall or use symbols or a communication system. For example, holding up an empty cup to request more juice may be both physically easier than activating an electronic device and cognitively easier than locating a symbol in an array.

Reinforcement rate is particularly important in teaching anew method of communication. Immediacy of reinforcement would suggest that aided communication devices be present and available for use by children throughout the day. If not, children may simply ignore a communicative opportunity rather than tolerate the delay in reinforcement resulting from finding and using the AAC device.

Reinforcement quality relates to the desirablity of the reinforcer. Simply put, when one event or object is preferred over another, the preferred one has a higher quality of reinforcement.

These variables usually do not function in a vacuum, but interact with each other. An AAC user has to determine the most efficient response for the message he or she wishes to send. The notion of efficiency depends on the demands of the communicative context and would support training multiple ways of communicating so that different options are available to a child.

Vocabulary

Although augmentative and alternative communication (AAC) systems offer increased opportunities for children with severe communication impairment to participation in activities in their home, school, and community, without the appropriate vocabulary, AAC systems will not be effective (Fallon, Light, & Kramer Paige, 2001). An initial vocabulary for young children should be meaningful, motivating, functional, and individualized, be appropriate to a child's age, gender, background, personality, and environments, and be able to support a range of communicative uses and intentions. This necessitates a detailed understanding of a child's most frequented contexts and the communication expectations of those settings and an appreciation of the individual child's own style of communication.

When selecting vocabulary, SLPs should be mindful of the need for two types of words:

- A core vocabulary of words commonly used in a given situation, such as common verbs and greetings.
- A fringe vocabulary of words specific to an individual or activity, such as the SLP's name, song words for "circle time," and favorite treats.

Core vocabulary is generally stable across people and contexts and generative in nature, consisting of words that can be combined into longer uttterances. Several potential core vocabulary lists exist and can be accessed easily by typing "core vocabulary" into your computer's search engine. Even so, core vocabulary should be adapted to the individual child.

Fringe vocabulary is activity-specific and infrequently used in other environments and contexts. Examples of fringe vocabulary might include action words such as *paint, dance*, and *color* that only occur in certain contexts.

There are three main approaches to selecting vocabulary for children: developmental, environmental, and functional, none of which are mutually exclusive. A developmental approach involves the use of vocabulary lists developed from studies of typically developing children and may not be appropriate for children with developmental disabilities. In contrast, an environmental approach is based on an ecological inventory, in which words are identified for specific communication environments. Finally, a functional approach is pragmatic in nature, and vocabularies are identified based on expressed communication functions such as requesting.

Several ecologically sound and individualized methods can be used by SLPs for fringe vocabulary selection. These include

- conducting a survey of the environments and activities in which a child needs to communicate.
- using a communication diary to record a child's attempted interactions.
- compiling a list of words and phrases thought to be potentially useful to a child.
- completing a caregiver vocabulary selection questionnaire similar to that for other nonsymbolic children.

A fine example of a questionnaire is presented in an article by Fallon, Light, and Kramer Paige (2001).

Children are most apt to communicate if they have vocabulary that allows them to do the things they want to do. In other words, they need to be able to request and discuss things they enjoy whether foods or games. Potential words should be selected based on the extent to which they enable a child to talk about the things in the environment and to use each symbol to express a variety of intentions.

New vocabulary items are often learned by TD children within the context of events and activities. This is the perfect vehicle for introducing new symbols in AAC as well. It's important, therefore, that parents and teachers use the AAC system when conversing with a child user.

SLPs should work closely with the family to select vocabulary and contexts that reflect the family's culture. For example, eating utensils may be inappropriate for Ethiopian American children while injera, a doughy flatbread used to bring food to the mouth, is not. The vocabulary should reflect food, clothing, and celebrations from the child's world. Representations should also depict the child's cultural background in skin color, facial features, and clothing, to mention just a few.

In part, the words we each use to communicate reflect our individual nature. The ECI team should select vocabulary the enables a child to express that unique personality as well.

Early words or symbols are usually learned during routines in which a child matches messages to functional goals within the interaction. AAC intervention with young children should include teaching new concepts and words by actually using them, rather than waiting for a child to demonstrate understanding first. We know from TD children that words are often learned within routines and scripts that provide a supportive environment for early production of words and phrases that a child may not fully understand. By experiencing a word within a routine, the child forms an activity-based concept to which the label may be attached.

Generalization: Role of the Environment

One of the biggest concerns, an issue I have stressed and will continue to emphasize throughout this text, is generalization of newly learned AAC skills to different use environments. In order for generalization to occur, it must be actively promoted from the onset of the intervention process rather than as a later add-on. Short of this, SLPs are left with a "train and hope" approach, in which, unaware of the variables that affect generalization, they "hope" that it will occur.

Research data indicate that intervention most often focuses on changing the behaviors of AAC users rather than that of partners (Schlosser & Lee, 2000). For children using AAC, most communication partners may have only marginally higher, if not lower, AAC competency. This results in a situation in which the educational needs of a child developing AAC may co-exist with similar educational needs among professionals, staff, and caregivers.

The effectiveness of an augmentative communication system depends on the commitment of all communication partners. SLPs must consider not only the needs and abilities of a child with CI when designing an AAC system but also the needs, preferences, and interactional styles of these communication partners. For example, given the imprecision and inherent slowness of some children using AAC, partners tend to

- dominate communicative interactions.
- take the majority of conversational turns.
- ask primarily yes/no questions.
- provide few opportunities for an AAC user to initiate conversations or to respond.
- interrupt frequently.
- focus on the AAC device or technique instead of the child or the child's message.

In response, AAC users may respond by playing an increasingly passive role,

- initiating few interactions and responding only when required to do so.
- producing only a limited range of communicative function, such as answers to yes/no questions.
- using restricted linguistic forms, such as one-word responses.

This situation is less than optimal and works against language and communication development for a child.

Obviously, the key to changing a child's role to a more active one is changing the behaviors of a child's communication partners. For a child's partners this means learning to facilitate interactions and to use strategies to better support the communication of the child using AAC. Four interactional skills have been identified as intervention targets for the communication partners (Kent-Walsh & Light, 2003):

- Extending conversational pause time or expectant delay by initiating eye contact with the child.
- Being responsive to communicative attempts.
- Using open-ended questions.
- Modeling of AAC system use.

Following instruction, communication partners can learn to lessen conversational dominance and to provide more turns for the AAC user. In turn, conversational participation, turn-taking, and the range of communicative functions of AAC users increase.

Intervention goals related to participation or involvement in life situations are more directly related to a child's communicative functioning in the family than are goals that are focused on execution of an AAC task such as using a new scanning technique (Granlund, Bjorck-Åkesson, Wilder, & Ylven, 2008). It is sometimes assumed that more immediate goals, such as improving intelligibility of AAC system use, will affect overall participation in interactive contexts. In fact, outcomes in one area of AAC intervention do not necessarily affect other areas of functioning (Lund & Light, 2006). If we hope to improve participation within family life, we should directly target this area of functioning and not just hope it will occur. In general, children with better AAC outcomes tended to have more supportive family environment than those with less positive outcomes (Hamm & Mirenda, 2006).

Parents and other family members can be taught techniques to support their child's communication. These include (Light & Drager, 2005):

- Planning together with the SLP to integrate the AAC system into the natural environment.
- Identifying varied communication opportunities within each context.
- Modeling AAC and speech.
- Learning to wait and to anticipate the child's communication.
- Responding to the child's communication attempts in meaningful ways:
  - Responding in a timely and positive manner when a child attempts to communicate
  - Fulfilling the child's intent, such as providing a requested toy
  - Expanding through AAC and speech to the child's message
  - Replying conversationally
  - Modeling correct forms of immature or incorrect child behaviors
  - Expanding on the child's message

Beginning with the facilitator's current strengths, the SLP can gradually build new knowledge and skills through a combination of explanation, modeling, practice, monitoring, and feedback. It's important to be mindful of family needs and comfort level and not to introduce too many new things at once. The last thing a family needs is a time-consuming burden, such as endless drills involving AAC.

Summary

To be truly useful with young children, AAC technologies will need to be redesigned to increase their appeal, expand functions, and reduce the learning demands (Light & Drager, 2002). For example, the appeal for young children may be increased by (Light, Drager, & Nemser, 2004)

- integrating play into both AAC design and intervention.
- providing meaningful fun contexts for interaction and intervention.
- expanding output options to include voice or animation.
- enhancing aesthetics to resemble toys in color and design.
- providing options for personalization.

These modifications cannot be accomplished at the expense of ease of learning. At present, learning AAC systems is extremely challenging for young presymbolic children, especially given the need to attend to and interact with communication partners at the same time (Light, Parsons, & Drager, 2002). Add to this, the dynamic nature of communication and you get some idea of the challenge for a young child with communication impairment.

Conclusion

As you can see, working with young children with CI and LI is a challenging task, especially if the child does not seem to be interested in or motivated to communicate. Given the complex world of infants, toddlers, and preschoolers, an SLP can hope to accomplish very little seeing a child an hour or even a few hours each week. It's sad to report, but given recent funding cutbacks, intervention may be even more limited. My grandson was being seen once a month! In my book, that's criminal. If the SLP does not enlist the aid of parents and family members, teachers and classroom aides, and childcare providers, he or she is missing a valuable opportunity to provide effective intervention in a functional manner that fosters communication and language growth.

Assessment of Preschool and School-age Children with Language Impairment

Chapter 4

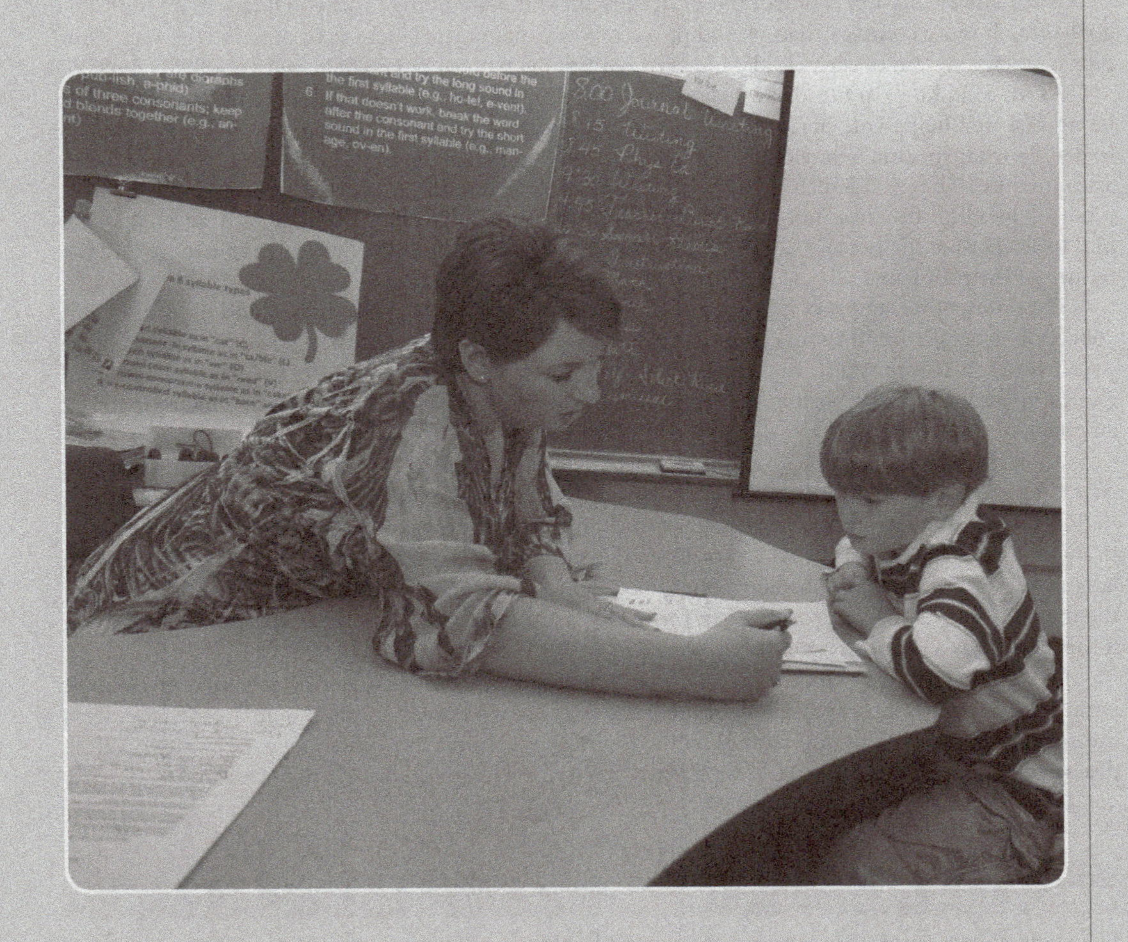

Still feeling overwhelmed by the list of possible disorders associated with LI? Here's some comfort. First, as an SLP, you won't be solely responsible for designating a child as one thing or another. For that type of diagnosis, you'll be on a team with other knowledgeable professionals. Ideally, your team will conduct a thorough assessment, weigh all the information, and make thoughtful and appropriate recommendations for intervention. Second, as you acquire more experience and become more skilled, you'll learn to recognize patterns of behavior and signs that indicate the presence or certain underlying disorders. In the last analysis, however, nothing is a substitute for the data you systematically gather through an individualized, well-designed, thorough assessment of a child's communication skills and deficits.

No clear line exists between assessment and intervention. Both are part of the intervention process, and portions of each are found in the other. Ideally, assessment and measurement are ongoing throughout intervention. No clinical goal should be determined or modified without first obtaining data on the communication performance of a child.

Adequate evaluation is one of the most difficult and demanding tasks you'll face as an SLP. The goal—much more complex than providing a score or a diagnostic label—is to describe the very complex language system of each child and his or her unique pattern of language rules and behaviors.

As an SLP, keep in mind the *why, what,* and *how* of assessment. Considering why a child is being assessed helps you clarify the purpose of the assessment. This clarity, in turn, enables you to decide what specific behaviors to assess and the best evaluative methods to use. The reasons for assessment can be grouped as (a) identification of children with potential problems, (b) establishment of baseline functioning, and (c) measurement of change. Baseline functioning enables an SLP to determine the present level of performance, the extent of the language impairment, and the nature of the problem.

The data-gathering process is scientific in nature in that it must be unbiased and objective. This collection process should be precise and measurable, with very little intrusion by an SLP's premature conclusions. It is important, however, not to lose the child in the mass of data you'll collect, and clinical intuition is an important factor when summarizing data and determining which aspects of language to evaluate.

It may be helpful to consider assessment procedures as existing along a continuum from formal, structured protocols to informal, less structured approaches. In general, the more structured the elicitation session, the less variety of structures and meanings expressed by the child. Language elicited in more structured tasks is usually shorter and less complex, especially with younger children, than language sampled in less controlled situations. Generally, the more specific the information desired, the more structured the approach. Even formal tests or portions of tests, however, can be used in an informal way as a probe of specific behavior.

In this chapter, we explore the differences between psychometric and descriptive assessment paradigms and describe a combined, or integrative, approach that attempts systematically to address the shortcomings of both approaches while describing a child's use of language in context. While discussing the integrated approach, we'll apply it to typical language impairment cases.

Psychometric versus Descriptive Procedures

The goals of communication assessment are to identify and describe each child's unique pattern of communication behaviors and, if that pattern signifies a language impairment, to recommend treatment, follow-up, or referral. Through this process, an SLP determines

- whether a problem exists.
- the causal-related factors.
- the overall intervention plan.

TABLE 4.1 Comparison of Norm Referencing and Criterion Referencing Measures

Norm Referencing	Criterion Referencing
The purpose is to identify individuals performing at various levels.	The purpose is to describe specific levels of performance.
Address a broad spectrum of content.	Address a clearly defined specified aspect of language.
Items distinguish among individuals.	Items cover aspects of language.
Performance is summarized using comparisons such as percentile or standard scores.	Performance is summarized meaningfully using measures such percent correct.

Information adapted from McCauley (1996).

There are two major philosophical approaches to this task. The *normalist* philosophy is based on a norm, or average performance level—usually a score—that society considers typical functioning. In contrast, the *neutralist*, or *criterion-referenced*, approach compares a child's present performance to his or her past performance and/or is descriptive in manner. The features of each approach are presented in Table 4.1.

The two methods are not mutually exclusive. For example, the results of normative testing can be reinterpreted to provide more descriptive information. Test items on which a child is unsuccessful can be probed to determine other methods that result in a correct response.

More descriptive approaches, such as language sampling, can highlight the individualistic nature of a child's communicative functioning. In contrast, psychometric normative testing imposes group criteria on an individual, thereby obviating an assessment of the individual. Each method of assessment has its strengths and weaknesses, as well as possible applications within the clinical setting. These are described in the following sections.

Tests are usually standardized and normed. **Standardized** means that there is a consistent or standard manner in which test items are to be presented and child responses consequated. For example, the test manual may direct an SLP to give the following instructions:

> I am going to read a sentence to you. When I'm finished, I want you to select the picture that best illustrates what I have said. Listen carefully, because I can only read each sentence once.

The test is to be administered in this manner.

Most standardized tests are also **normed**, which means that the test has been given to a group of children that supposedly represent all children for whom the test was designed and scores determined for typical functioning. Ideally, the norming group has the same characteristics as the children for whom the test is designed. In other words, gender, racial and ethnic, geographic, and socioeconomic differences present in your children are also represented in the norming group in the same proportions. Even these constraints do not ensure that the test will be appropriate, especially with children from culturally and linguistically diverse backgrounds. Usually, children with LI are rarely included in the norming group.

Traditional language assessment procedures heavily emphasize the use of standardized psychometric or norm-referenced tests. This situation is reflected in the fact that more than 100 norm-referenced language assessment tools are commercially available. In general, there are very few standardized measures for toddlers and adolescents and an abundance of measures for preschoolers and early-school-age children.

Ideally, a standardized test has demonstrated reliability and validity. **Reliability** is the *repeatability of measurement*. More precisely, reliability is the accuracy or precision with which a sample of language taken at one time represents performance of either a different but similar sample or the same sample at a different time. Very limited samples of language usually result in unstable or undependable scores. Thus, a test must include enough language to be reliable yet not unwieldy.

One measure of reliability is **internal consistency.** Internal consistency is the degree of relationship among items and the overall test. If a test has high internal consistency, children who score well or poorly overall should tend to have the same performance on individual items and to perform similarly among themselves.

Measures of reliability include *test-retest reliability, alternate-form reliability*, and *split-half reliability*. In test-retest reliability, a child is administered the same test with a time interval between each administration. With alternate forms, a child is administered equivalent or parallel forms of a measure. Finally, a test may be divided into equivalent halves. In each case, the two test scores are compared and the consistency of scores measured. This value is expressed as a reliability coefficient or as a standard error of measure (SEm). The closer the reliability coefficient to a value of 1 and the lower the standard error, the more reliable is the measure. In other words, a reliability coefficient of .84 indicates greater reliability than one of .62. SEm will be discussed in more detail later. These values are discussed in each test's manual.

In addition, an SLP is concerned with the probability of two judges scoring the same behavior in the same manner. This value is called **interjudge reliability**. As a group, scoring procedures that use a definite criterion, such as accepting only specific responses as correct, are more reliable than those that use scaled scoring, such as grading responses (1–5) by their degree of correctness. Graded scores can have increased reliability if each score has definite criteria or if the tester has received specific training.

Validity is the effectiveness of a test in representing, describing, or predicting an attribute of interest to the tester. In short, it is a measure of the test's ability to assess what it purports to assess. The tester is interested in measuring all of the attribute being tested but nothing other than that attribute. For example, if a test of receptive language abilities requires a child to respond verbally or to use expressive language, it goes beyond the stated domain of the attribute being tested.

Professionals should be cautious when choosing tests. Few language screening tests, for example, meet criteria for validity or provide information to enable SLPs to determine validity.

To test language knowledge, test designers must select concrete performance tasks. These tasks, in turn, can become the defining features of the entity supposedly being measured. It's important to remember that tests do not represent the overall attribute or behavior but are merely samples. From the samples, testers make inferences about the overall attribute or behavior. If the samples are not valid measures, the inferences will be incorrect.

Validity is not self-evident and must be proven. Three types of evidence are criterion validity, content validity, and construct validity. **Criterion validity** is the effectiveness or accuracy with which a measure predicts performance. This usually is calculated as the degree to which a measure correlates with some other suitable measures of success assumed to be valid.

Content validity is the faithfulness with which the sample or measure represents some attribute or behavior. In other words, the sum of the tasks involved should define or constitute, at least in part, the attribute or behavior being measured. Measures should reflect the professional literature, research, and expert opinion on the constitution of the attribute or behavior tested.

Finally, **construct validity** is the extent to which a measure describes or measures some trait or construct. Professionals are interested in the significance of results and in how precisely the measure notes individual or group differences. Construct validity usually is determined by comparing the measure with other acceptable measures assumed to be valid. If a child failed one language screening test but passed the other, it may indicate that the tests assessed different aspects of language.

Normative tests help the SLP determine how a child's performance, in the form of a score, compares with that of children who supposedly possess the same characteristics. Most frequently, tests are used to determine average and less-than-average performance and the need for intervention services. Although normative tests may be good for measuring isolated skills, they provide very little information on overall language use.

Psychometric Assessment Protocols

Although normed tests are potentially valid, reliable, and precise in measurement, it is difficult to find a language test that is acceptable in all three ways. In addition, normed tests do not easily accommodate cultural and individual variation, nor do they begin to provide a true picture of the richness and complexity of the child's communication behavior. By their nature, tests are less complex than the language being assessed. Language is multidimensional and its use individualistic, making it difficult to measure.

Test Differences

Language assessment instruments differ widely even when purported to measure the same entity. Even tests that seem to be significantly correlated, suggesting an interrelationship, may seem less so when subtests or various portions of tests are compared. In addition, tests can differ markedly in their levels of difficulty, yielding different results for the same child for the same skill.

Tests should be researched carefully by SLPs before being used. In the following section we explore some of these differences, specifically test content, and some of the common misuses of tests. Finally, the variables that should be considered in test selection are discussed.

Content

The major criticism of existing instruments is the inadequacy of the content covered in both breadth and depth. Two issues relative to content validity—relevance and coverage—must be addressed in test construction. Content relevance is the precision with which a certain aspect of language is delineated or defined. This is necessary to determine the dimensions of that aspect to test.

A child's knowledge of language, called *competence*, is measurable only as test behavior or *performance*, which is affected by the speed of responding and the complexity of the task. Thus, poor performance may indicate an underlying deficit or difficulty with the assessment procedure rather than a language problem.

Content coverage is the completeness with which an aspect of language is sampled. Theoretically, coverage of language features should reflect general use. If coverage is inadequate, more subtle language impairments may go undetected.

Testing produces data on minimal portions of behavior, thus reducing language to simple, possibly irrelevant dimensions that may not reflect the qualities of a child's language overall. By fragmenting language into observable and measurable features, tests tend to emphasize structural components of language form that are easy to observe. Although structured testing may reveal the child's ability to use language in the test context, it may also reveal very little about the child's language as it is needed and used in everyday communication. For example, a child may use interrogatives throughout the day to obtain information, desired objects, and needed assistance but may be unable to form interrogatives in isolation when given a group of words to include. In addition, the test situation may be so foreign to a child or that child's everyday communication environment that it influences the language the child produces. Performance may be affected also by factors as diverse as a child's state of health on the day the test is administered, attention level and comprehension of the instructions, and perception of the test administrator.

Misuse of Normative Testing

Norm-referenced tests should be used with caution. The best advice is to be an "informed clinician" and a wise consumer. SLPs should also be mindful of the possible misuse of these instruments, such as

- use of scores as a summary of a child's performance.
- use of inappropriate norms.

- inappropriate assumptions based on test results.
- use of specific test items to plan intervention goals.
- use of tests to assess therapy progress.

Let's discuss each briefly.

Misuse of Scores

When does difference become disorder? Where do we draw the line? Are the 1 percent of the population who are blood type B-negative considered deviant or just different? How do we decide?

The most frequently used score on standardized measures is the mean, or average, score. Test makers assume that the average score for a sample population is the "normal" score for the larger population. When plotted, the total number of individuals receiving each score will form the familiar *bell-shaped curve*, represented in Figure 4.1.

It is important to recall that a wide scoring area about the mean, called one standard deviation, also is considered to fall within the normal range. Approximately two-thirds of the population should score within 1 standard deviation on either side of the mean score. Nearly one-third of the population, approximately 16 percent above and 16 percent below, fails to fall within this range. Perhaps two standard deviations is a better index of deviancy, leaving approximately 3 percent of the population above and 3 percent below. Is this too restrictive? Another possible index is the 10th percentile, the lowest 10 percent of the norming sample. Children who score at or below the 10th percentile are often considered to be other-than-normal. An SLP must decide where "non-normal" or disorder occurs.

Scores at either end of the distribution represent a quantitative difference that can be called, *exceptional* or *other-than-normal*. Obviously, the boundary is relative and somewhat arbitrary. Tests offer guidance, but an SLP must decide when the difference is so great as to impair an individual.

The use of test scores imposes some constraints that may be overlooked. First, numbers establish equalities and inequalities. For example, 2 is twice 1 and half of 4. It would seem, therefore, that a child with a score of 4 correct has twice the skill of one with a score of 2, but this is a measure of the number of responses, not their quality. Some test items are more difficult than others.

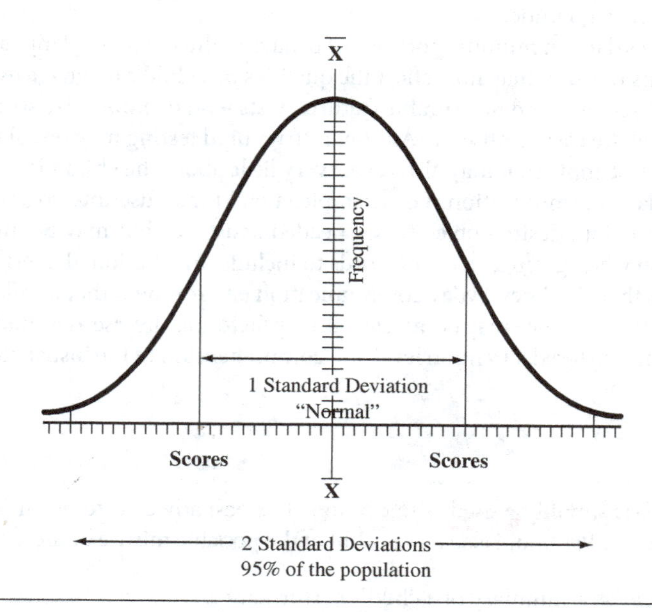

FIGURE 4.1 Parameters of the normal distribution.

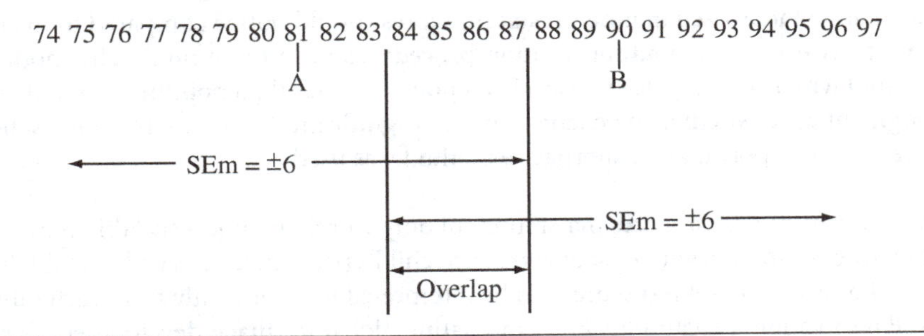

FIGURE 4.2 A comparison of scores using standard error of measure.

Second, all test items are assumed to be of equal importance because each has the same weight. If there is one item each for the verb to *be* and past-tense *-ed*, they each receive the same score even though they are not of equal importance developmentally.

Scores imply some standard of performance when in fact there may be none, except the numerical score. The equality of scores does not translate to an equality of behavior and offers an inadequate description of that individualistic behavior. A child who achieves the same score as a younger child may not make the same kinds of errors. Two children with the same error scores even on the same items could have answered very differently.

As an SLP, you should habitually check the *standard error of measure* (SEm) in the test manual for information about the confidence of test scores. Because tests are less than perfectly reliable, a certain amount of error is reflected in each score. The larger the SEm, the less confidence one can have in the test's results.

The SEm can be added to and subtracted from a test score to establish a band of confidence or where you can be most sure that the score resides. For example, assume that a child received a score of 75 on two different tests with confidence intervals of 2 and 6, respectively. On the first test, the child's error-free, or true, score is most probably 73–77; on the second, it is 69–81. The SLP can have more confidence that the score of 75 on the first test is closer to the child's actual performance.

SEm values also may mean that scores that seem very different actually overlap, as shown in Figure 4.2. Child A received a score of 81, and Child B received a score of 90. An SEm of 6 applied to each score results in an overlap. Therefore, the children's actual abilities may be much more similar than the test scores alone indicate.

My remarks are cautionary and do not mean that you should avoid testing. Quantification or use of scores is not inherently bad as long as measurement is meaningful and functional and reflects accurately the entity being evaluated. It is important that test designers define the entities being tested and provide a rationale in the test manual for the tasks selected. SLPs should read, understand, and evaluate the manual and be knowledgeable about test construction and administration. Evidence-based practice requires that the professional literature about a certain test be studied thoroughly before the test is used.

Inappropriate Norms. The norming sample should represent the population for whom you are using the test. Otherwise, the norms are inappropriate and should not be used. This situation occurs most frequently with children with culturally linguistically diverse, rural, or lower socioeconomic backgrounds. In these cases, local norms may need to be prepared by an SLP by following the norming procedure described in the test manual. Some test manuals, such as those for the Test of Language Development–Intermediate (TOLD-I) and the Clinical Evaluation of Language Functions (CELF), explain this process in detail.

Finally, we cannot assume that norms are stable. They change over time. In addition, changes in the format of the test, such as offering it on computer, may also change the norms. If a test is given in an other-than-standardized manner, resultant scores should not be compared to the test's norms. There may be occasions when administration procedures need to be minimally modified, such as allowing a child with cerebral palsy to use a head pointer rather than pointing by hand, and it is your clinical judgment as to whether the changes are nonsignificant. If you use the norms, however, you should state in your report that an alternative method was used.

Incorrect Assumptions. Test scores may represent only scores and not actual differences in linguistic ability. Therefore, as an SLP, you must analyze each child's performance in order to obtain descriptive information. For example, subtest scores can be interpreted independently from each other.

An SLP also should be cautious in extrapolating global language development from scores on language tests, especially those that sample only one or two aspects of language. For example, while the Peabody Picture Vocabulary Test (PPVT) is an excellent receptive vocabulary test, it does not address other aspects of language or indicate overall language use.

Identifying Intervention Goals. A thorough description of a child's behavior is needed before an SLP can identify areas needing intervention. Individual test items or subtests do not provide an adequate sample of that behavior. Because test items represent only a small portion of language, they do not provide enough information on which to base therapy goals. At the very least, more than one psychometric assessment procedure should be used because of the variability of some children across tests. The more test scores available, the more reliable the assessment. Only through the use of a number of different assessment protocols can the SLP hope to determine intervention objectives.

Measuring Therapy Progress. The continued use of a norm-referenced test to assess therapy progress may result in a child's learning the test, thus producing artificially high results. Widely spaced testing or the use of different forms of the same test or of different but highly correlated tests may better demonstrate changes in behavior over time. Criterion-referenced tests and other descriptive measures, explained later in the chapter, are more appropriate for measuring individual progress.

Variables in Test Selection

As an SLP, you should be a wise consumer of assessment materials and should base test selection on several factors. Of particular interest are test reliability and validity, discussed previously. Even language tests that meet very stringent psychometric or measurement criteria may not be very precise discriminators of impaired and nonimpaired language.

Before using any test, an SLP should check the characteristics of the test by examining the test manual. The results for any child must be weighed against the tests accuracy in four areas:

- Correctly detecting impairment that is present (a true positive result).
- Detect impairment when it is not present (a false positive result).
- Correctly identifying typical language (no LI) (a true negative result).
- Identifying child as having typical language when LI is present (a false negative result).

If, for example, a test has a high false positive rate, the SLP must consider the accuracy when a child is found to have LI. In this situation, it's easy to see the value of giving more than one test. Not every test manual will give all four values.

Other considerations in test selection include appropriateness of the test for a particular child, the manner of presentation and comprehensiveness, and the type and sensitivity of the test results. A test should be appropriate to the child's age or functioning level. In addition, the norming population should be sufficiently large and varied to include representatives of the child's racioethnic and socioeconomic background. If the child is from an identifiable group, you should check to see whether the norming information gives data by such groups.

Appropriateness may relate also to manner of presentation, the number of items, and the content coverage discussed previously. Some children perform better under certain conditions than under others. For example, children with LD can perform better if visual input accompanies the verbal.

Some tests offer a computerized version for children with motoric problems or those who may perform better on this format. Although it is still in its infancy, some professionals are exploring the provision of language assessment via the Internet (Waite, Theodoros, Russell, & Cahill, 2010). Although some language tests yield virtually the same scores whether administered by an online or face-to-face SLP, these results will vary across children.

The type of result, whether percentage, percentile, or age equivalent, is also a practical consideration in test selection. Depending on the test, the interpretive value of such scores may be very limited.

When given a choice of different tests, SLPs display a remarkable similarity in the relative importance they attach to different measures. Familiarity with the test procedure, overall opinion of the measure, and clinical experience are all factors in test or task selection and in the relative importance attached to data obtained from different measures.

Summary

Perceptive professionals have decried overdependence on and poor interpretation of the results of testing. Although standardized tests, especially those in language, frequently have been much maligned, SLPs often are required to incorporate standardized and normed results into their assessments. It is important for you as a future SLP to recognize that tests are informative, but not the be-all and end-all of evaluation. Awareness of a test's shortcomings can greatly aid the interpretation of a child's performance.

Norm-referenced approaches offer "canned" assessment with little consideration for the individual needs of the child with whom they are used. It is all too easy for assessment procedures to take priority over the child. Tests are a *priori* and product oriented, offering little information on the appropriateness of the features being tested. Test results, in turn, offer little assistance in identifying individual problems and in planning intervention.

Although norm-referenced tests play an important role in identifying children with LI, they should not be the only tools used. While use of these tests has led to much discussion, the related issue of cutoff scores for identification has been addressed less vigorously. Simply using a –1 *SD* or even a –2 *SD* criterion without considering other factors, such as cultural and linguistic diversity, may be doing a disservice to children (Oetting, Cleveland, & Cope, 2008; Spaulding, Plante, & Farinella, 2006). At the very least, SLPs should consider test results from a combination of measures. For example, one study found that in evaluating oral story comprehension, a combination the Joint Story Retell task and the Expectancy Violation Detection task (Dempsey, Jacques, Skarakis-Doyle, & Lee, 2002; Skarakis-Doyle, 2002), and the use of comprehension questions resulted in 96 percent accurate identification of children with LI (Skarakis-Doyle, Dempsey, & Lee, 2008).

The issue of testing is central to the purpose of assessment. Data gathered in an assessment should be relevant to the initial clinical complaint, to the determination that a problem exists, to individual differences and individual processing, to the nature of the problem, to prognosis, to intervention implications, and to accountability. Otherwise, it is just a numbers game. Although norm-referenced tests seem appropriate for determining if a language impairment exists, they are inconsistent in determining the specific area(s) of deficit required for intervention.

Descriptive Approaches

The descriptive approach, usually based on observation and a conversational sample of a child's language, is a widely taught method of defining children's communicative abilities. Unfortunately, because of time constraints the method may be used less frequently than normative testing in actual practice. Descriptive approaches have the potential of allowing SLPs to regard the language process while maintaining contextual integrity and individual differences.

Spontaneous sampling is an indicator of a child's overall language functioning rather than as a device for noting specific language problems. More specific data can be obtained by probing the child's knowledge. In general, data from language samples correlate significantly with results from elicited imitation and sentence completion tasks; however, the syntactic structural patterns can vary widely.

The advantages of the descriptive approach are that an SLP can apply his or her own theoretical model to the assessment process and can probe and assess areas that seem most handicapping to a child. Thus, the clinical process can remain flexible and attuned to the client's needs. To do this, an SLP must understand the complex interaction of constitutional—biological, cognitive, psychological, and social—and environmental forces.

A language sample has several advantages over more formal structured-response testing, which, as we've discussed, reveals little about the use, content, and form of a child's language as needed and used in daily living. Some language features are more sensitive to the linguistic and extralinguistic factors of conversational give-and-take.

The disadvantages of the descriptive approach are

- the level of language expertise needed to elicit and analyze a child's language.
- the amount of time needed to collect and analyze the child's language.
- the reliability and validity of the sample. Although a number of descriptive protocols exist, an SLP may not feel sufficiently well versed in all aspects of language to choose those appropriate for each child.

In addition, a large caseload may preclude the use of lengthy descriptive procedures. Finally, as in psychometric testing, the SLP may not elicit a reliable or valid sample of a child's usual language usage.

Reliability and Validity

Language samples are more susceptible than standardized measures to SLP bias, especially when used to assess intervention effectiveness. An SLP must attempt to analyze the language sample in the most objective manner possible. Objective descriptions of the actual behaviors observed are generally more reliable than subjective judgments of the causes or reasons for these behaviors. One way to increase reliability is to separate the actual events from inferences based on these events and to base decisions on the data from these events.

Reliability across observations can be increased by taking the following three precautions:

1. *Define the behaviors to be observed as explicitly as possible, and train observers to ensure good inter- and intraobserver reliability.* The selection of behavior categories to be observed will affect the validity of the observation. For example, it may be easier and more accurate to identify certain gestures than to record their intentions. Accuracy can be controlled by making comparisons between the ratings of two observers. This type of analysis helps sharpen definitions and to highlight possible areas of confusion.
2. *Make judgments on only one type of behavior at a time.* This procedure may require the use of videotaping or digital recording so that a language sample can be replayed often for additional judgments on other behaviors.

3. *Do not make summation judgments while observing "online."* It is too easy for preconceived notions of the child to influence our interpretation. Judgments about overall behavior are best made after assessing the accumulated data.

Some threats to validity are found within the sample itself. For example, preschool children vary in their attentiveness and disposition to talk moment by moment. The possible threats to validity in a speech sample, even with older children, are *productivity*, or the amount produced; *intelligibility*, or the amount understood by the listener; *representativeness*, or the typicality of the sample; and *reactivity*, or the response of the child to differing stimuli.

Productivity

The uncommunicative child or the child who says very little will not give an SLP a productive sample from which to work even though such a sample may reflect accurately the child's typical output. The child may have little language with which to talk. The key to greater production is for the SLP to plan a variety of elicitation tasks that serve the purpose of gathering the sample. Avoiding yes/no questions in favor of "Tell me about . . ." techniques is more likely to yield longer responses.

Intelligibility

Intelligibility is the amount of agreement between what a child intended to say and what the SLP interpreted from the sample. If much of the sample is unintelligible, few utterances will be suitable for analysis. In general, intelligibility can be increased with increased SLP control over the content of the child's utterances. In short, the SLP who knows the topic can determine more easily what the child said.

Representativeness

A sample should represent a child's typical behavior. This may not occur if the language sample is collected in an atypical context, for example, a clinical room with an unfamiliar SLP as the conversational partner. Three issues are relative to the representativeness of the conversational sample: *spontaneity, variability of context, and stability of the structure/function sampled.*

Spontaneity is increased if the child is allowed to establish the topic and/or the activity. Interesting and varied stimulus materials can provide an excellent basis for spontaneous conversation and can elicit a variety of forms and functions.

Variability in the context and stimulus items will elicit a greater variety of child behaviors theoretically more representative of the child's everyday behavior. Data collected in a variety of settings, with a variety of partners, and on a variety of child-based conversational topics ensures versatility. Because quantity and complexity vary with the task, no individual task is likely to yield a representative sample of a child's language.

Unrepresentative samples may reflect other-than-normal usage by a child. In this situation, the structures or functions sampled may vary widely from one situation to another. Everyday situations are most likely to elicit typical use and thus provide some stability across situations.

Some discussion has concerned whether SLPs should try to elicit typical or maximum production from a child. This debate is fueled by the often-reported gaps between what children with LI are capable of doing with their language and what they typically do. An SLP must decide on the appropriate tasks to use. For example, storytelling tasks yield longer utterances, while picture interpretation tasks elicit greater language quantity. Various elicitation tasks will be discussed in detail in Chapter 6.

Reactivity

A child's reaction to the techniques and the materials also will affect the overall validity of the sample produced. Sampling conditions and the nature of the content or stimuli available can greatly affect the sample. A directed condition, such as one in which an SLP uses a questioning technique, allows the examiner more control over the content being discussed and may, in turn, increase intelligibility. Unfortunately, this improved intelligibility may sacrifice productivity and representativeness. In general, too much control restricts a child's output. Sentence-building tasks in which a child is asked to "Make a sentence with the word X" elicit the least typical language and very short sentences.

Words or structures divorced from dialogue, as in the previous example, require high-level meta linguistic skills and thus are difficult for a child with LI. Even though the more open-ended conversation may be more representative, it is usually less intelligible and may be difficult for some children with LI. For example, children with LD exhibit as much difficulty with conversations as with other assessment protocols.

Although specific stimulus items may increase intelligibility by controlling the topics discussed, the child may develop or already have a stereotypic pattern of responding to the item. For example, a doll may elicit a "baby talk" style.

The items chosen and the directions given also may affect the validity of the sample. For example, pictures can be used to elicit language, but the instructions given to a child often affect the quantity of language produced. The directive "Tell me about this picture" elicits less language than a more directive style, such as the following:

> I'd like you to make up a story from this picture. I want you to tell me a whole story that has a beginning and an end. Start with "Once upon a time" and tell me the whole story.

The best advice for any SLP is to remain flexible in order to shift between different contexts and different content and to elicit the kinds of language behavior desired. As an SLP, you should have a variety of stimulus materials and be skillful in discussing a range of topics potentially interesting to a child.

Summary

Descriptive approaches are not without problems. Although they are potentially more representative of a child's everyday performance than formal testing, this potential is not guaranteed. In addition, descriptive approaches require that an SLP have considerable knowledge of language and of the variables that affect children's language performance. Skillful manipulation of these variables by an SLP can enhance the potential intervention value of descriptive methods.

An Integrated Functional Assessment Strategy

Speech-language professionals usually suggest a combined assessment approach. The purpose of an assessment should influence its design. Almost universally, SLPs would agree that no single measure or session is adequate. This allows for multiple assessment of language features and behaviors in a variety of relevant contexts.

Specific social behaviors may be context dependent. For example, parent and teacher perceptions of specific social behaviors in children with autism spectrum disorders (ASD) do not always agree (Murray, Ruble, Willis, & Molloy, 2009). Parents seem to note more initiating interactions, while teachers note responding behaviors and maintaining interactions. It's important, therefore, that SLPs use a multi-informant approach when attempting to describe the social abilities of children with ASD.

The SLP must consider the following several child variables in designing and implementing the assessment process:

- Chronological and functional age
- Background information, such as vision, hearing and health concerns and/or other handicapping conditions

- Cultural and linguistic background
- Cognitive functioning
- Interests and materials available
- Activity level
- Ability to attend to stimulus items

The SLP readily adapts the methods to each child and is mindful that children will respond differently to different adults. Caregiver concerns must also be taken into consideration.

The overall social interaction might also be of interest. One tool for rating social interaction is a handheld computer using the Social Communication Coding System (Olswang, Svensson, Coggins, Beilinson, & Donaldson, 2006). The Social Communication Coding System consists of six behavioral dimensions: prosocial/engaged, passive/disengaged, irrelevant, hostile/coercive, assertive, and adult-seeking behaviors coded for frequency of occurrence and duration.

A combined or integrated assessment approach provides the most thorough individualized method of evaluation and might include a referral, questionnaire and/or caregiver interview, an environmental observation, an SLP-directed formal psychometric assessment, and a child-directed informal assessment consisting of a conversational sample from the child. The actual components will differ with each child. Each component is discussed in the remainder of this chapter.

At each diagnostic step, objectives should be derived from the information collected to this point. Thus, each step becomes more focused, and the possible language problems are highlighted. Figure 4.3 presents a possible stage process of collecting data. At each stage, the process becomes more focused. The following discussion deals with a number of assessment steps, both formal and informal, that are aspects of an overall integrated functional model.

Questionnaire, Interview, and Referral

Caregivers—parents, teachers, and others—are central to a functional assessment and intervention process. Teachers, discussed in Chapter 12, can be a valuable referral source and should be encouraged to be alert for children with potential language problems. Some children in the schools will

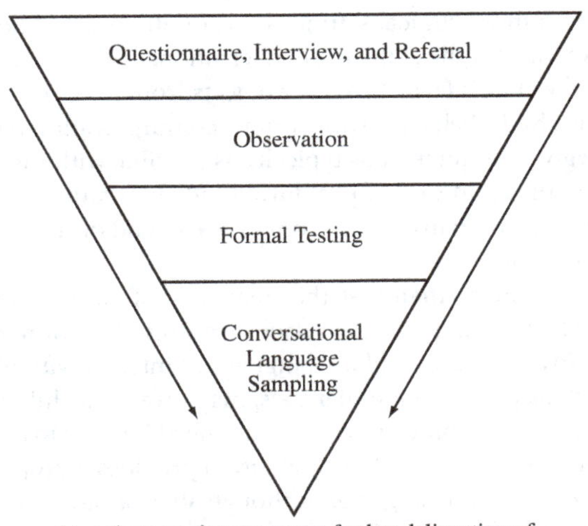

FIGURE 4.3 A model of the assessment process.

also be identified by screening tests. Parents and medical professionals can also be effective referral sources for children with more severe LI; however, they are less reliable in identifying mild impairment (Conti-Ramsden, Simkin, & Pickles, 2006). This is especially true for children with SLI who, by definition, lack other obvious disabilities.

A caregiver interview or questionnaire can be a valuable source of initial information on client functioning and on the perceived problem from the caregiver's perspective. Caregiver expectations for a child also provide an indication of a caregiver's willingness and perceived need to work with the child. Caregivers should be encouraged to ask questions and to participate fully.

With very young children, caregivers can be a source of information for difficult-to-test behaviors. For example, vocabulary checklists completed by parents correlate well with other measures of vocabulary. In fact, parental reports on the size of their 2-year-olds' vocabulary correlate well with the results of language screening tests (Klee, Carson, Gavin, Hall, Kent, & Reece, 1998). In other more open-ended estimates of oral language, such as judging intelligibility, parents are less accurate.

In face-to-face interviews it is best to ask questions of caregivers in a straightforward manner, with no hesitation that might signal embarrassment or discomfort. The SLP avoids tag questions (e.g., "You don't . . . , do you?") that seek agreement, rather than confirmation or information. Responses are treated matter-of-factly with little comment that might discourage a caregiver from talking. The SLP is interested in the child's prenatal, perinatal, and postnatal medical history, family medical and educational history, the child's educational and social history, and descriptions of the child's behavior. A list of possible language questions is presented in Table 4.2.

Caregiver responses are analyzed and hypotheses are formed before deciding on the strategy for the remainder of the assessment. Potential language problems are researched thoroughly.

Observation

To gain the most natural interaction, you'll want to observe caregiver(s) and peer(s) with the child as conversational partners in such everyday settings as the home and the classroom. In the classroom, an SLP might observe the child participating in a number of activities. This situation is not always possible. Time may not permit observation alone. In this case, an SLP may wish to observe closely while collecting a language sample and may form tentative hypotheses for later confirmation from the analyzed sample.

If observation occurs in a more clinical setting, appropriate toys and both structured and nonstructured activities are provided for the child and conversational partner. Caregivers are encouraged to use familiar objects and the child's favorite toys or objects from home or the classroom. Ideally, as an SLP, you will observe the child's behavior with various communication partners.

The SLP instructs caregivers to interact as typically as possible with the child. It is essential that caregivers not quiz or direct the child to perform during the observation. Optimum performance is attained if the SLP unobtrusively remains in the room or leaves and observes from outside via observation windows or video monitors.

The style of interaction is more than just the frequency of various forms of behavior. More important are the ways in which a child uses the various features of his or her linguistic interactional style. The key question is, How does the child use language to interact with others?

Routine situations, such as play with familiar toys, may provide a child with a scaffold or frame within which language processing becomes automatized. The SLP needs to assess the child's familiarity with the situation and the degree to which that situation provides a prop for the child's language. Atypical situations will not elicit typical language. Although atypical situations may be useful vehicles for enhancing some children's language performance, they can also suppress it and will not usually yield a representative sample of a child's language.

The INREAL/Outreach Program of the University of Colorado recommends an observation strategy called SOUL. The acronym stands for *silence, observation, understanding,* and *listening.* The

TABLE 4.2 Interview or Questionnaire Format

Questions relative to language uses:
How does the child let you know items desired? What does the child request most frequently?
What does the child do when requesting that you do something?
When wanting you to pay attention?
When wanting something?
When wanting to direct your attention?
Does the child ask for information?
How does the child express emotion or tell about feelings?
What emotions does the child express?
Does the child make noises when playing alone? Does the child engage in monologues while playing?
Does the child prefer to play alone or with others?
Does the child describe things in the environment? How?
Does the child discuss events in the past, future, or outside of the immediate context?
Questions relative to conversational skill:
When does the child communicate best?
How does the child respond when you say something? How does the child respond to others? Does the child interact more readily with certain people and in certain situations, and if so, with whom and when?
With whom and when does the child communicate most frequently?
Does the child initiate conversations or activities with you and with others? What is the child's most frequent topic?
Does the child join in when others initiate conversations or activities?
Does the child get your attention before saying something to you?
How does the child do this? Does the child maintain eye contact while talking to you?
Does the child take turns when talking? Does the child interrupt? Are there long gaps between your utterances and the child's responses? Will the child take a turn without being instructed to do so or without being asked a question?
When the child speaks to you, is there an expectation of a response? What does the child do if you do not respond?
When the child responds to you, does the response usually match or is it relevant to what you said?
How does the child ask for clarification? How frequently does this occur?
If you ask the child for more information or for clarification, what happens? Does the child demonstrate frustration when not understood?
When the child asks for or tells you something, is there usually enough information for you to understand?
When the child tells you more complex information or relates an event or a story, is it organized enough for you to follow the train of thought?
Does the child have different ways of talking to different people, such as adults and small children? Does the child phrase things in different ways with different listeners? Is the child more polite in some situations?
Does the child seem confused at times? What does the child do if confused?
Questions relative to form and content:
Is the child able to understand simple directions?
Does the child know the names of common events, objects, and people in the environment? What types of information does the child provide about these (actions, objects, people, descriptions, locations, causation, functions, etc.)?
Does the child seem to rely on gestures, sounds, or the immediate environment to be understood?
Does the child speak in single words, phrases, or sentences? How long is a typical utterance? Does the child leave out words? Are the child's sentences complex or simple? How does the child ask questions?
Does the child use pronouns and articles to distinguish old and new information?
Does the child use words for time, such as tomorrow, yesterday, or last night? Does the child use verb tenses?
Can the child put several sentences together to form complex descriptions and explanations?

Source: Compiled from Brinton & Fujiki (1989); Lund & Duchan (1993); and Spinelli & Terrell (1984).

TABLE 4.3 Features to Note While Observing the Child

Form of language. Does the child use single words, phrases, or sentences primarily? Are the sentences of the subject-verb-object form exclusively? Are there mature negatives, interrogatives, and passive sentences? Does the child elaborate the noun or verb phrase? Is there evidence of embedding and conjoining?
Understanding of semantic intent. Does the child respond appropriately to the various question forms (what, where, who, when, why, how)? Does the child confuse words from different semantic classes?
Are there frequent fillers or empty words (*thing, one, that*)?
Are relational words, such as prepositions and conjunctions, used correctly?
Language use. Does the child display a range of illocutionary functions, such as asking for information, help, and objects; replying; making statements; providing information? Does the child take meaningful conversational turns? Does the child introduce topics and maintain them through several turns? Does the child signal the status of the communication and make repairs?
Rate of speaking. Is the rate inordinately slow or fast? Are there noticeable or lengthy pauses between the caregiver and child's turn? Are there noticeable or lengthy pauses between the child's adjacent utterances? Does the child use fillers frequently or pause before producing certain words? Are there frequent word substitutions?
Sequencing. Does the child relate events in a sequential fashion based on the order of occurrence? Can the child discuss the recent past or recount stories? Are sequential sentences cohesive and easy to follow?

adult remains *silent* for periods of time, assessing the situation before talking. *Observation* of a child's play and interactions with other people occurs prior to forming hypotheses. Understanding is the insight into a child that comes from the distillation of data collected during observation. Finally, listening requires total involvement by an adult and the use of responses appropriate to the functioning level of the child.

As an SLP, you'll obtain some notion of what to observe from the caregiver interview. Reliability of observation is increased if your descriptions detail as closely as possible the actual observed behavior. Inferences and hypotheses come later. It is best if the observation is taped or digitally recorded for later referral. Handheld computers also have been shown to be an effective and reliable way to collect language data in situations where it is used, such as in the classroom (Olswang, Svensson, Coggins, Beilinson, & Donaldson, 2006).

Table 4.3 is a list of some features that an SLP might observe. This list is not exhaustive. Each category is discussed in some detail in Chapter 7, where we consider the analysis of a conversational sample. The purpose of observation is to note within the larger scope of interaction the language characteristics to be tested, collected, and analyzed later in the assessment.

Reliability of observation is not fortuitous. SLPs should train together thoroughly so that their observations are as accurate and as objective as possible. This accuracy and objectivity can be accomplished by repeated observation and rating of recorded samples by more than one SLP. Ratings then can be compared, discussed, and modified in light of reexamination of the samples.

Formal Testing

Within an evaluation session or sessions, a change to more formal testing tasks might be accomplished through the use of a nontreatening receptive task, possibly one requiring only a pointing response. Such a task allows a child to become accustomed to an SLP's direction. An annotated list of several current tests is presented in Table 4.4.

TABLE 4.4 Helpful Hints for Language Testing

Test	Description	Comments
Carrow Elicited Language Inventory (Carrow, 1979)	Consists of 52 sentences that the child repeats Contains scoring/analysis form and verb protocol Ages 3 to 7-11	One of only a few tests that are normed for 3-year-olds. It scores the number or errors rather than the number of correct responses. The norms are tricky, because older children tend to modify the sentences to make them conform more closely to speech, e.g., substituting "doesn't" for "does not." Test should be audio-recorded for accuracy in scoring, but you can gain a quick idea of a child's performance by marking each sentence as the child repeats it. The total errors can be quickly counted for an approximate error score. While easy to administer and a bear to score, the analysis yields vital information on language form.
Comprehensive Receptive and Expressive Vocabulary Test, 2nd edition (Wallace & Hammill, 2002)	Test of receptive and expressive vocabulary via pointing to pictures named and providing definitions Ages 4 to 89-11	Expressive vocabulary definitions are sometimes unusual when testing children with LI. Be prepared to have to interpret whether a response is correct or incorrect, even though the developers have tried mightily to anticipate responses. My favorite wrong answer for cider was "Her lunch was *inside her.*"
Fullerton Language Test for Adolescents, 2nd edition (Thorum, 1986)	Overall language test with subtests in syntax, morphology, semantics, and syllabication Ages 11 to adult.	Very difficult adolescent test. I question the value of the Syllabication subtest for students of this age. The Morphology Competency subtest is extremely difficult to score because the examiner must decide on the correctness of the response with very little guidance.
Peabody Picture Vocabulary Test, 4th edition (PPVT) (Dunn & Dunn, 2007)	Child or adult points to one of four pictures named Ages 2–6 to 89–11	Be careful not to overextrapolate from the results. The test, despite its claims, merely measures a client's ability to match a picture with a name. It tells us nothing about depth of understanding or definitions. Nouns are overrepresented despite that this type of word becomes a smaller portion of our lexicons as we mature.
Test of Adolescent and Adult Language, 4th edition (Hammill, Brown, Larsen, & Wiederholt, 2007)	Overall language test with subtests in written and spoken language in syntax and semantics Individual or group administration Ages 12 to 24-11	Good general test; easier than the Fullerton. Sentence Combination subtest will be very difficult for clients with auditory working memory problems. Spoken Analogies subtest is related more to cognitive abilities than language abilities.

(*Continued*)

TABLE 4.4 *(Continued)*

Test	Description	Comments
Test of Auditory Comprehension of Language, 3rd edition (TACL-3) (Carrow-Woolfolk, 1999a)	Consists of three subtests: Vocabulary, Grammatical Morphemes, and Elaborated Phrases and Sentences Ages 3 to 9-11	Often a child will pass the first two subtests but fail the third. This occurs with children who have language form difficulties and/or auditory memory problems. Norms are available by subtest, so to shorten the test, you might wish to give only this subtest. Extremely distractible children may need to be reminded to look at all the pictures. Although this violates test norms, remember that the test was not normed on children who are other than typical. Report your findings, and note that this score was only attainable with reminders to stay on task. (After all, are we measuring language or distractibility?)
Test of Language Development–Intermediate, 4th edition (Hammill & Newcomer, 2007)	General language test with several subtests covering semantics, morphology, and syntax Ages 8 to 17-11	Good overall test. Some of the two-word descriptors used in the picture vocabulary subtest are unnecessarily difficult. The Word Ordering subtest will be especially difficult for children with poor auditory working memory. While the task is fun to do, I question its relevance to the real world. When was the last time someone approached you and said, "Party fun was the"? The Malapropisms subtest is fun to give as long as you don't fall over the errors and give them away, but again I'm not positive of its relevancy.
Test of Narrative Language (Gillam & Pearson, 2004)	Assesses narrative skill in three modes: no pictures, single pictures and sequential pictures Assesses both literal and inferential comprehension Ages 5 to 11-11	Good overall measure of an area that may be difficult to assess through sampling and is difficult to analyze. Systematic data collection method.
Word Test Elementary, 2nd edition & Word Test Adolescent, 2nd edition (Bowers, Huisingh, LoGiudice, & Orman, 2004a, 2004b)	Comprehensive test of word associations, synonyms, semantic absurdities, antonyms, definitions, and flexible word use Ages 6 to 11-11 & 12+	Thorough evaluation of the mental mapping networks in which words are stored. The adolescent test is greatly improved over the previous edition. The developers have done a nice job of anticipating responses to the definition subtests. You'll still receive some weird ones.

Assessing All Aspects of Language

It is important that the SLP make a thorough assessment of all aspects of language. This task may necessitate more than one evaluative session. Only rarely is a language impairment limited to one aspect alone. Should this be the case, however, testing of all aspects confirms the absence of problems and provides a holistic image of the child's language. Even when problems in a single area are suspected, more than a single test should be used in order to best describe the child's language deficit. Issues relative to each aspect of language are discussed in the following section.

In an assessment, it is difficult to measure the degree of a child's developing language knowledge. Currently, tests are designed to measure a child's response as all or nothing, correct or incorrect. The physical act of responding rests upon the more subtle retrieval and preparation of linguistic material for this act. Formulation of an utterance is not an insulated process. Language production relies on the same types of knowledge as language comprehension (Bock, Dell, Chang, & Onishi, 2007).

Pragmatics. The pragmatic difficulties of children with ASD or TBI may be missed on traditional tests, which tend to focus mostly on linguistic structure and meaning rather than on pragmatic language use (Anderson, Lord, & Heinz, 2005; Bishop & Baird, 2001; Young et al., 2005). In fact, most of the common assessment instruments used by SLPs fail to measure pragmatic skills at all. This poses a special problem for high-functioning children with ASD who may score within normal limits on traditional language measures although still in need of intervention for dysfunctional social language skills that are evident in conversation and in the classroom (Young et al., 2005).

Pragmatic language has proven difficult to assess. Because pragmatics is defined as a context-dependent behavior, the rigid structure of most formal language tests fails to measure a speaker's adjustment to changing circumstances. In addition, the clear instructions in a concrete context, such as a standardized testing situation, may enable children with pragmatic difficulties to perform much better than they do in a naturalistic setting. Although some pragmatic tools, such as the Test of Pragmatic Language (TOPL; Phelps-Terasaki & Phelps-Gunn, 1992), do exist, they may fail to capture the full range of deficits of some children, such as those with ASD.

The TOPL samples typically developing pragmatic behaviors. After exposure to pictures depicting common social situations and to a brief description, the child is asked to produce a response for one of the characters. Verbal cues include such questions as "What do you think the boy is saying?" A child's response is scored as appropriate or inappropriate.

An alternative to clinician-administered, standardized pragmatic assessments is subjective interpretative parent/caregiver assessment of a child's language based on instances of language usage observed in the home. Such assessment may represent a child's typical level of functioning more than the child's performance on a one-time test procedure. In addition, some behaviors may be difficult to elicit in test situations.

The Children's Communication Checklist–2 (CCC–2; Bishop, 2003, 2006) is an example of a parent/caregiver assessment tool. Respondents are asked to rate the frequency with which a described behavior occurs, such as repeating memorized language. The CCC–2 asks about a range of clinically significant pragmatic impairments that other formal standardized pragmatic test instruments, such as the TOPL, fail to measure (Adams, 2002). As such, the CCC–2 appears to identify pragmatic impairment in children with ASD with age-appropriate language form better than the Test of Pragmatic Language does (TOPL; Volden & Phillips, 2010).

Semantics. Although children with LI have a range of semantic difficulties with acquisition, storage, and retrieval, most formal assessments are limited to receptive and expressive vocabulary. Few standardized tests assess multiple aspects of semantic knowledge. At the very least, we are interested in word knowledge, novel word learning, word categories, figurative language, multiple meanings, and word-finding.

When does an SLP know that a child has learned a word? Tests typically assume an all-or-nothing phenomenon in which a child either does or does not know the meaning. In reality, acquisition of word knowledge is a gradual process that may continue through the lifetime of an individual. An individual child's success or failure on a test item may be dependent on several factors, such as the type of task or the manner of cuing. Testing tasks are often contrived, out of context, and highly literate.

Testing of semantic abilities often is confined to picture identification, word definitions, and word categories. Of interest are a child's comprehension and production vocabularies. Comprehension vocabulary usually is measured by having a child point to a picture that best represents the word produced by the test administrator. Such tests tell an SLP very little about the frequency of use or the depth or breadth of a child's understanding of the concept named. Comprehension of longer utterances usually is assessed by having a child follow simple commands or again point to pictures.

When a word is not fully understood by a child, he or she may rely on other comprehension strategies based on linguistic features, such as word order, or on nonlinguistic features, such as the position or size of stimulus items in the picture. During testing, an SLP should note behaviors such as locational preferences in pointing responses and verbal comments that accompany responding and may indicate what influences the child's behavior.

Expressive or productive vocabulary usually is tested by having a child name pictures or supply a definition. Scoring may be of a correct-incorrect or scaled (0-1-2) type. The latter allows for partially correct responses but may be extremely difficult to judge. Descriptions by the SLP of the type of definition given by a child can be valuable in determining the maturity of the child's lexicon. Early definitions usually rely on use, as in *An apple is something you eat.* These are followed developmentally by descriptions, then use in context, adding synonyms and explanations, and finally, conventional definitions. The entire developmental process takes years to accomplish.

The Diagnostic Evaluation of Language Variance (Seymore, Roeper, & deVilliers, 2003), a criterion-referenced tool, includes a subtest of novel word learning. SLPs also may wish to develop their own evaluative instruments (Brackenbury & Pye, 2005). For example, incidental learning can be examined using either unknown words or nonsense words within contexts in which the referent or entity referred to is present but not directly defined. Follow-up testing can determine if the word was learned.

A number of factors, such as word length, syllable structure, and familiarity of consonant clusters, influence phonological working memory, where words are held while processing meaning. For this reason, an SLP should design informal measures only if she or he has researched this area thoroughly (Brackenbury & Pye, 2005). Typically, phonological storage and processing are assessed through nonword repetition tasks such as those found in the Children's Test of Nonword Repetition (Gathercole & Baddeley, 1996).

Several assessment instruments have subtests of semantic categories and relational words, such as prepositions. Sorting and labeling tasks and following directions, can be used in informal assessment.

Categorical understanding is assessed by asking the child to supply an antonym or a synonym, to name related words in a category, or to identify the category. Thus, category membership and related words, not just simple word meaning, should be tested with all children in late elementary and high school. Word-association tasks such as naming another member of a category (zoo animals) may be ineffectual in differentiating children with LI and those without. Responses are dependent more on the familiarity of the category and the number of responses possible.

Other semantic-related tasks include stating similarities and differences, telling all one knows about a word, detecting semantic absurdities, explaining figurative language, and noting multiple meanings. Each task requires different abilities, including determining the task demands, focusing on critical semantic dimensions, and interpreting cues, that can be complicated by word-retrieval difficulties.

Little is known about word-retrieval processes. Children with LD or TBI exhibit word-finding and word-substitution difficulties. Late elementary school children with LD exhibit more visually related word-substitution errors, such as saying *sheet* for *cape* and *net* for *screen*. than do TD children. Additional word-finding substitutions found in children with LD include functional descriptions, *such as book holder* for *shelf.*

Diagnostically, use of these word-finding strategies indicates that a child comprehends the word but has difficulty retrieving it. Although testing may reveal a deficit in naming skills, such tests rarely indicate the nature of the deficit. Identification of the word-retrieval strategies of these children may aid in the design of remediation techniques directly related to these strategies.

Word-finding difficulties can be assessed formally with measures such as the Test of Word Finding, Second Edition (TOWF-2; German, 2000), and informally using a similar format. It is important to distinguish between those words unknown to the child and those known but difficult to retrieve. Usually, the referents of unknown words cannot be identified by a child through pointing when their names are presented. In contrast, if a child can identify referents receptively but not name them on a different occasion, word-retrieval problems may be present. In informal assessment, especially in severe cases, such as the initial stage of recovery from TBI, it may be useful to begin with common everyday objects and actions in the environment.

One method for attaining more information from tests is a double-naming technique. In this procedure, a standard naming test is administered twice. The results are examined to identify error response groups that occur once and twice. The errors that occur on both administrations require further analysis.

The SLP can administer a number of prompts with the double-error words to determine whether the errors indicate word-finding difficulties and to identify naming strategies. In this procedure, cues can be administrated in the following order (Fried-Oken, 1987):

1. *General question.* The child is asked a general, open-ended question, such as, "Can you think of another word for this?" or "What is this again?" that provides no additional linguistic information.
2. *Semantic/phonemic facilitator.* Two cues, based on additional semantic and phonemic information, are administered. The order of presentation varies, but the SLP should record carefully the order and the response. The semantic cue describes the object's function, provides a categorical label or states the location. For example, if the picture shows a sofa, the SLP might say, "It's something you sit on," "It's a piece of furniture," or "You find it in the living room." The child's response to each type of semantic prompt should be noted.

   The phonemic cue includes the initial phoneme of the desired label ("The word starts with a /_/.") This type of cue requires certain metalinguistic skills of a child in order to use the information given.
3. *Verification.* If a child is still incorrect, the SLP provides the correct label and asks whether the child has ever seen this object before in order to verify whether the word is in the child's repertoire.

The child's responses and the cues are analyzed to determine the qualitative nature of the errors and the child's naming strategy. Possible naming strategies of 4- to 9-year-old children, regardless of whether you use this assessment method, are listed in Table 4.5.

Syntax. Syntactic testing can be extremely complicated because of the complexity and diversity of the syntactic system. SLPs may wish to use entire test batteries or portions of several tests. The latter strategy is recommended for in-depth probing of potential problem areas. Naturally, when tests are used in a nonstandard manner or test items are combined from several tests, the norms can no longer be used. Results must be described accurately and interpreted in light of the tasks involved.

There is considerable variability across tests in the length of individual syntactic items, the structures tested, and the type of testing tasks used. Test tasks are as diverse as highly unnatural ones, such as word ordering or unscrambling and sentence assembling, and more natural tasks such as sentence combining. Many mirror the highly decontextualized tasks found in school, such as fill-in-the-blank, but do not reflect everyday language use.

A thorough language assessment should include evaluation of both comprehension and production. Although the receptive procedures used and the structures assessed vary widely across tests, the common element is that a child demonstrates understanding—usually by pointing to a picture or following directions—while producing only minimal language, if any.

Syntactic production typically is tested by using structured elicitation, a sentence imitation format word-ordering, or correction-judging. In structured elicitation, a child might be asked to describe a picture, following a model by the test administrator. The model sentence establishes the sentence form to be used (*she is running*) but differs from the desired sentence by the structure being tested (*she will run*).

In sentence imitation, a child gives an immediate repetition of the test administrator's sentence. The underlying assumption of elicited imitation procedures is that sentences that exceed a child's working memory will be reproduced according to a child's own linguistic rule system, which the

TABLE 4.5 Naming Strategy Hypotheses: Target word is *SHOE*

Child's Behavior	*Possible Naming Strategy*
Child says, "Chew."	Word association may be phonological
Child says, "Show."	Word association may be phonological
Child says, "Boot" or "Sneaker."	Word association may be categorical or semantic
Child says, "Heel."	Word association may be part/whole
Child says, "Foot" or "Walk."	Word association may be functional
Circumlocution	
Child says, "Looks kind of like a car."	Child is using perceptual circumlocution
Child says, "You wear it."	Child is using functional circumlocution
Child says, "It has holes and strings."	Child is using descriptional circumlocution
Incorrect or non-answer	
Child says, "Sky."	Unrelated. Probe to see if there is a hidden or unperceived relationship.
Child says, "Thing" or "That."	Nonspecific
Child says, "I don't know."	Comment
Child does not respond.	Non-response
Child mimes putting on a shoe	Gestural response

One misnomer doesn't mean that the child has word-finding difficulties and does not establish a pattern. Always probe behind the child's response. Naming strategies are a key to the way in which a child organizes her world.

Information taken from Fried-Oken (1987)

child must use as a processing aid. Theoretically, the child's sentence should be very similar to the one the child would produce spontaneously.

The validity of elicited imitation has been questioned. Although the performance of children with LI on elicited imitation tests can be enhanced by the addition of contextual cues, such as pictures or object manipulation, their imitations are still simpler than their spontaneous language production.

Because the relationship between elicited imitation and spontaneously produced language is a very complex one, SLPs are advised to use elicited imitation results with caution and to rely on the data from spontaneous samples when the two differ. Elicited imitation responses should be analyzed for the specific ways they differ from the model. Such analysis is much richer than simple correct/incorrect scoring. Don't accept an incorrect response at face value. You need to understand what a child is doing before you can attempt to modify her or his behavior. For example, the child's response may be incorrect because it was not an exact imitation, but the child may have retained the correct meaning. Other than exact sentence imitation responses may

- maintain the intended meaning.
- change the intended meaning.
- omit a word or phrase.
- substitute a word or phrase.
- add a word or phrase.
- change the word order.
- produce an ungrammatical sentence.

In addition, the SLP should note the influence of sentence length, which may be related to the child's working memory.

Constructing sentences from a list of words also relies heavily on working memory. In addition, the task is one that is never performed in real life, and we should question its applicability.

Finally, tasks requiring the judging of grammatical acceptability are of two varieties. The first merely asks for a judgment while the second requires the child to fix the errant structure. While the second is more difficult, they both require metalinguistic skill, which does not begin to form until around age 5. These types of task, as well as making judgments of similarity and difference, are inappropriate for preschool children.

Morphology. Morphological testing usually focuses on bound inflectional morphemes, such as plural -s or past tense -ed. Most tests emphasize suffixes, such as tense markers, plurals, possessives, and comparators, because of their high usage and relatively early development. In general, children with good spoken and written language abilities have more morphological awareness and do better on such tests.

Suffixes can be divided into two types: inflectional and derivational. *Inflectional* suffixes indicate possession, gender, and number in nouns; tense, voice, person and number, and mood in verbs; and comparison in adjectives and do not change the part of speech of the base. For example, a noun can be made plural with the addition of the -s marker, but the noun remains a noun.

The second, larger category, derivational suffixes, is ignored in most tests. *Derivational* suffixes have a smaller range of application and many more constraints and irregularities than inflectional suffixes. Application may be unpredictable, as with *-tion*, which can be added to some but not all nouns. Also, morpheme meaning can be somewhat unclear, as with *-ment* in *apartment*. It's estimated that more than 80 percent of multimorpheme words do not mean what the constituent parts suggest. The development of derivational suffixes is related to oral language production abilities, reading level and exposure, derivational complexity, and metalinguistic awareness.

The two most common expressive test formats for morphology are *cloze*, or sentence completion, and sentence imitation. Most cloze procedure test items give the root word and require the child to respond with the root plus a suffix, as in *teach* and *teacher*. Tests use either actual words or nonsense words. The rationale for nonsense words is that their use will not bias performance by previous exposure. In general, tests using nonsense words are more difficult for young children and those with either ID or LD. Other testing tasks might include judgments of relatedness of words, such as *hospital* and *hospitable*, ability to deduce meaning from component parts, and ability to form words in different and changing linguistic contexts.

Although several tests have morphological portions or subtests, most have too few items and too narrow a scope to provide much valuable information. In addition, prefixes and derivational suffixes are included on only a few tests.

Written Language. A written sample should also be collected, especially if a literacy-specific learning disorder is suspected. It should include first drafts of expository writing, narrative fiction, and nonfiction. The SLP can evaluate the sample for phonological and linguistic awareness; word boundaries; vocabulary and usage; ability to communicate thoughts precisely, sequentially, and systematically; generation and organization of ideas; morpheme usage; syntactic usage, semantic awareness, and word associations, such as opposites and synonyms; and handwriting. This assessment will be discussed in Chapter 13.

Test Modification

As mentioned previously, tests can be modified to provide the information desired by an SLP. For example, as an SLP, you may wish to test a child's pronoun use in depth. No test is available that adequately assesses only these structures. You might construct your own assessment tool from items of other tests. This type of locally prepared test may be very useful for thorough assessment. Obviously, test standards of administration have been violated and the norms would be invalid. Occasionally, published tests include subtest norms. In this case, a subtest may be administered in its entirety as directed in the instructions, and the norming information would be applicable.

Test administration may be modified also for the child who cannot perform as required or for further investigation of the child's response strategies. For example, use of pictures or repetition of instructions may enhance the performance of some children. It is important to remember that nearly all tests are designed for TD children. The child with ID or cerebral palsy is at a very distinct disadvantage. In such cases, description of a child's ability under modified conditions may be much more useful for intervention than a score. Adherence to prescribed test procedures is more likely to result in a measure of that child's limitations.

Testing procedures may be modified through the use of multiple sessions, increased time to respond, and increased trials. For children with attentional difficulties, an SLP might enlarge materials, use a penlight or pointer, highlight certain information, verbally remind the child to attend, additional practice, or have the child repeat the test cue prior to responding.

The performance of children with motor problems, ASD, or LD might be affected also by visual or auditory distractions, placement of materials, temperature, lighting, light and dark contrasts, and positioning. Children who perseverate may need to be reminded that the correct answer for one item is not the same for another. Children with memory problems may need to have cues repeated, to repeat cues aloud themselves, or to have cues broken into easily processible units.

Finally, children with TBI may need a longer time to respond. The SLP also should test beyond base and ceiling scores to identify "islands" of learning. Other modifications for children with TBI may include reduction of distractions, different response modes, enlarged print and reduction of print per page, simplified instructions, substituting multiple choice questions to facilitate recall, giving multiple examples, providing breaks when fatigue is evident, and darkening lines or print in visual displays.

Sampling

Conversational sampling has the potential for providing the most accurate description of the child's language as it is actually used in conversational exchange. Although sampling usually includes freeplay and unstructured conversation, it also may include structured conversation and probing of language features noted in observation and testing. In the next several chapters, we discuss the best ways to maximize the information from this source through design of collection situations and analysis methods.

Assessment for Information-Processing Deficits

As mentioned in Chapter 2, Children with a variety of disorders exhibit difficulty processing verbal information. Although questions about cognitive functioning should be answered by a team that includes at least a neurologist, a psychologist, and an SLP, probing by the SLP can answer some questions and suggest alternative methods of intervention. Standardized testing will provide some insight but is no substitute for comprehension and production of language in real-life contexts.

Of most importance are changes in performance under varying task demands. The SLP can assess a child's performance by varying the speed of information using both familiar and unfamiliar words and structures (Ellis Weismer & Evans, 2002). Usually there is a tradeoff between accuracy and timing.

In addition, the SLP should use the test-teach-retest form of dynamic assessment, the most ecologically sound manner for assessing cognitive functioning (Gillam et al., 2002). Discussed in more detail in Chapter 5, dynamic assessment is concerned with the child's ability to learn rather than his or her level of past learning. For example, in the teaching phase, the child may be taught to identify the main idea in a paragraph or to interpret a comment, conversation, or narrative. In the retest phase, the SLP focuses on the kinds of change and the effort required. Of interest throughout are the child's ability to attend, perceive, and recall information, understand explanations, relate past information to new, infer, and generalize.

Many measures of language have inherent working memory (WM) demands. SLPs should consider the storage and processing requirements of language assessment tools and consider how these demands may influence a child's performance. Tasks that require a child to hold onto multiple pieces of information and engage in a mental activity require WM. An example would a language subtest in which the child must remember a random list of words while forming them into a coherent English sentence. By analyzing the pattern of a child's error breakdowns observed or performing a task analysis, an SLP can make standardized testing more informative (Ellis Weismer & Evans, 2002). If the SLP supposes that the test results may indicate a possible WM deficit, she or he can assess further to see if this may be the case.

Given the significant role working memory (WM) plays in language acquisition and learning, SLPs should include some measure of WM in a thorough language assessment, especially for children with SLI. This may be warranted, especially if memory is a concern, as in children with TBI, if memory difficulties have been implicated by other testing or observation, or if the SLP wants to consider the underlying factors that may contribute to language or academic difficulties (Boudreau & Costanza-Smith, 2011).

A central task to assessing the language performance of children with SLI and other disorders is determining to what extent a child's language and academic problems are related to deficits in linguistic knowledge, deficient WM abilities, slower processing speed, or a combination of these and other factors. Performance on standardized tests may be affected by poor general processing abilities. WM, especially phonological short-term memory (PSTM), plays a predominant role in children's performance on standardized language measures, thus explaining the poor language test scores of children with SLI (Leonard, Ellis Weismer, et al., 2007; Montgomery & Windsor, 2007). Although standardized language tests seem especially taxing of PSTM abilities for children with SLI, they are not for age-matched TD peers.

WM capacity is assessed using a variety of tasks. Listening span is measured by having children listen to sets of sentences that increase in number. They are then asked to respond to the correctness of each sentence, a processing task, and to recall as many sentence-final words as possible, a storage task. For example, a sentence set may consist of "Apples are *blue*" and "Birds can *fly*." A child would be expected to note that apples are not blue but birds do fly and to recall the words *blue* and *fly*. In another task, children count groups of dots while remembering the number of dots on each group. In a third, called operation span tasks, children perform multiple arithmetic problems, store the answer to each or a word presented after each problem, and then recall all these at the end of the set.

Nonword repetition (NWR) tasks are designed to measure phonologic processing efficiency independent of lexical knowledge (Gillam et al., 2002). PSTM is required to repeat a nonword, because a child must maintain an accurate phonological representation of unfamiliar phonologic information in memory. On both the Children's Test of Nonword Repetition (CNrep; Gathercole & Baddeley, 1996) and the Nonword Repetition Task (NRT; Dollaghan & Campbell, 1998), a child is required to repeat lists of nonwords, which vary in both the number of nonwords and the number of syllables represented in the nonword. The CNRep is more sensitive in identifying phonologic memory deficits in children with SLI (Archibald & Gathercole, 2006a). An increasing number of standardized language tests are including an NWR task. Although the Nonword Repetition Test (NRT; Dollaghan & Campbell, 1998) is widely recommended as an assessment tool for schoolage children with SLI, its use with preschool children is questionable, resulting in many false positives, meaning that children are misidentified as having LI when they do not (Deevy, Wisman Weil, Leonard, & Goffman, 2010).

In the competing language processing task (CLPT; Gaulin & Campbell, 1994), an experimental task developed to assess WM span in children, a child is presented with a sentence and asked to assess its truth by verbally stating whether it is true or false while simultaneously holding the last word of each sentence in WM. At the end of each set of one to six sentences, the child is asked to recall the last word of each sentence in the group in order. Performance in comprehension and/or final word retention will decline when the two tasks conjointly exhaust the available WM resources. The Clinical Evaluation of Language Fundamentals–Fourth Edition (CELF–4; Semel, Wiig, & Secord, 2003) includes a WM index that is based on two subtests: Number Repetition and Familiar Sequences.

Any diagnosis should be based on inclusionary and exclusionary criteria. In addition, assessment of memory impairment should be made independent of other cognitive abilities (Gathercole & Alloway, 2006). Inclusionary criterion includes poor performance on a standardized memory task, irrespective of IQ. Exclusionary criteria for SLI include the absence of hearing and articulation deficits. A variety of standardized tools and informal methods for assessing WM are presented in Table 4.6.

TABLE 4.6 Standardized Tools and Informal Assessment Methods of WM and Processing Speed

Assessment Tool/Method	Characteristics	Aspect of WM
Automated Working Memory Assessment (AWMA; Alloway, 2007)	Ages 4 to 22 years Subtests on digit, word, nonword, and block recall, and visual matrix memory or visual STM	Verbal STM Visuospatial STM Verbal WM capacity Visuospatial WM capacity
Children's Test of Nonword Repetition (Gathercole & Baddeley, 1996)	Ages 4 to 8 years	Verbal STM
Clinical Evaluation of Language Fundamentals, Fourth Edition (CELF–4; Semel, Wiig, & Secord, 2003)	Ages 9 to 21 years Sentence Repetition task reliably identifies children with SLI and memory deficits Understanding Spoken Paragraphs Rapid Automatic Naming	 Verbal WM capacity Verbal WM capacity Word level processing speed
Nonword Repetition Task (Dollaghan & Campbell, 1998)	Nonstandardized	Verbal STM
Rapid Automatized Naming and *Rapid Alternating Stimulus Tests* (Wolf & Denkla, 2005)	Ages 5 to 19 years Letters, numbers, colors, objects,	Word level processing speed
Test of Narrative Language (Gillam & Pearson, 2004)	Ages 5 to 11 years Perform a pattern analysis to determine the nature of child's errors	Verbal WM capacity
Test of Word Finding, Second Edition (German, 2000)	Ages 4 to 13 years Picture naming, sentence completion and category naming	Word level processing speed
Working Memory Rating Scale (Alloway & Archibald, 2008)	22-item behavior-rating scale for use by teachers Correlates with AWMA	Verbal STM
Working Memory Test Battery for Children (Pickering & Gathercole, 2001)	Ages 5 to 15 years Subtests of verbal STM: Digit recall word list matching, word list recall, and nonword repetition. Block recall and mazes memory. Listening span, backward digit Verbal WM capacity recall, and counting span.	Verbal STM Visuospatial STM

Information taken from Montgomery, Magimairaj, & Finney (2010) and Boudreau & Costanza-Smith (2011).

Few tests are designed to assess the speed of input and/or output processing, but some standardized language tests measure the rate and accuracy of lexical access and retrieval. Unfortunately, beyond the word level, there are no standardized tests for the speed at which a child can process language.

It is never sufficient with any child to accept test scores at face value. An SLP can perform careful analyses of children's performance on other standardized language tests to hypothesize on the effects of WM abilities on poor language performance. Inability to recall a list of words in order to find a common category or to recall a sentence for sentence imitation can greatly influence performance. By informally manipulating factors such as the number of units to be recalled, an SLP can determine whether WM was a contributing factor. For example, in narrative retelling, poor memory may be inferred based on a child's performance on various probe questions, while story retelling can be evaluated for responses that indicate a loss of information. Other informal assessment techniques might include an SLP systematically varying her or his speaking rate as well as volume and complexity while presenting language information. This will enable the SLP to observe the degree to which memory and comprehension of material are affected by input rate. On the output side, systematically varying the time children have to complete language production tasks, such as single word retrieval, sentence production, narrative, description, and explanation, may document how children manage multiple memory and language demands. In this way, the SLP may gain a sense of the conditions under which children have trouble coordinating their language and memory (Montgomery et al., 2010).

Conclusion

There is no one way to assess children with LI. A combination of interviewing, observation, testing, and sampling/probing offers a holistic approach that can incorporate not only the child but also significant others and familiar communication contexts.

It's important as you move through an assessment not to become too absorbed in the minutia of various isolated language features. This "forest for the trees" approach can result in missing the holistic nature of the child's communication system.

Once all the data is assembled, final analysis begins. More data may be needed. If collection can be characterized as somewhat scientific in its approach, analysis, while similar in nature, requires more of the artist in each SLP, as he or she paints an individual portrait of each child with LI. More of this in Chapters 6 through 8.

Chapter

5

Assessment of Children with Culturally and Linguistically Diverse Backgrounds

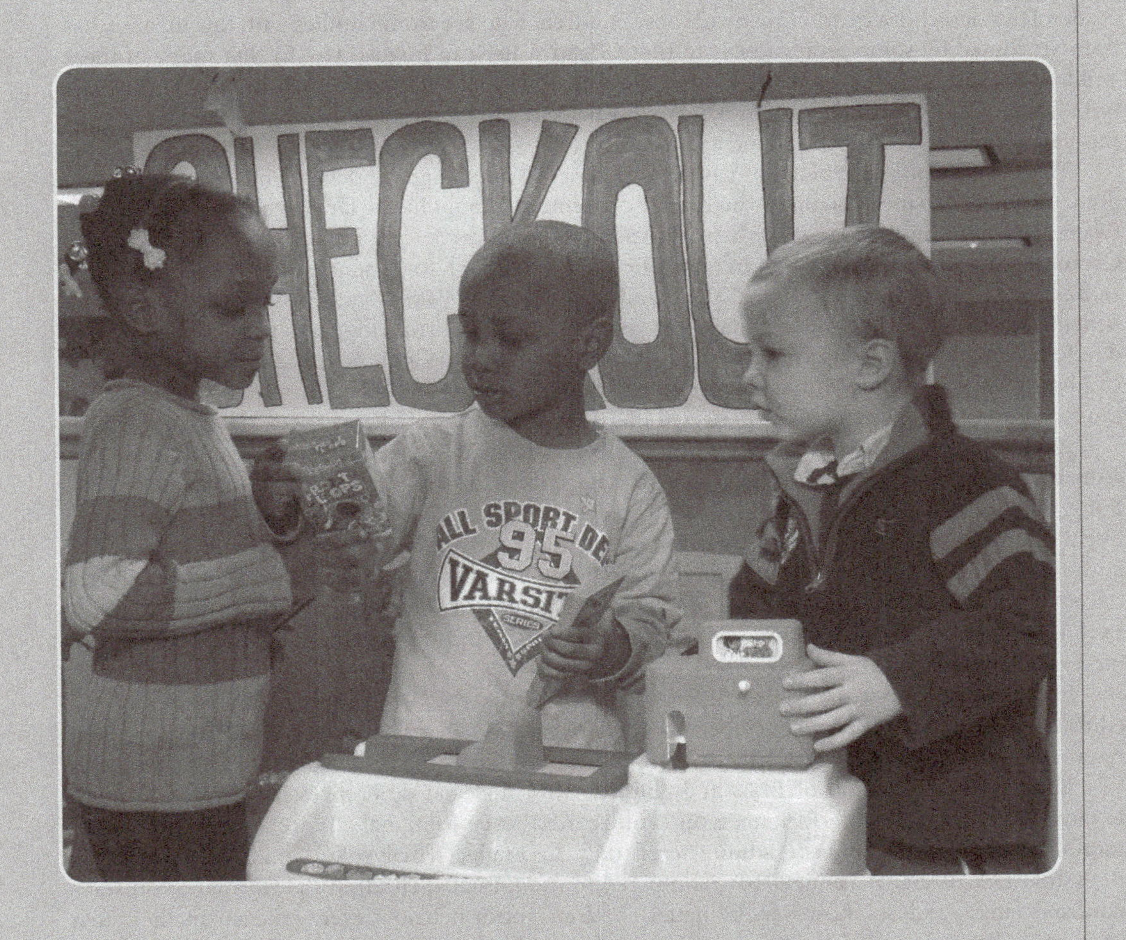

Language differences, such as dialects or the influence of a first language on a second, are not disorders. Such differences are valid rule-governed linguistic systems in and of themselves. A child learning a nonstandard dialect of American English or learning American English as a second language may also exhibit language disorders, such as LD, SLI, or any of the others discussed in Chapter 2. The task for you as an SLP is to separate these natural differences from disorders.

According to a 2008 U.S. Census Bureau report, 21 percent of the U.S. school-age population speak a language other than English at home. This figure is expected to double by 2030 (Davis & Bauman, 2008). Approximately one-third of these children are English language learners (ELLs). Seventy-nine percent of the bilingual and ELL children in the United States speak Spanish as a home language (Goldenberg, 2008; U.S. Department of Education, 2008). There are also large numbers of Asian American and some Native American children for whom English is a second language.

African American (AA) children, as the second largest minority racial group in the country, make up approximately 17 percent of the children enrolled in public schools (Fry, 2007). The reported academic underachievement of many of these children, who are from families with low income, has been attributed by some professionals to the African American English (AAE) that many of these children bring to school, which differs from the majority American English dialects used for instruction. Those AAE-speaking children who are bi-dialectal are better able to navigate the language of the classroom when they go to elementary school.

There is a strong link between language experience and language development in young children. Compared to monolinguals who receive concentrated input in one language, bilingual children receive less input in each language being learned. They also have less practice using each language. Given this situation, bilingual children may be at increased risk for language delay (Kohnert, 2008; Kohnert, Yim, Nett, Kan, & Duran, 2005; Paradis, 2007). On the other hand, possible developmental benefits may accrue from dual language use. Switching between two languages may possibly confer developmental advantages on some bilingual children (Bialystok, Craik, & Luk, 2008a). For example, children who were bilingual from birth demonstrate advantages in executive function compared to monolinguals and children newly immersed in a second language (L2).

Any assessment of children with culturally linguistically diverse (CLD) backgrounds must recognize the relationship between the risk for language impairment and socioeconomic status (SES). For example, children in the United States who speak Spanish as their first language (L1) are more likely to come from low-SES backgrounds (Krashen & Brown, 2005). Socioeconomic status (SES) and maternal education level influence language development in a number of ways. Higher maternal education is associated with better vocabulary development, language comprehension, and narration. In contrast, children from low-SES backgrounds with poorer maternal education have an increased incidence of LI (Schuele, 2001).

ELLs and children with dialectal differences are more likely to be identified as in need of special education services (de Valenzuela, Copeland, Qi, & Park, 2006). In general, these children are overrepresented as having LI, while majority dialectal English-only speaking students are underrepresented.

The higher proportion of ELLs and children with dialectal differences in special education is most likely related to performance on standardized tests. Bilingual children score lower than monolingual children on tests administered only in English (Bialystok, Craik, & Luk, 2008b; Bialystok, Luk, Peets, & Yang, 2010). Compared to monolingual children's performance on standardized language tests, however, bilingual children perform below average, even in their first language.

Clearly, there is a critical need to develop language assessment measures appropriate for these children. As mentioned, assessment in only one language underrates bilingual children's overall language ability. It is important that an SLP be able to distinguish between a disorder and a difference that may be the result of interaction of the native language with English or of non-majority dialects with the majority dialect. SLPs must appreciate the rule-governed nature of native languages and dialects and know their contrastive features. Elective speech and language services may be provided to those children whose parents desire more standard production of English. It is important for an SLP to remember, however, that dialects of English that reflect the influence of the native language on English are not disorders.

Assessment and intervention with ELLs should be conducted in the native language as mandated by federal law (PL 94-142 and PL 95-561), legal decisions (*Diana v. Board of Education*, 1970; *Lau v. Nichols*, 1974; and *Larry P. v. Riles*, 1972), and state educational regulations. Adequate service delivery by an SLP requires native or near-native fluency in both languages and ability to describe speech and language acquisition in both languages, to administer and interpret formal and informal assessment procedures, to apply intervention strategies in minority language, and to recognize cultural factors that affect service delivery to the CLD community.

Language testing should establish language dominance and the most appropriate language for intervention. One error often made by inexperienced SLPs is to assume that the native language (L_1) is dominant. Young children may lose L_1 as they begin to acquire a second language (L_2), which in this case is American English.

State of Service Delivery

Although the demographics of the United States are changing, the overwhelming majority of SLPs will continue to belong to the majority culture for the foreseeable future. Approximately one in three SLPs has some bilingual clients, but more than 80 percent of these professionals do not feel confident in their abilities to serve these clients. It's estimated that only 2 percent of certified members of ASHA are able to provide services in languages other than English (Langdon & Cheng, 2002). Inadequacies include a lack of academic preparation and unfamiliarity with different languages and/or cultures and a lack of appropriate assessment tools, Let's discuss these briefly.

Lack of Preparation and Unfamiliarity with Different Languages and Cultures

Most academic programs offer little preparation for working with children with CLD backgrounds through either coursework or practicum. Until this deficiency changes, it is the responsibility of each SLP to educate him- or herself through continuing education. The following are some ways to interact more with culturally diverse populations:

- Work alongside a bilingual speech-language pathologist as an assistant.
- Take a foreign language course and/or a course in cultural diversity.
- Join cultural organizations and attend cultural festivals.
- Become a Big Brother or Big Sister or volunteer to work with culturally diverse youth.
- Volunteer in organizations such as Habitat for Humanity.
- Join organizations, such as National Coalition Builders Institute, that foster cooperation and understanding.
- Join church groups that foster interactions with inner-city churches.
- Go out of your way to introduce yourself to individuals from other cultures.

Becoming familiar with another culture and another language requires shedding many preconceived notions and becoming culturally aware. This requirement is followed by education about particular languages and cultures and about language development among children with CLD Backgrounds. It is extremely difficult to become fluent in a second language as an adult or from classroom instruction. Therefore, one method for an SLP to use to overcome linguistic deficits is language interpreters. This alternative is discussed at the end of this section.

Growth of Awareness

All aspects of our lives are overlaid by culture. It affects our institutions and the way we act and think. **Culture** is a shared framework of meanings within which a population shapes its way of life. Thus, culture is what one needs to know or believe to function acceptablely in a particular group culture has been shaped by the population's history and evolves as individuals constantly rework it and add new ideas and behaviors. As such, culture includes, but is not limited to, history and the explanation of natural phenomena; societal roles; rules for interactions, decorum, and discipline; family structure; education; religious beliefs; standards of health, illness, hygiene, appearance, and dress; diet; perceptions of time and space; definitions of work and play; artistic and musical values, life expectations, and aspirations; and communication and language use. Culture interacts with language to influence cognitive and affective processes and the interpretation of behavior.

Each culture has a unique outlook. It is essential for SLPs to recognize that culture is pervasive and diffused throughout their own lives. Therefore, culture influences the way each SLP views other cultures.

SLPs from the majority culture in the United States typically have Euro-centered standards. These standards will influence each SLP's decisions about LI, although these standards may not apply within other cultures. For example, Vietnamese culture is much more tolerant of speech and language diversity than is U.S. majority culture. Likewise, the Navajo culture values a quiet, introspective persona, which may seem withdrawn by U.S. majority standards. Language differences affect much more than language form, including rules for appropriate interaction in specific contexts, awareness of content information required in different situations, appropriate structures for participation, and communication styles.

Words and concepts also are related culturally. For example, the word and the concept *crib* are not found in Korean. Table 5.1 offers other examples of cultural variants. Although SLPs cannot know all cultures, they can become increasingly culture sensitive. It is important to respect other

TABLE 5.1 Cultural Variants That May Influence Assessment

Concept	Other Cultures*	Majority U.S. Culture
Achievement	Cooperation and group spirit. Accept status quo. Manual labor respected.	Emphasis on competition and success. Define self by accomplishments. *To the victor go the spoils.*
Age	Elders are revered. Growing old is desirable.	Youth is valued.
Communication	Respectful, avoid eye contact, loudness for anger. Silence means boredom. Nonlinguistic and paralinguistic important.	Casual, direct eye contact, loud voice acceptable. Silence means attentiveness. Emphasize verbal.
Control	Fate.	Free will.
Education	Formal for few. Entrance into mainstream society. Elders, peers, and siblings are teachers. Active, physical learning. Spontaneous, intuitive. Testing not integral.	Universal, formal, verbal. Key to social mobility. Teacher is authority. Classroom passivity rewarded. Reflective, analytical. Tests are part of learning.

(*Continued*)

TABLE 5.1 *(Continued)*

Concept	Other Cultures*	Majority U.S. Culture
Family	Extended, kinship important, more varied, elder or parent centered. Male or female dominated.	Nuclear, small, contractual partnership, child centered.
Gender/role	Males independent, pampered. Females have many home responsibilities.	Relative equality.
Individuality	Humility, anonymity, deference to group.	Individual makes own life. Stress self-reliance.
Materialism	Excessive accumulation is bad, status ascribed.	Acquisition, symbol of success and power.
Social interaction	Contact, physical closeness. Kinship more important than friends.	Noncontact, large interpartner distance. Large group of friends desired.
Time	Enjoy the present, can't change future. Little concept of wasting time. Flexible.	Governed by clock and calendar, punctual, value speed, future oriented. Time is money. Scheduled.

*No specific culture.

cultures and to recognize that no one culture is the standard. Many traditional notions of the U.S. majority culture are inappropriate in our global environment.

The following are guidelines for interacting with children from different cultures.

- Each encounter is subject to the cultural rules of both participants.
- Children perform differently because of their unique cultural and linguistic backgrounds.
- Different modes, channels, and functions of communication may evidence differing levels of linguistic and communicative performance.
- Cultural norms should be considered when evaluating behavior and making determinations of LI.
- Possible sources of conflict in assumptions and norms should be identified prior to an interaction and action taken to prevent them from occurring.

Learning about culture is ongoing and should result in constant reevaluation and revision of ideas and in greater sensitivity.

The subjective nature of the assessment process is undeniable. You and the child each bring your cultural assumptions. To make sense of our behaviors, we must view them against the background of culture.

Education in Language, Culture, and Language Development

Sensitivity by SLPs is not enough. You must educate yourself about the dialects, languages, and cultures of the individuals you serve and about the process of dialect and second-language learning.

Typically, SLPs make two common errors in evaluating the language of children with CLD backgrounds. Either children are identified incorrectly as having a language disorder, or those with a disorder are missed. For example, African American children from rural Alabama who speak the African American English dialect common to that area continue to delete final consonants beyond the age at which middle-class European American children do. An SLP who is unaware of this difference might conclude, incorrectly, that these children exhibit a disorder.

Cultures. The breadth of cultural diversity is beyond the scope of this text. Suffice it to say that each SLP should become familiar with the cultures that he or she serves. Reading and observation are both essential methods of learning. An SLP must remember that cultures are not monolithic and that there is much heterogeneity, especially in the Latino American population.

The need for professionals to understand and appreciate the beliefs and values of families with CLD backgrounds is critical. One study found that both parents and Head Start staff were unaware of their differing assumptions about education, parenting, child learning, and disability (Hwa-Froelich & Westby, 2003). Of particular importance are differences in child-rearing practices, family structure, attitudes toward LI and intervention, and communication style. Variants of communication style include nonlinguistic and paralinguistic characteristics, such as eye contact, facial expression, gestures and intenation; intercommunicant space and the use of silence and laughter; pragmatic aspects, such as roles, politeness and forms of address, interruption rules, turn taking, greeting and salutations, the ordering of conversational events, and appropriate topics; and the use of humor. It is best if an SLP is somewhat cautious at first, until he or she has a sense of cultural expectations.

Cultures differ in their beliefs about health, disability, and causation. A great deal of discomfort may surround disorder and intervention. Families will be surprised by the extent of their expected role in functional intervention.

Dialects and Language Learning. It is not possible to learn all of the dialects or languages one might encounter, especially in large metropolitan areas. Therefore, each SLP should attempt to learn the contrastive influences of other languages and dialects of children she or he serves. Common phonological, syntactic, and morphological contrasts are found in Appendix A. SLPs can also learn high-usage words and forms of greeting used in these language communities.

Earlier language research focused not on the typical language development patterns of African American children but on how their development differed from other groups of children, particularly white middle-class children who were regarded as the prototypical normative group. As the U.S. population has changed, there has been a recognition of cultural and linguistic diversity and a shift in the study of child language acquisition from a *deficit* to a *difference* perspective (Stockman, 2007). Empirical evidence legitimized AAE as a linguistic system. Researchers began to focus on the typical language development patterns of AAE-speaking children and on variation based on different demographic characteristics of African American children.

Not all children with different dialects are the same. Each child's language will differ with the specific dialect spoken and the maturity of language and dialect development. Although data are limited, we know that children learning African American English show only minimal evidences of their dialect by age 3. Earlier development is closer to the middle-class standard. By age 5, however, most African American English forms are being used, at least in part.

Findings in the speaking and writing of third- and eighth-grade speakers of African American English (AAE) suggest that during this period in writing development speakers of AAE learn to dialect switch in their writing (Ivy & Masterson, 2011). Although third graders have comparable use of dialect in spoken and written modalities, a difference in use between the modalities is found by eighth grade. In general, eighth graders use more dialectal features in speaking than writing.

Awareness and discrimination of dialects appear to increase slowly throughout elementary school while actual production gradually shifts to more standard use (Isaacs, 1996). Interestingly, speaking a minority dialect does not seem to influence the ability to comprehend the majority dialect.

The challenge of accurate assessment is further complicated by the large numbers of African American children who live in economic poverty relative to their percentage of the U.S. population. Poverty limits access to adequate healthcare and other resources that maximize developmental potential. As a result, these children may be more prone to developmental delays than the general population.

One subgroup of low-SES families is those who are homeless. Within the last twenty years in the United States, the percentage of families who are homeless has increased to approximately 40 percent of the total homeless population of more than 2 million individuals (U.S. Conference of Mayors, 2003). Nearly three-fourths of these families are headed by a single parent, usually a mother (Lowe,

Slater, Wefley, & Hardie, 2002; Weinreb, Buckner, Williams, & Nicholson, 2006). These parents experience many stressors associated with bureaucratic challenges, shelter living, self-expectations, and the stress related to the stereotypes of women in shelters as unfit mothers even though they overwhelmingly care deeply about their children and wish to be good parents. Preschool children who are homeless are at risk for a combination of language, learning, or cognitive delays that later negatively impact school achievement (O'Neil-Pirozzi, 2003).

In general, African American English (AAE)–speaking children reared in poverty tend to use majority American English morphological markers, such as past tense-*ed* (*walked, jumped*) and passive particle (*eaten, chased*), less frequently than middle-class African American children (Pruitt, Oetting, & Hegarty, 2011). The weakness in morphological marking is related to the general vocabulary weakness of these children and may reflect the relatively impoverished language environment of children raised in poverty. Although children who speak AAE use morphological markers variably, none of their performance suggests LI (Pruitt & Oetting, 2009). In fact, their performance is distinctly different from children with LI.

When assessing a child who uses AAE, the SLP must be aware of multiple layers of dialectal use that can affect pronunciation, grammatical rules, and word usage. A child may be erroneously judged as having delayed or disordered language. This outcome is likely to occur when the child exhibits a high density or rate of AAE use (Stockman, 2010). As a consequence, children who speak AAE are either overdiagnosed with speech-language delay or disorder because of AAE is considered to be disordered or underdiagnosed because observed differences are attributed to dialect use.

Second Language Learning

Children in the United States who are bilingual Spanish-English or who use Spanish only may perform very differently even from each other. These differences may reflect U.S. regional differences, country of origin, or dialectal or socioeconomic differences.

In general, second-language learning is more difficult than first-language learning, which for most children is fairly effortless. A language assessment must distinguish between those errors that reflect this difficulty and those that represent an LI.

Most children are sequential bilingual learners: The first language (L_1) has reached a certain level of maturity before acquisition of the second language (L_2) begins. Sequential learning may maximize the interference between the two languages. **Interference** is the influence of one language on the learning of another. For example, the English /p/ is difficult for Arabic speakers but not for Spanish speakers because of L_1. Children who learn L_1 at home and are not exposed to L_2 (English) until school move toward L_2 dominance in middle school, but the transition occurs earlier in comprehension than in production, suggesting interference in production (Kohnert & Bates, 2002).

The monolingual model of development is inappropriate when describing second-language learning. Likewise, rate of learning is a poor index because of the many variables that affect second-language learning.

Preschool children will have an immature L_1 when introduced to L_2. The result may be that a child fails to reach proficiency in either language. A child may be delayed in development of L_1 after exposure to L_2 if the second language is dominant in the culture. This situation is rarely considered in language assessments. In general, competence in L_2 is related to the maturity of L_1. The more mature a child's use of L_1, the easier it is to learn L_2.

Initially, a child in preschool may be silent for a while on exposure to L_2 and appear to have an LI. It takes time for a child to decipher the new linguistic code. Older children possess metalinguistic skills that aid in this deciphering process.

School-age children exposed to L_2 may appear to have LD. The decontextualized language of the classroom may be especially difficult. If exposure to L_2 does not occur until after age 6, it may take five to seven years to acquire age-appropriate cognitive and academic skills. The result is that in the United States many children have never fully developed L_1—often Spanish—and are deficient in academic use of English (L_2). L_1 may exhibit arrested development or be lost if it is not used, is not valued by the child, is discouraged by the parents, or is considered less prestigious.

Factors that affect L_2 competency are individual characteristics, such as intelligence; learning style; positive attitude about one's self, one's own native language, and the target language; extrovertism and a feeling of control; a lack of anxiety about L_2 learning; and home and community characteristics, such as parental and community attitudes and the level of literacy in the home. Low socioeconomic status alone is not a negative factor but may be paired with poor literacy or poor L_1 use in the home and/or little opportunity to converse one-on-one with mature L_2 users.

In general, L_1 forms a foundation for the learning of L_2. What a child knows from one language is transferred to the other. This may be general knowledge about sentence construction and parts of speech or similar language processes if the languages are similar. Of course, interference also can occur, but its effects are usually minimal. A poor base in L_1 usually leads to difficulties in L_2.

Languages other than English are devalued in the United States. This is the result of racial and ethnic discrimination and has resulted in a bilingual educational policy that sends a very clear message on the relative value of English. The result is weakened linguistic and ethnic ties. The most common educational paradigm is a transitional bilingual program in which a child receives two or three years of bilingual education prior to placement in a monolingual English classroom. The not-so-subtle message is that English is better. Long-term maintenance programs that attempt to continue use and development of L_1 are rare. A period of even three years is insufficient for the child to attain academic proficiency in English.

It is important that an SLP recognize the process of sequential bilingual acquisition. This is a dynamic process in which a child's language is changing. Performance may vary widely within and across ELL children. Therefore, language assessments need to be tailored individually to each child.

Lack of Appropriate Assessment Tools

We can expect the performance of children with CLD backgrounds on formal tests to be affected by cultural differences. Negative listener or tester attitudes also affect children, causing poor performance. The result is lower expectations and inappropriate referral or classification.

Few nonbiased standardized language tests are available for evaluating children with CLD backgrounds. Tests are typically unique to one culture or language. Spanish versions of most tests fail to consider dialectal differences and are normed on monolingual children (Gutiérrez-Clellen & Simon-Cereijido, 2007). In two judicial decisions regarding placement of Mexican American and African American children in classes for children with ID (*Diana v. State Board of Education*, 1991; *Larry P. v. Riles*, 1984), the courts ruled that judgments made on the basis of responses to tests whose norming populations are inappropriate for these children are discriminatory.

Many of the English-based tests widely used by SLPs are normed on population samples with a disproportionately high number of middle-class, European American, English-only children. Tests may yield lower scores for lower socioeconomic groups and for African American children. Some test items may be culturally biased against certain children. A critical need exists for nonbiased language testing for children of color, especially those from lower socioeconomic backgrounds (Rhyner, Kelly, Brantley, & Krueger, 1999). Having said all this, when we survey SLPs, we find that most use formal, standardized English tests to assess bilingual children (Caesar & Kohler, 2007).

In general, poor performance leads to lower expectations. It is inappropriate to compare many bilingual children with LEP to native speakers of English. The use of chronological norms is especially questionable, given the great variety in developmental rate among CLD populations. The child with limited English does not have language similar to a native speaker of English of a certain age. The problem becomes deciding what standard to use.

Two promising tools for identifying language impairment in U.S. Spanish-English bilinguals are the Bilingual English Spanish Assessment (BESA; referenced in Peña, Gillam, Bedore, & Bohman, 2011) and the Bilingual English Spanish Oral Screener (BESOS; referenced in Peña et al., 2011).

Both measures are currently under development. In preliminary studies (Peña et al., 2011), although bilingual children score significantly lower than their functional monolingual peers, they are no more likely to fall in the at-risk range.

Overcoming Bias in Assessment of ELLs

The challenge in a communication assessment of ELLs is to differentiate difficulties that result from experiential and cultural factors from those that are related to language impairment. Both groups may have some language difficulties. ELL adolescents in need of intervention exhibit greater difficulty expressing themselves, establishing greetings and opening and maintaining a conversation, listening to a speaker, and cueing a listener to a topic change.

Both cultural and linguistic factors influence performance in an assessment. These may lead to misinterpretations and miscommunication. An SLP must be careful not to stereotype behavior and draw incorrect and unfair conclusions. For example, Latino American children may seem uncooperative and inattentive, when, in fact, their behavior signifies different concepts of time, body language, and achievement.

An SLP can avoid biasing data interpretation by asking the following questions:

- Are there other variables, such as limited exposure to English or contextual factors, that might explain the child's difficulties with English?
- Are the problems related to English language learning or dialectal differences?
- Are similar problems exhibited in L_1?
- Can the problems be explained by cultural difference?
- Is there any consistency in linguistic problems that might suggest an underlying rule?
- Can the problems be explained by any bias related to personnel, materials, or procedures?

An SLP should interpret the child's performance in light of the intrinsic and extrinsic biases inherent in the assessment process. Intrinsic biases, such as knowledge needed and normative samples, are part of the test, while extrinsic biases, such as sociocultural values and attitude toward testing, reside in the child. When groups of minority children score similarly to the norming population—as on the Communication and Symbolic Behavior Scales (Wetherby & Prizant, 1993)—it suggests a less biased assessment device. On the other hand, scores of low-income African American children on the Preschool Language Scale (Zimmerman, Steiner & Pond, 2002) suggest that, even though the test is generally nonbiased, some items should be interpreted with caution because they are problematic for these children (Qi, Kaiser, Milan, Yzquierdo, & Hancock, 2003).

Language use patterns of both a child and an SLP and the language-learning history of that child also may influence the assessment. Communication and interactive style are culture bound.

Bias can be overcome by

- identifying variables that might affect the assessment.
- analyzing tests and procedures for content and style. For example, the Fluharty Speech and Language Screening Test accepts an /f/ for /θ/ substitution on *teeth* as dialectal, but in New Orleans, African Americans substitute /t/ to produce *teet* (/tit/). In addition, simply asking children to repeat what the SLP says may go against the cultural norm. Some African American children are not expected to imitate adults.
- taking variables into account and changing assessment procedures.
- using dynamic assessment techniques.

Each child's level of acculturation will differ with the age of the child and the extent of exposure to both cultures.

Use of Interpreters

The accuracy of testing with ELLs may be increased by using interpreters who speak the child's primary language. When an interpreter is not available, family members can aid the SLP.

All children perform significantly better with familiar examiners. This finding suggests the use of interpreters familiar with both the language and the culture of a child and his or her caregivers.

An SLP must recognize the limitations of the process and must select and train the interpreter carefully. They must work together as a team with mutual respect. Three factors seem critical in the use of interpreters: selection, training, and relationship to the family and community. Let's say a little more about each one.

Selection

Selection should be based on a potential interpreter's linguistic competencies, ethical and professional competencies, and general knowledge and personality. An interpreter should possess a high degree of proficiency in both L_1 and English, be able to paraphrase well, be flexible, and have a working knowledge of developmental, educational, and communication terminology.

Ethical and professional competencies should include an ability to maintain confidentiality, a respect for the feelings and beliefs of others and for the roles of professionals, and an ability to maintain impartiality. Confidentiality is especially important if the interpreter is a resident of the immediate geographic area served.

Finally, it is very desirable for the potential interpreter to have a knowledge of child development and educational procedures. Personal attributes include flexibility, trustworthiness, patience, an eye for detail, and a good memory.

Training

Training must include the critical factors of assessment and intervention, including procedures and instruments. The interpreter must understand the importance of exact translation from L_1 to L_2 and the reverse.

Preassessment training must include the elements of a thorough assessment and the methods of specific test protocols, including technical language. Rapport-building strategies and questioning techniques also should be taught.

Prior to each evaluation of a child's language, the SLP and the interpreter should review each case and the assessment procedures; practice pronunciation of the name, introductions, questioning, and nonlinguistic aspects of the interaction; and discuss the topics to be introduced. During the evaluation, the interpreter can interact with the child and caregiver(s) while the SLP records the data and directs the process. In the post-assessment interview with caregivers, the interpreter will convey the results of the evaluation as they are reported by the SLP.

Relationship with Family and Community

Prior to the assessment, the interpreter should try to get to know the caregiver(s) and child. It is very important that the interpreter convey the confidentiality of the proceedings, especially if the interpreter is from the community. During the assessment, the interpreter is to translate exactly. The SLP can aid this process by keeping interactional language simple and use of professional jargon to a minimum. It is the interpreter's responsibility to ensure that the caregivers thoroughly understand the process and the results and recommendations.

Summary

Working through interpreters can be difficult and does not address some of the other problems in assessment of ELLs. The following list contains suggestions for working successfully with an interpreter. The SLP should

- meet regularly and keep communication open and the goals understood.
- have the interpreter meet with the child and caregiver(s) prior to an interview to establish rapport and to determine their educational level, attitudes, and feelings.
- learn proper protocols and forms of address in the native language.
- introduce himself or herself to the family, describe roles, and explain the purpose and process of the assessment.
- speak more slowly and in short units, but not more loudly.
- avoid colloquialisms, abstractions, idiomatic expressions, metaphors, slang, and professional jargon.
- look directly at the child and caregiver(s), not at the interpreter. Address remarks to the caregiver(s).
- listen to the child and caregivers to glean nonlinguistic and paralinguistic information. What is not said may be as important as what is said.
- avoid body language or gestures that may be misunderstood.
- use a positive tone that conveys respect and interest.
- avoid oversimplification and condescension.
- give simple clear instructions and periodically check the family's and child's understanding.
- instruct the interpreter to translate the client's words without paraphrasing.
- instruct the interpreter to avoid inserting her or his own word or ideas in the translation or omitting information.
- be patient with the longer process inherent in translation.

Although these suggestions will not ensure success, they may lessen some friction that potentially could disrupt effective delivery of services.

Overcoming Bias in Assessment of African American Children

The research on African American children's language has helped in developing more culturally sensitive clinical procedures. As a result, SLPs have recognized the need for more options in assessing children's spoken language.

In the past, the norm-referenced standardized tests used to identify children with LI often did not include AA children in their normative samples or included them in such small numbers as to be inconsequential. When compared to norming samples that were overwhelmingly majority dialectal speakers, AAE speakers performed poorly. Now that African American children are included in tests' normative samples, some groups of children have continued to obtain below-average scores while others have not (Champion, Hyter, McCabe, & Bland-Stewart, 2003; Qi, Kaiser, Milan, & Hancock, 2006; Qi et al., 2003; Thomas-Tate, Washington, Craig, & Packard, 2006). This indicates that African American children are a heterogeneous group.

The challenge in an assessment is to distinguish differences due to normal dialect use from those that are due to LI. Most standardized tests were not designed to make such a distinction.

Measures to counter negative bias in existing standardized tests may include (Stockman, 2010)

- creating local norms for evaluating African American children's test responses.
- comparing the performances of a child and his or her parent on the same test.
- embedding test items in more familiar tasks or thematic contexts.
- using community judgments of typical use.

These modifications may not please those who prefer the use of a standardized test method. An alternative is the Diagnostic Evaluation of Language Variation (DELV; Seymour, Roeper, & de Villiers, 2003), a norm-referenced standardized test designed to assess both those who speak AAE and those who speak "Mainstream American English." Designed for children ages 4;0–9;11, the DELV yields performance profiles in syntax, pragmatics, semantics, and phonology.

Alternative assessment approaches may include spontaneous oral language sample analysis and procedures that measure learning potential. Spontaneous speech is natural, authentic, readily accessible to observation, and implicitly sensitive to linguistic differences because speakers choose their own words and how they are said. Much of this text will be devoted to a discussion of language sampling techniques.

An SLP can use analysis techniques that have been adapted to take AAE grammatical patterns into account or those that look for development of phonologic, morphosyntactic, semantic, and pragmatic performances that are noncontrastive in AAE and the majority dialect (Stockman, 2008; Stockman, Karasinski, & Guillory, 2008). Some measures of spontaneous speech performance, such as length of communication units, can help to identify LI.

Similar to standardized tests, samples attempt to describe a child's existing language status, which reflects past learning. An SLP is left with the question of whether a child's performance reflects limitations on the child's language experiences in the environment or the child's inadequate ability to learn from those language experiences.

An SLP's use of dynamic assessment and fast-mapping strategies can minimize the effect of past learning experiences on current performance by evaluating a child's ability to learn from new linguistic input. The dynamic assessment approach relies on a mediated test–teach–retest strategy explained in more detail later in this chapter.

Fast-mapping assessments were based on a child's quick incidental learning of words seen during typical development. TD children learn most words without deliberate instruction from caregivers, and this learning can occur with very little input. Novel-word learning is less dependent on prior experience than typical vocabulary testing. For example, TD middle- and low-income 2-year-old African American children do not differ significantly on fast-mapping novel word tasks, although they differ significantly on the norm-referenced standardized tests of receptive and expressive vocabulary (Horton-Ikard & Weismer, 2007). Similar results are reported when African American children's performance is compared with other racial and ethnic groups (Rodekohr & Haynes, 2001).

An Integrated Model for Assessment

In language assessment, language is often treated as an autonomous cognitive ability divided into many components. Language is not viewed as holistic.

It seems more appropriate to use an integrated approach for children with CLD backgrounds, one that uses the child's natural environment and that depends on descriptive analysis, rather than on normative test scores. Such an assessment would focus on the functional aspects of language and on flexibility of use.

The overall question would be: "Is this child an effective communicator in his or her communication environment?" It follows then that the criterion would not be norm referenced, but communication success referenced. Data could be collected in natural settings as a child converses with his or her natural conversational partners, parents, teachers, and peers.

Assessment would begin as mentioned in Chapter 4 with data gathering. This collection process might include screening all children for other-than-English and for dialectal use. The Expressive Vocabulary Test (Williams, 1997) is a screening measure that has been reported to be culturally fair and appropriate for use with African American children (Thomas-Tate et al., 2006).

This step may be followed by referral information from classroom teachers on children experiencing academic difficulty. A teacher checklist of the child's language functions, a questionnaire, and/or caregiver interview might follow. Parents can be a valuable source of information. Not surprisingly, Spanish-speaking parents are as accurate in reporting the expressive vocabulary and grammar of their toddlers as monolingual English-speaking parents (Thal, Jackson-Maldonado, &

Acosta, 2000). Parental reports of bilingual children's vocabulary and word combinations are consistent with sampling findings (Patterson, 2000).

The data collection stage is particularly important for ELLs. Many variables affect second-language development and are of interest. In addition, seemingly simple information such as age—Is the child age 1 at birth or a year later?—is culturally dependent and can greatly affect determinations of impairment.

Considerations for ELLs include the degree of exposure to English-speaking peers, self-esteem, personality (introverted vs. extraverted), motivation to learn English, family attitude toward English, ethnic community's view of education, the socioeconomic status of the family and of English-speaking peers, and the process of learning a second language. The same child may appear very different depending on the stage of English development.

Four measures may be especially important in discriminating predominantly Spanish-speaking children with LI from those developing typically. These are parental reporting, a family history of speech and language problems, the number of errors per T-unit, and the mean length of T-units. A T-unit is a main clause and phrasal or clausal embedding attached to it. T-units will be discussed in more detail in Chapter 7.

Language assessments should occur where a child and her or his caregivers are most comfortable, such as the home. Parents, especially recent immigrants, may speak little or no English. A properly trained interpreter can be very helpful in obtaining needed information. Occasionally, older siblings have sufficient English skills to answer questions or to translate for their parents. Table 5.2 contains possible questions to be asked in an interview for both ELLs and children with dialectal difference.

Observation should occur in several settings with different conversational partners, topics, and activities. This tactic will give an SLP some idea of the extent of bilingualism and possible language and communication difficulties.

In addition to verifying demographic information, an SLP should observe the child in the classroom and with peers and caregivers. Of interest is the child's language use, academic strengths and weaknesses, and learning style.

Data collection and observation would be followed by testing and language sampling. The following five guidelines should be considered prior to using standardized tests with children from CLD backgrounds:

1. What is the relationship of the norming population and the client? Are enough minority children included to give a fair representation? Are separate norms used for different minority groups?
2. What is the relationship of the child's experience and the content areas of the test? Items using farm content, for example, may have little relevance for children in the inner city.
3. What is the relationship of the language and/or dialect being tested and the child's language and/or dialect dominance? This issue is critical in determining language impairment. The determining factor should be the child's ability to function within her or his own linguistic or dialectal community.
4. Will the language of the test penalize a nonstandard child by use of idiomatic or metaphoric language?
5. Is the child penalized for a particular pattern of learning or style of problem solving?

Test scores should not be taken at face value. For example, the omission of some morphological endings by bilingual children is similar to the error pattern of children with SLI, leading to possible misdiagnosis (Paradis, 2005). Although differences do exist, they are often subtle and require great care when examining assessment results. When bilingual Spanish-English children who are typically developing (TD) and those with LI are compared on use of English past tense, different error patterns emerge (Jacobson & Schwartz, 2005). In addition to scoring lower with regular past-tense *-ed* on real

TABLE 5.2 Interview Questions for Children with CLD Backgrounds

Demographic
How long has the family been in the United States?
In which country were the parents born? From which country did the family immigrate?
How much contact does the family have with their native country? Is there any plan to return?
* How long has the family been in this community?
Is the family connected to a large community from their native country?
Family and Childrearing
* How old is the child? What is the child's general health?
* Which family members live in the household? Number of siblings? Other individuals?
In what cultural activities does the family participate?
* Who is primarily responsible for the child? *Who else participates in caregiving?
* Approximately how much time do the child and caregiver spend together on a typical day?
* With whom does the child play at home?
* How much education do family members have? In what language?
* Are there scheduled meals? *What types of foods usually are eaten?
* Is there an established bedtime?
* Does the child misbehave? How? How is the child disciplined? Who disciplines?
Are any television shows (radio shows, videos) in the native language? If so, how often does the child watch such shows?
* Are stories read or told to the child? If so, in what language? How often?
* Are there books, magazines, or newspapers in the home? In what language?
* At what age did the child begin school? *Has the child attended school regularly? *How many schools has the child attended? What language has been used in the classroom?
Attitudes and Perceptions
* Is blame assigned for the child's problems or condition? To whom or what?
* How does the family view intervention? Is there a feeling of helplessness?
How does the family view Western medical practices and practitioners?
Who is the primary provider of medical assistance and information?
* From whom does the family seek assistance (organizations and individuals)?
* What are the general feelings of the family when seeking assistance?
* Does one family member act as the family spokesperson when seeking assistance?
* How is the child expected to act toward parents, teachers, or other adults? Adults toward the child? Are there any restrictions or prohibitions, such as the child not making eye contact or not asking questions?
* How important are English language skills? How much English is used at home?
Language and Communication
What language is spoken in the home? Between adults? Between caregivers and the child? Between the children? When playing with neighborhood friends? Other caregivers and the child?
What language is used in community activities, such as church, Girl Scouts, and team sports?
At what age did the child begin to learn English? Where and how?
* At what age did the child say the first word? Use two-word utterances?

*Applicable to both LEP and dialectally different children.

and nonsense verbs and with irregular past tense verbs, bilingual children with LI made significantly more omission errors, while TD children made overgeneralization errors (*eated, sitted*).

All is not lost. American English standardized tests can be used with modified procedures to enhance a child's performance. Modifications may aid an SLP in describing a child's language and communication skills. Obviously, the scores from such testing would be invalid, although the descriptive information may be invaluable. If reported, the scores must be qualified by a description of the modified procedures.

Dual sets of norms—those from the test and locally prepared ones—can also be used to compare the performance of children with CLD backgrounds to that of the standard group and of their peer group, but they must be used cautiously because most likely the test will still be in majority

American English. It seems more appropriate to measure a child's performance in his or her dialect and compare this performance to that of other children also using that dialect. Unfortunately, we have very little data on this development and even fewer tests.

Parents, who presumably speak the same dialect, may be used as referents when very little normative data are available. A language test can be given to both the parent and the child. Once enough data has been gathered, the SLP can compare the child's performance with that of the adult. Assuming the adult has no language impairment, child use that reflects parent use but that differs from majority American English would represent a dialectal difference, not a disorder. For example, omission of final plosives found in African American English would result in omission of the regular past tense marker *-ed*. Just testing the child, an SLP might assume that the child does not have past tense. Parental omission would confirm a dialectal difference.

Some tests have been normed on population samples from different languages, such as children speaking English and Spanish, by using English and a Spanish translation. Results of translated tests must be used very cautiously because they assess structures important for speakers of English and ignore those of the other language. For example, *hitting* something with a stick in English is *sticking* in some Spanish dialects, but that verb is not used with other types of hitting.

The standardized norms from such translated tests could be used to identify children with language differences. Children who exhibit LI relative to their peer group could be identified by use of the peer group norms. Even this peer procedure may bias results, given the diversity of some populations, such as Latinos. Norms for all speakers of a language fail to consider dialectal variations. Other variables, such as socioeconomic status, family grouping, length of time exposed to English, and quality of L_1 used at home, affect the child's performance.

The differences found between majority and minority children on knowledge-based tests are not found on process-based evaluations. It may be possible to reduce bias in language testing of children with CLD backgrounds by using methods and tools that emphasize processing abilities, such as memory and perception, rather than language experience and knowledge. Process-based tests can be useful in distinguishing LI from experiential difference. Processes are the mental operations required to manipulate linguistic material. Testing might include such tasks as nonword vocal repetition, completion of two language tasks simultaneously, and following directions. To ensure that past learning is minimized, tasks should be completely novel, and task-related vocabulary and grammar should be familiar or, if not, reviewed prior to testing.

Because the manner of a child's development of two languages and the child's environment interact, it is important to assess ELLs in both languages. Each child's language skills must be compared to sociolinguistic factors such as the following:

- Age at exposure to each language
- Extent of exposure to each language
- Ability to use each language
- Comparative linguistic structure of the two languages
- Individual child differences (Goldstein, 2006)

Assessment in both languages is especially important for preschool and kindergarten children in order to evaluate development in each (Hammer, Lawrence, & Miccio, 2007).

A child's phonological repertoire can be an important determiner of morphological use. It is important, therefore, in an assessment to know the phonological properties of both languages of a bilingual child.

The languages used in testing and the manner of their presentation differ with each child and the purpose of the evaluation. It is important to establish the primary language, language dominance, and language proficiency in both languages. Testing in both L_1 and English seems essential for assessment of language impairment. In fact, federal law requires bilingual testing before such determinations are made. Successive testing in the stronger language, followed by the weaker, results in the best performance, especially for young children with monolingual L_1 homes, although simultaneous testing may be best for children who exhibit poor competence in both languages or who speak a combined $L_1 - L_2$ language, such as "Spanglish."

The mode of administration and scoring can greatly change the reported responses of bilingual children on vocabulary assessment. The number of correct responses increases as SLPs move from monolingual to bilingual administration and from monolingual scoring to conceptual scoring in which the child is credited for different aspects of meaning (Bedore, Peña, Garcia, & Cortez 2005). If, for example, a Spanish-English-speaking child is shown a picture of housecat, she might respond with "cat" or "gato" or with both words. That is one aspect of the definition, the entity's name. If the child adds, "It's like *leon* [lion] in jungle," she has added a new aspect to the definition and demonstrated conceptual knowledge. This example is very simplistic. Conceptual knowledge can be assessed using questions such as the following in response to objects and pictures.

Tell me three things about . . .

Describe what an X looks like.

This is Rosa. Tell me what she looks like.

What shape is X?

What do you do with X?

What is the difference between X and Y?

What are they going to do?

Normative testing should be supplemented by probing. Children with CLD backgrounds score lower on knowledge-based testing, such as that found in normative procedures, but the same on process-based assessments, such as comprehension and production of real conversations. Both Latino and African American children's standardized vocabulary test scores increase significantly from pre- to posttest after they are exposed to test-taking strategies (Peña, Iglesias, & Lidz, 2001). As you might suspect, typical language learners obtain significantly higher posttest scores than do atypical ones. These outcomes suggest that learning mechanisms are more likely intact for TD children but not for atypical ones.

Assessment of bilingual children is an important but often less-than-accurate process. Unfortunately, bilingual children are often diagnosed with LI although they may simply have had fewer opportunities to learn English than their English-speaking monolingual peers. Dynamic assessment shows promise as an effective method for identifying bilingual children with LI.

Dynamic assessment tasks are appropriate and deemphasize grammar in favor of ability to communicate and learn. Tasks are interactive, focused on learning, and yield information on learner responsiveness.

Dynamic assessment is based on the educational notion of *zone of proximal development* (Vygotsky, 1978), or the difference between a child's current performance on a task and the amount of guided assistance needed by the child to be successful. Thus, in dynamic assessment an SLP is interested not only in a child's performance but also in the best way to facilitate learning and in the child's ability to respond to learning. The three primary methods are "testing the limits," graduated prompting, and test-teach-retest (Gutierrez-Clellan, & Peña, 2001). In testing the limits, an SLP probes behind a child's response using elaborative feedback and verbal explanations by a child to determine his or her understanding of the task and the way in which he or she arrived at the response. For example, a child may have interpreted the word *buoyancy as boy-in-seat* (Peña, 2002).

Graduated prompting is a method of probing a child's readiness for learning. By subtly manipulating the prompts given to a child, the SLP determines the level of support needed by a child in order to be successful. In essence, the SLP is trying to bridge the gap between what a child knows and the requirements of the task.

In a test-teach-retest format, an SLP becomes an active agent of change. Focusing on "how" rather than "what" children learn, language-neutral dynamic tasks can provide a nonbiased assessment (Lidz & Peña, 1996). The initial test establishes a baseline measure, then during teaching the SLP supports learning and discovers how modifiable a child is and how a child responds to adult support. The method of teaching called *mediated learning experience* (MLE) is an individualized approach to the response and strategies used by a child and includes explaining the importance of the learning and giving evaluative feedback (Peña, 2002). Several types of mediation are possible, including the following:

- Informing a child of the purpose for the interaction and attempting to maintain a child's involvement
- Focusing a child's attention on important features and helping a child understand their importance and relevance
- Bridging concepts and learning beyond the immediate context by relating specifics of the task to other experiences
- Encouraging a strategic, deliberate approach to problem solving and manipulating a task to help a child be successful

The focus is not simply on what a child learns but also on how a child learns. An example of MLE is presented in Table 5.3. In retesting, or posttesting, children with LI usually demonstrate little change (Peña et al., 2001).

One dynamic assessment technique approach that shows promise involves a 30 to 40-minute word-learning session (Kapantzoglou, Restrepo, & Thompson, 2012). Results indicated that TD children made associations between the phonological and semantic representations of the new words more rapidly than children with LI and demonstrated greater *modifiability* or ability to change and work more independently. Target words, real or nonsense, can be taught using a structured play activity in which the child is provided with as much support as is necessary to produce the novel word. Adult feedback is adjusted to the child's responses (Peña et al., 2001). The SLP records the amount of support the child needs to produce the novel word.

The SLP is also interested in the way in which a child thinks that results in the answers the child gives. This requires probing of a child's responses. One method of testing or probing that circumvents an SLP's inability to speak the native language and the affects of delayed English acquisition is the *invented rule*. For example, an invented rule might state that /i/ is added to a noun to mean a portion of that noun, as in book and book-/i/. This procedure can be taught through modeling using pictures to illustrate and can be tested with novel objects or pictures. Naturally, the same picture of objects would not be used for both testing and training to enable the SLP to assess learning and generalization. Possible pictures to be used for testing or training are presented in Figure 5.1. For example, the SLP says, "This is clock; this is _____ (clocky)." Modeling would be a two-step process:

"This is X, X," as the speech-language pathologist points.

"This is X-/i/, X-/i/," as the speech-language pathologist points.

As the model is repeated several times with a few items, the child repeats the SLP's production of the noun and the noun plus /i/. Testing would follow a cloze procedure:

"This is Y, Y. This is _____."

Again the SLP would point to pictures illustrating the meaning. Of interest is whether a child can abstract a language rule and then apply it to novel situations, certainly an important skill for language learning.

TABLE 5.3 Examples of Mediated Language Experiences (MLE)

Introduction
Today we're going to play with some special toys and use them in special ways. While we're using the toys we'll think about the actions we do with each and the different names we use. Now, what are we going to be talking about? [Child response]
Um-hm, and why do you think it would be important to be able to name the different actions that we can do? [Child response]
Good, so we can explain our actions to other people. Can you think of anything else? [No response]
Do you ever ask for some help from your mother? [Child response]
And . . . [Child response]
Yes, of course, we can use actions to ask others to help us. Suppose I called your mother and said, "Dad!" [Child response]
You're right, it would be the wrong name. To help people understand us, we call things by their right name. I know that you have a dog. What's his name? [Child response]
Okay, if I called him something else, would he answer? [Child response]
No. So names are important. We call actions by their right name too. I have a whole box full of different objects. Some tell us what we do with them. Here's one your mother uses. It's called an iron. And what do we do with it? [Child response]
Right, we iron, we iron clothes. That was a hard one. How should we name the actions that go with each object? [No response] Would it help to name the object? [Child response]
Okay, let's begin that way. Suppose that you know the name of the object but not the name of the action? [Child response]
Well, I could tell you but can you think of a way to show me what you know? [Child response]
Good, you could show me by doing the action. Then together we can figure out the name of the action, maybe from the object used or their might be other ways to remember. . . . [Lesson continues]
Within lesson
Now we've named all the actions. Some objects have more than one. Let's try something else. You name the action and I'll name the object. Only one rule, you cannot repeat an action. If you can't think of the action, act it out and I'll try to help. . . . [Continues]
Do you know how to play Simon Says? [No response] Well, in this game you get to be the queen and you tell me what to do. Let's use your name: "Catalina says, 'Eat!'" [SLP pretends to eat in a very sloppy manner. Child laughs.] Now you try one. . . . [Continues]
Wow, that was fun. What a busy queen you are! Look at this. I have a book full of actions. Let's see if we can describe what's happening in the book. . . . [Continues]
Conclusion
You worked really hard today. Do you remember what we learned? [Child response]
Why are action names important? [Child response]
And what did you do when you couldn't think of the action word? [Child response]

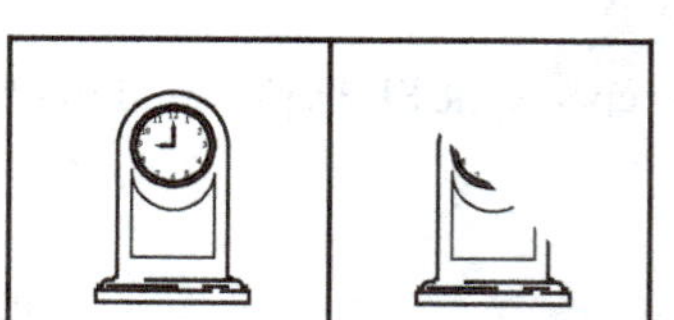
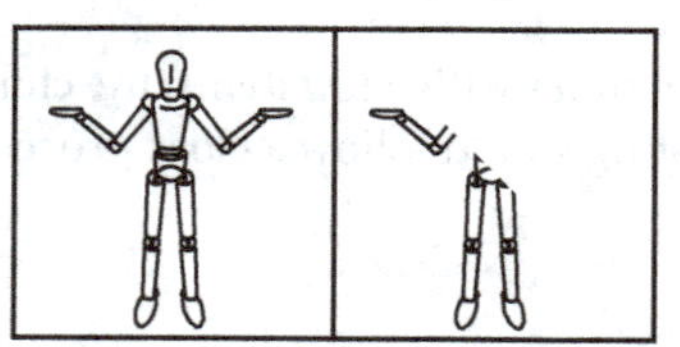
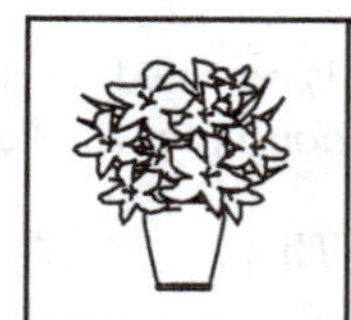
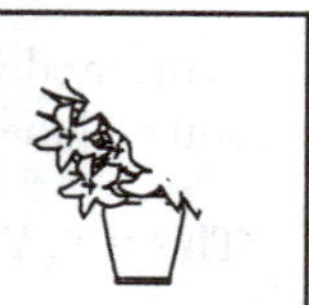

FIGURE 5.1 Possible format for invented rule assessment.

Structured tasks designed by an insightful SLP can also provide more flexibility than standardized tests and may be effective assessment vehicles. In a structured format conceptual knowledge can be probed using linguistic terms in either language that facilitates the child's response.

Throughout this text, I stress the need for alternatives to standardized testing, such as language sampling. For children with CLD backgrounds, language sampling and ethnographic interviewing are essential parts of any language evaluation (Battle, 2002). Although useful, language samples are not guaranteed to be nonbiased. All interactions are culturally based and have the potential of biasing results against a child. Members of the community or family should aid the SLP in analyzing a child's language sample.

Sampling should be based on the realistic demands of a child's communication contexts, such as the classroom. In this setting, a sample should reflect the contextual, performance, and instructional constraints of the situation. A child can then be measured against the minimal competency needed to function within that context. That's a functional assessment.

Of course, children's responses will differ with the task used to elicit language. For example, based on the type of narrative eliciting task, bilingual Spanish-English 4- to 7-year-old children's narratives will differ in both the amount of each language produced and the amount of language mixing (Fiestas & Peña, 2004).

Family and community members can aid an SLP in assessing performance, especially with a language sample. For example, Head Start teachers and aides, many of whom usually come from the local ethnic community, can be asked to judge children with poor language and those with typically developing language. The poor-speech samples can then be analyzed, and a set of community standards derived.

Similar but more stringent *social validation* has been accomplished by using direct magnitude estimates (DME) of subjective judgments. In DME, stimuli are scaled by assigning numerical values to them on the basis of their relative magnitude along some continuum. Each child's language speech sample is rated against a standard, the language of a child with no language impairment. If raters listen to several children and score them against a taped standard, they can begin to form a continuum of performance. For stability of scoring, at least ten listeners are required. Performance of a single child can be compared over time to measure improvements and can be compared with others by using the same dialect to assess overall performance.

Obviously, child-centered sampling has the potential of reducing the impact of biases found in testing. Performance will vary across different language tasks. For example, 4- to 6-year-old speakers of African American English (AAE) use more AAE forms on picture description tasks than in free play (Washington, Craig, & Kushmaul, 1998). Because even heavily dialectal speakers use dialectal forms on only about 20 percent of words, sample analysis should focus on nondialectal components (Craig & Washington, 2002). The shared features of AAE and Standard American English may be more diagnostically important in assessing language impairment among African American children speaking AAE.

Summary

Despite the incredible difficulties inherent in assessing children with CLD backgrounds, there is hope. The same integrated, functional methodology proposed for native speakers of English can be used with some modifications with these children as well. With sensitivity, unbiased administration of testing, and sampling within the everyday context of a child, a fair and meaningful assessment can be accomplished.

Conclusion

Unfortunately, sometimes a battery of readily available tests is given to every child regardless of possible language impairment. This passes for an individualistic and thorough assessment. As with intervention, assessment procedures must be designed for the individual client. Standardized tests are only a portion of this process. Language tests are only aids to an SLP and cannot substitute for the informed clinician.

A thorough assessment includes a variety of flexible procedures designed to heighten awareness of the problem and enables an SLP to delineate more clearly the language abilities and impairments of the child with a CLD background. For training to be truly functional, a thorough description of a child and that child's language must be made.

Chapter

6

Language Sampling

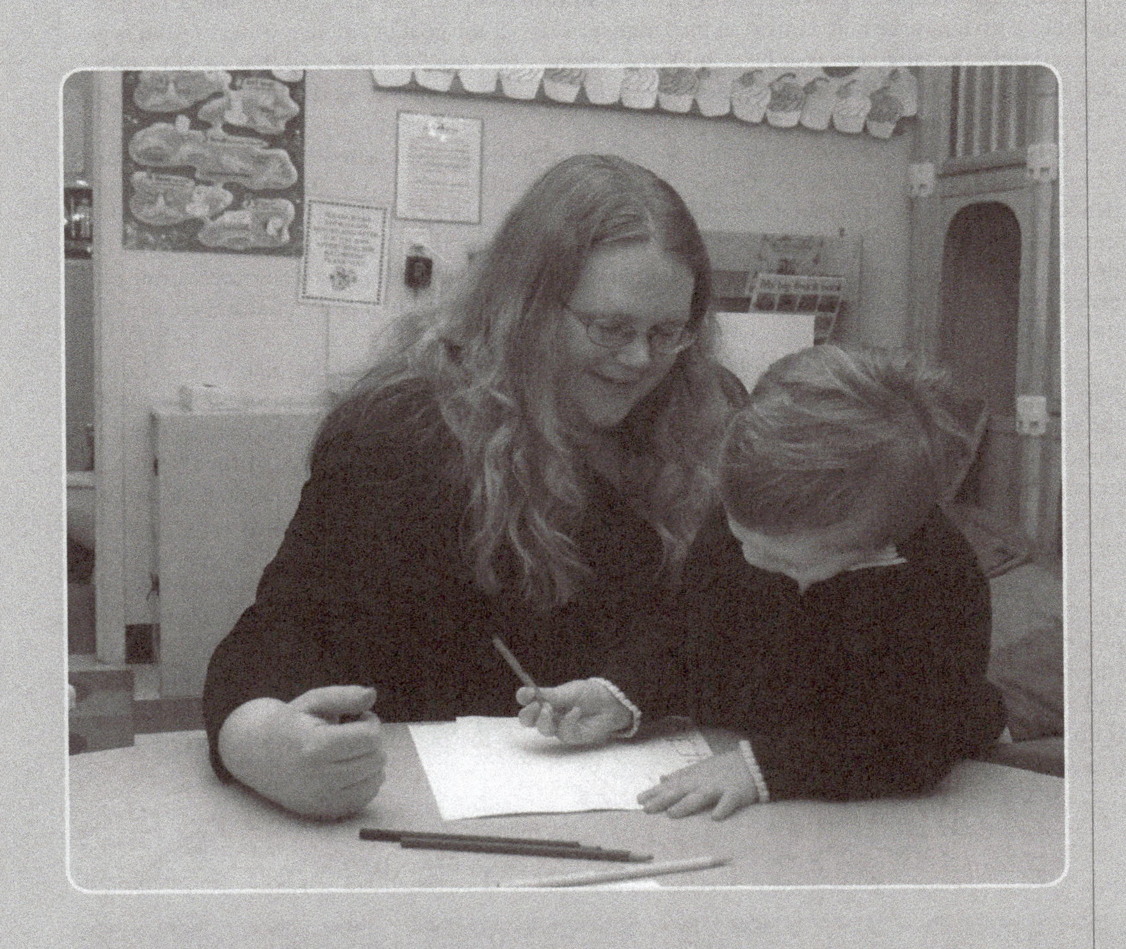

Although standardized tests of language often figure prominently during evaluations, heavy reliance on such measures for evaluation and treatment is not without its problems. First, many school districts require universal cutoffs of −1.5 or −2.0 Standard Deviations below the mean for a child to qualify for services. When a universal cutoff criterion is applied, a child with LI has about a 50–50 chance of being identified, depending on the test (Spaulding et al., 2006).

Second, tests are inadequate for identifying intervention goals. Standardized tests are designed to be efficient rather than to assess the entire range of skills that might need treatment. The necessity of assessing skills with one or two items provides insufficient opportunities for a child to demonstrate mastery or need. Although tests are useful for assessing global change, they miss many small or subtle behaviors.

Third, standardized tests offer a highly restricted measure of language that is very different from a child's typical communication interactions. Environmental cues for typical performance, such as toys and objects and the child's typical conversational partners, are missing.

Language sampling provides more specific information for planning intervention because it includes both language and context of the language's use. If the goal of language intervention is generalization to the language used by a child in everyday situations, it is essential that an SLP collect a language sample that is a good reflection of that language in actual use. And that's what we're going to learn to do in this chapter.

It is important that some portion of the sampling be accomplished in real communication situations (Olswang, Coggins, & Timler, 2001). In general, the cognitive and linguistic processing demands of contrived situations have been shown to be less than in real-life interactions. With the increased demands and multiple cues of natural situations, the language performance of many children with LI will deteriorate. As demands increase, the cognitive and linguistic resources available to process them are stretched. If we are going to program for use within a child's natural communication contexts, then we must assess within those same contexts.

Good language samples do not just occur. They are the result of careful planning and execution. An SLP can design the assessment session so that the context fits the purpose of collecting the sample. The result is usually a combination of free or spontaneous conversation sampling and some evocative techniques. Both are essential and will be explained fully later in the chapter. For example, children with autism perform poorly on both standardized tests and spontaneous language samples (Condouris, Meyer, & Tager-Flusberg, 2003). With these children, evocative techniques may be crucial.

You'll need to make several decisions before collecting the sample. After studying the interview, observational, and testing results, an SLP decides the context, participants, materials, and conversational techniques to be used. It should be remembered that "there is no way to 'make' children talk . . . [the SLP] can only make them want to talk by creating a situation in which there is a reason to talk and an atmosphere that conveys the message that . . . [the SLP is] interested in what they have to say" (Lund & Duchan, 1993, p. 23). In this chapter, we'll cover the planning, collection, recording, and transcription of conversational samples.

Planning and Collecting a Representative Sample

Several issues are of importance when planning and collecting our language sample. Among the most prominent are the representativeness of the sample and the effect of the conversational context. In addition, collection of several language forms and functions may require the use of evocative techniques. All of these issues are important.

Representativeness

Representativeness or typicalness can be addressed by ensuring spontaneity and by collecting samples under a variety of conditions. Spontaneity can be achieved if a child and a conversational partner engage in real conversations on topics of interest to the child. To ensure spontaneity, you can follow the (LCC)^3 formula for (a) *less clinician control,* (b) *less clinician contrivance,* and (c) a *less conscious child* (Cochrane, 1983).

An SLP's control of the context should be weak so as not to restrict a child's linguistic output in quantity or quality. Although there is some indication that SLP style has little effect on gross measures, such as average or mean utterance length, more subtle measures may be affected to a greater degree. Control devices, such as the use of questions and selection of topics by the SLP, may cause a child to adopt a passive conversational role and contribute little.

A child's communication can be influenced by the adult communication partner's language. For this reason, the SLP needs to refrain from leading the interaction or providing excessive support. He or she should (Rollins, McCabe, & Bliss, 2000)

- offer minimally invasive responses, such as "Oh, I see, tell me more about that."
- ask open-ended questions, such as "What else happened?" or "What happened next?"
- use topic-continuing questions on the content of the child's previous utterance.

When a child does not participate freely and willingly, other, more structured approaches may be required. For example, you can elicit longer and more complex language from young children with picture interpretation tasks than with imperatives or story recitation. In storytelling, the use of pictures can enhance the length and complexity of the sample, especially if an SLP gives cues, such as "Tell me a story about this picture. Begin with 'Once upon a time.' " The least spontaneous condition involves the specific linguistic tasks of answering questions or completing sentences. The effects of each technique will vary with each child. An SLP can relinquish some control by placing these tasks within a less formal or play format. Less control ideally means a more typical as representative sample.

The sample will be less contrived if the SLP follows the child's lead and adopts the child's topics for conversation. More contrived situations, such as "Tell me about this picture" or "Explain the rules of Monopoly," do not elicit spontaneous everyday speech.

Finally, if a child is less conscious of the process of producing language, the sample will be more spontaneous. Asking a child to produce sentences containing certain elements, for example, makes the linguistic process very conscious and may be very difficult, especially out of context. Although a child may not be able to produce a sentence with *has been* on demand, the same child may be able to relate the story of the three bears with "Someone *has been* sleeping in my bed." The former task requires metalinguistic or abstract linguistic skills that may be beyond the child's abilities.

A child's caregivers can offer suggestions to the SLP on contexts to help obtain a representative sample. It may be desirable for caregivers to serve as partners, especially with young children. After the sample has been collected, caregivers can review the data and comment on the typicality of their child's behavior.

A Variety of Language Contexts

The sampling environment can contribute to representativeness if there is a variety of contexts, including various settings, tasks, partners, and topics. Context is dynamic and complex, and the effects are very individualistic. One child may respond well to a certain toy and partner, while another child does not. Contextual variables include the task or purpose of the activity, the opportunities to use language, the extent of ritualization in the event, the amount of joint attending, and the responsivity of the partner.

The task itself, as previously noted, can affect both the number and length of the conversational interactions. For example, young children are more referential, attempting to focus the listener's attention in free play, and are more information seeking in book activities. Similarly, parents are influenced by context and engage in more conversation when playing with dolls than they do with cars and trucks.

The opportunities to use language will vary and may need to be provided. Although specific elicitation tasks, described later, may work for older children, they may not be effective with toddlers.

Two aspects of context are structure and predictability. *Structure* is the amount of adult manipulating of materials and evoking of particular utterances. *Predictability* is the familiarity of the overall task and materials. In general, children will produce a greater frequency and diversity of language features in low-structure situations and more new features in predictable ones. Free-play sampling contexts have both low structure and predictability. Possibly in such low-structure contexts, children assume that the adult knows very little about the situation and needs an explanation. In restrictive, planned contexts, children may assume that the adult knows more, and thus children say less.

An attentive, responsive partner can elicit more language from a child. In joint, or shared, attention situations, children produce more extended conversation and are best able to determine the meanings and intentions of the partner. Similarly, timely responses by a partner increase a child's understanding.

Variety ensures that the sample will not be gathered in one atypical situation. Instead, variety can reflect a sampling of the many interactional situations in which a child functions. Although variety is desirable, it is not always practical, especially in the public school setting. Audio samples collected by the parent or teacher can provide an acceptable substitute.

Settings and Tasks

Although it's one thing to say that you should design the elicitation context for the language you desire, doing that is quite another thing and there is little evidence-based guidance beyond an SLP's clinical instinct. The task can be especially difficult if the SLP is attempting to use a context that is naturalistic, one in which the child can play freely and express his or her interests, ideas, and emotions without adult directives. While a naturalistic elicitation context is the most desirable, it is also the most unpredictable.

A number of studies have examined the effect of context on children's language, especially syntax, and have reported that linguistic complexity is related to characteristics of the elicitation context, but results are inconclusive. Comparisons across studies are also problematic because of uncontrolled differences in these studies.

The best sampling context is a meaningful activity containing a variety of elicitation tasks. In general, a child who is more familiar with the situation will give the most representative sample. Familiar routines provide a linguistic and/or nonlinguistic script that guides a child's behavior. For young children, play with familiar toys and partners is one of these routine situations. Language is a natural part of many routine events.

Preschool and Early School-age Children Sampling Contexts

As an SLP, you'll need to decide whether you want a child's typical or optimal production. Some possible elicitation contexts for preschool and young school-age children include the following:

- *Free play.* Free-play is a situation in which toys with a variety of cars, trucks, and vehicles or a doll house with dolls and furniture are available to encourage expression accompanying play.
- *Script-play.* In script-play, children are free to talk within tasks designed for enactment of familiar experiences, such as a trip to the market or to McDonald's.

- *Conversation.* Conversations can vary in the amount of adult control, but most frequently the adult attempts to follow the child's lead and maximize the child's talking with prompts, such as "What happened next?" and "Tell me more."
- *Elicited description* is more directive than the first three and asks children to describe an ongoing action sequence for the examiner who cannot see the actions.
- *Story retelling.* Story telling can be the most directive. This is especially true if the child is recounting a story from a book that the child can see. On the other hand, narratives of non-present books or of movies can be more open-ended.

In general, children engaged in free play produce more utterances than those telling stories. While both story generation and conversation result in more complex sentence structure than free play overall, there are differences by age (Southwood & Russell, 2004). Younger preschool children around age 3 produce a greater proportion of complex sentences in the free-play and script-play contexts. In contrast, older preschoolers of approximately age 5 produce a greater proportion of complex sentences while engaging in script-play and retelling stories (Klein, Moses, & Jean-Baptiste, 2010). As might be expected, the type of complexity of these utterances will also vary with age. The differences in play and language behaviors of children with LI in various play situations with assorted partners emphasize the need to evaluate these children in multiple play and conversational situations with several different partners (DeKroon, Kyte, & Johnson, 2002).

Conversations can be elicited using introductions such as the following:

- Tell me about . . . (your family, your birthday party, your favorite movie).
- Do you have any . . . ? Tell me about your . . . (pets, your brother, your sister). Tell me about how you take care of them.
- Tell me about the things you do . . . (in school, on the soccer team, in scouts).

There are additional ideas in the fine writings of Evans and Craig (1992), Miller and Iglesias (2006), and Southwood and Russell (2004).

In contrast to conversational language sampling, narratives elicit extended discourse, requiring prior planning and organization of information. For these reasons, narratives are more likely to challenge a child's language system to use advanced language structures, text structures, and literate-style language (Southwood & Russell, 2004). These advanced language skills are more likely than conversation to reveal an older school-age child's linguistic limitations.

Although story generation elicits longer utterances than either free play or conversation, the context of story generation varies. While TD children in kindergarten and second grade provide more information when they are retelling a story than when telling the same story from pictures alone, the use of pictures in narrative elicitation tasks seems to increase average utterance length for adolescents with Down syndrome who need the extra input (Miles, Chapman, & Sindberg, 2006; Schneider & Dubé, 2005). For some children at least, wordless picture books seem to be a good resource for eliciting narratives. Narratives can be elicited using the following starters:

- Do you know the story of . . . (any popular children's book)? Tell me the story.
- Your mom said that your really liked the movie . . . . I didn't see that one. Tell me the story.
- Look at this [wordless picture] book for a minute. Do you understand the story? Tell the story.

Do some research beforehand to find out from parents or teachers about the child's favorite book, movie, or TV show.

Direct questions elicit the greatest number of different words (Gazelle & Stockman, 2003). Although question type does not seem to influence mean length of utterence (MLU) in toddlers, preschoolers respond with more multiword utterances following conversationally open-ended

(*What should we do next?*) and topic-continuing questions (de Rivera, Girolametto, Greenberg, & Weitzman 2005).

Settings should not be too contrived. Familiar, meaningful situations with a variety of age-appropriate and motivating activities provide greater variety and thus are more representative. Good settings for preschoolers include the free play mentioned earlier, snack time, and show-and-tell. School-age children can be sampled during group activities, class presentations, conversations with peers, and field trips. Generally, a child involved in some activity produces more language than a child who is watching others or conversing about pictures. It is better if the sample consists of at least two different settings in which different activities are occurring.

The challenge for an SLP is to find a collection technique that strikes a balance. Too highly structured methods often are not representative. Free play, although low in structure, may be time-consuming and result in variable unreliable data. For older children, an interview technique may be an effective alternative. For 8- to 9-year-old children with SLI, the interview technique yields more and longer utterances, more complex language forms, more temporal adjacency and semantic contingency, and more reliable, less variable results than free play.

Conversational sampling should be authentic and functional. Authenticity comes from the use of real communication contexts in which the participants convey real information. Functional sampling is most concerned with the success of a child with LI as a communicator. Success can be measured by effectiveness in transmitting meanings, fluency or timeliness, and appropriateness of the message form and style in context.

The materials used should be interesting, age appropriate, and capable of eliciting the type of language desired. Interest can be piqued if a child is allowed to choose from a preselected group of toys or objects. Parents also can bring their child's toys from home in order to increase the validity of the sample.

The selection of clinical materials can affect the pragmatic performance of young children by modifying the physical context in which the sample is collected. When no toys are present, children are more likely to initiate memory-related topics. Toys with construction properties, such as Legos, Play Doh, or clay often remove the conversation from the present and are more likely to elicit more displaced topics, especially while objects are being constructed. On the other hand, toys that encourage role-play elicit more verbalizations or vocalizations about the objects, events, and actions performed. Compared with construction-type toys, a toy hospital elicits more discussion of the here and now and more fantasy topics and is more conducive to sociodramatic play and verbal representations of events and actions.

In general, children around age 2 respond well to blocks, dishes, pull and wind-up toys, and dolls. Children around age 3 prefer books, clothes, puppets, and such toys as a barn with animals or a street with houses and stores. These toys encourage role-playing and language production. Kindergarten and early elementary school children respond best to toys with many pieces and to puppets and action figures. Finally, older children usually converse without the use of objects and can be encouraged to talk about themselves and their interests or to provide narratives. Narratives, a special type of language production, are discussed in more detail in Chapter 8.

Toys also can assist in eliciting specific linguistic structures. For example, children are more likely to produce spatial terms in play with objects than in conversation. Object movement and manipulation can serve as nonlinguistic cues for a child. Because children's cognitive knowledge and linguistic performance of spatial relationships may differ markedly, manipulation of toys can also aid an SLP in assessing a child's comprehension. The toys and positions should be varied so as not to suggest answers to children.

If certain language features are desired, an SLP must increase the probability of their occurrence by adding more structure. With school-age children, discussion, rather than conversations based on pictures or toys in context, yields more mature language as measured by clause structure complexity, the ratio of hesitations to words, and grammatical and phonemic accuracy.

Adolescent Sampling Contexts

As children progress through the early school years, they are expected to use different text-level communication genres. In school, children are exposed to expository discourse, an advanced form consisting of a monologue providing factual descriptions or explanations of events. Examples of expository discourse include sharing a news event, explaining the rules of a game, or comparing two events. This discourse genre may be particularly helpful in revealing a child's ability to use complex language structures.

In order to produce expository language, a child needs advanced cognitive abilities and exposure to decontextualized language that contains advanced linguistic structures (Nippold, 2004). In school, children are exposed to expository language through nonfiction books or teacher explanations. By third and fourth grade children are expected to be able to learn new information through reading. In addition to exposure, a child needs the opportunity to use the more advanced linguistic structures characteristic of this type of discourse.

Research into expository discourse of school-age children has shown that expository discourse improves with age (Berman & Verhoeven, 2002; Nippold, Hesketh, Duthie, & Mansfield, 2005; Scott & Windsor, 2000; Westerveld & Moran, 2011). With increasing age, children show a gradual increase in overall length of their language samples, utterance length, and clausal density. Early detection of children with language deficits in expository discourse may help guide our intervention and prevent some of the problems children face in expository writing tasks in later school years.

Expository discourse can be elicited in several different ways (Berman & Verhoeven, 2002; Nippold, Hesketh, et al., 2005; Scott & Windsor, 2000), such as asking a child to

- explain or describe a procedure.
- provide a summary of a short descriptive film.
- discuss the issue of interpersonal conflict after watching a short video.
- describe a favorite game or sport.

For example, in the favorite game or sport task, a child is asked to name his or her favorite game or sport and explain why. The SLP then asks the child to explain the game or sport, using prompts such as "I am not too familiar with the game of [..]." Finally, the child was asked what a player should do to win a game of [..].

Because of the more complex language required in peer conflict resolution, these problems hold promise as a language sampling and intervention milieu for adolescents (Nippold, Mansfield, & Billow, 2007). A peer conflict resolution task consists of a set of hypothetical peer conflicts read aloud by the SLP. After an adolescent has retold the scenario, the SLP poses a series of questions concerning the nature of the problem, how it might be resolved, and what the likely outcome might be. Possible questions might include (Nippold, Mansfield, & Billow, 2007):

- What is the main problem?
- Why is that a problem?
- What is a good way for *Person A* to deal with *Person B*?
- Why is that a good way?
- What do you think will happen if *Person A* does that?
- How do you think they both will feel if *Person A* does that?

Responses by adolescents include more complex utterances than testing alone may elicit.

A teen should be allowed to take as much time as necessary to finish the explanation. The SLP should demonstrate interest in the explanation, using neutral feedback, such as "uh-huh." For specific information regarding the expository procedure, you should see Nippold, Hesketh, et al. (2005).

Conversational Partners

Because the SLP is interested in a child's use of language, the conversational dyad of the partner and the child is important. This is evident in the conversations of adolescents. When teens talk to peers, they ask more questions, obtain more information, shift to more new topics, use more figurative expressions, and make more attempts to entertain than when they talk with their families (Nippold, 2000). Partners influence all aspects of communication.

Conversational partners for young children should be carefully selected and instructed in their role. As noted in Chapter 3, it is especially important to use familiar conversational partners with children under age 3 because these children often respond poorly to strangers.

With preschool and school-age children familiar conversational or play situations attain the most typical spontaneous sample in which a child converses as naturally as possible. Interaction may involve one adult or child or a small group of children engaged in sharing, playing, or working in the home or the classroom.

A child should be assessed across several familiar persons with different interactive styles. Peer interaction usually involves more equal status between participants than do adult–child interactions. Adults tend to guide and control the topic when conversing with children. As one might expect, these two conditions can result in very different interactive styles for a child.

The language performance of children below age 3, of minority children, and of children with LD may deteriorate in the presence of an authority figure such as an unfamiliar adult. This does not mean that you cannot act as a conversational partner. In many ways, as an SLP, you may be the best conversational partner because of your knowledge of language and of interactions.

The SLP and all other participating adults need to be mindful of the inherent problems in adult–child conversations and act to reduce the authority figure persona. The adult can accomplish this by accepting the child's activity, agenda, and topics and by participating with the child. The best way to attain a semblance of equal authority is for you and the child to engage in a play interaction. Instead of being directive, the SLP comments on and participates in their ongoing shared activity. With young children, participation may necessitate using the floor for play.

As the conversational partner, an SLP can set the tone of the interaction by being nondirective, interesting, interested, and responsive. The SLP should respond to the content of the child's language, not to the way it is said. At this point, the purpose is to collect data, not to change behavior. Our goal is *collecting, not correcting.*

By manipulating the situation skillfully, an SLP can probe for a greater range of information. Initially, interaction may be dampened because you're not the child's usual communication partner. Therefore, it is important for the SLP to get acquainted slowly and in a nonthreatening manner. This task is best accomplished by meeting a child on his or her terms through play and by following the child's lead.

SLPs possess the clinical skill to elicit a variety of functions, introduce various topics, and ask questions about experiences. Role-play, dolls, and puppet play provide information about a child's event knowledge in a range of situations. There is the potential to elicit a greater variety of language than might be possible when the child and parent communicate.

Children who are reluctant to talk to adults may be more willing to interact with a puppet or a doll. I have found that small animals, such as guinea pigs, make excellent communication partners for children. For example, after explaining to a child that I must leave to run a short errand, I introduce the guinea pig and ask the child to talk to it so that it will not get lonely. The child is observed via one-way glass or on a monitor and his or her language recorded while I'm absent.

Despite conventional wisdom, neither the race of the conversational partner nor the race depicted in stimulus materials seems to affect language performance as measured by response length and response latency. This is not to say that all children, particularly children with CLD backgrounds will be unaffected. SLPs should be aware of potential difficulties and should approach each child with an open mind. Racial incompatibilities should not be expected, but all SLPs should be conscious of this potential.

Topics

Children have a wide variety of interests, and the conversational partners must be careful to enable a child to talk about them. Children are more spontaneous and produce more language when they are allowed to initiate the topics of discussion.

An SLP should be prepared to shift topics as readily as activities. Expect to be conversant in topics of interest to children, such as school activities, holidays, movies, television programs, fads and fashions, videogames, and music.

Summary

Child variables, such as recounting recent past experience and being in a good mood, can greatly affect language sampling, because in these situations the child is often the initiator and because there are few performance constraints. To get the most representative sample possible, therefore, an SLP should use familiar situations, persons, and tasks or topics. Representativeness is enhanced if the conversational sample is collected in more than one setting, with different conversational partners and tasks or topics in each. Guidelines are summarized in Table 6.1.

It may be helpful to think of interactional situations along a continuum from relatively nondirected or free to more controlled or scripted. Such toys as a dollhouse, a farm, action figures, bubbles, or dress-up clothes are rather open-ended, especially when a partner has suggested, "Let's talk and play with these things." Books offer more control and can be used to elicit particular words, forms, and narratives. Familiar routines, such as doing the dishes, also can be used, along with such cues as "What are you going to do now?" to elicit more specific behavior. Interviews, picture labeling, and responding to questions offer the most control but at the sacrifice of spontaneity and representativeness. These latter techniques are more appropriately considered evocative techniques used to elicit specific behaviors.

Table 6.2 presents contextual variables that can be manipulated in an assessment to influence a child's performance. Each variable can be modified to offer minimal or maximal contextual support.

Sampling should engage children in challenging interactions that stretch their language and reveal deficits. This requires a range of interactive situations and discourse types, including conversation, play, narration, and expository or factual/causal communication.

It may seem obvious, but we should note that while increased structure within the sampling task may be necessary to obtain certain information, it comes at the expense of spontaneity and typical

TABLE 6.1 Ensuring Representativeness in a Language Sample

*Keep it spontaneous with
• Less clinician control
• Less clinician contrived
• Less conscious child
Have a variety of
• Settings and tasks
• Conversational partners and topics

*Source: (LCC)[3] from Cochrane (1983).

TABLE 6.2 Continuum of Contextual Support

Minimum Contextual Support	Maximum Contextual Support
Naturalistic interaction	Controlled and contrived interaction to elicit particular structures or behaviors
No prompts, toys, props, or activity	Familiar activities, toys, props, and routines providing scripts
Conversational partner is SLP	Conversational partner is parent, other adult, or child familiar with child
Novel activity	Familiar activity or routine
Indirect language modeling	Elicited utterances and imitation
Neutral responses, such as "Oh" and Um-hm"	Turnabouts and questions

Source: Information taken from Coggins (1991).

performance. In addition, at some point, the entire interaction slips from conversation into probing or informal testing. Probing a child's knowledge certainly has its place in an assessment as another informal data-gathering technique, but it shouldn't be confused with conversational language sampling. As an SLP, you need to be aware of when you cross that line.

Evocative Conversational Techniques

Although the sample should represent everyday language use, free samples may have limitations, such as low frequency or nonappearance of certain linguistic features and conversational behaviors. Absence or low incidence does not mean a child lacks these features or behaviors. Therefore, it may be necessary to supplement the sample with evocative procedures specifically designed to elicit them. Test protocols also might be modified to obtain more structured samples.

As an SLP, you may need to plan both the linguistic and nonlinguistic contexts for elicitation of various functions and forms. This requires some forethought. For example, infinitive phrases not only are difficult for children with LI, but they also require specific evocative techniques (Eisenberg, 2005). Infinitives come in two varieties, noun-verb-*to*-verb (*John wants to go*) and noun-verb-noun-*to*-verb (*John wants Fred to go*). An SLP can use play with dolls or puppets and have a child complete sentences within the play in the following manner:

> The cat says, "Can I eat?" The cat wants . . . . You finish the story. The cat . . . ?
>
> The boys says to the girl, "Swim with me." The boy asks . . . . You finish the story. The boy . . . ?

Early developing infinitives accompany verbs such as *ask, forget, go* (*gonna*), *have* (*hafta*) (*gotta*), *like, need, say, suppose, tell, try, use, want.*

At first, some procedures may seem stiff and formal, even forced. Initially, you may need to role-play the sampling situation and memorize conversational openers and replies. Once familiar with the many ways of eliciting a variety of functions and forms, an SLP can relax and use the techniques more naturally as opportunities arise within the interaction.

Specific tasks that are within a child's experience also can be used to elicit specific language forms. This approach allows a broad range of pragmatic functions to occur. For example, a mock birthday party can be used to elicit plurals, past tense, and questions. The SLP might elicit plurals by saying the following:

> Today is X's birthday. Let's have a party. What are some things we'll need? (Or, Here are some things we need. What are these?)

TABLE 6.3 Situations with the Potential to Elicit a Variety of Language Functions

Dress-up	Role-playing
Playing house or farm	Playing school
Dolls, puppets, adventure or action figures	Acting out stories, television shows, movies
Farm set or street scene	Imaginary play
Simulated grocery store, gas station, fast-food restaurant, beauty parlor	Simulated TV talk show

In this way, the child's utterances are placed within context in which they make sense. Within the same situation, past tense might be elicited by dropping dishes and asking what happened or by reviewing whether you did everything to get ready ("Okay, now tell me what *you* did to get ready for the party. *I* washed the dishes"). Finally, questions can be elicited by a party game variation of Ask the Old Lady.

> Let's play a question game. This is X (puppet, doll, action figure). I want you to ask X some questions about his birthday party. I wonder how old he is. You ask him.

The child may need a demonstration before being able to complete the question task.

Specific procedures and activities can be used to elicit a variety of communication intentions, examples of presupposition, and the underlying social organization of discourse within a variety of situations. Table 6.3 lists examples of situations that each elicit a variety of language functions. In addition, SLPs are interested in ways to elicit various semantic and syntactic features. These elicitation techniques are presented in the following section.

Intentions

Most utterances clearly demonstrate the speaker's intent. "What time is it?" demonstrates a desire for information. However, the relationship is not always so obvious. "What time is it?" might be used as an excuse. For example, the speaker who does not wish to do something and knows that time is limited might use this utterance to establish the time factor for other people.

> Well, I don't know . . . , it's getting late. What time is it? Oh, well, I really better be going.

Utterances also may express more than one intention. For example, the speaker might respond to a piece of art with "What do you call that *thing*?" Here, the speaker requests information and also makes an evaluation.

Some intentions are responsive in nature, for example, answering a question or following a directive or request for action. In addition to a child's production level of such requests, it is helpful to know the child's level of response.

With responsive functions, an SLP must not interpret noncompliance as noncomprehension. A child simply may not want to comply or may choose to ignore the request. My granddaughter at age 6 was especially good at ignoring. Come to think of it, so was her mom! An SLP first should be certain that the child can perform the behavior requested. The ages at which children comprehend different levels of requests are listed in Table 6.4.

It might be helpful for the SLP to use two children in an ask-and-tell situation so that each child can act as a model for the other. In a similar manner, an SLP and child can switch roles as questioner (or director) and respondent.

TABLE 6.4 Age and Comprehension of Requests

Age in Years	Comprehension
2	I need a ______. Give me a ______.
3	Could you give me a ______? May I have a ______? Have you got a ______?
4	He hurt me. (Hint) The ______ is all gone. (Hint)
4½	Begin to comprehend indirect requests: Why don't you ______ or Don't forget to ______. Mastery takes several years.
5	Inferred requests in which the goal is totally masked are now comprehended. In this example, the speaker desires some juice: Now you make breakfast like you're the mommy.

Source: Information from Ervin-Tripp (1977).

These are just a few suggestions for eliciting a variety of communication intentions. An SLP must note the type of intentions displayed, their forms, the means of transmission, and the social conventions that affect these means. For example, some situations may call for the use of nonverbal means; others may not. The following are a broad range of intentions and accompanying activities that may elicit language functions or intentions within a conversational or situational context.

Answering/Responding. An SLP asks a child a variety of questions while engaged in play ("Where shall we put the houses?" "Who is that?" "What's in his hand?") and notes the type of question and the expected response. Some question forms may be easier or more difficult for a child to respond to.

Calling/Greeting. An SLP leaves and reenters the situation, role-plays people entering and leaving a business, calls on the telephone, or uses dolls, puppets, or action figures to elicit greetings. If the SLP turns away from the child with a favorite toy, the child also may call.

Continuance. Continuance is turn filling that lets a speaker know that a listener is attending to the conversation. Typical continuants include "uh-huh," "yeah," "okay," and "right." These can be observed throughout the session. The SLP notes when the child seems to rely on this function, rather than contribute anything new or relevant to the conversation.

Expressing Feelings. An SLP models feeling-type responses throughout the play interaction. Dolls, puppets, or action figures are described as having certain feelings and the child is asked to help. For example, the SLP could say, "Oh, Big Bird is sad. Can you talk to him and make him feel better?"

Hypothesizing. An SLP poses a physical problem for a child, such as, "How can we get everyone to the party on time?" or, "How can we get Leonardo out of the cage?" The child proposes solutions to the problem.

Making Choices. An SLP presents a child with alternatives, such as, "I don't know whether you'd rather have a peanut butter sandwich with jelly or fluff."

Predicting. In sequential activities or book reading, an SLP can ponder, "I wonder what will happen now" or, "I wonder what we'll do next."

Protesting. An SLP can elicit protesting by putting away toys or taking away snacks before the child is finished. When a child requests an item, an SLP can hand the child something other than what was requested.

Reasoning. An SLP attempts to solve a problem, such as, "I wonder why the boy ran away" or, "I wonder what we did wrong."

Repeating. An SLP should note the amount of repetition of self and of the partner. This can take the form of empty comments in a conversation in which a child adds no new information, for example:

Adult: Did your class go to the zoo yesterday?
Child: Yeah, zoo.
Adult: What did you like best? The monkeys?
Child: Monkeys.
Adult: Monkeys are my favorite too. They're so funny.
Child: Monkeys funny.

Replying. An SLP should note occasions when a child responds to the content of what the SLP has said. Unlike answers, replies are expected but not required. This behavior is one of the mainstays of conversation as each speaker builds on the comment of the previous speaker.

Reporting. Reporting can include several functions, such as declaring or citing, detailing, or naming/labeling.

Declaring/Citing. While engaged in an activity, a child spontaneously comments on the present action. The SLP can model this behavior ("Car goes up the ramp") but not attempt to cue a response because declaring/citing is spontaneous. The SLP also can engage in unexpected or unusual behavior and await the child's comment.

Detailing. An SLP presents a child with two objects of different size or color. If the child takes one and says nothing, the SLP models ("I'll take the little one" or "Here's a green truck") and presents other objects later. The SLP does not attempt to cue a response because detailing is also spontaneous.

Naming/Labeling. An SLP presents a novel object or points to pictures in a book and remarks, "Oh, look." If the child does not label the object or picture, the SLP models the response ("Look. A clown.") and goes on. The child may do so on subsequent exposure to other novel objects. The SLP does not cue a response because labeling like the other forms of reporting should be spontaneous.

Requesting Assistance/Directing. An SLP presents interesting toys in a way that requires adult help to open or use, such as

- placing objects in clear plastic containers or drawstring bags that require help to open.
- giving the child one portion of a toy while keeping the other on a shelf.
- letting windup toys run down.

The SLP makes such comments as, "I wish we could play with this; it would be fun," "Oh, we could use more parts," or "Gee, we need to fix that." In another situation, the child helps two puppets or dolls solve a problem in which one will not share a special toy with the other. The SLP also can present the child with situations that require a solution, such as toys with missing pieces. During interactions the SLP should note self-directing or self-talk accompanying play. This behavior can be modeled for the child, but it should be spontaneous on the child's part.

Requesting Clarification. This intention can be elicited when an SLP mumbles or makes an inaccurate statement.

Requesting Information. An SLP places novel but unknown objects in front of a child. Naming the object correctly is the naming labeling function and the SLP should confirm the child's name. If the child labels incorrectly, the SLP says, "No, it's not an X," "No, can you guess what it is?" or "How can we ask what it's called?" The responses "What's that?" or "What?" and those with rising intonation ("Frog?") should be considered requests for information. The child can also be directed to ask others.

Requesting Objects. An SLP exposes the child to enticing objects or edibles that are just out of reach. The SLP also might direct the child to use an object not present in the situation or not in the expected location. If prompting is required, the SLP can ask, "Do you have the scissors?" When the child answers negatively, the SLP can direct the child by saying, "Ask Sally if she does."

Requesting Permission. An SLP hands an interesting object to a child and says, "Hold the X for me." The technique is more effective if the SLP uses a nonsense name for the object. The SLP then awaits a response from the child, such as, "Can I play with X?" or just, "Play X?"

An even more effective technique is to keep the object hidden in an opaque box. The SLP peeks into the box and tells the object that it can come out to play when someone wants to play with it. If necessary, a puppet can model the requesting behavior desired.

Presuppositional and Deictic Skills

Whereas intentions are noted at the individual level, other linguistic aspects, such as presupposition and deixis, underlie the entire conversational interaction. **Presupposition** is the speaker's assumption about the knowledge level of the listener and the tailoring of language to that supposed level. **Deixis** is the production and interpretation of information from the perspective of the speaker. When a speaker says, "Come here," this must be interpreted as a point close to the speaker, not as a point with reference to the listener. Deictic terms include, but are not limited to, *here/there, this/that, come/go, and you/me.*

Presuppositional and deictic skills can be assessed in *referential communication tasks*. In classic referential tasks, one partner describes something or gives directions to the other partner, who is usually on the other side of an opaque barrier or unable to see the speaker (see Figure 6.1). Variations include blindfold games or telephone conversations. Deixis can be elicited by using object-finding tasks in which the child directs the conversational partner toward a hidden object.

In these tasks, an SLP must be alert to the use of direct/indirect reference. In direct reference, the speaker considers the audience and clearly identifies the entity being mentioned. Indirect reference typically follows direct reference and refers to entities through the use of pronouns or such terms as *that one*. A child with poor presuppositional skills may use indirect reference without prior direct reference.

Additional presuppositional information can be gathered by varying the roles, topics, partners, and communication channels available in the sampling situation. Roles can be varied so that a child has an opportunity to act as listener and speaker. Assessment of both roles is essential. For example, a child with LD generally will ask few questions for clarification even when he or she has little understanding of what has been said. As speakers, these children make limited use of descriptors, provide very little specific information, and are less effective than children developing normally.

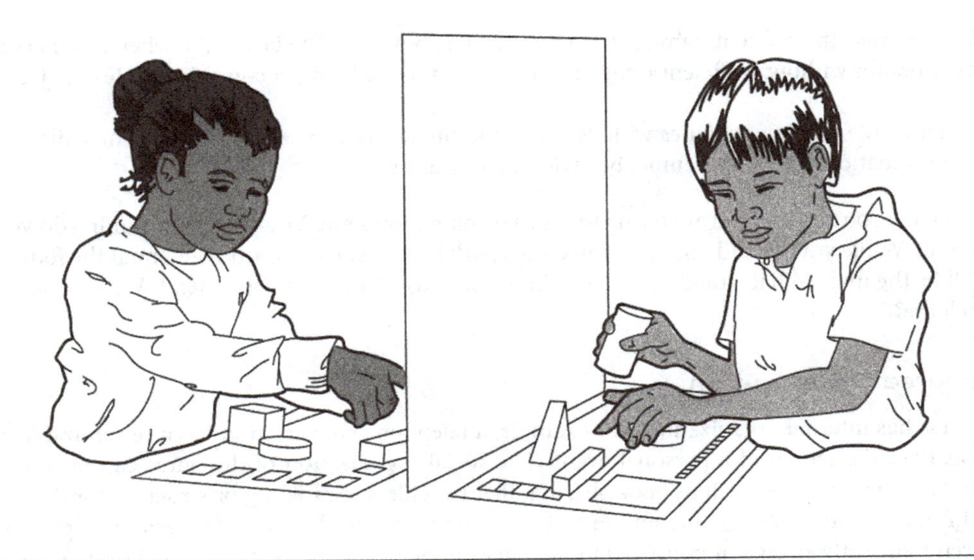

FIGURE 6.1 Barrier tasks.

The choice of topics also can influence presuppositional behavior and provide for a variety of role taking. Children can be asked to describe events about which the SLP or partner is ignorant (e.g., a family outing). In this situation, the child must determine the amount of information necessary for the listener to understand the topic.

As the number of communication channels decreases, a speaker is forced to rely more heavily upon the remaining ones. For example, the use of a telephone requires the speaker to rely almost exclusively on the verbal communication channel. This situation is a challenge even for some non-impaired language users.

While gathering the language sample, an SLP can manipulate channel availability systematically. During play, I sometimes turn or look away and then ask the child to describe what he or she is doing. Barrier games or blindfold games with the child in charge may also elicit interesting information; however, role-playing with the telephone is more realistic.

Several other activities can be used to elicit presuppositional skills. Of interest is whether a child can encode the most informative or uncertain elements in a situation. In general, human beings tend to comment on entities that are new, changing, or unexpected. In the sampling situation, novel items can be introduced. The SLP must attend to the child's behavior to see whether the child refers to the novel stimulus.

I know of one clinic where a kitten is abruptly introduced into the sampling situation. The SLP says nothing but waits to see whether the child will comment and in what manner.

In general, young children with LI encode novel information less frequently than do children developing typically. Older school-age children with LI tend to use more pronouns with less identification of the referent than do TD children.

Games and stories can elicit indirect/direct reference. For example, a story can be told and then questions asked to elicit indefinite and definite articles and/or nouns and pronouns. The child can also retell a story to a second child who has not heard it. Any portion of extended discourse, such as describing a movie, explaining how to accomplish a task, or telling a story, will provide valuable clinical data.

The SLP is interested in both the lexical items used and the ambiguity of the referent. Of interest is the number of times the child mentions the referent by name or by the use of pronouns. Some children overuse the referent name ("The boy . . . , The boy . . . , The boy . . ."), whereas others rely on the pronoun without sufficient return to the referent name to avoid confusion ("He . . . , He . . . , He . . .").

Finally, role-playing activities with very specific situations also can be helpful. The child in the following situation faces very definite behavioral constraints.

> Imagine you and a friend are trying to find a drinking fountain. You see a man coming down the street. While your friend remains seated on a park bench, you try to find out about the fountain. I'll be the man. What would you say? (Child responds.) Now, I'm your friend. What would you tell me?

Discourse Organization

Discourse has internal organization. For example, a telephone conversation has a recognizable pattern, as does the telling of a personal event. The social organization of discourse can be assessed within familiar activities, such as book sharing, that provide a scaffolding or structure for dialogue. An SLP may be interested in the amount of social and nonsocial speech. For example, preschool children frequently engage in nonsocial monologues in play, in contrast to older children, who participate more in dialogues or in social monologues. This change signals a growing awareness of the social nature of speech and language use.

An SLP can provide opportunities for a child to initiate conversation, to take turns, and to repair in response to self-feedback or the feedback of others in different situations. Turn taking may need to begin at a physical level with some reticent children. In conversation, an SLP might even say, "Now it's your turn," and point to the child initially. By failing to respond to the child or by responding inappropriately, mumbling, failing to establish a referent, misnaming, or providing insufficient information, an SLP may elicit requests for clarification from a child.

Semantic Terms

Relational terms, such as *in front of*, *more/less*, and *before/after*, are especially difficult for children with LD and LI. These children often use comprehension strategies that have several implications for assessment. For locational terms, these strategies may include probable location, physical properties of objects, and preferred location. Adjectival relational words, such as *big* and *little*, may be comprehended by using either a preference for amount or word synonymity. With temporal terms, strategies may include sequential probability and order-of-mention or main-clause-first. Each of these strategies is explained below.

It is easier for children to comprehend locational terms and to follow locational instructions when familiar objects are combined in familiar, predictable, or probable ways, such as juice in a cup. Levels of comprehension can be determined by using both the usual context and a neutral context in which object placement is not so predictable, such as block and cup.

The physical properties of an object can also influence responding. For example, a child's rule may be, *Containers are for* in, *and surfaces are for* on. Square containers can be turned on their sides by the SLP and used for both *in* and *on*.

Some objects are fronted or have an obvious front, such as a TV, while others, such as a wastebasket, are not. This characteristic affects comprehension and production of such terms as *in front of* and *behind*. In general, these terms are easier to use with fronted objects than with nonfronted objects. In addition, some young children interpret *behind* to mean *hidden from view by*. Obviously, *in front of* and *behind* must be assessed with fronted and nonfronted and small and large objects.

With deictic terms, young children may employ either a child-centered or speaker-centered strategy, preferring that location as the reference point. Assessing contrastive terms, such as *here/there*, with different speakers may help determine if such preferences exist.

Adjectival terms, such as *more/less, long/short*, and *big/little*, may be interpreted by the child using a preference for a greater-amount strategy in which a child usually chooses the largest one when in doubt. Assessing both words of the pair in different contexts and in different word order may help an SLP understand a child's errors.

Similarly, height of the objects used affects comprehension of such words as *big, tall, top, young*, and *old*. Preschoolers often equate *big* with *tall* and *old* and *little* with *short* and *young*. Objects can be placed so that their heights are similar by using stands of different heights.

Some children use a strategy in which they interpret contrastive terms such as *big* and *little* to be synonymous or assign the meanings to similar terms. In the latter, *big* becomes synonymous with *tall, wide*, and *thick*. Object dimensions can be controlled so that, for example, the widest objects are not always the biggest overall.

Finally, as mentioned, temporal sequential terms, such as *before* and *after*, may be interpreted by using a most probable, order-of-mention, or main-clause-first strategy. In the most probable strategy, a child trusts experience. Among preschoolers, this is the most widely used strategy with familiar, real-world sequences. Order-of-mention, or the first-action-mentioned-occurred-before-the-second, is also popular among preschoolers, while children over age 5 often use the main-clause-first strategy in which the main clause of the sentence is assumed to have occurred first. For example, in the sentence "After we finish school, we can go to the rec center," a child may assume the rec center occurs first. Sequential terms should be note when used as both prepositions, as in *after school*, and conjunction, as in *she did X after she did Y*.

Language Form

An SLP can manipulate the context to elicit particular forms. For example, the objects and the verbal routines chosen for play may facilitate the use of pronouns or prepositions. Specific syntactic forms, such as verbs, and morphological markers, such as the regular past-tense -ed, also can be elicited in creative ways. Some intentions discussed previously in this chapter, such as requesting information, have specific linguistic forms. A few elicitation methods for specific structures are listed in Table 6.5.

Language Sampling of Children with CLD Backgrounds

It is even more important that the language of children with CLD backgrounds be collected in several different contexts. Code switching and differing language and dialect use in context is extremely important information for determining the effectiveness of a child as a communicator.

Sampling should occur in monologue and dialogue situations in both languages or dialects. Monologue activities might include static, dynamic, and abstract tasks. Static tasks describe relationships among objects in the context and might include directing others to perform a task or describing entities by location, size, shape, or color. Dynamic tasks describe changes over time as in narration. Finally, abstract tasks might include opinion-expressing tasks, such as stating or justifying a position.

Dialogue situations should include a variety of partners because of the special constraints that each imposes on a child with a CLD background. At least a portion of the sample should include a parent, sibling, or peer as a partner. The classroom is especially important because of the academic difficulties these children may encounter.

In each context, different conversational partners can pose communication problems for a child. Change and problem solving encourage communication and enable an SLP to determine the effectiveness of the child as a communicator. In addition, such situations can offer clues to the learning style of the child. Guidelines for collecting a language sample from children with CLD backgrounds are presented in Table 6.6.

TABLE 6.5 Elicitation of Language Features

Feature	Elicitation Technique
Word classes (nouns, verbs . . .)	Pull object from a bag and name it. (Nouns) Identify actions in pictures, such as sports. (Verbs) Ask specific *Wh-* questions: *What's that?* (Nouns); *What's he doing? What will (did) she do?* (Verbs); *Where's X? When's X?* (Prepositions); *How does he feel (look, smell)?* (Adjectives); *How did she do X?* (Adverbs); *Whose X is this?* (Possessive pronouns)
Sequencing preposition and conjunctions	Tell me how to . . . (make a cake, play *Chutes and Ladders*, talk about your favorite movie)
Comparatives	Pull items from a bag and tell how they differ from some reference item or from the last item. (*This one's longer.*)
Adjectives	Play "I spy." (*I see something and it's X.*)* Offer choices with similar objects and ask "Which one do you want?" (*The green one.* Or *The big one.*)
Verb tenses	*Tell me what we're we going to do? . . . doing? . . . did?*
Plural *–s* marker	*Let's play camping (birthday party, grocery store)! What do we need to play?* Play with Legos or Mr. Potatohead or make crafts and request pieces. (*I want the stickers.* Or *Can I have Mr. Potatohead's ears?*)
Possessive pronouns	Pull objects with known owners from a bag and name the owner (*That's John's*). Play dress up or with action figures or dolls and have child identify what goes with whom (*That's X-Man's backpack*).
Complex sentences	*Your mom says you play soccer. That sounds exciting. But I've never played. Can you tell me how to play?*
Yes/no questions	Play "Twenty Questions" (Is it . . . ?).

Source: Information from Crais and Roberts (1991) and my own clinical experience.

*Also a good eliciter of pronouns.

TABLE 6.6 Guidelines for Language Sampling with Children from CLD Backgrounds

Observe the child in various communication contexts, especially low-anxiety, natural communication environments.
Observe the child with speakers of both languages or dialects. Language mixing during collecting may confuse the child.
Record conversations with the child's family for comparison.
Explore with the family the child's communication in the home and community environment.
Use culturally relevant objects to stimulate conversation. Pictures should contain members of the child's racial/ethnic group.
Avoid the tendency to "fill in" for the child's communication gaps. Observe the child's strategies for getting the message through.

Note:
- Language uses and purposes. How flexible is the child's system?
- Success at communicating. Are certain content and situations more successful?
- Communication breakdowns. Where do they occur? With whom?
- Strengths and weaknesses. What strategies are used to compensate for weakness?
- Anxiety and frustration.

Recording the Sample

Optimum number and length found in various studies range from one 175-utterance sample to two 100-utterance samples. Although short 1- and 2-minute samples are reliable for measures of verbal productivity and fluency, including total number of words (TNW) and number of different words (NDW) produced in the entire sample, children's use of grammatical errors is difficult to determine in schooage children, and measures of general performance, including mean length of utterance (MLU), were not reliable (Tilstra & McMaster, 2007). In contrast, in a narrative retelling task with English language learners (ELLs) who speak both Spanish and English, short narratives averaging 4 minutes in length are reliable in TNW, NDW, MLU, and words per minute (WPM) (Heilmann et al., 2008).

While some professional literature suggests lengthy samples, these are very time consuming and not feasible in most clinical settings. The time demands of recording, transcribing, and analyzing 100 child utterances is one of the biggest barriers to the clinical use of language sampling and analysis (LSA). How much language sampling is enough? The impact of sample length may vary as a function of the sampling context. When we compare 1-, 3-, and 7-minute samples, we find that many language sample measures are quite consistent across all three. Measures of productivity, lexical diversity, and utterance length are the most reliable measures when shorter samples are compared with longer ones (Heilmann, Nockerts, & Miller, 2010).

Occasionally, children fall into repetitive patterns of responding, such as naming pictures in a book. This kind of activity provides very little variation in a child's behavior. It is best either to limit this type of interaction or not to use it for analysis. If, on the other hand, a child frequently exhibits perseverative or stereotypic patterns, they should be recorded for analysis, saved for supporting data, or commented on in the assessment report but possibly not included in the sample for analysis.

A language sample can be recorded permanently by using an analog or digital recording device such as your MP3 player for listening or transferred to a computer. Audio recording is essential because the interaction must be reviewed repeatedly for information.

Language samples can be recorded directly into your computer. This requires a sound card that enables CD-quality recording, an unobtrusive unidirectional external microphone, and an audio recording software program, such as *Audacity*, found at http://audacity.sourceforge.net/download.

When recording onto a computer, it is recommended that audio be recorded onto the internal hard drive. If hard drive space is limited, burn the file onto a CD or move it to an external hard drive. Files stored externally can also provide a backup (Hammett Price, Hendricks, & Cook, 2010).

Although videorecording can be intrusive, it yields the best data for describing the verbal and nonverbal behaviors observed. You could even use your webcam if you have recording software. The alternatives to videotaping are not as reliable and thus increase the variability in the behavior recorded. Even if video is used, you may find a simultaneous audio recording helpful for transcribing the speech and language portion. The following recording methods are listed in order of decreasing desirability:

1. Simultaneous video and audio recording.
2. Simultaneous audio with SLP descriptions of nonlinguistic behaviors recorded in one device and the linguistic interaction in the other.
3. Simultaneous audio recording and written-data recording on time sheets (see Table 6.7). Having more than one observer may help ensure that no behaviors are overlooked and may increase the reliability of description of those that are observed. Writing data as the interaction progresses is extremely tedious but necessary for some analysis.

It is important for later transcription that different data collection methods begin at the same time. This should be accomplished as unobtrusively as possible. A cough or some similar signal by the SLP can alert observers that recording has begun but hopefully not alert the child being recorded.

TABLE 6.7 Time Form for Recording the Nonlinguistic Context

			Minute 2
Time (sec.)	Child's Behavior	Partner's Behavior	Other
0			
.			
.			
.			
.			
10			
.	*Looks at partner*		
.			
.	*Points to truck*		
.			
20			
.			
.	*Reaches for truck*		
.		*Hands truck*	
.			
30			
.			
.			
.	*Pushes car*		
.			
40	*Looks at partner*		
.			
.	*Points to gas station*		
.			
.		*Moves car to gas station*	
50			
.		*Moves car to gas station*	
.			
.			
.			
60			

Transcribing the Sample

The conversational sample is transcribed as soon after recording as possible. This timeliness ensures that you bring to the task as much memory of the situation as possible.

The format of the transcript varies with the purpose of the assessment. For most purposes, the type of format shown in Table 6.8 is suggested. There are situations, however, in which the SLP is only interested in the child's utterances.

Unfortunately, at present, there are no programs that can transcribe language samples automatically. Probably the simplest way to transcribe is to type the child's utterances into a text file or word processing document while listening to the recorded sample using an audio player or computer.

Transcription may be sped up by using free, downloadable, and user-friendly software, such as *Transcriber* (Barras, Geoffrois, Wu, & Liberman, 1998–2008). This software will allow you to divide

TABLE 6.8 Possible Transcription Format

			Minute 2
Time (sec.)	**Child's Utterances**	**Partner's Utterances**	**Nonlinguistic**
0			
		What do you need now?	
10			
	Can I have the truck?		*C looks at partner*
			C points to truck
20		*Which one?*	
	That one		
			C reaches for truck
		Oh, the red one	*P hands truck*
		Okay	
30		*Now can we go on vacation?*	
	Bro-o-om		*C pushes car*
40	*We need gas first*		*C looks at partner*
			C points to gas station
		Well then	
		I'll drive my car over, too	*P moves car to gas station*
50			
			C moves car to gas station
		What else do we need?	
	Gotta get soda and chips		
60			

the audio stream into utterance segments that you can listen to any number of times while transcribing without removing your hands from your keyboard. *Transcriber* displays the transcript in the top portion of the screen and the waveform in the bottom.

To segment into utterances, you press enter on the keyboard while listening to the audio file. After each utterance of the audio file is segmented, you can listen to each one individually using a simple keystroke as many times as necessary to transcribe it. The "export-to-text" feature generates a text file that can then be used for analysis. You can download *Transcriber* at www.nch.com.au/scribe/index.html.

There are a number of available computer software programs for accurately and efficiently analyzing a language sample (Long, 2001; Long & Channell, 2001). These include

- CLAN program (MacWhinney, 2000a, 2000b).
- Computerized Profiling (Long, Fey, & Channell, 1998).
- SALT (www.languageanalysislab.com; Miller & Iglesias, 2006).

The SLP transcribes the linguistic behavior of both the child and the conversational partner, along with the nonlinguistic behaviors of each. The timesheet format in graphically Table 6.8 enables the SLP to graphically evaluate delays or latencies on the part of the child.

All of the child's utterances, including false starts, nonfluencies, and fillers, are transcribed. Although these linguistic elements may not be used for calculation of utterance length, they are extremely important in determining language and communication difficulties.

All utterances of the conversational partner(s) also are transcribed. These are important in assessing the manner and style of the conversational partners. The SLP is interested in the amount of control and the amount and type of talking exhibited by the partner.

Determining utterance boundaries is often difficult. This is not an exact science, and the artistry of an SLP is needed at this point. An *utterance* is a complete thought that is divided from other utterances by sentence boundaries, pauses, and/or a drop in the voice. Table 6.9 contains examples of utterance boundaries.

TABLE 6.9 Utterance Boundaries

A sentence is an utterance.

Mommy went to the doctor's tomor . . . yesterday.

Run-on sentences with *and* should contain no more than one *and* joining clauses.

We went in a bus and we saw monkeys and we had a picnic and we petted the sheeps and one sheep sneezed on me and we had sodas and we came home.

Utterances:

1. We went in a bus and we saw monkeys.
2. (And) we had a picnic and we petted the sheeps.
3. (And) one sheep sneezed on me and we had sodas.
4. (And) we came home.

Other complex or compound sentences should be treated as one utterance.

He was mad because his mommy spanked him because he broke the lamp and spilled the doggie's water.

Imperative sentences are utterances.

Go home.

Pauses, voice drops, and/or inhalations mark boundaries.

Eat (pause and voice drop) . . . chocolate candy.

Two utterances: Eat. Chocolate candy.

Eat (momentary delay) . . . chocolate candy.

One utterance: Eat chocolate candy.

Situational and nonlinguistic cues help to determine boundaries.

Eat (hands plate to partner insistently) . . . chocolate candy (points to candy dish).

Two utterances: Eat. Chocolate candy.

Want (reaches unsuccessfully) . . . mommy (turns to look).

Two utterances: Want. Mommy.

Want mommy (reaches unsuccessfully).

One utterance: Want, mommy.

The linguistic context also helps.

Partner: Well, what do you want?

Child: Candy (pause) . . . you get it.

Two utterances: Candy. You get it.

Declaring sentences to be utterances is easy. Most of what is said, however, is not in complete sentence form. For example, the response to a question often omits shared information and might consist of such responses as "No," "Cookie," and "Okay." Each of these is a complete utterance. Longer responses, such as "No, later" or "No, let's go later," are also single utterances. This determination might change if the child were to respond with a pause and a drop in the voice after "No." "No (pause and drop voice). Let's go later." Now there are two utterances.

Partial sentences or phrases, nonfluent units, and run-on sentences are even more difficult. A partial sentence might consist of the child pointing to an object and saying, "Doggie." This would count as an utterance. Parts of sentences may be strung together, as in the following exchange in which the child makes an internal repair:

Partner: I like to play mommy.
Child: No, you not . . . me the . . . you baby.

The entire unit is an utterance and will be analyzed in different ways by using all or part of what the child said.

For run-on sentences, the SLP can follow the general rule that allows two clauses to be joined together in a sentence with *and*. In the following example, sentence/utterance boundaries have been marked as they might be on a transcript:

> [I went to the party, and we ate pizza] [(and) We played games, and I won a prize] [(and) We had cake and ice cream.]

Division can be aided by the child's pauses and breath patterns. Children in the late preschool years often make long strings of clauses with *and* meaning *and then*. Counting these as a single utterance inflates the mean utterance length. Young children are less likely to form run-ons with other conjunctions. Once the sample is transcribed, it can be analyzed.

The use of computerized analysis programs, such as the Systematic Analysis of Language Transcripts (SALT), requires a consistent transcription format (Miller & Chapman, 2003) (see Appendix B). This format will include not only the utterances but also the symbols for the program to aid it in identifying morphological markers and syntactic categories. Usually, multiple analyses can be performed without reentering the transcript or with only minor changes to accommodate different transcription conventions and analytic capabilities.

Collecting Samples of Written Language

With school-age children and adolescents, an SLP also will want to collect samples of their written language. Underlying language processes make it imperative that an SLP sample all modalities. Collection and analysis of written samples is explained in more detail in Chapter 13.

If a teacher suspects that a child has a language impairment, he or she should contact the school's SLP, who can ask the teacher to compile a portfolio of the child's written work. It should include first drafts of both narrative and expository writing.

In addition the SLP should elicit a written sample as he or she observes the child. In addition to the writing, the child's general demeanor, the presence of frustration, the amount of help needed, and the look and quality of the finished product will be of interest.

The child's written language can be compared to the spoken sample for similarities and differences. Of particular interest will be language features noted in the language of older children, such as cohesive devices, noun and verb phrase structure, illocutionary functions, vocabulary and word relationships, conjoining and embedding, along with spelling and penmanship. These will all be discussed in later chapters.

Conclusion

Collecting a representative language sample that demonstrates a child's diverse abilities is a difficult task. Careful planning and execution are required, as are exacting methods of recording and transcription. Although these procedures may seem difficult and time-consuming initially, they can be accomplished easily and relatively quickly with practice. A properly planned and executed sampling and a thorough transcription will yield an abundance of linguistic and nonlinguistic information.

Guides for collecting a language sample include the following:

- Establish a positive relationship with the child before recording the language sample.
- Reduce your authority-figure persona to ensure more participation by the child. A child is more likely to respond naturally with someone who is an equal.
- Be unobtrusive while collecting the sample so that the child is less conscious of the process.
- The conversational partner should keep talking to a minimum. Although SLPs abhor a vacuum, when possible you should wait out the child when possible.
- Avoid yes/no questions and constituent questions (e.g., *what's that*?) that require only a one-word response from the child. Ask process rather than product questions (e.g., *how do you do that*?)
- Follow the child's lead in play and in the selection of topic. Determine the child's interests before beginning the collection process. Select those materials at the child's interest level that are likely to stimulate interest.
- If the child does not talk or responds in a very repetitive or stereotypic manner, model responses for the child or have another person model.
- Collect more than one sample.

Only through sampling the child's linguistic abilities in a conversational context can the SLP gain insight into how a child's language works for that child. This is the first step in designing intervention that is relevant to the child and thus more likely to generalize to use environments.

Chapter

7

Language Sample Analysis

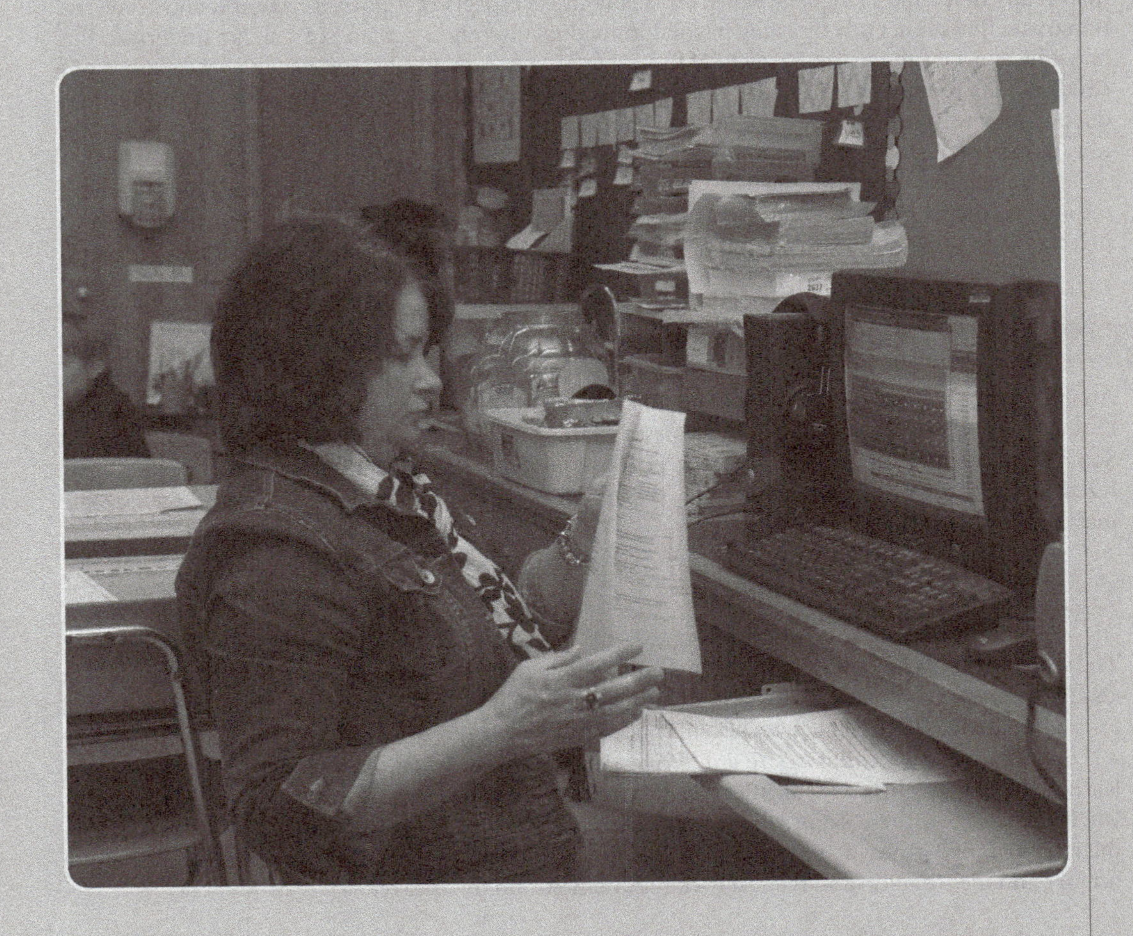

You probably analyzed a language sample in your language development course . . . and hated it! That may be because you found it extremely challenging. After all, you'd never done it before. But it may also reflect the global nature of the assignment: Analyze for everything! While I'll be reviewing many of the analyses possible with a sample, please remember that if we follow the model introduced in Chapter 4, by the time we get to sample analysis, hopefully, we have some idea what we're looking for and this fact can greatly shorten the process. Let's begin.

Language is complex, and the analysis methods used with a conversational sample reflect this complexity. You were afraid I'd say that, right? For this reason, analysis of a language sample should not be a fishing expedition for possible problems. Language analysis is best used to explore certain aspects of a child's behavior brought into question through other data collection methods.

Traditional analysis has focused exclusively on the utterance or sentence as the unit of analysis. Although this type of analysis is appropriate for many language features, it may not be the best way to assess behaviors that transcend these units. To analyze language only at the utterance level is to miss many of a child's language skills, especially those aspects that govern cohesion and conversational manipulation. Only by going beyond individual utterances can an SLP gain an understanding of a child's use of the many language skills required to communicate. For example, an analysis of a child's use of pronouns necessitates crossing utterance boundaries in order to describe the child's introduction of new information (*. . . a doggie*) and reference to old or established information (*He . . .*) that may have been introduced by the child or the conversational partner.

In this chapter, we explore analysis across utterances and partners, by communication event, and at the utterance level, noting the adjustments a child must make to meet conversational demands. Table 7.1 presents some types of analyses possible across utterances and partners and by communication event.

Across Utterances and Partners

Analysis at the utterance level reveals much about a child's discrete, finite language skills but may obscure a child's knowledge of the "big picture," the cohesion that threads through conversations. Some linguistic devices serve this cohesive purpose, and larger units than the utterance must be analyzed to assess their development. Other devices vary across whole conversations, and one sample may be very different from another.

Stylistic Variations

The style of talking, whether formal, casual, or varied in other ways for the situation, usually does not change utterance by utterance. Rather, it is a manner of talking with a specific language partner or in a specific situation. Different styles also may be seen in role-play.

As early as age 4, children use a different style of talking when they address younger children learning language. This style resembles *motherese* or *parentese*, the stylistic changes made by parents when they address these same younger children. Mature language users have a variety of styles at their disposal and can switch styles with little effort. Such variation requires a speaker to consider the listener and the situation and the resultant requirements on the speaker.

Register

Style switching, the move from one style or register to another, must be judged against the age, gender, and language ability of the speaker and the listener. Styles differ according to role-taking characteristics, dialectal variations, amount of politeness, and conversational control.

Conversational roles can be established by the topics chosen, vocabulary (*dear, sir, honey*), pronunciation, and the discourse style (formal, casual, playful, etc.) selected. Usually, the more dominant partner takes longer turns and asks more questions. The degree of politeness also varies. In general,

TABLE 7.1 Types of Analysis

Across Utterances and Partners	By Communication Event
Stylistic Variations	Social Versus Nonsocial
Register	Conversational Initiation: Method, Frequency, and Success Rate
Interlanguage and Code Switching	Topic Initiation: Method, Frequency, Success Rate, and Appropriateness
Channel Availability	Conversation and Topic Maintenance: Frequency and Latency of Contingency
Referential Communication	Duration of Topic: Number of Turns, Informativeness, and Sequencing
Presuppositional Skills: What Is Coded and How	Topic Analysis Format: Topic Initiation; Type of Topic; Manner of Initiation, Subject Matter, and Orientations; Outcome; Topic Maintenance: Type of Turn; and Conversational Information
Linguistic Devices: Deictics, Definite and Indefinite Reference	Turn Taking: Density, Latency, and Duration
Cohesive Devices	Overlap: Type, Frequency, and Duration
Reference: Initial and Following Mention	Signals
Ellipsis	Conversation and Topic Termination
Conjunction	Conversational Breakdown
Adverbial Conjuncts and Disjuncts	Request for Repair: Frequency and Form
Contrastive Stress	Conversational Repair
	Spontaneous Versus Listener-Initiated
	Strategy and Success Rate
Analysis at the Utterance Level	
Use	Form
Disruptions	Quantitative Measures
Illocutionary Functions and Intentions	Mean Length of Utterance
Frequency and Range	Mean Syntactic Length
Appropriateness	T-units and C-units
Encoding	Syntactic and Morphological Analysis
Content	Morphological Analysis
Lexical Items	Syntactical Analysis
Type-token Ratio	Noun Phrase
Over-/Underextensions and Incorrect Use	Verb Phrase
Style and Lexicon	Sentence Types
Word Relationships	Embedding and Conjoining
Semantic Categories	Computer-assisted Language Analysis
Intrasentence Relationships	
Figurative Language	
Word Finding	

speakers are more polite when in the less dominant role or when requesting something that belongs to or is controlled by the other partner, who may be unlikely to grant the request.

Children with LD often fail to use registers based on differing situational variables. Data suggest that these children do not adjust to different speakers or may adjust in different ways from TD children. Children with LD may fail to recognize the characteristics of different settings. Other children with LI may not be able to discriminate dominant from nondominant roles and the language form that goes with each. The most frequent problems with register include providing insufficient information for the listener, not knowing when to make a statement, asking inappropriate questions, giving insufficient reason for the cause and effect of a situation, and not adjusting register to the speaker. It may be especially difficult for a child who has been abused to express feelings and emotions. These expressions may be very direct.

When we study a sample to determine the stylistic variations present, the value of collecting language samples in two very different but client-appropriate situations is apparent. An SLP can look for a child's modifications in politeness, intimacy, and linguistic code based on the age, status, familiarity, cognitive level, linguistic level, and shared past experience of the listener. Of interest is the attention given to the listener's characteristics. In addition to noting stylistic variations, the SLP looks for inappropriate styles—those that are too formal, too casual, or include excessive swearing, for example.

The SLP might also note features such as differing utterance length with various partners. Other variations include vocabulary and topic. More subjective indices include intonational patterns and the use of attention-getting and maintaining devices.

Interlanguage and Code Switching

With ELLs, it is important to establish patterns of language use in both L_1 and L_2. Two possible patterns are called interlanguage and code switching. **Interlanguage** is a combination of the L_1 and L_2 rules, plus ad hoc rules from neither or both languages. This "hybrid" language may vary among children and within an individual child across situations. Usually, interlanguages are transitional in nature, but some features may stabilize as a permanent form, especially if there is little motivation to change. Of interest are the rules used by the child and any situational variables.

Linguistic **code switching** is the shifting from one language to another within and/or across different utterances. A complicated, rule-governed behavior, code switching does not signal poor language skills, although it may be used by children when they have inadequate English skills. As with interlanguage, code switching is influenced heavily by contextual and situational variables. For example, the Spanish-speaking storyteller might use English when referring to Anglos and Spanish when referring to Latinos. Code switching follows agreed-upon community rules and usually occurs to enhance meaning, emphasize a change of topic, and convey humor, ethnic solidarity, and attitudes toward the listener.

The SLP should note uses of interlanguage and code switching, along with sampling variables such as the situation and the partner(s). It is especially important to identify patterns that may impede the transmission of meaning or interrupt communication.

Channel Availability

Most children below age 11 experience less communication success when they do not visually share the communication environment with their listener, as when on the phone. As the number of communication channels decreases, a child with LI should have increasing difficulty communicating. In fact, children with LD often have great difficulty if forced to rely solely on the verbal channel. The SLP should note in the sample the relative success of the child's communication efforts as the number of channels varies.

Referential Communication

Referential communication is the ability of a speaker to select and verbally identify the attributes of an entity in such a way that the listener can identify the entity accurately. To succeed, the speaker must be able to determine what information the listener needs, deliver that information in a specific manner, make comparisons, and use feedback on message adequacy and breakdown. While "He has brown hair" fails to communicate the referent, "The only boy in my history class has brown hair" succeeds.

Referential communication includes directions, explanations, and descriptions. These are three essential aspects of classroom discourse, and their impairment may contribute to the academic difficulties of children with LD.

Presuppositional Skills

Presupposition is a speaker's assumptions about both the context and the listener's knowledge that, in turn, influence the speaker's utterances. The speaker must take the conversational perspective of the listener(s) and determine what information to communicate and its form.

For most children, the ability to consider a partner's perspective is well established by age 10. Production requires knowing how and when to provide information. Children with LD have poor referential skills and are less likely to adjust to the listener and more likely to provide ambiguous and insufficient information.

As an SLP, be alert to the informativeness of a child's utterances and to the social context. The following questions can be applied to the sample.

- What does the child choose to encode?
- Does the child encode what is novel or merely comment on what is already given?
- Does the child encode new information gesturally, linguistically, or both?
- Are messages informative, vague, or ambiguous?
- Are different referents clearly established?
- Does the child talk differently about things present in the context and things that are not?

Noninformative language can take several forms. Table 7.2 presents forms and examples seen in children with LI. These types of noninformative language may be especially relevant to the language of children with TBI and LD. The SLP can rate utterances to determine the strategy used by the child.

Linguistic Devices

Several linguistic devices are used to mark informativeness, including deictics and direct/indirect reference. Both of these devices can be used to note referents internal or external to the conversation; other cohesive devices, listed in Table 7.3, establish relations entirely within the discourse.

Deictics. As mentioned in Chapter 6, deictic terms are linguistic elements that must be interpreted from the perspective of the speaker in order to be understood as the speaker intended. The use of deixis is based on the *speaker principle*, in which the referential point shifts as speakers change, and on the *distance principle*, in which referents are coded by their distance from the speaker.

Words with deictic meanings appear in several word classes, including personal pronouns (*I/me* and *you*), demonstrative adjectives (*this, that, these,* and *those*), adverbs of time (*before, after, now,* and *then*), adverbs of location (*here* and *there*), and verbs (*come* and *go*). A child's behavior, especially the errors, should be analyzed to determine confusion or overreliance on one principle or one aspect of a principle.

TABLE 7.2 Types of Noninformative Language

Empty phrases (common idioms, such as *and so on* and *et cetera, excetera*)
Indefinite terms and highly nonspecific nouns (*one, thing, that*)
Deictic terms (*this, that, here, there*)
Pronouns used without antecedent nouns
Comments on task instead of stimulus
Neologisms (*Oh, you know the one that you fly in*)
Paraphrases
Repeated words or phrases
Personal value judgments about the stimulus (*That's pretty dumb*)
Use of *and* alone
Conjunctions *but, so, or,* and *because* alone

TABLE 7.3 Cohesive Devices Used in English

Relation	Explanation	Example
Reference	Initially, the entity is named and may use the indefinite article (*a/an*). Subsequent mention may use a pronoun, words such as *this, that,* and *one*, or use the definite article (*the*) with the noun.	*John* went looking for *a car*. He found *one* in the city. I want to buy *a coat*, but *that one* I saw last night is too expensive.
Ellipsis	Subsequent sentences omit redundant or shared information.	Who *ate all the cookies?* I did [eat all the cookies]. I would like to *make a phone call*. May I [make a phone call]?
Conjunction	Conjunctions join clauses to express additive, causal, and other relationships.	We went to the circus, *and* I saw elephants. John's angry *because* I drank his soda.

Definite and Indefinite Reference. A mature language user is able to mark specific (definite) and nonspecific (indefinite) referents by manipulation of definite (*the*) and indefinite (*a/an*) articles. The speaker must consider what the listener knows about the topic under discussion.

Article use can be especially difficult for a child with LI. In part, this difficulty may reflect the use of articles in English to mark new and old information also. The tendency for children with LI is to overuse the definite article the. Each article present in the sample can be analyzed for appropriate referential use. Note that Asian American ELLs may omit articles reflecting nonuse in many Asian languages.

Cohesive Devices

Conversational *cohesion*, how language hangs together, can be a useful analysis tool. Cohesion can be expressed through both syntax and vocabulary. For example, a pronoun or a demonstrative, such as *this* or *that*, can refer to the referent, which was identified previously in the conversation. *Conjoining*, the connection of phrases, clauses, and sentences through the use of such conjunctions as *and, because*, and *if*, also is used for cohesion. The major cohesive devices used in English are listed in Table 7.3.

The most frequent problems of cohesion relate to providing redundant information, deleting necessary information, using unclear and ambiguous reference, sequencing old and new information, and marking old and new information with articles and pronouns. In short, errors usually reflect including or excluding information or confusing new and old information.

Reference

Reference is a linguistic device used continuously in conversation to keep information flowing and to designate new and old information. In the process, new information is stated clearly and then subsequently implied by the referral to it as old information, one utterance presupposing the other. We'll explore all this in the following section. Some children with language impairments, such as children with ASD, have difficulty marking new and old information.

An SLP can note the method of introducing new information and the use of following mention. Speakers should ensure that listeners can easily determine relationships.

Initial Mention. In initial mention, mature speakers establish mutual reference clearly, especially if the entity mentioned is not present. Generally, the referent name is stressed and preceded by the indefinite article (*a/an*). In English, the referent often is placed at the end of the sentence, the most salient position. The following are examples of the introduction of new information:

Did you see *John at the party*?

We went to a *circus* yesterday.

In addition, referents that are present may be pointed to or handled. Young children tend to rely more on these nonlinguistic behaviors to establish new referents.

Children with LD or ASD have difficulty with new information. As speakers, they may not identify new information for the listener. As listeners, these children may have difficulty identifying the new information but will ask few questions to clarify.

Children with word-finding difficulties or poor vocabularies may use empty words, such as *that, one*, or *thing*, that do not help clarify the referent. These children may rely on the immediate context and use pointing to specify the referent that their nonspecific vocabulary failed to identify.

Following Mention. In following mention, previously identified referents often are moved to the initial position in English sentences and may be referred to by the use of the definite article (*the*) or a pronoun. "Did you see John at the party?" might be followed by "*He was* so thrilled." Pronoun use is appropriate when the referent is unambiguous or clearly identified. The pronoun should be in close proximity so that there is no confusion as to which noun it refers.

An SLP is interested in the way a child introduces new information and refers to that information later. Also of interest is any confusion with article and pronoun use. It is not uncommon for a preschool child or a child with LD to introduce new information with "She did it," leaving the listener to determine who *she* is and what *it* is.

Ellipsis

Ellipsis is a process in which redundant information is omitted. For example, the response to "What do you want?" is "Cookie," which omits the shared information "I want."

Elliptical fragments are used frequently to keep the conversation moving smoothly and rapidly, but they are missed if linguistic analysis concentrates solely on full sentences or fails to look across partners. Children with LI may not realize that information is shared or may assume that it is shared when it is not. Either assumption interferes with the flow of conversation.

Conjunctions

Conjunctions, such as *and, then, so, and therefore*, are used to connect thoughts. Although preschool children have several conjunction-type words in their vocabularies, they rarely use them to join clauses.

Just as conjunctions can be analyzed at the utterance level because of their use in linking clauses, conjunctions can be analyzed across utterances, as in the following exchange.

Parent: We had a great day at the zoo. I liked the monkeys best.
Child: *And* feeding the deer babies.

Analysis at the level of the child's utterance alone would miss the child's considerable skill.

Adverbial Conjuncts and Disjuncts

Adverbial conjuncts and disjuncts are conversational devices used for cohesion. *Conjuncts* are intersentential forms that express a logical relationship, such as the conjunctions *then* or *so*. Conjuncts are of two types: *concordant*, such as *similarly, consequently*, and *moreover*, and *discordant*, such as *nevertheless, rather*, and *in contrast*. *Disjuncts* are used to comment on or to convey the speaker's attitude toward the topic and include words and phrases such as *honestly, frankly, perhaps, however, yet, to my surprise, it's obvious to me that*, and the like.

Conjuncts and disjuncts develop rather late in childhood and, therefore, may be good measures of adolescent language. By age 12, children use only an average of 4 conjuncts per 100 utterances. In contrast, adults average 12 conjuncts per 100 utterances. Children between ages 6 and 12 use conjuncts infrequently and rely most frequently on *then*, so, and *though*. Adolescents use the same conjuncts but also use *therefore, however, rather*, and *consequently* most accurately in both their reading and writing. Comprehension seems to be better than production although similar.

Contrastive Stress

Contrastive stress or emphasis can be used to negate or correct the message of a conversational partner. For example, if one speaker said, "Jose brought the cookies," the other might correct, "*Mary* brought the cookies." Again, an SLP must transcend the traditional utterance-level analysis.

Communication Event

The term **communication event** can represent an entire conversation or a portion thereof that includes one topic. For purposes of our discussion, we use the larger definition and include within it a conversation that comprises one or more topics.

Usually, a shared or negotiated agenda(s) occurs within a conversation. Utterances within the event support this agenda. The teenager who wants to be granted a privilege, such as getting to use the family car, is polite, and each utterance supports this agenda.

The social organization of discourse consists of the two roles of speaker and listener. The effective communicator has the ability to function in and contribute to the conversation by assuming responsibility for both roles. Assessment variables that might measure a child's ability to participate effectively are the amount of socialized speech and a child's adaptive style; conversation and topic initiation, maintenance, and termination; the completeness, relevance, and clarity of a child's behavior; on-topic exchanges and turn taking; and conversational repairs. We'll discuss all of these.

Analysis occurs at two levels: the molar and the molecular. At the *molar level*, an SLP evaluates each behavior for appropriateness or inappropriateness within the conversational context. Inappropriate behaviors may indicate problem areas for further assessment. At the *molecular level*, an SLP is interested in the *frequency, latency, duration, density*, and *sequence* of the child's behaviors.

Decisions of appropriateness may be facilitated through the use of a modified ethnographic technique similar to that used in anthropological studies. Using an expository form of writing, an SLP attempts to describe each child utterance with reference to form, content, and use, discourse relations, code switching, learning and cognitive style, and the partner's arrangement and selection of nonlinguistic strategies, materials, and procedures. Thus, each utterance is given a reference frame in which to judge appropriateness. Table 7.4 provides a sample of a dialogue and the accompanying ethnographic analysis. Ethnographic techniques are especially important when assessing children with CLD backgrounds.

Frequency data will reveal inordinately high- or low-frequency features and information on the range of features. *Latency*, the span of time when an individual does not engage in behavior, is also important. Pauses and hesitations may reveal difficulty decoding the preceding utterance or forming a response. *Duration* is the length of time that a child and a partner are engaged in a certain behavior, such as conversational gaze or conversational turns by both partners. *Density* is the number of behaviors within a certain period of time. Of interest are the density of different conversational topics or specific linguistic structures, such as questions. *Sequence* includes the order of events within a topic or conversation. A child exhibiting difficulty with sequencing of a conversation may not understand the rules of conversational participation.

TABLE 7.4 An Example of Ethnographic Analysis

Language Sample	Ethnographic Analysis
Child: What's that? *Partner:* That's a "Thing-a-majibit." *Child:* What it do?	Child does not seem to know the identity of an object and inquires as to its name with an appropriate *wh-* question addressed to the partner. The partner supplies an appropriate answer but does not elaborate. The child seeks such elaboration by asking a second *wh-* question in which he omits the auxiliary verb. Other sentence elements are included in the proper adult word order.
Partner: What do you think it does? *Child:* On the table.	The partner does not answer the question but responds with a second *wh-* question in order to have the child guess at the function from its appearance. The child responds inappropriately to the partner's question, either ignoring the content of the question or miscomprehending the meaning of the *wh-* word.
Partner: YES, on the table. What about "On the table?" *Child:* On the table.	The partner does not pursue the question by restating or reformulating it. Instead, the partner confirms the child's utterance and asks a third *wh-* question incorporating the child's utterance. Again, the child does not respond to the content of the partner's question but repeats the previous utterance with no additional information to aid the partner's understanding.

Social versus Nonsocial

Social speech is speech addressed explicitly to and adapted for a listener. It is characterized by explicitness and clarity, repairs of breakdowns, and an obligation for a listener to respond. Social communication includes dialogues and social monologues addressed to a listener or uttered for the mutual enjoyment of both the speaker and listener. A lecture or recounting a story is a social monologue. The speaker adapts the explicitness of the message for the listener and repairs breakdowns. The speaker's message is delivered as if the speaker expects a listener response.

In contrast, *nonsocial speech* is not addressed explicitly to a listener, and the listener has no obligation to respond. An important measure of communication is the percentage of the child's utterances or the amount of total talk time that can be characterized as social.

Although preschoolers produce many asocial monologues accompanying their play, the amount of time spent in this type of production decreases with age. School-age children developing typically produce very little nonsocial speech. In general, children's communication becomes more interpersonal as they mature. In contrast, the speech of some children with ASD may contain many asocial monologues.

Conversational Initiation

The most efficient way to initiate a conversation is to gain your listener's attention, greet the listener, and clearly state the topic of conversation or some opener, such as, "Guess what happened to me yesterday?" or "Where have you been? I haven't seen you in ages." Openers set the tone of the conversation and the subsequent turns. Opening and closing a conversation is one of the pragmatic problems most frequently encountered in children with LI. Children with ASD may initiate very little conversational behavior. Of clinical interest is how a child initiates the conversation and how successful he or she is in having the conversation continue.

Method

It is best to get a potential listener's attention before initiating a conversation. This usually is accomplished by eye contact and a greeting. A child with LI may begin without any greeting or may interrupt an ongoing conversation with, "Hey." While in a classroom recently, I become aware that a preschooler was talking to my butt. He had neither sought my attention nor offered a greeting. Some children use the same opener repeatedly (e.g., "Guess what?"), whatever the conversational context. Data may need to be collected over a wide variety of situations or by parental or teacher report to discern a pattern.

Frequency and Success Rate

Children who are withdrawn or unsure of the conversational expectations may initiate conversations only rarely. Instead, they adopt a more passive, responsive role. In contrast, other children may interrupt frequently and attempt to initiate conversation indiscriminately. Of interest to an SLP is the density of initiations, or the number of initiations over a given time. Obviously, this figure will change with the situation.

The success rate of children in initiating conversations is also significant. Although children may attempt to begin conversations frequently, they may be ignored or mocked, depending on the audiences they choose. Children who are socially inappropriate may experience more than their share.

Topic Initiation

Once a conversation has been initiated, the participants negotiate the topics. **Topic** is subject matter being discussed. The process begins with one partner introducing a topic; the other partner agrees to adopt that topic by commenting on it, disagrees by changing the topic, or ends the conversation. Mature speakers identify the topic clearly by name and, if in the immediate context, by pointing. Preschool children and those with LI rely more on nonlinguistic cues, such as pointing to and holding or shaking objects.

In general, children with LI are less adept than both their age-matched and language-age-matched peers in their ability to direct the conversation by introducing topics. This lack of ability might reflect difficulty introducing topics clearly and/or these children's limited lists of potential topics.

Method

An effectively initiated topic is identified clearly. Generally, the speaker provides information the listener needs to identify referents and their relationships. Topics are negotiated between speakers, and even when explicitly stated, topics are based on the shared assumptions of each participant.

In general, the less sure a speaker is that a listener knows the topic, the longer the speaker will take to introduce it. In return for the introduction, listeners assure speakers that they understand, or they ask for clarification when they do not understand.

Topics typically are changed by stating a new, often related, one. Although we don't possess much normative data, we know that between seventh and twelfth grade the number of abrupt topic shifts in an adolescent conversation decreases from 3.19 to 1.44.

A child with LI may not establish topics, preferring to adopt those of others. If a child does introduce topics, there may be little or no background information to aid the listener. A child with LI may have a very restricted set of conversational or topic openers or may rely on a stereotypic utterance (e.g., "Guess what?"). Children with emotional difficulties may continue the conversation with the assumption that the listener has been privy to this information. As mentioned previously, children with word-finding difficulties or poor vocabularies may rely on nonspecific nouns, such as *one* or *thing*. Nonspecific verbs, such as *do* and *get*, also may be used frequently. "I did that one" may not get the topic off to a roaring start.

A child's responses to the openers of others may be nonexistent or noncontingent/off-topic. The child with LI may not be able to identify the topic or to determine what response is required.

Both the linguistic and nonlinguistic aspects of a sample should be analyzed. The nonlinguistic aspects, such as eye contact, regulate the linguistic ones and are significant in the regulation of turn initiation and termination, topic choice, and interruptions.

Frequency and Success Rate

As with conversational initiation, the density and success rate of topic initiation are noteworthy. In general, less dominant speakers will introduce fewer topics and will be less successful in having their topics adopted by their partners. Lack of success also may indicate problems with topicalization, such as establishing and commenting on, marking changes in, and maintaining the topic for a sufficient length of time. Related factors to be evaluated are the articulation clarity, degree of completeness, and form of the topic statement; social adaptation of a child's language style; degree of content relevance to the ongoing activity and to listener interests; use of eye contact; and physical proximity.

Appropriateness

The appropriateness of a topic is determined by the context. Some topics, such as the weather, are always appropriate, whereas others, such as age, income, or sexual behavior, are appropriate only in limited contexts.

As an SLP, you'll be interested in determining a child's favorite topics and in assessing their appropriateness in context. Although some topics will work in one context, they are inappropriate for others. Some children with LI have only limited topics or perseverate on a few regardless of the context. I worked with two brothers with ASD who seemingly could talk only about mathematics. A third child with severe LD seemed limited to discussing—Excuse me—throwing up, a topic with little appeal.

Conversation and Topic Maintenance

Once a topic is introduced, speakers comment, each sentence reflecting the general discourse topic. In effective conversations, the participants seem to adhere to four principles: stay on topic, be truthful, be brief, and be relevant.

Each partner depends on a response's *contingency*, or relatedness to the preceding utterance. Each response adds new information on the topic. The topic is mentioned frequently enough to enable both participants to recall it as the conversation progresses, because the topic becomes less specific with each subsequent reference.

Topic continuance may be signaled by maintenance devices, such as *now, well, and then, in any case, next*, so, followed by *I* (*you, we, they*) (did something). Some devices, called *continuants*, maintain the conversation but add little if any new information. Examples of this behavior are *yeah, uh-huh*, and *okay* when used as a signal that the listener is paying attention. Other maintenance devices are repeating a portion or all of the previous utterance.

Children with LI tend to engage in fewer and shorter interactions than do children developing typically. The most frequent pragmatic problems for children with LI include connecting discourse cohesively, listening and responding to a speaker, knowing when to take a turn, and knowing how to ask and answer questions.

The difference between the turn-taking skills of children with LI and of those without widens as language becomes increasingly more complex. Children with ASD may not respond to initiations, while other children with LI may overuse turn-fillers or acknowledgments (*uh-huh*) to keep the conversation going even when their comprehension is lacking.

Frequency of Contingency

Semantically contingent utterances relate to or reflect the meaning of the prior utterance. Thus, a contingent utterance maintains the topic of the previous utterance and adds to it in some way. For example, in response to the utterance, "We went to Captain Jake's for dinner last night," a second speaker might make the contingent remark “Oh, did you enjoy the food?” A noncontingent remark would be “My uncle lives on a farm.”

In general, children with LI are less responsive than are their age-matched TD peers. Instead these children may respond to questions with stereotypic acknowledgments (*uh-huh, yeh*) and with nonspecific requests for clarification (*what, huh*).

The frequency of contingent behaviors by a child and caregiver also is of interest. The child who exhibits few contingent utterances may prefer to initiate new topics instead. The SLP can note the percentage of a child’s utterances that are on-topic, the relevance of the child’s questions, and the child’s nonverbal responses, such as following directions or looking at something that was mentioned.

A large percentage of off-topic responses may indicate a semantic disorder characterized by difficulty in identifying the topic of discussion. A listener’s ability to identify a topic subsequently affects comprehension of comments made about that topic. Imagine responding to “what do you think?” when you can’t identify what’s being discussed.

The SLP should look for an underlying contingency that may not be readily obvious. Children with LD may assume that their partners know the underlying relationship and, therefore, may only include unshared information.

Of particular interest are the child’s responses to questions. Such responses should be appropriate to the question. For example, the question “Why is the man eating?” might elicit the following responses from different children:

1. Food.
2. Because.
3. He has to.
4. So he won’t be hungry.
5. He’s hungry.

The first answer is inappropriate although functionally accurate. It does not answer the question, but tells what the man is eating. The second and third responses are appropriate but too brief to be accurate. The fourth and fifth answers fulfill appropriateness and accuracy criteria.

If an answer does not fulfill both appropriateness and accuracy requirements, it is in error and may indicate any number of possible breakdowns in the communication process. I worked with a child with a severe emotional disorder who gave extremely inappropriate replies to emotional or personal questions, although her responses to factual questions were usually both appropriate and accurate.

A child with LI may not understand what the questioner desires or may not realize that a reply is required. The question form and the specific *wh-* question type also may be confusing. Some *wh-* question forms seem easier than others. Three groupings, from easiest to most difficult, are as follows:

Easiest	What + be, which, where
	Who, whose, what + do
Most difficult	When, why, what happened, how

This order suggests a hierarchy for both analysis and intervention. In addition, it is easier for children to respond to questions referring to objects, persons, or events within the immediate setting.

Latency of Contingency

When a child makes a contingent response, there should be little delay or latency between his or her turn and the preceding speaker’s turn. Preschoolers and children with LI may allow long gaps to develop without any of the apparent embarrassment found among adults when there are long unfilled pauses. A noticeable latency prior to a child’s response may indicate word-finding difficulties, lack of comprehension, or difficulty forming a reply.

Latency is an important measure for both contingent and noncontingent utterances, whether adjacent or nonadjacent. Adjacent utterances are spoken as sequential behaviors by the same speaker. A nonadjacent utterance crosses conversational turns and is an utterance or turn of one partner followed by an utterance or turn of the other. Definitions and examples of these categories are presented in Table 7.5.

Duration of Topic

A topic is sustained as long as each conversational partner cares to continue and can contribute relevant information. The number of turns taken on a topic is a function of the particular topic and partners involved, the conversational context, and the conversational skill of each participant.

Number of Turns on a Topic

The SLP is interested in the number of turns taken by a child and a partner on a given topic and in the manner of changing topic. In general, a greater number of turns will occur in an adult–child conversation if the child, rather than the adult, initiates the topic. Topics that are sustained longer than others may suggest the child's interest or knowledge or both.

Below age 3, children rarely maintain a topic for more than two turns. In general, preschoolers take very few turns on a single topic unless enacting scenarios, describing events, or solving problems. More turns generally will be produced when the preschool child is directing the partner through a task or when the child is telling a story. Although the number of turns increases slightly with age, a great increase does not occur until mid-elementary school.

Informativeness

Each turn should add to the conversation by confirming the topic and contributing additional information. Children who have difficulty identifying the topic or determining what is expected of them conversationally may repeat or paraphrase old information, overuse continuants, or circumlocute. Circumlocution occurs when a child is unable to identify the topic or retrieve needed words and thus talks around the topic in a nonspecific manner. The SLP can rate each utterance for its contribution to the topic being discussed.

Sequencing

Once a topic is introduced, a sequence of conversational acts follows. In general, more specific information is introduced until a natural termination or a change in topic occurs. Answers or replies

TABLE 7.5 Definitions and Examples of Utterance Pairs

Types	Definitions	Examples
Contingent	The utterance of one speaker is based on the content, form, and/or intent of the other speaker.	S_1: What do you want for lunch? S_2: Peanut butter. S_1: I hope I don't miss my plane. S_2: Don't worry. Every flight is delayed.
Noncontingent	The utterance of one speaker is not based on that of the other.	S_1: What do you want for lunch? S_2: Gran'ma gots a new car.
Adjacent	Utterances spoken sequentially by the same speaker.	We went to the zoo. I saw monkeys and elephants. But my favorite part was petting the sheeps.
Nonadjacent	Utterances spoken sequentially by different speakers. The utterances may be contingent or noncontingent.	S_1: Here comes the school bus. S_2: Yukk, I was hoping he'd get a flat tire. (Contingent)

follow questions; comments or questions follow comments. New information is introduced and later referred to as old information. A lack of sequencing may indicate a semantic disorder or a pragmatic disorder characterized by a lack of presuppositional abilities. Further analysis of conversational turns is discussed later in the chapter.

Topic Analysis Format

Several topic analysis formats have been proposed. Each addresses different aspects of topic initiation, maintenance, and change. These are presented in Table 7.6. Topic initiation analysis may include the type of topic, the manner of initiation, the subject matter and orientation, and the outcome. Topic maintenance analysis may consider the type of turn and the ability of the client to further the conversation with the addition of new conversational information.

Topic Initiation

Topic initiations occur when the topic of discussion is changed in some way. Utterances on that topic express concepts subsumed by that topic. Each new topic and directly related utterances can be identified on the transcript.

Type of Topic. Each topic can be rated according to its novelness. Some children have a limited range of topics in their repertoire. Possible rating categories may include *new, related, reintroduced*, and *rolling*. New topics would be those appearing in the conversation for the first time and not linked to the immediate preceding topic. Related topics would be linked directly to the previous topic. Reintroduced topics would have appeared in the conversation previously but prior to the immediate preceding turn. Finally, rolling topics are initiated in sequence with no opportunity for the listener to maintain the preceding topic or the first of the consecutive ones to be introduced. In addition, the SLP could check with the caregivers to determine whether any of the topics introduced by the child are habitual ones. Table 7.7 presents examples of different types of topic initiation.

Manner of Initiation. The manner of topic initiation might include *coherent changing, noncoherent changing, branching*, and *shading*. Coherent changing occurs when one topic is terminated and a following topic's content is not derived from the immediate preceding topic. Noncoherent changing occurs with the absence of topic termination and/or an utterance signaling transition to a new topic. Branching occurs when the topic being discussed serves as a source for a new topic. Shading differs from branching in that shading is a change of focus on the same topic, rather than a discrete topic change. Table 7.8 presents the different manners of initiation.

Subject Matter and Orientation. The *subject matter* is the content of the topic initiation. Two broad analyses might consist of judgments of appropriate versus inappropriate topics for the communication context. Orientation might include topics about self, a shared experience or interest with the listener, or a topic seemingly unrelated to the listener or a shared interest. If the topic is always the speaker or always unrelated, then serious communication problems may exist.

TABLE 7.6 Analysis Aspects of Topic

Topic Initiation	Topic Maintenance
Type of topic	Type of turn
Manner of initiation	Conversational information
Subject matter and orientation	
Outcome	

TABLE 7.7 Types of Topics Initiated

Topic Type	Example
New	*Partner:* Uh-huh, and what else did you see at the zoo? *Child:* Mommy got a new car.
Related	*Partner:* I like monkeys too. What else? Were there any clowns at the circus? *Child:* I don't like clowns. They're scary. *Partner:* Clowns are scary? Why do you think clowns are scary?
Reintroduced	*Child:* And Ernie spilled s'ghetti all over Bert. *Partner:* Was Bert angry? *Child:* Uh-huh. And . . . and Ernie .?. . And Ernie laughed. *Partner:* Poor Bert. That would be yukky. What else happened on *Sesame Street?* *Child:* Big Bird and Little Bird singed a song. *Partner:* Can you sing it for me? *Child:* Uh-huh. I don't like s'ghetti on me.
Rolling	*Partner:* Oh, tell me the story. *Child:* Okay. This little girl .?. . Can you come to my birthday party? I got a new bike yesterday. Do you live here?

TABLE 7.8 Manner of Topic Initiation

Manner of Initiation	Example
Coherent changing	*Child:* And he chased the dinosaur away. *Partner:* What a great story. Anything else to tell? *Child:* I have a new baby.
Noncoherent changing	*Child:* Let's have toast for breakfast. *Partner:* Let me fix it. *Child:* Those are supposed to go down. *Partner:* You do this one, and I'll do the other one. *Child:* I'm gonna have a bowl of . . . What's that? I think it's a fireman hat. I wanta be a fireman. *Partner:* May I wear it?
Branching	*Partner:* There, I'm gonna make some eggs. *Child:* I don't like eggs. *Partner:* No, why don't you like eggs? *Child:* I want some?. . . some juice. I like juice. *Partner:* What kind of juice do you want?
Shading	*Partner:* Let's have toast. *Child:* Where's the toaster? *Partner:* I'll cook the toast. *Child:* I'll butter it. Where's the knife? *Partner:* You have to find the knife. *Child:* It too sharp for toast.

Outcome. Outcomes may be rated as successful or unsuccessful. Success is dependent on the manner of initiation, the subject matter, and the form of the initiation. Success occurs when the conversational partner acknowledges the speaker's topic in some way, responds, repeats, agrees or disagrees, or adds information to maintain the topic. Nonsuccess includes no response, an interruption, initiation of a new topic, or a request for repair. Although there are many variables related to success, the percentage of time that a child is successful can be an important descriptive index.

Topic Maintenance. Topic maintenance would be analyzed in all turns subsequent to topic initiation. Each turn can be analyzed on the basis of the continuous or discontinuous nature of the turn and on its informativeness.

Type of Turn. Turns may be classified as continuous or discontinuous on the basis of their linkage or nonlinkage to the topic (see Table 7.9). Continuous turns continue the topic in some way. Discontinuous turns—ones not linked to the current topic—include new topic initiations, off-topic responses, monologues, and evasion, including inappropriate silence.

Analysis includes the frequency and range of each type of turn and the average number of turns per topic. The percentage of continuous versus discontinuous turns also would be valuable data as a descriptive value although no norms exist.

Conversational Information. Turns might be analyzed for the extent to which they contribute to the development of the topic by adding relevant, novel information. Those adding new information include topic incorporation, such as unsolicited conversational replies that add more information or requests for new information, and answers and replies to questions that contain new information. Other turns—such as acknowledgments; requests for repair; partial, whole, or expanded repetitions; responses to requests or questions that do not contain new information; emotional responses; and agreement or disagreement—add no new information to the conversational exchange. Problematic turns include word searching, incoherent utterances, ambiguous utterances, and incomplete turns. Examples of conversational informativeness are included in Table 7.10.

TABLE 7.9 Continuous and Discontinuous Turns

Type of Turn	Example
Continuous	*Partner:* What's that? *Child:* A cowboy hat. *Partner:* Put it on. *Child:* No, it's too hot for a coat. *Partner:* We have to make some bread for dinner. *Child:* Okay, I'll help.
Discontinuous	*Partner:* Do you want to hold the baby? *Child:* I'll eat my cupcake now. *Partner:* What else happened at school? *Child:* I don't like my baby brother.

TABLE 7.10 Informativeness of Turns

Informativeness	Example
New information	*Partner:* Where's Mary? *Child:* She's sick today. *Partner:* We're going to the zoo tomorrow. *Child:* Monkeys live in the zoo.
No new information	*Partner:* And cowboys ride horsies too. *Child:* Ride horsie. *Partner:* Let's play with the stove. *Child:* What?
Problematic	*Partner:* What should we play now? *Child:* A . . . a . . . with a . . . a . . . with a . . . you know. *Partner:* Who's your teacher? *Child:* At school.

The SLP can calculate the percentage of turns contributing novel information and thus furthering the topic. Other types of turns may indicate possible problem areas. Specific strategies used by children should be investigated by analyzing the form of the utterances being used.

Summary

The topic analysis categories presented in this section overlap and are not always mutually exclusive. More than one turn type and informativeness category may be present in a turn. A possible analysis format is presented in Table 7.11. Each type of analysis gives an SLP an additional tool for sorting the child's language data.

TABLE 7.11 Possible Format for Rating Topics and Turns

	Turns																			
Categories	1	2	3	4	5	6	7	8	9	10	11	12	13	14	15	16	17	18	Total	% of Total
Topic Initiation																				
Type of topic																				
New																				
Related																				
Reintroduced																				
Rolling																				
Manner of initiation																				
Coherent change																				
Noncoherent change																				
Branching																				
Shading																				
Subject matter																				
Appropriate																				
Inappropriate																				
Orientation																				
Self																				
Shared																				
Unrelated																				
Outcome																				
Successful																				
Unsuccesful																				
Topic Maintenance																				
Type of turn																				
Continuous																				
Discontinuous																				
Conversational information																				
New information																				
No new information																				
Problematic																				

Turn Taking

Turn taking is an excellent vehicle for evaluating the interactional framework of a listener and a speaker. The unit of analysis is the dyad (both partners) and the interaction.

The minimum number of turns to complete an exchange is three. The person who begins the exchange must have a second turn before an interaction has occurred: for example,

Speaker 1: We just returned from Florida.
Speaker 2: Oh, did you go to Disney World?
Speaker 1: No, we were in Fort Lauderdale. Ever been there?

Each full conversational turn consists of three elements: an acknowledgment of the preceding utterance, a contribution by the present speaker, and an indication that the turn is to be shifted. In the preceding example, the previous turns are acknowledged by *oh* and *no*. Indications of turn allocation may consist of questions, intonational markers, and pauses.

An SLP can mark each exchange on the transcript, numbering it *turn 1, 2, 3*, etc. In other words, a child's ability to initiate, add to, and terminate exchanges can be noted. Of particular interest are eye contact, turn allocation signaling, and the location and cause of exchange breakdown. In addition, an SLP can indicate the frequency, variety or range, and consistency of a child's communication. Within each turn, the SLP notes the presence or absence of the three aspects of a full turn and the average amount of time spent in a turn. The SLP also can examine the effects of adult behaviors on the child's conversational turns and later can help adults develop more facilitative styles.

Turns may be classified as *obligation, comment, or reply*. An obligation is initiated by the speaker and demands a response. In contrast, a comment does not require a response. A reply can be to either an obligation or a comment. The percentage of each category may indicate active and passive speakers, those that initiate and those that respond.

All responses to obligations can be analyzed further as *adequate, over-adequate, inadequate*, and *ambiguous*. Adequate responses give only the information requested; they are appropriate for the request. Over-adequate responses give more than requested, while inadequate do not give enough. Ambiguous responses are unclear. Examples are given in Table 7.12.

TABLE 7.12 Types of Turns

Turn Type	Example
Obligation	Do you want some cookies? What time is it? What's that?
Comment	I really love to ski. I saw horses in the parade.
Response to comment	(Comment: This dessert is great!) It's an old family recipe.
Response to obligation	(Obligation: How old are you?)
Adequate	I'm 25.
Over-adequate	I'm 25, and I have a master's degree.
Inadequate	I go to college.
Ambiguous	None of your business. Guess.

Density

We might be interested in the density of turns within each conversation and on various topics. A low density may indicate that a child's conversational partner dominated the conversation by taking very long turns, relinquishing them to the child only occasionally, or that the child was very reticent. Children with ASD may take relatively few verbal turns, thus leaving the partner to fill the void. In contrast, if a child talked for lengthy turns, the density also would be low because the listener would have little chance to reply.

Oddly enough, the rate of interrupting increases during the teen years, but the purpose changes. Increasingly, speakers interrupt not to disrupt or change the topic but to move the discussion forward to facilitate communication.

Latency

An SLP can summarize the overall contingent and noncontingent latencies of a child. Longer periods and/or the continual use of fillers and interjections may indicate difficulties with topic identification or word finding.

Duration of Turns

There is no ideal length for a turn, although most listeners know when a turn has continued for too long. We all know at least one incessant talker who does not know when enough has been said. A child who talks incessantly may be exhibiting a semantic disorder of not knowing what information is needed to close the topic, a pragmatic disorder of not knowing the mechanisms for closing a turn or topic, or a processing problem of not being certain what information was conveyed.

The SLP is interested in the average length of the child's and the partner's turns. Different situations, partners, and topics may yield clinically significant differences in the length of these turns.

Type of Overlap

Most turns will be nonsimultaneous. However, overlap or simultaneous speech can be very revealing. In general, overlap is of two types: *internal* and *initial.* Sentence internal overlaps are used to complete the other speaker's turn and secure a turn. This ability requires a high level of pragmatic-linguistic knowledge. A child with LI may interrupt internally, indicating a lack of understanding of the process and may add new information or change the topic, rather than complete the other speaker's utterance.

Sentence initial overlaps result when a listener interjects between sentences to secure a turn. This interjection may occur when the listener is unsure of the speaker's intention to continue or when the listener wants to gain a turn at speaking. Continual overlaps of this type may indicate a breakdown in turn taking as a result of the behavior of one or both partners. In contrast, a low incidence of interrupting, as noted among some children with SLI, may indicate passivity or an inability to initiate a "turn grab."

Frequency of Overlap. Although it may seem counterintuitive, data indicate that, as a group, children with LI exhibit less simultaneous speech in their conversations. Although children with LI may be responsive, many are passive in initiating interaction or turn taking.

Duration of Overlap. The adult rules for turn taking state that when an overlap in turns occurs (when two speakers speak at once), one speaker will withdraw. Young children or children with LI may continue to talk or try to outshout their partners. Some children withdraw habitually. The SLP should try to determine whether the child in question is more likely to withdraw or to continue talking.

How Signaled? Changes in turn are signaled very subtly. A child with LI may miss such signals. Occasionally, such a child will respond only to questions, knowing that in this situation a response is required. Other children lack a basic understanding of the expectation to reply within a conversation. Still others cannot decipher the language code efficiently enough to respond.

Conversation and Topic Termination

Conversations or topics are ended when no new information is added. In the case of a conversational termination, the topic is not changed. As with the opening of a conversation, there are often adjacency pairs, such as "Bye, see ya"—"Have a nice day" or "Thank you"—"You're welcome."

Preschool children or those with LI may end the conversation abruptly when they decide it is over, occasionally just exiting the conversational context. Children with LD may not prepare the listener for the termination of the conversation by signaling with body language—for example, becoming restless, looking away, or looking at a watch. In the opposite extreme, children with LD or emotional disorder may be unable or unwilling to end the conversation and may perseverate or continue to ask questions that have been answered previously.

Topics usually are terminated by shifting to another related topic. For more mature language users, this process is accomplished by *shading*, in which the speakers shift to another aspect of the topic or to a closely related topic, as in the following exchange:

Speaker 1: I biked along the canal path yesterday.
Speaker 2: Oh, I love to bike there at this time of year.
Speaker 1: I didn't know you bike. What sort of bike do you have?
Speaker 2: I have an inexpensive 12-speed.
Speaker 1: I have a 21-speed?. . .

The original topic of the canal bike path slid into the topic of bicycles.

Whether topics are shaded or are changed abruptly, there is normally some continuity, and the new topic is stated clearly. When there is little left to discuss on a given topic, the conversation shifts. The SLP notes the method the child uses to terminate and change topics and to terminate conversations.

Conversational Breakdown

For intervention purposes, an SLP's analysis of the language of children with LI is an attempt, in part, to find where they are ineffectual, where they fail to communicate. It is important for an SLP to determine where these breakdowns occur and how a child attempts to repair them. The SLP should try to determine the number of conversational breakdowns and describe the cause of breakdown, the repair attempt, the repair initiator, the repair strategy, and the outcome.

Requests for Repair

Requests for repair, called *contingent queries*, signal the listener's attentiveness or understanding and skill in addressing the point of conversational breakdown. Conversations may be maintained by use of simple unspecific contingent queries, such as *Huh?*, *What?*, and *I don't understand*. In general, young children use unspecific requests. More mature speakers try to specify the information desired. Requests for repair may seek repetition of the preceding utterance, confirmation, or clarification.

Appropriate requests for repair and responses by the conversational partner demonstrate an awareness of the cooperative nature of conversation. Not only must a child attend to the partner's message, detect misunderstandings, and initiate an appropriate request, but he or she also must possess the knowledge and willingness to use clarification strategies to aid the partner's comprehension.

A child who continually responds with *Huh?* or *What?* may not be attending to the conversation or may have difficulty understanding. The SLP is interested in the degree to which a child requests additional information toward maintaining the conversation and in the form of these requests.

A child with LI may be unaware that communication breakdown has occurred. The SLP can hypothesize about the child's awareness of misunderstanding and confirm the hypothesis through manipulation of utterances addressed to the child. In general, children first gain awareness of breakdowns caused by unintelligible words. The order of breakdown awareness development is

unintelligible words.

impossible commands.

unrealistically long utterances.

unfamiliar words.

question or statement without an introduction and ambiguous, inexplicit, and open-ended statements.

Frequency and Form. In general, preschool children and those with LI, such as those with LD, tend to blame themselves, rather than the speaker, for misunderstanding. Thus, these children use fewer requests for repair than might be expected, especially given the greater likelihood of communication breakdown. The requests produced tend to be less specific, reflecting the difficulty encountered with these forms. In short, as listeners, children with LD do not accept the responsibility to signal miscomprehension, even when taught the procedures for doing so. Instead, these children assume that the speaker will be unambiguous, informative, and clear.

Children's strategies can be assessed in different contexts, such as familiar topics, unfamiliar topics, and contrived pragmatic violations, by the SLP. For example, the SLP can assume the child does not understand from nonverbal behavior, such as a quizzical look. A request for information may or may not follow.

Although there are no norms for the frequency of repair requests, general guidelines do indicate a change in both the frequency and type of contingent query with age. The earliest requests for repair are repetitions of the partner's utterance with rising intonation (*Doggie go ride?*) or nonspecific requests for repetition (*What?*). With age, requests become more specific and increase in frequency, although both vary according to the conversational partner. With an adult partner, 24- to 36-month-olds use approximately seven requests an hour, and 54- to 66-month-olds use approximately fourteen. When the partner is a familiar peer, the mean rate for 36- to 66-month-olds increases to thirty per hour.

Conversational Repair

Conversational repair may be spontaneous or in response to a request for repair. Preschool children spontaneously repair very little. Even in first grade, children spontaneously repair only about one-third of their conversational breakdowns. Young children or children with LI often do not attempt to repair communication breakdowns.

By age 2, most children respond consistently to neutral requests, such as "What?", although they are more likely to respond if the conversational partner is an adult rather than another child. Two-year-olds also tend to overuse "yes" and thus confirm interpretations even when incorrect, possibly because nonconfirmation requires clarification on their part. By age 3 to 5, children respond correctly, even to specific requests, about 80 percent of the time regardless of the partner. Most 10-year-olds are able to determine communication breakdown and repair the damage. Although children with LD at that age can identify faulty messages, they do not seem to understand when to use these repair techniques.

Repair can provide valuable information about communication breakdowns. Breakdown can occur for a number of reasons, including lack of intelligibility, volume, completeness of information, degree of complexity, inappropriateness, irrelevance, and lack of mutual attention, visual regard, or mutual desire. As might be expected, children with LI experience a greater number of breakdowns than do age-matched TD peers.

Repairs usually focus on the linguistic structure or on the content or nature of the information conveyed. Extralinguistic signals, such as pointing, may be used to clarify. These strategies are not mutually exclusive. In general, successful outcome is related to the explicitness and appropriateness of the repair strategy chosen.

When a child repairs spontaneously, the nature of the original error and the repair attempts should be noted. The SLP scans the transcript for all fillers, repetitions, perseverations, and long pauses. All of these may indicate word-finding difficulties on the child's part. The original error or repair attempt may be based on any number of relationships with the intended word or phrase, as noted in Table 7.13.

Spontaneous versus Listener-Initiated. An SLP is interested in the percentage of conversational repairs that are either self- or listener-initiated. Usually, listeners signal a breakdown with facial expression, body posture, and/or a contingent query.

Strategy. Immature speakers usually respond to listener-initiated requests for repair by restating the previous utterance. Continued requests also may result in children providing additional information, although children with LI seem less flexible in the use of this strategy.

More mature speakers usually give additional information or reformulate, rather than repeat the utterance. When requested to clarify, children with LI tend to respond less frequently and with less complex responses than do their peers developing typically. The responses of children with LI usually consist of repetition with little new information included to aid comprehension. Children developing typically seem to have a greater range of repair strategies at the same age.

An SLP can prepare a list of the various types of requests for clarification and use them in conversation with a child. Of interest is the child's rate of responding to various requests and the nature of the child's responses.

Frequency of Success. An SLP is interested in how successfully a child identifies breakdowns, repairs them spontaneously, and follows listener requests. In general, children with LI make more inappropriate responses to listener requests than do age-matched TD peers. For assessment purposes the responses of the listener determine the child's success.

TABLE 7.13 Relationship of Word-Finding Errors and Repair Attempts to the Intended Word

Association	Example
Definition	*the thing you cook food on* for *stove*
Description	*the long skinny one with no legs* for *snake* *book holder* for *bookend* *fuzzy* for *peach*
Generic (less specific)	*do* for more specific verb *hat* for *cap, bonnet, scarf,* etc. *thing* or *one* for name of entity
Opposites	*sit* for *stand*
Partial	*ball . . . big ball . . . red ball* for *big red ball*
Semantic category	*stove* for *refrigerator* (both are *appliances*)
Sound	*toe* for *tie* (initial sound similar) *goat* for *coat* (rhyme)

Within Utterances

Now, let's consider the analysis of language that can be accomplished within utterances by noting significant aspects of use, content, and form. These aspects were outlined in Table 7.1.

Each utterance can be analyzed within use, content, and form categories following a variety of analysis formats. Individual utterances can yield the frequency and range of various features. Some data will be descriptive, whereas other data will be more normative. This situation reflects the research information available and the type of analysis desired.

A number of computer-assisted and unassisted language sample analysis methods are available. Several are listed in Table 7.14. Although each method yields different data, none presents a total

TABLE 7.14 Language Sample Analysis Methods

Unassisted Methods

Pragmatics

Adolescent Conversational Analysis (Larson & McKinley, 1987)
Assessing Children's Language in Naturalistic Contexts (Lund & Duchan, 1993)
Clinical Discourse Analysis using Grice's framework (Damico, 1991a)
Language functions (Boyce & Larson, 1983; Gruenewald & Pollack, 1984; Prutting & Kirchner, 1983, 1987; Simon, 1984)

Syntax/Morphology

Assessing Children's Language in Naturalistic Contexts (Lund & Duchan, 1993)
Assessing Language Production in Children: Experimental Procedures (J. Miller, 1981)
Developmental Sentence Analysis (L. Lee, 1974)
Guide to Analysis of Language Transcripts (Stickler, 1987)
Index of Productive Syntax (IPSyn) (Scarborough, 1990)
Language Assessment, Remediation, and Screening Procedure (Crystal, Fletcher, & Garman, 1976, revised 1981)
Language Sampling, Analysis, and Training: A Handbook for Teachers and Clinicians (Tyack & Gottsleben, 1977)

Semantics

Profile in Semantics-Lexical (PRISM-L) (Crystal, 1982)
Analysis of Propositions (APRON) (based on Johnston & Kamhi, 1984; Kamhi & Johnston, 1992; Lahey, 1988)

Narratives

Narrative level (Larson & McKinley, 1987)
Story grammar analysis (Garnett, 1986; Hedberg & Stoel-Gammon, 1986; Roth, 1986; Westby, 1984, 1992; Westby, VanDongen, & Maggart, 1989)

Classroom-based

Classroom Script Analysis (Creaghead, 1992)
Curriculum-Based Language Assessment (N. Nelson, 1994)
Descriptive Assessment of Writing (Scott & Erwin, 1992)

Computer-Assisted Methods

Syntax/Morphology

Automated LARSP (Bishop, 1985)
Computerized Language Analysis (CLAN) (MacWhinney, 2000b)
Computerized Profiling (Long & Fey, 1988, 1989)
DSS Computer Program (Hixson, 1983)
Lingquest 1 (Mordecai, Palin, & Palmer, 1985)
Parrot Easy Language Sample Analysis (PELSA) (Weiner, 1988)
Pye Analysis of Language (PAL) (Pye, 1987)
Systematic Analysis of Language Transcripts (SALT) (J. Miller & Chapman, 2003)

picture of a child's language. In general, the more normative the results, the less descriptive and prescriptive, and vice versa. A few of the more widely used analysis methods are described in more detail in Appendix B. We'll be discussing a more generic analysis method borrowing useful portions from several places.

Language Use

At the utterance level, an SLP can analyze the breakdowns that occur and the intentions of individual utterances.

Disruptions

Communication breakdown or disruption can occur for many reasons. The amount and type of disruption will vary with the language task, topic, and partner(s). In general, more breakdowns occur in narration than in conversation. In addition, the longer the utterance, the more breakdowns present. Disruptions tend to occur at the developing edge of the child's language where production capacity is "stretched" and there's increased risk of processing difficulty. These utterances are of particular diagnostic significance (Rispoli & Hadley, 2001). Children with LI experience more disruptions than TD children.

The frequency of disruptions is inversely related to subjective impressions of communicative competence. More disruptions are equated with less competence. In addition, disruptions can be a valuable clue to a child's process of forming an utterance and to the level of cognitive and linguistic demands made on the speaker. Obviously, this type of analysis is not needed for all children with LI but may be helpful for those with word-finding problems or with "tangled," slow, or too long utterances.

Analysis requires that an SLP transcribe all words and word portions and all speechlike vocalizations. Pauses of 2 seconds or more also should be noted. Pauses should be obvious on a timed transcript format, as suggested in Chapter 5. All **mazes** should be identified. Mazes are language segments that, like physical mazes, disrupt, confuse, and slow movement—movement of the conversation in this case. Mazes may consist of silent pauses, fillers, repetitions, and revisions. Traditional syntactic analysis occurs after most mazes are eliminated and only well-formed utterances remain, thus depriving an SLP of data on communication breakdown.

Intentions

At the individual utterance level, pragmatic analysis can describe the intentions expressed and understood. The appropriateness and form of these intentions are also of interest. Although there is little normative data on the sophistication of intention form, each intention can be analyzed for its form and means of transmission.

Frequency and Range. Very little normative data are available on the frequency and range of intentions. This paucity reflects the contextual variability of intentions and the lack of agreement by professionals on the intentions expressed at various ages. Intentions are heavily influenced by and heavily influence the conversational context.

A number of taxonomies of intentions are available, reflecting different ages and contextual situations. I have attempted in Tables 7.15 and 7.16 to demonstrate possible changes over time. As an SLP, you may wish to develop a taxonomy based on one or a combination of the available taxonomies.

The range of intentions becomes wider and more complex with increasing age. In addition, with maturity, a child may express multiple intentions within a single utterance. Thus, a more mature speaker's ability to express different functions is more flexible.

TABLE 7.15 Intentions of Children

Early Symbolic (below age 2)	Symbolic (age 2–7 years)
Dore (1974), Owens (1978)	R. Chapman (1981), Dore (1986), Folger & Chapman (1978)
Requesting action	Requests (for) Action/assistance/objects Permission
Regulation Protesting	Regulation Protesting and Rule setting
Requesting information	Requesting information
Replying Continuants Comments	Replying Acknowledgments Qualifications Agreements Comments Assertives
Naming	Identifications and descriptions
Personal feelings	Personal feelings Statements, reports, and evaluations Attributions/details Explanations Hypotheses and reasons Predictions
Declarations Choice making	Declarations Procedurals Choice making and claims
Answers	Answers Providing information Clarification Compliance Conversational organization
Calling/Greeting	Attention getters and speaker selection Rhetorical questions Clarification requests Boundary markers Politeness Exclamations
Repeating	Repetitions
Practicing	Elicited imitations

Note: As children become older, they add new functions and continue to diversify those they already possess.

After selecting the most comfortable taxonomy or combination of taxonomies, an SLP can rate each utterance of a child and conversational partner for the intentions expressed. Of interest are the conditions under which each intention occurred, possible environmental cues, and the discourse demands, such as the type of discourse (dyad, group) and nature of the task (motor, verbal, visual, or tactile).

The normative data available, though only limited, do demonstrate that within a conversation, partners use a wide range of intentions; no intention predominates unless warranted by the situation.

TABLE 7.16 Intentions and Age of Mastery

Prior to 24 months	Answering/Responding Continuance Declaring/Citing Making choices Naming/Labeling Protesting/Denying Repeating
24–36 months	Calling/Greeting Detailing Predicting Replying Requesting assistance/Directing Requesting clarification Requesting information Requesting objects
After 36 months	Expressing feelings Giving reasons Hypothesizing

A child developing typically will initiate conversation and reply to the initiations of the partner, seek information and provide it, ask for assistance, and volunteer information. In contrast, some children, such as those with ASD, may initiate communication only rarely and respond with minimal replies.

Occasionally, adults or children fall into perseverative patterns of communicating, for example, a parent who constantly quizzes her or his child to name the pictures in a book or a child who keeps repeating a pleasing or tantrum phrase. Such behavior can skew the data or allow one type of intention, such as answers, to predominate. These patterns should be noted during conversational sample collection, and the situations gently changed. The use of different situations and different partners may ensure a better distribution of intentions.

Some children use only a limited range of illocutionary functions. If this persists across a number of situations and partners, the SLP can be reasonably certain that this narrow range of functions represents the child's typical behavior.

Appropriateness. A very narrow intentional range may indicate inappropriate use of language. The question of appropriateness must be judged against other factors, such as age, race or ethnicity, region of the country, socioeconomic status, gender, and, most important, the communication context.

The language sample can confirm the caregiver's observation that "John seems to ask questions all the time, even when he knows the answers." Although the observation may not be unfounded, only data from the language sample or systematic observation can offer concrete proof.

Encoding. Intentions can be analyzed by using a means of transmission format, such as verbal/vocal/nonverbal. The transition from linguistic through paralinguistic to nonlinguistic can be used to describe a hierarchy of competency or effectiveness based on a child's developmental level. The nonlinguistic context and behaviors of the conversational partners must also be transcribed to make this information available.

In general, a child with poor linguistic skills will rely on other than verbal means of communicating intentions. Although some very sophisticated information can be communicated nonlinguistically, as in an extended *pause,* less mature language users tend to depend on nonlinguistic and paralinguistic means more than do mature users. As with the various intentions expressed, a range of transmission means should be exhibited by the child and partner.

If a child uses an augmentative form of communication, the form of AAC should be specified along with other means, such as physical manipulation of an object, physical manipulation of a partner, gestures, and vocalization and verbalization. Two children described as nonverbal may have very different means of communicating their intentions.

Content

The understanding of word meanings and word relationships is affected by many factors, such as age, gender, and regional and racial/ethnic differences. To know a word is to know more than just what it identifies or its definition. It means a child understands that word's relationship to similar words of meaning and sound and to words of an opposite meaning and understands the semantic class into which the word can be placed.

Meaning extends beyond the word, however, and larger units of analysis, such as the phrase or sentence, also must be considered. What is said—for example, "Don't hit me"—may be very different from the intended message, which might be "Go away, I don't understand what you want."

Obviously, all of this information cannot be ascertained from a brief language sample. Word understanding is complicated and can be assessed across several sessions by playing games like Simon Says directing a child through a series of tasks or matching tasks. The SLP can make statements in which words obviously are used incorrectly in order to judge the child's reactions. Word games that solicit definitions or antonyms also can provide valuable information. Sorting and categorization tasks can be part of a play situation and can provide information on the child's ability to categorize and classify. The child can be asked to name the members of a category or to deduce the category name from a list of members. The SLP can play the "fool" and make ridiculous comparisons ("A mouse is bigger than an elephant") or silly pairings ("The comb goes between his toes") to gauge the child's reactions.

Vocabulary abilities are strongly related to reading comprehension. Reading and writing analysis is discussed in Chapter 13. The child with semantic difficulties also may exhibit academic and reading failure, especially with comprehension.

Although children with LI and with LD usually do not have difficulty with referent-symbol tasks, such as matching names to pictures, they may have difficulties with double meanings, abstract terms, synonyms, and nonliteral interpretation. In addition, the physical setting can be especially important for children with LI because they depend on the context for support. The child may understand a word only given certain physical situations or contexts.

It may be best to assess definitions in formal decontextualized activities, such as testing, but word use in conversations, where context can influence behavior, can also indicate correct usage. Between ages 5 and 10, the nature of definitions changes from functional to categorical and more elements are added. By second grade, 49 percent of definitions include categorical membership, such as *an apple is a fruit*, increasing to 76 percent by fifth grade.

Multiple definitions are more difficult to interpret in a decontextualized or isolated format because of the use of context to disambiguate. In general, sentence format aids performance but this varies with word type. Words with multiple definitions appear frequently in school texts. For example, 72 percent of the 9,000 most frequent words in one elementary reading series had multiple meanings.

Lexical Items

Obviously, there are several levels of semantic analysis relative to individual words and relations between words and larger units. Norms are difficult to establish, especially for older school-age children and adolescents because of the individualistic nature of lexical growth. In addition, increases in vocabulary occur at a slow and steady pace into adulthood. School-age children and adolescents exhibit semantic development in the following areas:

- Comprehension of literate verbs, such as *interpret* and *predict*
- Comprehension of textbook terms, such as *invertebrate* and *antecedent*
- Comprehension of adverbs of magnitude, such as *slightly* and *unusually*
- Comprehension of adverbial conjuncts, such as *meanwhile* and *conversely*
- Comprehension of sarcasm based on its linguistic aspects, as well as intonation
- Comprehension of slang terms used by peers, such as *phat*
- Comprehension of complex proverbs
- Comprehension of complex metaphors
- Explanation of infrequently occurring idioms, such as *to vote with one's feet*
- Explanation of ambiguous messages
- Definition of abstract concept words, such as *courage* and *justice*

Type-Token Ratio. The **type-token ratio (TTR)** is the ratio of the number of different words to the total number of words. The number of different words (NDW) in a sample of fixed length is strongly correlated with age and measures of semantic diversity. Significantly lower values than those in Table 7.19 might suggest retrieval problems or poor vocabulary.

The total number of words (TNW) also increases steadily with age and is a general measure of verbal productivity. Although a general measure of ease of language use, TNW also is affected by other factors, such as motor ability and word retrieval. For these reasons, the validity of TNW as a measure of preschool language development has been questioned by some professionals. (Values of TNW for a 20-minute sample are listed in Table 7.19)

As a quantitative measure, TTR has had a checkered past of professional acceptance. This uncertainty reflects recognition that the value may vary widely with the language sample size. In general, less variability is found across larger samples of 350 words or more. Multiple settings and more representative samples would yield theoretically more stable values, although there may be great situational variability for an individual child.

Children between ages 2 and 8 demonstrate TTRs of 0.42 to 0.50. Children who receive values greater than 0.50 have greater variability and flexibility in their language, whereas those below 0.42 tend to use the same words over and over again. Very low values may indicate perseverative or stereotypic behavior, word-retrieval problems, or restricted vocabulary. ELLs also may score lower because of their lack of English vocabulary.

Children with poor vocabularies or word-finding difficulties may use empty words, rather than more specific words that are not at their disposal. Some children with word-finding problems exhibit word-finding difficulties both on structured naming tasks and in spontaneous samples. Other children have difficulty only on structured naming tasks, although they produce relatively less language in spontaneous samples than do TD children.

Speakers should possess a variety of words for describing sensory experiences, such as sight (*clearly*), sound (*loud*), smell (*stunk*), and feelings (*happy, tired*). They should be able to describe the environment in terms of time (*at five o'clock*) and location (*in front of*). Entities should possess physical qualities, such as shape (*sort of round*), size (*big*), number (*two, many, few*), substance (*metal, wood*), and condition (*new, ragged*). There should be terms for relationships, such as comparisons (*bigger than, as big as*) and qualifications (*nearly, not quite, only, enough*); and verbs for describing actions (*run, jump, eat*), states (*am, is, are*), and sensory processes (*feel, hear, see*). Finally, the speakers should be able to describe causation (*because . . .*) and motivation. As noted previously, these terms develop slowly. The full range is characteristic of the mature speaker.

Deictic terms, or terms that must be interpreted from the perspective of the speaker (e.g., *here, there, this, that, come, go*), offer a special problem for the child with LI. The shifting reference that occurs with each speaker change contributes to the child's difficulty. Children with LLD, ASD, or emotional disturbances may lack either the listener or speaker perspective. These children also may refer to themselves by name and may echo the utterances of others.

No one measure, such as type-token ratio, should be used in isolation. This is especially true for children from CLD backgrounds. Although type-token and its component parts, total number of words and number of different words, can be used to differentiate the narratives of typical language from impaired language for monolingual children, they do not do so for bilingual Spanish-English preschool children (Muñoz, Gillam, Peña, & Gulley-Faehnle, 2003). Other measures, such as syntactic accuracy, may be more appropriate.

Over-/Underextensions and Incorrect Usage. An SLP should note all inaccurate uses of words that indicate some variation between a child's meaning and the conventional one. In general, meanings mature from the concrete, personal, experiential ones found in preschool children to the shared, conventional, abstract ones of adults.

Some children use words incorrectly because they do not know the shared conventional definition. Others use word substitutions that are incorrect. For example, a recent letter from a young adult with LD included the following:

> I wish I could write as good as you. You know where to put paragraphs and how to use *punctuality* [my italics] right.

Because I am usually late, I assume he meant *punctuation*. Further testing by an SLP can reveal the basis of a child's substitutions. The child may miss the target word slightly, as in the above example, or may have word-finding difficulties, resulting in word substitutions.

ELL children may use English words in either very restricted or overextended ways. Restricted use may be limited to specific features of a word or to word-for-word transfer in which the word has only the meaning of its L_1 equivalent. In the latter, for example, the English *for*, which is *para* in Spanish and has slightly different syntactic uses, might be used only where *para* would be used.

Style and Lexicon. Children begin to use different styles of talking relatively early. Analysis across utterances and partners might highlight a conversational style shift. These changes can be analyzed further for the vocabulary used in different styles.

Slang is important for adolescents. A teen with LI may seem odd in peer situations because he or she underuses or overuses adolescent slang or uses it inappropriately. Although difficult to assess because of its changing nature and subgroup use, slang is, nonetheless, extremely important. In brainstorming sessions, TD teens can suggest vocabulary targets for assessment and training.

The child's literate vocabulary, consisting of words primarily used in common academic contexts, is also important. A good, literate lexicon is needed to achieve academic success, especially among adolescents. Possible lexical items are *analyze, criticize, deduce, define, infer, interpret, predict, remember*, and *understand*. Classroom teachers can suggest other useful literate terms.

Word Relationships

Each word in a language is related to other words. These relationships consist of word associations (e.g., *salt and pepper* or *king and queen*), synonyms, antonyms, and homonyms. Some of these associations are expressed in a conversational sample, whereas others need to be probed by an SLP. These associations reflect underlying cognitive organizational strategies.

Semantic Categories. Semantic categories, such as agent, action, and location, are the earliest word classes children use. Several categorization schemes attempt to describe the semantic classes of young children and adults. Table 7.17 is a composite of the range of semantic categories expresssed by late preschool and school-age children.

TABLE 7.17 Semantic Categories

Semantic Function	Description	Example
Action	The predicate expresses action with a transitive or intransitive clause.	We *grew* pumpkins and squash. (Transitive) He *swims* daily. (Intransitive)
State	The predicate makes a statement about the way things are with a transtive, intransitive, or equative clause.	I *want* a hot fudge sundae. (Transitive) Tigers *look* fierce. (Intransitive) My sister *is* now at Harvard. (Equative)
Agent or actor	Animate instigator of action. Sometimes inanimate, especially if natural force. Usually the subject but may also be passive complement.	*Mike* threw the ball. *Termites* destroyed our cabin. *Wind* blew down the trees. The *cat* chased the dog.
Instrument	Usually refers to the inanimate object used by the actor to effect the action stated in the verb. The actor is usually not stated but may be.	The *axe* split the wood. The building was erected by a *crane.* She used the *baseball bat* with great skill. The shaman kept rhythm on his *drum.*
Patient	The entity on which an action is performed. The patient may be a direct object in transitive clauses or the subject in intransitive clauses.	Mike threw the *ball.* *The lighthouse* withstood the hurricane.
Dative	The animate recipient of action. Usually the indirect object but may also be the direct object if it does not undergo any action but receives something.	Father bought *mother* a bouquet of roses. Our mascot brought *us* good luck. He built a treehouse for his *daughter.* I loved that *movie.*
Temporal	Fulfills the adverbial function of time in response to a *when* question. May also be the subject of a sentence or a complement.	I'll see you *later.* We'll meet at *four o'clock. Then,* I'll know. *Tomorrow* is a holiday. It is *time to leave.*
Locative	Fulfills the adverbial function of place in response to a *where* question. May also be the subject of a sentence or a complement.	Some of us looked *in the old log.* I knew it was right *here.* *Chicago* is indeed a windy city.
Manner	Fulfills the adverbial function of manner in response to a *how* question.	We stalked the big cat *carefully.* He worked *with great skill.*
Accompaniment	Fulfills the adverbial function of *with* X in response to *with whom* or *with what* questions.	He swam *with his sister.* She left *with Jim.* He hunted *with his dogs.*
Empty subjects	Serve a grammatical function.	*It* was sunny. *There* may be some rain.

Semantic knowledge, the underlying concepts, may be a better framework than language form for assessment children with minority dialects, including African, Latino, and Asian American English and Appalachian English. The adequacy of the semantic knowledge of these children is often questioned on the basis of the form of their language. It is assumed, incorrectly, that minority dialect speakers acquire concepts later than do speakers of dialects closer to the majority dialect.

Intrasentence Relationships. In addition to an interest in a child's word meanings and relationships, an SLP can investigate other relationships expressed in the sentence through the use of conjunctions, negatives, and prepositions and various sentence forms, such as passive voice.

Conjunctions. Four types of conjunctive relations are expressed in conjoined sentences: additive, temporal, causal, and adversative. In the *additive* form, two clauses with no dependent relationship simply are joined to one another. In the sentence "Julio ate pie, and Brigid drank coffee," neither event depends on the other for its existence.

In the *temporal* form, one clause depends on the other to precede or follow or occur at the same time. In "I'm going to the store before I go to the party" or "I'll rake the leaves while you finish painting the trim" the timing of the clauses is clearly stated.

Causal conjoining implies a dependency in which one clause is the result of the other, for example, "I went to the party because I was invited." The preschool child may use because alone or at the beginning of a clause, as in "Cause I want to," although true causal conjoining occurs much later (see Table 7.25).

Finally, in *adversative* conjoining, one clause contrasts with information in the other, as in "I read the article, but I was unimpressed." One clause opposes or negates the other.

Negatives. Negatives may be expressed in several ways and develop at different stages. The four mature negative forms include (a) *not* and *-n't;* (b) negative words, such as *nobody* and *nothing;* (c) the determiner *no* used with nouns; and (d) negative adverbs, such as *never* and *nowhere*. Again, the more mature language user should have a variety of forms. Those used by the child can be compared with the developmental data available in Table 7.25.

Prepositions. Prepositions are some of the hardest working and most versatile English words. They can be used to mark location (*in the box*), time (*in a minute*), or manner (*in a hurry*) to fill adjectival and adverbial functions and to make figurative expressions. These small, often unstressed words may be misinterpreted or misunderstood by children with LI and those who are ELLs. A strategy they use is overreliance on one form. As mentioned previously, an SLP examines the sample for the breadth of use.

Passives. In general, children with LI exhibit difficulty interpreting sentences in which the information might be interpreted in a reverse manner. For example, a passive sentence, such as "The cat is chased by the dog" might be interpreted incorrectly as "The cat chased the dog" by using a agent-action-object interpretation strategy. Children with LI have difficulty interpreting the grammatical functions of words and integrating grammatical and semantic information.

Figurative Language

Nonliteral meanings used for effect are characteristic of school-age and adult language. Examples include metaphors, similes, idioms, and proverbs. For the purposes of analysis, jokes and puns also can be considered figurative language. Figurative language occurs frequently in oral conversation and written texts and interpretation of idioms is highly correlated with reading ability.

Children as young as 3½ are able to comprehend some idioms, especially the more literal ones. In general, figurative interpretation increases with increasing age. Individual interpretive ability is related to each person's world knowledge.

An SLP can consider the range of figurative language used. Some children overrely on well-worn phrases and expressions, with little knowledge of their actual meaning. Such expressions as these can be probed by an SLP to determine a child's actual knowledge.

Analysis of figurative language is especially important for ELLs. Idiomatic expressions may be interpreted literally and/or based on cultural interpretation.

Word Finding

Word-finding difficulties are an impaired ability to generate a specific word that is evoked by a situation, stimulus, sentence context, or conversation. In Chapter 4 we discussed a method of probing for word-finding difficulties and strategies. Earlier in this chapter we noted that latency may signal such difficulties. Other symptoms include frequent pauses, repetitions, circumlocutions, fillers, nonspecific words, frequent pronouns, and high usage of cliches and routinized expressions, such as *you know*. Inaccurate naming may be analyzed using the strategies presented in Table 4.5.

Word-finding difficulties relate to several aspects of the target words, such as word frequency, age of acquisition, familiarity, and lexical neighborhood (German & Newman, 2004). Neighborhood density, or the number of words that differ from the target word by only one sound, is particularly important. Words such as *rat* have many neighbors: *cat, bat, fat, gnat, sat, hat, mat, rap, ran, rot, wrote/rote, write/right, rate*, and so on. The neighborhood is very dense. Both children and adults find it easier to produce and remember words that are phonologically similar to words already known. If neighbors are high-frequency words, recall is enhanced even more. In contrast, word substitutions tend to be words that have a higher frequency, are learned earlier, and also reside in dense neighborhoods with other high-frequency words. Blocked words, or those a child is unable to retrieve, tend to reside in sparse neighborhoods. Phonological errors tend to occur on rare words and those whose neighbors contain lower frequency, uncommon phonological patterns.

Other variables include the context, syntactic requirements, type of stimulus and manner of presentation, priming, and use of categories. In general, sentence contexts are easier than picture ones, which, in turn, are easier than definitions. Formulation of more difficult sentences, however, interferes with word recall, probably because of the greater cognitive energy needed to form the sentence. Priming results when preceding words aid recall. Finally, use of subordinate categories can aid word recall.

The effect of these variables can be very important and difficult to assess in a language sample. It is important, therefore, to use familiar partners, topics, and situations to facilitate retrieval and to probe word recall.

Form

Language form includes syntax, morphology, and phonology, or the means used to encode the intentions and meanings of a speaker. Even though most language analysis methods concentrate on this aspect of language, little normative data is available. The task is partially normative and partially descriptive, involving both quantitative and qualitative analysis. Several available analysis methods are described in Appendix B. A discussion of phonological analysis is beyond the scope of this text.

Quantitative Measures

Quantitative measures include mean length of utterance (MLU), mean syntactic length (MSL), T-units and C-units, and the density of sentence forms. Each is discussed in some detail.

The SLP must be cautious with all word and morpheme counts. Careful editing of utterances is required so that interjections, false starts, fillers (*you know*), imitations, and the like are not included in the count. Circumlocutions, or talking around an unretrievable word, actually may increase the length of the child's utterances. It is recommended that an SLP follow consistent rules for counting. For example, incomplete words, nonessential repetitions, revisions not containing a complete thought, unintelligible words and phrases, and fillers should be offset in brackets and not counted. These structures are retained, however, for disruption analysis.

Quantitative measures may present some problems. In general, there can be wide variability across children and situations. In addition, many values change only slowly with age. Still, average words per sentence values increase from 7 to 14 between third and twelfth grade.

Combinations of quantitative data may yield better information than individual bits of information. For example, MLU, percentage of utterances containing one or more errors of morphology or syntax, and chronological age seem to be optimal for predicting clinical diagnosis of SLI. Structural errors might include word misordering; omission or incorrect use of a morpheme; omission of articles, auxiliary verbs, or contractions; use of telegraphic speech; or incorrectly selected negatives.

Mean Length of Utterance. *Mean length of utterance* is the average length in morphemes of the speaker's utterances. Up to an average of 4.0, MLU is considered a good measure of language complexity although not all linguists agree. The reliability of MLU has been questioned and the values have been found to vary in response to SLP input, but MLU has been shown to be both a reliable and valid measure of general language development through age 10 for children with SLI (Rice, Redmond, & Hoffman, 2006).

Although there is less variability in MLU above 4.0, a value reached by the TD child at around age 4, MLU continues to increase with age. At lower MLUs, new structures added to the child's utterances increase the complexity of those sentences. After this level of development, much of the growth in complexity is the result of internal reorganization of utterance form, rather than addition of new structures. This explanation of the relationship between length and complexity is extremely simplified, and there are many related factors.

To calculate MLU, an SLP divides the language sample into utterances. It is best not to include in analysis the portions of conversation that occurred while the child was adjusting to the partner or to the situation. The number of morphemes in each utterance is counted and totaled for the entire sample. Rules for counting morphemes on the basis of the order of development with nonimpaired children are included in Table 7.18. Brief rationales for these rules are included where appropriate.

The total number of morphemes for the entire sample is divided by the number of utterances from which it was derived to determine the MLU. This value then can be compared to the age data in Table 7.19. It is obvious from the table that a wide variability and a wide range of ages are considered within the normal range. Even so, the need to collect a typical sample is very important. If data have been collected in two or more settings, the MLUs from each can be compared to assess the stability of the overall data.

Although age and MLU are correlated as shown in Table 7.19, some interesting data suggest cautious acceptance of this correlation. First, the relationship of rate of MLU change and age is not a constant. Second, some language impairments are not evidenced by delays in MLU as might be expected.

Using 200-utterance language samples, we find a similar age progression in MLU words and morphemes. In addition, there is a persistently lower level of performance for children with SLI (Eisenberg, McGovern Fersko, & Lundgren, 2001; Rice, Smolik, et al., 2010). If a child falls below one standard deviation and we're reasonably sure that we have captured his or her typical peformance, we should consider that the child has a possible LI.

As with any single measure, MLU alone is a poor diagnostic tool, and the validity and reliability of results will vary with the sample size (Eisenberg et al., 2001). Standard errors of measure may differ .19 at 18 months to .71 at 60 months based on a 50-utterance sample. Values are less for 100-utterance samples.

Nor is a low MLU necessarily indicative of language impairment. Utterance length may vary with the situation, and some children with LI, especially those with circumlocution or empty words, may have inflated MLUs.

It's easy to make some common errors when calculating MLU. The Kansas Language Transcript Database (Rice, Ash, et al., 2004) provides guidance for English anomalies. For example, you should not count two morphemes for seemingly plural nouns, such as *scissors* and *pants*, that have no singular equivalent.

Mean Syntactic Length. *Mean syntactic length* (MSL) is the mean length in words of all utterances of two words or more—those utterances with some internal grammar. This measure eliminates all one-word responses, such as yes/no answers. MSL seems to correlate more strongly than MLU with age. Values for MSL are listed in Table 7.19 (Klee, 1992).

T-Units and C-Units. Expressive language syntax of older children and adolescents can be measured in **T-units** (minimal terminal units), consisting of one main clause plus any attached or embedded subordinate clause or nonclausal structure (discussed in the following section). Thus, the unit has shifted from the utterance to the sentence. Any simple or complex sentence would be one T-unit, but a compound sentence would be two or more. For example, the sentences "I want ice cream" and

TABLE 7.18 Rules for Counting Morphemes Relative to the Speech of Preschool Children

Structure	Example	Count	Rationale
Each recurrence of a word for emphasis	No, no, no.	1 each	
Compound words (2 or more free morphemes)	Railroad, birthday	1	Compound words learned as a unit by preschoolers
Proper names	Bugs Bunny, Uncle Fred	1	Proper names, even those with titles, learned as a unit by preschoolers
Ritualized reduplications	Choo-choo, Night-night	1	
Irregular past tense verbs	Went, ate, got, came	1	Verb tense learned as new word by preschoolers, not as *verb* + *ed*
Diminutives	Doggie, horsie	1	Phonological form CVCV easier than CVC for preschoolers and does not denote smallness
Auxiliary verbs and catenatives	Is, have, do; gonna, wanna, gotta	1	Preschoolers do not know that such words as *gonna* are *going to*
Contracted negatives	Don't, can't, won't	1–2	Because negatives *don't, can't,* and *won't* develop before *do, can,* and *will,* count as one until the positive form appears. Then count the negative forms as two morphemes. All other negatives—*couldn't*—count as two.
Possessive marker (-*'s*)	Tom*'s*, mom*'s*	1	
Plural maker (-*s*)	Cat*s*, dog*s*	1	
Third-person singular present tense marker (-*s*)	Walk*s*, eat*s*	1	
Regular past tense marker (-*ed*)	Walk*ed*, jump*ed*	1	
Present progressive marker (-*ing*)	Walk*ing*, eat*ing*	1	
Dysfluencies	C-c-candy, b-b-baby	1	Count only the final complete form.*
Fillers	Um-m, ah-h	0	

*In the example "I want can . . . I want can . . . I want candy," only the last full reduction is counted, being three morphemes.

"I want the one that is hidden in the blue box" each constitute one T-unit with varying numbers of words and clauses. "I want the ice cream in the picture, and he wants a shake" consists of two main clauses and thus two T-units. Examples of T-units are given in Table 7.20.

The T-unit is more sensitive than MLU to the types of language differences seen after age 5, such as phrasal embedding and various types of subordinate clauses. Throughout the school years, a slow but regular increase occurs in sentence length in both oral and written contexts.

Children's language can be described in words per T-unit, clauses per T-unit, and words per clause. A gradual and progressive increase in words and clauses per T-unit and in words per clause in spontaneous speech occurs with increased age throughout childhood and adolescence, although the values change only gradually during early school years (see Table 7.21). The values for spoken words/T-unit and clauses/T-unit are similar for Spanish.

TABLE 7.19 Quantitative Measures of Language

Age in Months	MLU_w (SD)[4]	MLU_m (SD)	Range of Mean MLU[1]	MSL[2]	TNW[2] (20 *min.*)	NDW[2] (50 *utt.*)
18		1.1	1.0–1.2			
21		1.6	1.1–1.8	2.7	240	36
24		1.9	1.6–2.2	2.9	286	41
27		2.1	1.9–2.3	3.1	332	46
30		2.5	2.4–2.6	3.4	378	51
33 [30–35]	[2.91 (0.58)]	2.8 [3.23 (0.71)]	2.7–2.9	3.7	424	56
36		3.1	3.0–3.3	3.9	470	61
39 [36–41]	[3.43 (0.61)]	3.3 [3.81 (0.69)]	3.2–3.5	4.2	516	66
42		3.6	3.3–3.9	4.4	562	71
45 [42–47]	[3.71 (0.58)]	3.8 [4.09 (0.67)]	3.4–4.3	4.7	608	76
48		3.9	3.6–4.7	4.9	654	81
51 [48–53]	[4.10 (0.65)]	4.1 [4.57 (0.76)]	3.7–5.1	5.2	700	86
54		4.3	3.9–5.8			
57 [54–59]	[4.28 (0.72)]	[4.75 (0.79)]				
60		4.4	4.0–6.0			
[60–65]	[4.38 (0.63)]	[4.88 (0.72)]				
[66–71]	[4.47 (0.61)]	[4.96 (0.70)]				
[72–77]	[4.57 (0.66)]	[5.07 (0.75)]				
[78–83]	[4.70 (0.66)]	[5.22 (0.71)]				
[84–98]	[4.72 (0.83)]	[5.22 (0.91)]				
[90–95]	[4.92 (1.03)]	[5.35 (1.13)]				
[96–101]	[5.08 (0.84)]	[5.67 (0.97)]				
[102–107]	[4.99 (0.71)]	[5.51 (0.79)]				
108		8.8	7.2–10.4[3]			

[1]Combined data from four different studies (Klee, Schaffer, May, Membrino, & Mougey, 1989; J. Miller, 1981; Scarborough, Wyckoff, & Davidson, 1986; Wells, 1985).
[2]MSL (mean syntactic length), TNW (total number of words), and NDW (number of different words) extrapolated from tables in Klee (1992).
[3]From J. Miller, Freiberg, Rolland, & Reves (1992).
[4]Rice, Smolik, et al. (2010).

TABLE 7.20 Examples of T-Units and C-Units

Sentence Structure	Example	Number of T-units and C-units
Simple—one clause	They watched the parade on TV.	1 T-unit, 1 C-unit
Complex—embedded clause	Washington has the horse I want.	1 T-unit, 1 C-unit
Compound—conjoining of two or more clauses	*They went to the movie,* but *I stayed home.*	2 T-units, 2 C-units
	Mom went to work, I went to school, and *my sister stayed home.*	3 T-units, 3 C-units
Partial sentences		
Elliptical answers	(Who went with you?) Marshon.	1 C-unit
Exclamations	Oh, wow!	1 C-unit
Aphorisms	A penny saved.	1 C-unit

TABLE 7.21 T-Units and C-Units by Age and Grade

Units	Age 4	Age 6	Age 6-7*	Grades 3–4	Grades 6–7	Grade 9	Grades 10–12
Words/T-unit							
Spoken			8.67	7.8	9.7		11.4
Oral Spanish		5.64					
Written				9.5	9.4–11.8		10.6–14.3
Words/C-unit							
Oral					9.82	10.96	11.7
Oral AAE	3.14	3.81					
Written					9.04	10.05	13.27
Clauses/T-unit							
Spoken		1.26	1.33	1.31	1.5		1.5
Written				1.3	1.6		1.6–1.8
Subordinate Clauses/C-unit							
Spoken					.37	.43	.58
Written					.29	.47	.6
Words/Clause							
Spoken		7.14		7.75	7.26		8.82
Written							

Source: Adapted from Nippold, Mansfield, Billow & Tomblin (2008); Crowhurst & Piche (1979); Scott, Nippold, Norris, & Johnson (1992).
*Use expository task.

To calculate these values, the SLP divides the sample into sentences, each equaling one T-unit. The number of words and clauses then can be determined for each and divided by the number of T-units to calculate an average. The words per clause can be determined similarly.

It should be noted that the type of conversational task will influence some T-unit measures. Information-giving tasks increase the words and clauses per T-unit. In addition, T-unit values can be misleading because complexity and length are not directly related. For example, among adolescents, phrases may be used in place of subordinate clauses for conciseness, suggesting greater syntactic sophistication.

A variance of the T-unit is the C-unit. C-units are similar to T-units but also include incomplete sentences in answer to questions (Table 7.20). C-unit values are given in Table 7.21.

Although data are not complete, some values for T-units and C-units have been calculated for children speaking primarily African American English and Spanish. These are presented in Table 7.21 also. Children speaking AAE demonstrate infinitive phrase embedding and clausal embedding at an early age. Three-year-olds have one or more complex syntactic forms in 6.2 percent of their utterances, while 4-years-olds increase that to 11.7 percent (Jackson & Roberts, 2001). Additional values include mean number of morphemes per C-unit for AAE speakers (Craig, Washington, & Thompson-Porter, 1998):

Age	*Mean Morphemes/C-Unit*
4	3.48
5	3.76
6	4.24
Preschool	3.55
Kindergarten	3.98

Number of errors per T-unit was also found to be a significant value for predominately Spanish-speaking children (Restrepo, 1998). Five- to 7-year-old Spanish-speaking children developing typically made only .09 (S.D. = .05) errors, while those with LI made .39 (S.D. = .21).

Syntactic and Morphological Analysis

Many children with LI experience difficulty with syntax and morphology. For example, children who are mildly to moderately behaviorally disordered seem to have word-order difficulties.

Morphological Analysis. An SLP is interested in intraword development, as well as in sentence development. With preschool children, the SLP will want to analyze inflectional morphemes for correct production. These are listed in Table 7.22. Older children may use a variety of morphological prefixes and suffixes. A list of the more common prefixes and suffixes is included in Appendix C.

The percentage of correct morpheme use is determined by dividing the number of correct appearances by the total number of obligatory contexts. In obligatory contexts, the child might use the morpheme correctly, make an error substitution, or omit the morpheme. Table 7.23 presents selected portions of a language sample and the calculation of percentage correct for the regular plural marker.

The percentage correct yields only limited data. For example, an SLP who calculated only the percentage correct for past-tense *-ed* still would not know whether errors were related to nonuse of *-ed* where required or to use of *-ed* on irregular past tense verbs.

Morphological markers are applied to word classes. For example, the past tense marker *-ed* is confined to verbs. Therefore, an SLP should also note word classes in which errors occur. Occasionally, errors are confined to only one word class, such as verbs. Nouns would be affected by such markers as plural regular and irregular, possessive, and articles. Verb markers include third-person singular, past tense regular and irregular, present progressive, modals, *do* + *verb*, copula (*am, are, is, was, were*), and perfective (*have* + *be* + verb). Finally, adjective and adverb markers include, but are not limited to, comparative (*-er*) and superlative (*-est*) and adverbial *-ly*.

Pronouns offer a special case of morphological analysis because of the complex nature of the underlying semantic and pragmatic functions. If the child's strategy is "when in doubt, use the noun,"

TABLE 7.22 Inflectional Morphemes and Age of Mastery

MLU	Morpheme	Example	Age Range of Mastery* (in months)
2.0–2.5	Present progressive *-ing.* (no auxiliary verb)	Mommy driv*ing*	19–28
	Regular plural *-s*	Kitties eat my *ice* cream. Forms: /s/, /z/, and /Iz/ *Cats* (/kæts/) *Dogs* (/dɔgZ/) *Classes* (klæsIz), *wishes* (/wIʃIz/)	24–33
2.5–3.0	Possessive *'s*	Mommy's balloon broke. Forms: /s/, /z/, and /Iz/ as in regular plural I throw *the* ball to daddy.	26–40
3.0–3.5/3.75	Regular past *-ed*	Mommy pull*ed* the wagon. Forms: /d/, /t/, and /Id/ *Pulled* (/pʊld/) *Walked* (/wɔkt/) *Gilded* (/g I al d Id/)	26–48
	Regular third person -s	Kathy hits. Forms: /s/, /z/, and /Iz/ as is regular plural	26–46

*Used correctly 90% of the time in obligatory contexts.

Source: Adapted from R. Brown (1973); J. Miller (1981).

TABLE 7.23 Calculating Percentage Correct for Plural

Utterance	Correct	Incorrect	Type of Error
2. Want more cookies.	x		
3. Three cookie.		x	Omitted
4. No, one big cookies.		x	Placed on singular
22. Dogs.	x		
27. Give the pencils to me.	x		
28. I want two pencils.	x		
31. You color the foots.		x	Placed on irregular
48. What blue crayons?	x		
TOTAL	5	3	

$$\text{Percentage correct} = \frac{\text{Total of correct}}{\text{Total of correct} + \text{incorrect}} = \frac{5}{8} = 62.5\%$$

then it will be difficult to find errors in pronoun substitution. The types of errors, such as gender or word class, made may reveal the underlying rules that the child is using.

When analyzing the oral and written language of school-age children and adolescents, an SLP will want to note the scope of prefix and suffix use. In addition to inflectional suffixes, such as plural *-s* and past-tense *-ed*, derivational suffixes also should be analyzed. These suffixes, more common in written than in oral language, are used to change word classes, as in adding *-er* to a verb such as *teach* to create the noun *teacher*. The two most common derivational changes are from verbs to nouns (*paint* to *painter*) and from verbs to adjectives (*run* to *runny*).

Children with CLD Backgrounds. An SLP should be mindful of dialectal and bilingual variations. Even though a child omits a morphological ending, it cannot be assumed that the child does not understand or is not able to produce the morpheme. For example, children who speak African American English may omit some word endings for phonological reasons. Others are omitted because they are redundant, such as the plural *-s* when the noun is preceded by a number as in *ten cent*. The child's abilities must be established by the testing of both the marker and the concept associated with it.

The standard for comparison of children's performance is the communication community of each child. A child's language is impaired to the extent that he or she is unable to communicate effectively in that community. In general, dialectal variations develop by age 5, with a few noticeable at age 3.

Language sampling analysis of bilingual Spanish-English children should consider code switching, dialectal differences, English proficiency, and the effects of context on a child's language performance (Gutierrez-Clellen, Restrepo, Bedore, Peña, & Anderson, 2000).

The most frequent morphological errors of ELLs are presented in Table 7.24. Morphological markers often are omitted or overgeneralized. Some Spanish speakers lump English syllables together, decreasing intelligibility. A Cuban American friend calls me "Bobowens." This chunking may cause small units such as morphemes to be deemphasized or omitted.

Syntactic Analysis. Analysis also is accomplished at the intraclausal and clausal levels. For this type of analysis, it is best to exclude imitations, short answers to questions, and stereotypic or rote responses because these types of utterances are not usually clinically significant.

For analysis purposes, it is helpful to separate sentences and nonsentences. Sentences can be grouped for further analysis by length or structure. For example, declarative sentences can be categorized as subject-verb, subject-verb-object, subject-verb-complement, and multiple clauses, either embedded or conjoined. The form of a preschool child's sentences can be compared with normative

TABLE 7.24 Frequent Morphological Errors of English Language Learners (ELLs)

Morpheme	Type of Error	Possible Explanation
Articles	Omission or overgeneralization of *the*	Articles are used infrequently in many languages.
Auxiliaries and modals	Omission	Many languages do not have auxiliary verbs and rely on verb markers.
Contractions	Omission	Unstressed forms often omitted; a phonological error.
Copula	Omission	Unstressed forms often omitted.
Gerund	Omission of *-ing* ending	Many languages do not have this form.
Plural *-s*	Omission or error in agreement, as in *many tree*	Unstressed forms often omitted; used when other languages mark by adjective.
Possessive *-'s*	Omission or overgeneralization	Many languages use the *possession of possessor* form.
Prepositions	Substitution errors	Very complex system in English; multiple meanings of words.
Pronouns	Substitution errors, noun-pronoun agreement errors	Most languages do not have as many pronouns as English.
Regular past *-ed*	Omission or overgeneralization	Unstressed forms often omitted.
Third-person *-s*	Omission or overgeneralization	Exception to English rule of no person or number markers.

data, such as those in Table 7.25, to best determine the child's development, although descriptive data are also valuable. The SLP should note intrasentential noun and verb phrase development, sentence types, and embedding and conjoining. These and other sentence analyses are especially important for school-age children and adolescents.

The ELL child may not exhibit difficulty in a sentence-by-sentence analysis. Analysis of connected speech beyond the sentence may provide more insight. Word-order errors and cohesive difficulties become evident in analysis of units larger than the individual sentence.

Noun Phrase. Noun phrase elaboration is assessed by describing the number and variety of noun phrase elements. Analysis of noun phrases is especially appropriate for children in late childhood or adolescence. The order of the elements within the noun phrase is relatively fixed. The noun function is obligatory, and the other modifiers are nonobligatory. Some or all of these elements may be present in the noun phrase, as shown in Table 7.26. Some elements may be used in combination, whereas the use of others is more exclusive.

Initiators consist of a small core of words that limit or quantify the phrase that follows. Examples are *only, a few of,* and *merely*. Most of these words can serve also as adverbs. The SLP must be careful to identify the accompanying noun phrase in order to avoid adverb-initiator confusion.

Determiners come in many varieties and include, in order of mention, quantifiers; articles, possessive pronouns, and demonstratives; and numerical terms, such as *two, twenty,* or *one hundred. Quantifiers* include such words *as all, both, half, twice,* and *triple*. In combination with initiators, determiners can yield *nearly all, at least half,* and *less than one-third. Articles* include common forms such as *the, a,* and *an*. Possessive pronouns include *my, your,* and *their* and are used without articles. *Demonstratives* serve as articles but are interpreted from the perspective of the speaker as in *this, that, these,* and *those.*

TABLE 7.25 Preschool Language Development

MLU	Approximate Age	Sentence Types	Intrasentential/Morphology
MLU 1–1.5	12–21 mos.	Single words. *Yes/no* questions use rising intonation. *What* and *where.* *Negative* + X. Semantic word-order rules.	Pronouns *I* & *mine.* Isolated nouns elaborated as *art./adj.* + *noun.* Serial naming without *and.*
MLU 1.5–2.0	21–26 mos.	*S* + *V* + *O* appears. Negative *no* and *not* used interchangeably. *Yes/no* question form is *This/that* + *X*?	*And* appears. *In* & *on* appear.
MLU 2.0–2.25	27–28 mos.	*Wh-* question form is *What/where* + *noun*? *To be* appears as main verb*	Present progressive (*-ing*), no aux. verb mastered by 90%. Pronouns *me, my* & *it, this* & *that.* Nouns elaborated in object position only *[(art./adj./dem./poss.)* + *noun].*
MLU 2.25–2.5	28–29 mos.	Basic *SVO* used by most. Negative element (*no, not, don't, can't* interchangeable) placed between noun and verb.	*In/on* & plural *-s* mastered by 90%. *Gonna, wanna, gotta, hafta* appear.
MLU 2.5–2.75	30–32 mos.	*What/where* + *N* + *V*? Inversion in *What/where* + *be* + *N*?* *S* + *aux. verb* + *V* + *O* appears. Aux. verbs include *can, do, have, will.*	Pronouns *she, he, her, we, you, your, yours,* & *them.* Noun elaboration in the subject & object position *[art.* + *(modifier)* + *noun].* Modifiers include *a lot, some* & *two.* Select irregular past (*came, fell, broke, sat, went*) & possessive (*-'s*) mastered by 90%.
MLU 2.75–3.0	33–34 mos.	*S* + *aux. verb* + *be* + *X* appears. Negative *won't* appears. Aux. verbs appear in interrogatives: inverted with subject in yes/no type.	*But, so, or,* & *if* appear.

MLU	Approximate Age	Sentence Types	Intrasentential/Morphology
MLU 3.0–3.5	35–39 mos.	Negative appears with aux. verb + *not* (*cannot, do not*). Inversion of aux. verb and subject in *Wh*- questions.	Uncontractible copula (verb *to be* as *main verb*) mastered by 90%. Pronouns *his, him, hers, us,* & *they*. Noun phrase elaboration includes *art./dem. +adj/poss./mod. + noun.* Clausal conjoining with *and* appears. Clausal embedding as object with *think, guess, show, remember,* etc.
MLU 3.5–3.75	39–42 mos.	Double aux. verbs in declaratives. Add *isn't, aren't, doesn't,* and *didn't.* Inversion of *be* and subj. in *yes/no* interrogatives. Add *when* and *how* interrogatives.	Articles (the, a), regular past (-ed), & third person regular (*-s*) mastered by 90%. Infinitive phrases appear at end of sentence.
MLU 3.75–4.5	42–56 mos.	Indirect objects appear in declaratives. Add *wasn't, wouldn't, couldn't, shouldn't.* Negative appears with other forms of *be.* Some simple tag questions appear.	Pronouns *our, ours, its, their, theirs, myself, & yourself.* Relative clauses appear attached to object. Infinitive phrases with same subj. as main verb.
MLU 4.5+	56+ mos.	Add indefinite negatives (*nobody, no one, nothing*), creating double negatives. *Why* interrogatives appears in more-than-one-word interrogatives Negative interrogatives after 60 mos.	Irregular past (*does, has*), uncontractible auxiliary *to be* and contractible auxiliary *to be* and copula (*to be* as main verb) mastered by 90%. Remaining reflexive pronouns added. Multiple embedding; embedding + conjoining. Relative clauses attached to subj. appear.

*Copula

TABLE 7.26 Elements of the Noun Phrase

Initiator	+Determiner	+ Adjectival	+ Noun	+ Post-Noun Modifier
Only, a few of, just, at least, less , nearly, especially, partially, even, merely, almost	**Quantifier:** All, both, half, no, one-tenth, some, any either, twice, triple **Article:** The, a, an **Possessive:** My, your, his, her, its, our, your, their **Demonstrative:** This, that, these, those **Numerical Term:** One, two, thirty, one thousand	**Possessive Noun:** Mommy's, children's **Ordinal:** First, next, next to last, last, final, second **Adjective:** Blue, big, little, fat, old, fast, circular, challenging **Descriptor:** *Shopping* (center), *baseball* (game), *hot dog* (stand)	**Pronoun:** I, you, he, she, it, we, you, they, mine, yours, his, hers, its, ours, theirs **Noun:** Boys, dog, feet, sheep, men and women, city of New York, Port of Chicago, leap of faith, matter of conscience	**Prepositional Phrase:** On the car, in the box, in the gray flannel suit **Adjectival:** Next door, pictured by Renoir, eaten by Martians, loved by her friends **Adverb:** Here, there (embedded) **Clause:** Who went with you, that you saw
Examples				
Nearly	all the one hundred	old college	alumni	attending the event
Almost all of	her thirty..............................	former	clients	
Just	half of your	brother's old baseball	uniforms	in the closet

Adjectivals consist of nouns marking possession, as in *mommy's;* ordinals, such as *first, next,* and *final;* adjectives, such as *little, big,* and *blond;* and nouns used as descriptors, as in *hot dog* stand and *cowboy* hat. Thus, a speaker might say, "Brother's first little cowboy hat." The exact order of adjectivals in a noun phrase is more complex, requiring more explanation than space allows; however, most speakers recognize that "Cowboy little first brother's hat" is incorrect.

The *noun* function can be filled by subjective pronouns, such as *I, you,* and *they;* objective pronouns, such as *me, you,* and *them;* genitive pronouns, such as *mine, yours,* and *theirs;* simple singular and plural nouns, such as *boy, girls,* and *women;* and mass nouns that have no distinction between singular and plural, as in *sand, water,* and *police.* When a pronoun is used, the noun to which it refers usually has already been identified, and the noun phrase is relatively simple. The noun function also may be complex or may consist of a phrase, as in *Statue of Liberty, need to succeed,* and *city of Los Angeles,* or a compound, as in *Jim and Bob* and *duty and responsibility.* Finally, if the noun is understood by both the speaker and the listener, it may be omitted, as in the following exchange:

"What did you and Barb do last night?""(We) Went to that movie at the mall."

Post-noun modifiers may take many forms, including prepositional phrases (*in the gray flannel suit*), embedded clauses (*who lives next door*), adjectivals (*next door* and *driven by my mother*), and adverbs (*here* and *there*). Post-noun modifiers may be used singly or in combination—for example, "The man *who lives in the green house on the next* block bought all of the candy *that I was selling.*"

The development of elements of the noun phrase takes most typically developing children many years and continues into adolescence. As noted in Table 7.25, elaboration begins in isolation and then moves to the object position in the sentence before appearing in the subject position. This pattern is only the beginning of the development process; with increasing age, the child should use more and more noun elaborations. Table 7.27 offers some developmental guidelines from 50-utterance language samples. The most elaborated forms usually are produced in written language. An SLP is interested in the distribution of these elaborations in these positions and the average number of morphemes within noun phrases.

Children with LI can be expected to have simpler, less elaborated noun phrases. Pronouns offer a special problem. ELLs may exhibit confusion with modifier order and pronoun use.

Verb Phrase. As mentioned in Chapter 2, verb morphology is particularly difficult for children with SLI. Analysis of verb phrase construction and inflected morphology can be a useful measure for identifying 3½- to 6-year-olds with SLI.

Verb phrase elaboration consists of the verb and associated words, including noun phrases used as complements or as direct or indirect objects. An SLP is concerned with the verbs used and those that are missing or incomplete. Other elements of the verb phrase that are present or absent are also important and reflect the maturity of the speaker's language system.

TABLE 7.27 Development of Elaborated Noun Phrases

Age in Months	Number of Elements	Specific Elements
36	2	Noun, Article
48	3	Noun, Article
60	3	Noun, Article, Adjective, Post-noun prepositional phrase
72	3	Noun, Article, Adjective, Post-noun prepositional phrase
84	4	Noun, Article, Adjective, Post-noun prepositional phrase, Possessive pronoun, Quantifier

Source: Information from Allen, Feenaughty, Filippini, Johnson, Kanuck, Kroecker, Loccisano, Lyle, Nieto, Wind, Young, & Owens (In press).

Predicate or verb relationships take three forms: intransitive, in which the verb cannot take an object as in *she walks;* transitive, in which the verb can take an object as in *to her;* and equative, which consists of the copula (*to be*) plus a complement of a noun, adjective, or adverb as in *they are students, they are young,* or *they are late* respectively. Verb phrases can be described by the length and range of types, as demonstrated in Table 7.28.

Simple transitive (*Mommy throw*) and equative verb phrases (*Doggie big*) appear at an MLU of about 1.5. At this level, the verbs are unmarked for tense or person, and the copula is omitted. As language becomes more complex, verbs become marked, the copula appears, and intransitive verb phrases appear. By an MLU of 2.0-2.5, the progressive *-ing* marker and catenatives (*gonna, wanna, gotta, hafta*) appear. The perfective form (*have + verb*-en) and the passive voice begin to be used when the MLU reaches 3.0-3.5/3.75. Adverbial phrases also appear. Late childhood and adolescent language development is characterized by increasing verb complexity with the use of auxiliaries, (*do, have*) modals (may, *should*), and perfective forms, such as *have been going.* There is also increasing use of adverbs and adverbial phrases, such as prepositional phrases of manner (*in silence*), place (*in the city*), and time (*in a week*). In general, many children with LI exhibit these more complex structures but tend to use them less frequently than do children developing typically.

Tense markers are used to describe the temporal relationships between events. For example, if the event being described is taking place while the speaker mentions it, the speaker uses the present progressive verb form (auxiliary + verb-*ing*) to indicate an ongoing activity (*walking, eating*). In

TABLE 7.28 Elements of the Verb Phrase

Modal Auxiliary	+ Perfective Auxiliary	+ Verb to be	+ Negative*	+ Passive	+ Verb	+ Prepositional Phrase, Noun Phrase, Noun Complement, Adverbial Phrase
May, can, shall, will, must, might, should, would, could	Have, has, had	Am, is, are, was, were, be, been	Not	Been, being	Run, walk, eat, throw, see, write	On the floor, the ball, our old friend, a doctor, on time, late
Examples:						
Transitive (May have direct object)						
May	have				wanted	a cookie
Should	not		throw			the ball in the house
Intransitive (Does not take direct object)						
Might	have	been			walking	to the inn
Could			not		talk	with you
Equative (Verb *to be* as main verb)						
		is	not			a doctor
		was				late
		were				on the sofa
May		be				ill.

*When model auxiliaries are used, the negative is placed between the model and other auxiliary forms, for example, "Might not have been going."

contrast, the perfect form of the verb (have + verb-*en*) indicates that the action is being described in relation to the present. Thus, "I have been working here for two years" implies that this action is still occurring, whereas "I *have eaten* my dinner" implies that the action is now complete. Verb tense analysis can be accomplished in a form similar to that presented in Table 7.28. Table 7.25 identifies the ages at which most preschool children acquire auxiliary and modal auxiliary verbs.

Irregular past tense verbs are a special problem (Shipley, Maddox, & Driver, 1991). English contains approximately 200 irregular verbs. Although many are used infrequently, words such as *went, saw, sat*, and *ate*, are among the most frequently used verbs. Development begins in the preschool years and extends into adolescence. Their irregular nature precludes rule learning and generalization, and most acquisition is by rote. Some morphophonemic regularities do occur, however, and may influence the relative ease of learning. The least difficult verbs to learn are those that exhibit no change from present to past, such as *cut/cut* and *hurt/hurt*. The most difficult seem to be those with a final consonant change from /d/ to /t/, as in *build/built*. Other morphophonemic changes include internal vowel change (*fall/fell, come/came*), vowel change with added final consonant (*sweep/swept*), total change (*go/went*), and vowel change with a final dental consonant (*ride/rode, stand/stood*). Obviously, other factors, such as the concept expressed (semantics) and the sounds involved (phonology), also affect learning. Table 7.29 presents the ages at which 80 percent of children are able to use different irregular verbs in a sentence completion task.

Adverbs, like verbs, also can mark temporal relations. Temporal relations can be expressed between two events (*before, next, during, meanwhile*), with the continuation of an event (*for the past year, all week*), in the recent past (*recently, just a minute ago*), and with repetition (*many times, again*).

Verb aspect indicates temporal notions, such as momentary actions, duration, and repetition. Momentary actions are of short duration (*fall, break, hit*). In contrast, duration is marked by verbs of longer action with definite beginnings and ends (*sleep, build, make*). Phrases also may be used to convey a definite act (*sing a song*) and an act without a well-defined terminal point (*sing for your own enjoyment*). Still other verbs describe repetitive actions (*tap, knock, hammer*). All these characteristics affect verb learning.

The development of tense markers seems to be related to the temporal aspect of each verb. The SLP should investigate the relationship between tenses the child uses and the verbs to which these tenses are applied. No doubt, a full analysis will require something larger than a 50- to 100-utterance sample.

TABLE 7.29 Irregular Verbs and Age of Acquisition

Age in Years	Irregular Verbs
3:0 to 3:5	Hit, hurt
3:6 to 3:11	Went
4:0 to 4:5	Saw
4:6 to 4:11	Ate, gave
5:0 to 5:5	Broke, fell, found, took
5:6 to 5:11	Came, made, sat, threw
6:0 to 6:5	Bit, cut, drove, fed, flew, ran, wore, wrote
6:6 to 6:11	Blew, read, rode, shot
7:0 to 7:5	Drank
7:6 to 7:11	Drew, dug, hid, rang, slept, swam
8:0 to 8:5	Caught, hung, left, slid
8:6 to 8:11	Built, sent, shook

Source: Information taken from Shipley, Maddox, & Driver (1991).

Modal auxiliary verbs, such as *can, could, will, should, shall, may, might*, and *must*, are used to express the speaker's attitude. Syntactically, modals function in the formation of questions (***Can*** *we go tonight*?) and negatives (*I* ***shouldn't*** *go out in this weather.*) They are used also in such statements as "I *will* do it tomorrow." Modals represent a complex interaction of form, content, and use that is reflected in the slow rate of acquisition, which usually lasts from age 2 to age 8. Semantic categories of modals include wish or intention (*will, would*), necessity or obligation (*must, should*), ability or permission (*can*), certainty (*will*), and probability or possibility (*may, might*).

Those modals associated with action, such as *can* and *will* (ability, intention, and permission request), are acquired first. During the third year, the number of modals and the categories increases. After age 4, the child clarifies the different forms and their uses.

Children with LI rarely use modal auxiliaries, possibly because they lack the linguistic subtleties expressed. In general, children with LI have more difficulty with catenatives (*gonna, wanna*), modals, and auxiliary verbs than their language level would suggest. An SLP is interested in the range and frequency of the types of verbs a child exhibits.

Children with CLD backgrounds may also experience difficulty with verb tense and with auxiliary verbs. Irregular past tense verbs may exhibit substitutions (*I go yesterday.*) Verb endings may be omitted as a general phonological rule pattern. Verb-subject agreement is also difficult (*She go every day*).

When analyzing a sample, an SLP pays particular attention to the level of development, the range of semantic concepts, the variety of usage, and the types of errors. Variety of usage is noted with different pronouns, verb tenses, negative and positive statements, and sentence types.

Sentence Types. A single event may be described by the agent that originates the action, the action or state changes, and/or the recipient or object of that action. In English, the agent as a noun or a noun phrase is usually first, followed by the action word or verb, which in turn is followed by the recipient or object of that action in the form of a noun or a noun phrase ("John threw the ball" or "Mother will eat the cookie").

If the agent performs the action for the benefit of some other person, that beneficiary—the indirect object—either precedes or follows the noun phrase describing the object of the action. For example, in "He painted the picture *for mother*," *for mother* follows the object of the sentence. Likewise, we could say, "He painted *mother* a picture." Instruments used to complete the action usually are placed after the action and follow the preposition *with*, as in "He painted *with a brush*."

Sentences that differ from the predominant subject-verb-object English format may be difficult for the child with LI to decipher and form. Often, overreliance on the S-V-O strategy is not noted until the child begins school. The child with LI may resist rearrangement or interruption of this form and may attach other structures only at the beginning or the end. Yes/no questions may be asked with rising intonation, rather than through transformation of the subject and verb elements (*He is sick*? vs. *Is he sick*?). Passive sentences, which use an object-action-agent form, may be misinterpreted.

An SLP is interested in the range of internal sentence forms and in the different sentence types. Sentence types include positive and negative forms of the declarative, interrogative, and imperative. The range of sentence types and the maturity of form are of interest. For preschool children these are listed in Table 7.25.

Embedding and Conjoining. Finally, both embedding and conjoining involve relationships between clauses. In addition, embedding involves the relationships between phrases and clauses. It's sometimes difficult for students to identify multiclausal sentences as conjoined or embedded. I suggest that you refer to the excellent tutorial by Steffani (2007). Her descriptions and identification flowchart are extremely helpful.

Clausal embedding initially develops in the object position at the end of the sentence (Table 7.25). Called *object noun complements*, these dependent clauses take the place of the object following such words as *know, think,* and *feel* ("I know *that you can do it*"). Object noun complements using *that* ("I think *that I like it*") appear at an MLU of 4.0, most frequently following the verb *think*. By an MLU of 5.0–5.9, this type of embedding accounts for only 6 percent of children's two-clause sentences. Object noun complements using *what* ("I know *what you did*") account for 8 percent of these sentences.

Relative clauses attached to nouns develop next, beginning in the object position, as in "I want the dog that *I saw last night*." Finally, the relative clause moves to the center of the sentence, describing the subject, as in "The one *that you* ate was my favorite." During late childhood and adolescence, an increase occurs in relative clauses either attached to the subject or serving as the subject, as in "*Whoever wishes to go* should come to the office." This type of clausal embedding is more common in written language than in oral.

Relative clauses appear less frequently among preschoolers than other forms of clausal embedding, although by school age, 20 to 30 percent of two-clause sentences may be of this type. Relative clauses appear at about 48 months initially as post-noun modifiers for empty nouns, such as *one* or *thing*. The most common relative pronouns for preschoolers are *that* and *what*. During the school years, relative pronouns expand with the addition of *whose, whom*, and *in which*.

Phrases also may be embedded in clauses. As in clausal embedding, phrasal embedding usually develops initially at the end of the sentence.

An SLP is interested in the number and type of embeddings. Some developmental data are included in Table 7.25. The position of these embeddings within the sentence is also important, given the developmental significance of position.

Clausal conjoining appears relatively late in preschool development, although some conjunctions appear much earlier. Around 30 months of age, children begin to sequence clauses, using *and* as the initial word in each sentence ("And we saw ponies"). As noted in Table 7.25, *and* is also the first conjunction used to join clauses. At this point, *and* is used for sequential events and is interpreted as *and then*. Even among school-age children, 50 to 80 percent of all narrative sentences begin with *and*. With age and an increase in written communication, use of *and* decreases. Between ages 11 and 14, only 20 percent of spoken narrative sentences begin with *and*. In written narratives, the rate is only about 5 percent.

Other conjunctions may express a causal relationship (*because*), simultaneity (*while*), a contrasting relationship (*but*), and exclusion (*except*). Conjunctions generally develop in the following order: *and, because, when, if, so, but, until, before, after, since, although*, and *as*. The most frequently used conjunctions through age 12 are *and, because*, and *when*.

Early developing strategies that rely on the order of mention for interpretation may persist with a child with LI. Thus, a child ignores the conjunctions and their intended meanings. The sentences "Go to the market before you go to the movie" and "Go to the market after you go to the movie" may be interpreted as having the same meaning because of the order of the clauses.

An SLP is interested in the range and frequency of the conjunctions used and in the amount of conjoining present in the sample. This information is especially important with more mature speakers and is discussed in the following chapter on narratives.

An SLP also should note multiple embeddings and embedding and conjoining that occur within the same sentence. Again, this usage is much more characteristic of school-age language than of preschool language. The narratives of children ages 10 to 12 years are easily distinguishable from those of preschoolers by the presence of multiple embedding and conjoining within the same sentence.

Computer-Assisted Language Analysis

Because of its inherent slowness, conducting language sample analyses (LSA) by hand significantly limits the amount of data SLPs are able to extract from the sample. In contrast, a language sample analyzed with the aid of a computer program, such as SALT, can provide broad information on a child's language abilities. SALT is described in detail in Appendix B.

The availability of a wide range of software and hardware technologies increases an SLP's opportunities for using computer-aided language sampling and analysis (CLSA). In general, the accuracy of computerized analyses is greater than or equal to the accuracy of the analyses conducted by hand and much more time efficient (Long, 2001). In addition, given the sensitivity of CLSA, it can be used efficiently to measure changes over time in response to intervention.

One danger in both testing and CLSA is having the method of testing or analyses dictate or heavily influence identification and intervention. The danger always exists that the method used to assess a child's progress directly affects the goals that educators establish for a child and the methods they use to achieve those goals. When standardized measures are used to assess a child's language, SLPs may be much more likely to focus on the types of discrete skills that are on those measures and to teach them in contexts similar to what the children may encounter on the test. In other words, the very choice of a test or CLSA can have far-reaching effects on an individual child's identification and subsequent intervention with that child.

Although SALT is the most widely used computerized language analysis program, for a number of reasons, it does have some disadvantages. The advantages are as follows (Hammett Price et al., 2010):

- Developed in collaboration with SLPs working in schools, SALT was designed to be user friendly and to generate the types of data SLPs need.
- It has a strong normative database on children between ages 2;8 (years;months) and 13;3.
- SALT enables a clinician to compare a child's language sample to an earlier sample from the same child or to samples from children the same age or grade.
- The databases provide language sample comparison data in conversations and narrative retellings.
- SALT is available in both English and Spanish versions.

There are two disadvantages. The first is SALT's cost, which, although modest, compares favorably to many standardized language tests. Second, SALT is only available for use on computers with a Windows operating system.

The SALT databases of more than 6,000 typical speakers provide a useful tool for the clinical management of children with language impairment, correctly identifying 78 percent of children previously identified as having LI and 85 percent of TD children (Heilmann, Miller, & Nockerts, 2010).

Once mastered, CLSA is more efficient than analysis by hand; this efficiency increases as the complexity of analysis increases. Although CLSAs may quicken the analysis phase of sampling, they cannot replace the clinical intuition of the trained SLP. Nor can CLSAs fill the deficiency caused by a poorly collected sample. In addition, only the SLP can use the data generated to make clinical decisions.

Conversational Partner

Language does not occur in a vacuum. Children converse with many conversational partners, both at home and in school. Each partner helps form a dynamic context in which a child communicates and learns.

Parent–child interactions usually offer an example of a communication process finely attuned to the language skills of a child. Thus, the adult–child dyad represents a highly individualized learning exchange based on the interactional styles and skills of the two communicators.

Variables that affect language learning are complexity, semantic relatedness, redundancy, maternal responsiveness, and reciprocity. In general, maternal linguistic complexity seems to be related to the language learner's level of comprehension.

Semantically related utterances provide a contingency-based language-learning experience. The topic and subsequent content usually are derived from the child. Approximately 68 percent of a mother's speech is related directly to the child's verbal, vocal, and nonverbal behavior.

The mother's input tends to be highly redundant because it relates to ongoing contextual occurrences and attempts to explain, clarify, and comment on her child's experiences and behavior. In addition, the caregiver may repeat content several times in different forms.

Consistent maternal responsiveness teaches children that their responses and behavior have a predictable effect. One valuable lesson the child learns is that communication and communication partners are predictable.

Especially when working with preschool children, an SLP should observe the conversational behavior of the primary caregiver and determine the language learning contributions. Utterances can be rated as to semantic relatedness, redundancy, and reciprocity. From these data, the SLP can comment on the overall teaching environment provided by the caregiver's utterances and behaviors.

It's important to remember that being too directive or not responding in the most appropriate manner to enhance learning does not make a mom or dad a bad parent. By and large, parents of children with handicapping conditions face obstacles that you may not even be able to imagine at this point in your life. I credit parents for bringing their child to his or her present level of language functioning. I try to find where I can tweak the parent's behavior or teach new behaviors to help the child continue that progress. Parents can become important allies, and demonizing them doesn't aid this process.

Conclusion

A language sample is a rich source of information on a child and that child's conversational partners. Analysis may be accomplished at the individual utterance level, across utterance and across partner, and by conversational event. Analysis should not be attempted unless an SLP has a good understanding of the child's language and of the caregivers' concerns. Then a language sample would be analyzed to examine the portion of language in question. A conversational sample can be the best example of a child's actual language use in context.

Utterance-level analysis is most appropriate for language form. Analysis of larger units, such as turns and topics, gives an SLP information on the use of language in context and answers questions about the efficacy of a child's use of language to communicate. A caregiver's style is also of interest if an SLP hopes to employ the caregiver as a language facilitator.

Although a conversational sample is a rich source of data about children's language, analysis is time-consuming. SLPs should analyze only areas of suspected difficulty rather than attempt a blanket analysis. Of interest is the child's present communication system and the communication characteristics of the child's communication partners.

Chapter

8

Narrative Analysis

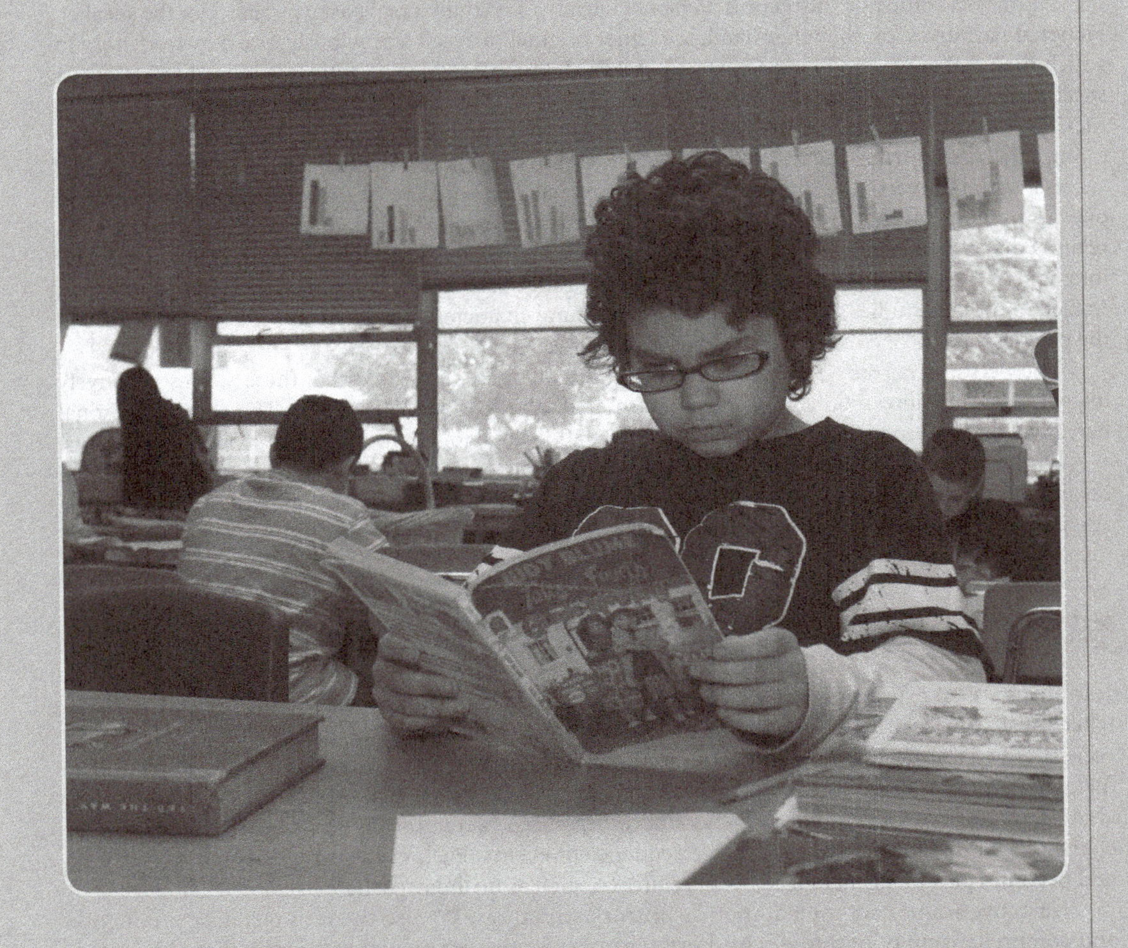

Narratives are a self-initiated, self-controlled, decontextualized form of discourse. As such, narratives are an important part of the language assessment, especially for school-age children and adolescents, because they provide an uninterrupted sample of language that the child or adolescent modifies to capture and hold the listener's interest. The narrative speaker is responsible for ordering and providing all of the information in an organized whole.

Although narration and conversation share many qualities, they differ in very significant ways. First, narratives are extended units of text. Second, events within narratives are linked with one another temporally or causally in predictable ways. Narratives are organized in a cohesive, predictable, rule-governed manner representing temporal and causal patterns not found in conversation. Third, the speaker maintains a social monologue throughout. The speaker must produce language that is relevant to the overall narrative while remaining mindful of the information needed by the listener. Fourth, narratives have an agentive focus. In other words, narratives are about agents—people, animals, or imaginary characters—engaged in events over time.

Narratives come in many genres. Personal narratives recount a real past experience of the speaker. Fictional narratives, on the other hand, are either original or recall a previously heard or read story in which the speaker was not a participant. A child's ability to produce narratives is related to his or her success in acquisition of literacy (Catts, Hogan, & Fey, 2003; Griffin, Hemphill, Camp, & Wolf, 2004; McCardle, Scarborough, & Catts, 2001; Scarborough, 2001; Tabors, Snow, & Dickinson, 2001). For example, a kindergartner's ability to recall narratives is one of the strongest single predictors of reading success. In the conversations of young children personal narratives are far more prevalent than fictional ones. This along with the extensive contextual support parents provide in early conversations for the relating of real past events suggests that personal stories are likely to be more useful to children in social interactions than fictional narratives and are a better gauge of narrative development than fictional ones. In fact, numerous studies have shown that the structural characteristics of narratives develop initially in the personal stories of children with and without LI (Kaderavek & Sulzby, 2000; Losh & Capps, 2003).

The personal narratives of children with LI are often so disordered that these stories negatively impact the social interactions of these children (McCabe & Bliss, 2004–2005). The shorter personal narratives of children with LI often omit key information and violate chronological sequences of events.

Oral and written narratives should form a portion of any child's language assessment. The results should be compared with a child's other linguistic abilities prior to making judgments on the adequacy of the child's language system.

Scripts and Narrative Frames

Narratives are an expression of the organization and interconnection of data in the brain. The storyteller must construct a context within which to relate events, both real and imaginary. Narratives consist of two frameworks, scripts and story frames (Naremore, 2001). Scripts consist of typical, predictable event sequences formed on the basis of experience, either real or vicarious. Scripts are not about any one experience but are generalized, organized hierarchically and causally, inhabited by characters, and containing a predictable sequence of events. Each event is represented in the brain and becomes part of a generalized event sequence, such as birthday parties.

Narrative frames are mental models of story structures. We use them to facilitate production and comprehension of narratives. In short, narrative frames are mental organizers that reduce processing demands.

The narratives of children with LI may break down because of linguistic difficulties or because the child doesn't know either the script or the narrative frame. If too much mental capacity is used for linguistic processing, the narrative frame and/or the script may collapse. In similar fashion, poor script knowledge or poorly formed narrative frames may require too much mental "energy," leaving the child little capacity for linguistic processing.

Prior to collecting a narrative, an SLP should attempt to determine if a child has script and narrative frame knowledge. Script knowledge can be assessed by inquiring about a child's experiences, routines, and event knowledge (Naremore, 2001). Assessment of the retrieval of script knowledge can be accomplished by asking a child to act out the script with toys, pictures, or other items. If the child is successful, the SLP attempts to have the child recite an event account with a cue such as "Tell me what you do when you do X" or "Tell me what happened one time when you did X." If the child needs more help, the SLP can ask a few questions to determine the setting, then begin as follows:

You ride the bus to school every day. Last week on the way to school, you . . .

Note that the focus is the child and the verb tense is present. You can assist the child with the event recount by saying, "And then" or "Tell me what happened next." The recount should have some logical organization.

Knowledge of narrative frames can be determined by discussing with a child the purpose of narratives and determining the child's experience with narrative frames, either at home or in school. The SLP is interested in the use of narratives at home and in story reading. Narrative frames will be analyzed in more detail after a few narratives have been collected.

Children will not possess scripts for all possible events. Nor will all children possess narrative frames. Cultural variations are to be expected and will be discussed at the end of this chapter. The SLP should be reasonably positive that the child possesses event and script knowledge and a notion of narrative frames prior to beginning a narrative collection and analysis.

Collecting Narratives

The quality of a narrative is influenced by the selection of appropriate stimuli and topics based on the age, verbal ability, interests, and gender of a child or adolescent. Stimuli may include objects or pictures used for original constructions and heard or read stories used for retelling. In general, the task used to elicit the narrative influences the speaker's adaptation to the listener.

There are many different types of stories and many different contexts within which to tell them. The story type and context affect the eventual narrative form produced. In general, maximally naturalistic topics and contexts elicit the most representative narratives. Other variables that may affect the narrative form are the story type, a child's experiential base, the task in which the narrative is told, the source of the narrative, the topic, the formal or informal atmosphere of the context, and the audiovisual support available.

Several oral and written narratives should be collected. The wide variation in narratives that can be produced by a single child within different contexts supports this notion. Prior to collecting, the SLP decides on the type of narratives desired and the stimuli to be used in their collection.

In general, fictionalized narratives may result in incomplete narratives with little emphasis on goals, characters' feelings or motivations, and endings. The pace, action orientation, and frequent commercial interruption found in television form a very different base for narratives than does experience or children's books.

The type of elicitation task will affect the child's performance. Books elicit descriptive information, whereas films elicit action sequences. Films also elicit more causal sequences in retelling than do oral stories. Pictures tend to constrain the form of the narrative and may lead to the production of additive chains (And this . . . and this . . .), although children with Down syndrome express more verbal content in narratives to wordless picture books than might be expected based on their formal test results (Miles & Chapman, 2002). Stories in response to pictures tend to exclude character information, internal responses, or intentions. Shared information may be omitted and new information treated as old even when the listener has not viewed the picture. In contrast, individual photographs or discussions of familiar events foster event chains.

Narrative retelling and recall can be used to determine a child's memory organization. In narrative retelling, the child listens to a well-formed story and then reconstructs the story orally or in writing. Retelling of short narratives even may serve as a screening tool with young elementary school children. At this age, children should be able to retell the story without deviating significantly from the original in sequence or content.

Children with LD perform much like younger children, recalling less of the stimulus story. In general, children with LI produce longer and more complete stories in retold narratives than in self-generated ones. Clause length is also greater in retold narratives.

A *minimal narrative* should consist of a sequence of two temporally ordered clauses. In addition, both events should be conveyed in the past tense. Although fictional narratives retold with wordless books are significantly longer than personal stories, they are more frequently not true narratives because they often become picture descriptions that are signaled by a lapse into present tense.

It is important to consider the amount of structure inherent in the stimulus and its effect on retold story construction. For example, nondescript dolls or puppets or sets of vehicles provide no structure. In contrast, a sequence of related pictures provides maximal structure. In general, the more structure found in the stimuli, the less structure the child must provide. The best stories, measured by the most complete episodes and the amount of information, occur when children retell a story without picture cues. Although pictures provide additional input, thus reducing the memory load, they provide no linguistic structure in and of themselves. The task then becomes one of story generation rather than retelling. One additional consideration is that/pictures may distract some children with LI.

In story retelling tasks, an SLP must also consider the comprehension skills needed to understand the story, the mode of presentation (oral or written), story length, a child's past experience with the story genre (e.g., fairy tale, mystery), the child's interest in the content, and the degree of story structure. In general, more familiar, more interesting, and more structured stories result in more complete, better organized retellings.

Well-formed stories should be chosen for retelling and should be modified to enhance clarity and organization. Stories can be rewritten to reduce complexity in their oral form and to summarize important sections. Subparts and transitions between parts of the narrative may need to be highlighted. Good narrative models often have repetitive elements.

Independent, self-generated narrative production requires a child to use her or his own organizational structure and narrative formulation. Narratives can be classified as fictional, personal-factual, or a combination of the two. Fictional or make-believe stories are good vehicles for preschoolers and may be stimulated by objects or pictures. The SLP should provide a model narrative, begin the story for the child, or ask the child to relate a story about the object or picture, beginning with, "Once upon a time . . ." This initial structure usually results in a more literate style.

Personal-factual narratives may be collected from conversation or prompted. This type of narrative is very common in preschool and early elementary school, especially in show-and-tell activities. Preschoolers naturally create these types of narratives in conversation with each other.

It may be helpful for the SLP to establish some common experience with the child and to share a narrative about this experience as an example for the child. To get a narrative, the SLP often has to give one. Using a combination of narration and probing questions, the SLP can tell a personal story related to a common event, such as going to the doctor, and prompt the child with leading questions to stir the child's memory of past events ("Have you ever been to the doctor?"). Experiential topics prompted in this fashion usually result in the longest and most complex narratives.

Topics such as a new sibling or a death usually result in very truncated narratives. Rather, the child can be prompted to relate the scariest or funniest thing that ever happened. In addition, the child might be asked to relate a favorite movie, television show, or story, although these prompts may elicit a sequential list of events.

You should add nothing to the child's narrative other than feedback in the form of "uh-huh," "okay," "yeah," "wow," or a repetition of the child's previous utterance. These neutral but enthusiastic responses will not influence the course of the story as others might. The narrative can be resumed or the child prompted to continue by such utterances as, "And then what happened?"

Stories are enhanced by familiarity with the listener and the location. The SLP should decide ahead of time on strategies for terminating rambling stories and for probing to elicit longer ones. A suggested guideline is not to expect children to engage in storytelling unless their MLU is 3.0 or more.

Narrative Analysis

Narrative analysis is a portion of an overall language analysis occurring at both macro (overall) and micro (finite) levels. Macrostructural analysis examines hierarchical organization, such as story grammar, while microstructural considers internal linguistic structures, such as dependent clauses and conjunctions.

The two levels of analysis are related. Children's lexical and grammatical growth plays an important role in the acquisition of narrative skill. In this process, linguistic forms take on new functions that aid in the organization of narratives. For example, narrative organization skills are positively related to advances in use of grammatical forms, such as verb tense, aspect, and voice, lexical forms, and lexico-grammatical features, such as relational words. Interestingly, children's ability to retell a story seems to be more strongly related to linguistic ability than nonverbal IQ (Bishop & Donlan, 2005). Complex syntax and the ability to relate causal concepts are influential in memory of events.

Given the relationship between microstructure and macrostructure, it should come as no surprise that children with language impairment have difficulty with both aspects of narratives (Manhardt & Rescorla, 2002; Pearce, McCormack, & James, 2003; Reilly, Losh, Bellugi, & Wulfeck, 2004). This difficulty, in turn suggests that these language deficits may be due to broader information-processing deficits, possibly reduced processing capacity (Boudreau, 2007; Colozzo, Garcia, Megan, Gillam, & Johnston, 2006). Given the use of narratives in conversation, a child's difficulty with narrative organization can have a serious impact on her or his everyday language use. This can further impact school performance because narratives are a major component of the school curriculum.

Macrostructural analysis can occur in several ways, such as narrative levels, high points, story grammars, and cohesive devices. *Narrative levels* are concerned with the structural relationship of the narrative parts to the narrative as a whole. Events may be seemingly unorganized or organized sequentially or by causality.

Narrative levels do not have a goal-based organization, whereas story grammars (what happens in the story) do. Narrative level analysis is most appropriate for the stories of 2- to 5-year-olds and for school-age children with limited verbal abilities; story grammar analysis is best for those over age 5. The narratives of preschool children may be evaluated also by using high-point analysis to determine the type of narrative structure.

Story grammars describe the internal structure of a story, including its components and the rules underlying the relationships of these components. By serving as a framework, story grammars may facilitate narrative comprehension and may be used to remember and interpret stories and to anticipate content.

Cohesion analysis describes the linguistic devices used to connect the elements of the text. In narratives, coherence, or making sense, is conveyed through cohesion. Inappropriate or inadequate use of cohesive devices results in a disjointed text that is difficult to comprehend.

From the analysis, an SLP should address the following questions:

- Does the narrative contain chains? If so, what type?
- Does the narrative follow the typical story grammar model? Is the story organized maturely?
- What are the guiding scripts of the narrator, and what do they reveal about the storyteller's knowledge of events and expectations?
- What linguistic means are used to create a cohesive unit?

In addition, the SLP is interested in the sensitivity of the narrator to the perceived needs of the listener.

Narrative Levels

Children use two strategies for organizing their stories: centering and chaining. *Centering* is the linking of attributes or objects to form a story nucleus. The links may be based on similarity or complementarity of features. Similarity links are formed by perceptually observed attributes, such as actions, characteristics, and scenes or situations. *Chaining* consists of a sequence of events that share attributes and leads directly from one to another.

Most stories of 2-year-olds are organized by centering. By age 3, however, nearly half of the children use both centering and chaining. This percentage increases, and by age 5, nearly three-fourths of the children use both strategies.

These organizational strategies can result in six basic developmental stages of story organization (Applebee, 1978), presented here in developmental order:

Heaps are sets of unrelated statements about a central stimulus. The statements identify aspects of the stimulus or provide additional information. The common element may be the similarity of the grammatical structure, for there is no overall organizational pattern.

Dogs wag their tails and bark. Dogs sleep all day. A dog chased a cat.

Sequences include events linked on the basis of similar attributes or events that create a simple but meaningful focus for a story. The organization is additive, and sentences may be moved without altering the narrative.

I *ate* a hamburger. And Johnny *too*. Mommy *ate* a chicken nuggets. Daddy *ate* a fries and coke.

Primitive temporal narratives are organized around a center with complementary events.

I go outside and swing. Bobby push swing. I go high and try to stop. I fall. And I start to cry. Bobby pick me up.

Unfocused temporal chains lead directly from one event to another, while linking attributes, such as characters, settings, or actions, shift. This is the first level of chaining, and the links are concrete. As a result of the shifting focus, unfocused chains have no centers.

The man got in his boat. He rowed and fished. He ate his sandwich. (Shift) The fishes swimmed and play. Fishes jump over the water. Fishes go to a big hole in the bottom. (Shift) There's a dog in the boat. He's thirsty. He jump in the water.

Focused temporal or causal chains generally center on a main character who goes through a series of perceptually linked, concrete events.

This boy, he found a jellybean. And his mother said not to eat it. And he did. And a tree growed out of his head.

Narratives develop the center as the story progresses. Each incident complements the center, develops from the previous incident, forms a chain, and adds some new aspect to the theme. Causal relationships may be concrete or abstract and move forward toward the ending of the initial situation. While young school-age children both with LI and without use scripts for familiar events in their narratives, children with LI often omit causal links to tie together the elements of the script (Hayward, Gillam, & Lien, 2007). There is usually a climax.

There was a boy named Juan. And he got lost in the woods. He ate plants and trees. And he was friends with all the animals. He builded a tent to live in. One day, he builded a fire, and the policemen found him. They took Juan home to his mommy and daddy.

Each narrative can be divided into episodes that are analyzed according to this scheme. Table 8.1 contains examples of narratives and their analysis by narrative level.

Cultural differences must be considered too. African American children often tell topic-associating narratives in which events that happened at different times and places may be combined around a central theme. The narratives of Japanese children may be succinct collections of experiences, rather than single detailed sequential events. Children from Latino cultures often do not relate sequential events.

High-Point Analysis

High-point analysis is a method for identifying narrative macrostructure. The high point, or most significant point of a narrative, is revealed not in the past events recalled, but in an event's meaning to the narrator. The accompanying structure has developmental significance.

It is best for high-point analysis to use narratives that describe events in which the narrator is present. An SLP should select the longest personal event narratives for analysis. Length and complexity have been shown to be related.

The evaluated high point is marked by children in many ways. These markings include paralinguistic features, such as emphasis, elongation, and use of environmental noises ("It went BOOM!"); and linguistic features, such as exclamations ("Wow!"), repetition, attention getters ("Here's the best part."), exaggeration, judgments, or evaluative statements ("It was my favorite."), emotional statements, and explanations.

Once he or she has identified the high point of the narrative, an SLP can analyze for narrative structure. Different types of structures are presented in Table 8.2. Next to each is the approximate age at which these structures are most common for Caucasian, English-speaking, North American children. You can use this table to determine whether the child is using narrative structures typical of his age group. After age 5, fewer than 10 percent of children produce one-event, two-event, leapfrog, and miscellaneous narratives. Obviously, a small sample of a few narratives will be needed for an adequate evaluation.

TABLE 8.1 Narrative-level Analysis

Example	Classification
Simple frames	
Granma lives on a farm. There are horsies and piggies. The cows moo. I can ride on the tire swing in a tree. And the calf licked me. That's all.	Sequence
Once there was two kids, Cassidy and . . . and Fred. Fred's a funny name. And they was fighting. Their mother said, "Why are you fighting?" Cassidy and Fred doesn't know why. They stop and be friends.	Focused chain
Complex narrative frame with episodic development	
The kids all went to Burger King on Halloween. Super Zhiming—that's me—got a cheese-burger. My sister got a Whopper. Mommy and Daddy got nuggets and (Sequence) *salad bar. They were eating when a big ghost came out of my milkshake. He threw milkshake on everyone and got them mad. Super Zhiming stuck the ghost with a fork. The ghost got flat. All the air came out. Daddy was so happy that he buyed ice cream cones for all the kids.*	Sequence Narrative

TABLE 8.2 High-point Narrative Structure

Narrative Structure	Characteristics	Expected Age in Years
One-event narrative	Contains one event.	Below 3.5
Two-event narrative	Contains two past events but no logical or causal relationship in the real world or in the narrative.	3.5
Miscellaneous narrative	Contains two or more past events that in the real world are logically or causally related.	Very low frequency at all ages (3.5–9)
Leapfrog narrative	Contains two or more related past events, but the order does not mirror the real-world relationship.	4
Chronological narrative	Contains two or more related past events in a logical or causal sequence without a high point.	Present at all ages (3.5–9)
End-at-high-point narrative	Contains two or more related past events in a logical or causal sequence with a high point but no following events (resolution).	5
Classic narrative	Contains two or more related past events in a logical or causal sequence with both a high point and a resolution.	6+

Source: Information from McCabe & Rollins (1994).

Variations are to be expected within and across children. Many young children will "test the waters" by stating the high point first ("I got stung by a bee") and then, if it is accepted, will proceed with the narrative. This is not an example of impaired narration and can be analyzed by using high-point analysis when the entire narrative is told.

Story grammar analysis, discussed in the following section, does little to differentiate the narratives of TD children and those with LI. High-point analysis tends to draw sharper distinctions. When we use high-point analysis, the oral personal narratives of early elementary school children with LI, while still below those of TD children, are more mature than their fictional narratives from pictures. In addition, the quality of these children's personal narratives is only minimally related to that of their fictional ones (McCabe, Bliss, Barra, & Bennett, 2008).

Story Grammars

Story grammars provide an organizational pattern that can aid information processing. The competent storyteller constructs the story and the flow of information in such a way as to maximize comprehension. A *story* consists of the setting plus the episode structure (story = setting + episode structure). Each story begins with an introduction contained in the setting, as in "Once upon a time in a far-off kingdom, there lived a prince who was very sad . . ." or "On the way to work this morning, I was crossing Main Street . . . ," or simply "We went to the zoo today."

An *episode* consists of an initiating event, an internal response, a plan, an attempt, a consequence, and a reaction. An episode is considered to be complete if it contains an initiating event or response to provide a purpose, an attempt, and a direct consequence (Stein & Glenn, 1979). Episodes may be linked additively, temporally, causally, or in a mixed fashion. A story may consist of one or more interrelated episodes.

The seven elements of story grammars occur in the following order (Stein & Glenn, 1979):

1. Setting statements (S) that introduce the characters and describe their habitual actions, along with the social, physical, and/or temporal contexts that introduce the protagonist.

2. Initiating events (IE) that induce the character(s) to act through some natural act (e.g., an earthquake), a notion to seek something (e.g., treasure), or the action of one of the characters (e.g., arresting someone).
3. Internal responses (IR) that describe the characters' reactions, such as emotional responses, thoughts, or intentions, to the initiating events. Internal responses provide some motivation for the characters.
4. Internal plans (IP) that indicate the characters' strategies for attaining their goal(s). Children rarely include this element.
5. Attempts (A) that describe the overt actions of the characters to bring about some consequence, such as attain their goal(s).
6. Direct consequences (DC) that describe the characters' success or failure at attaining their goal(s) as a result of the attempt.
7. Reactions (R) that describe the characters' emotional responses, thoughts, or actions to the outcome or preceding chain of events.

The two very different stories in Table 8.3 present examples of different story grammars.

TABLE 8.3 Story Grammar Examples

Narrative	Story Grammar Elements
I. Single Episode	
There was this girl, and she got kidnapped by these pirates.	Setting statement (S)
	Initiating event (IE)
So when they were eating, she cut the ropes and got away.	Attempt (A)
	Direct consequence (DC)
And she lived on a island and ate parrots.	Reactions (R)
II. Multiple Episodes	
Once there was this big dog on a farm.	Setting statements (S)
And he got hungry 'cause there wasn't enough food.	Initiating event$_1$ (IE$_1$)
The dog . . . his name was Max . . . was sad with no food, so his owner went to find some.	Internal response$_1$ (IR$_1$)
	Attempt$_1$(A$_1$)
He met a witch, but she wouldn't give him food 'til he killed a yukky toad.	Initiating event$_2$ (IE$_2$)
	Internal response$_2$ (IR$_2$)
He was scared but he decided to build a trap.	Internal plan$_2$(IP$_2$)
	Attempt$_2$(A$_2$)
He dug a hole and filled it with frog food.	Direct consequences$_2$ (DC$_2$)
The frog wanted to eat the man but got caught.	Direct consequence$_1$ (DC$_1$)
The man went back to the witch and she got some hamburgers for the man and the dog.	
And the man and Max ate hamburgers and were happy.	Reaction$_1$ (R$_1$)

There is a sequence of stages in the development of story grammars (Glenn & Stein, 1980). Certain structural patterns appear early and persist, whereas others are rather late in developing. The overall developmental sequence is as follows, although much individual variation exists:

Descriptive sequences consist of descriptions of characters, surroundings, and habitual actions. There are no causal or temporal links. The entire story consists of setting statements.

> This is a story about my rabbit. He lives in a cage. He likes to hop around my yard. He eats carrots and grass. The end.

Action sequences have a chronological order for actions but no causal relations. The story consists of a setting statement and various action attempts.

I had a birthday party. (S) We played games and winned prizes. (A) I opened presents. (A) I got balloons. (A) I blowed out the candles. (A) We ate cake and ice cream. (A) We had fun.

Reaction sequences consist of a series of events in which changes cause other changes, with no goal-directed behaviors. The sequence consists of a setting, an initiating event, and action attempts.

There was a lady petting her cow. (S) And the cow kicked the light. (IE) Then the police came. (A) Then a fire truck came. (A) Then a hook-and-ladder came. (A) And that's the end. (S)

Abbreviated episodes contain an implicit or explicit goal. At this level, the story may contain either an event statement and a consequence or an internal response and a consequence. Although the characters' behavior is purposeful, it is usually not premeditated.

There was a mommy and two kids. (S) And the kids baked a cake for the mommy's birthday. (S) They forgot to turn on . . . off the stove and burned the cake. (IE) The kids went to the store and buyed a cake. (C) The end. (S)

Complete episodes contain an entire goal-oriented behavioral sequence consisting of a consequence statement and two of the following: initiating event, internal response, and attempt.

This man was a doctor. (S) He made a monster. (IE) And it chase him around his house. (IE) He run in his bedroom. (A) He push the monster in the closet. (A) And the monster go away. (C) That's all. (S)

Complex episodes are expansions of the complete episode or contain multiple episodes.

Once there was this Luke Skywalker. (S) And he had to fight Darf Invader. (S/IE) They fought with swords. (A) And he killed him. (C) And he got in his rocket to blow up these kind of horse robots. (IE) And he shot them. (A) Then all the bad soldiers were killed. (C)

Interactive episodes contain two characters who have separate goals and actions that influence each other's behavior.

Sally never helped her mom with the dishes. (S) She got mad and said that Sally had to do it. (IE) So, Sally washed the dishes but she was mad. (IR) Then Sally dropped some dishes. (A) Then she dropped more. (A) And her mom said that she didn't have to do any more dishes. (C) And Sally watched TV every night after dinner. (S)

Specific structural properties associated with each structural pattern are listed in Table 8.4.

Although most narrative macrostructure measures are based on the components of story grammar, the coding of these components varies widely from those methods that identify their presence or absence (e.g., Miles & Chapman, 2002; Reilly et al., 2004) to those measures that use holistic judgments of the quality and developmental level of children's narratives. Simple story grammar coding procedures are more reliable across different analysts but may be limited in their ability to account for different qualitative aspects of a narrative, such as depth, especially for older school-age children and adolescents.

Children with LD produce fewer mature episodes than do their age-matched TD peers. In addition, children with LD make fewer complete setting statements and are less likely to include response, attempt, and plan statements in their narratives. Inter-episodic relations are also weaker in the narratives of children with LD.

Story grammar analysis alone may lack the sensitivity to differentiate children with LI from those without. Unfortunately, there is little normative data for clinical use. In general, children developing typically produce all of the elements of story grammar by age 10. Children's narratives can be used, however, to approximate their functioning level and to determine which structural elements

TABLE 8.4 Structural Properties of Narratives

Structural Patterns	Structural Properties
Descriptive sequence	Setting statements (S)(S)(S)
Action sequence	Setting statement (S) Attempts (A)(A)(A)
Reaction sequence	Setting statement (S) Initiating event (IE) Attempts (A)(A)(A)
Abbreviated episode	Setting statement (S) Initiating event (IE) or Internal response (IR) Direct consequence (DC)
Complete episode	Setting statement (S) Two of the following: Initiating event (IE) Internal response (IR) Attempt (A) Direct consequence (DC)
Complex episode	Multiple episodes Setting statement (S) Two of the following: Initiating event (IE_1) Internal response (IR_1) Attempt (A_1) Direct consequence (DC_1) Two of the following: Initiating event (IE_2) Internal response (IR_2) Attempt (A_2) Direct consequence (DC_2) Expanded complete episode Setting statement (S) Initiating event (IE) Internal response (IR) Internal plan (IP) Attempt (A) Direct consequence (DC) Reaction (R)
Interactive episode	Two separate but parallel episodes that influence each other

are present. Table 8.5 contains several narratives analyzed by story grammar structural pattern and narrative level.

Expressive Elaboration

Expressive elaboration occurs when the storyteller goes beyond information transmission and creates a pattern of theme, structure, story genre, and mood. The result is an interesting or well-crafted narrative. The skilled narrator selects words and sentence structure to attain his or her desired affect on the listener. For example, the narrator might withhold certain information in order to build suspense or choose words that create a specific illusion. Even real-life narratives may include fictionalized elements that increase listener interest.

While structural properties are essential for narratives, there are other areas of language that also contribute to development of narratives, including the use of literate language and cohesive devices. Literate language contains abstract language features commonly used by teachers and included in the curriculum (Westby, 2005). Features of literate language related to narrative competence include

- metacognitive verbs (*think, know, remember, forget*),
- metalinguistic verbs (*say, talk, tell, ask*).
- elaborated noun phrases (ENPs) (*the little girl in the car with her mom*).

These features appear in preschool and continue to develop into adulthood and are essential for relating the ordered relationships between events in complex narratives (Curenton & Justice, 2004; Nippold, 2007). Not surprisingly, these literate language features are used less frequently by children with LI (Greenhalgh & Strong, 2001).

TABLE 8.5 Story Grammar Analysis

Narrative	Story Grammar Elements	Structural Pattern	Narrative Level
I.			
We went to a farm.	(S)	Descriptive sequence	Unfocused temporal chain
I got to feed chickens.	(S)		
Then I saw cows in the barn.	(S)		
Cows give milk.	(S)		
Cows stay in the field all day and eat grass.	(S)		
At night they come in.	(S)		
II.			
There was this boy who lived in a city.	(S)	Reaction sequence	Focused temporal chain
And one day a giant bug got out of this place where they keep bugs.	(IE)		
And the boy got in an airplane and shot it.	(A)		
III.			
Once there was two boys.	(S)	Complex episodes	Narrative
One boy fell into a big hole with rats and he was scared.	(IE_1)		
His brother got a ladder but the rats ate it.	(IR_1)		
So, he threw his lunch in the hole.	(A_1)		
The rats ate it, too, and the boy climbed up a rope and was safe.	(DC_1/IE_2)		
	(A_2)		
	(DC_2)		
	(R)		

Note: Even though the third narrative possesses advanced structural properties, it demonstrates some pronoun confusion. The relationship of the boys is not established until the third utterance.

Literal language features are used in expressive elaboration in appendages, orientation, and evaluation (Ukrainetz et al., 2005). Appendages alert the listener that a story is being told or ended and consist of five categories:

- Introducer or opening elements (*One morning last week . . .*).
- Abstracts, which provide summaries of events prior to the narrative (*This is about what happened when I . . .*).
- Themes, which provide summaries within the narrative (*This is why I'm so grouchy today*)
- Codas, which are general observations that show the effect on the narrator or characters (*So I learned not to drive too fast*).
- Enders (*The end*).

Orientations are setting statements that often consist of ENPs and include

- names (*Jill*).
- relations, which describe roles or jobs (*my teacher*).
- personality attributes that persist throughout the narrative (*lazy*).

Finally, evaluation describes how the narrative and character perspectives are delivered. Evaluation consists of five categories:

- Interesting modifiers, which consist of most descriptive adjectives and adverbs, including ENPs.
- Expressions, which are multiword modifiers (*tired as a marathon runner*).

- Repetition of nouns, adjectives, or verbs (*walked and walked and walked*) for effect.
- Metacognitive internal state words, which reflect thoughts (*remembered*), feelings (*depressed*), reactions (*surprised*), intentions, and physical states (*tired*).
- Metalinguistic dialogue words (*So she said . . .*).

By age 9, all typically developing children should exhibit some expressive elaboration in their narratives. Naturally, these vary by type of elaboration, so several narratives are required for a full picture of a child's abilities. Table 8.6 presents narratives with varying types of expressive elaboration.

Quantitative Measures

Several microstructural measures vary significantly with age. These are total number of words (TNW), number of different words (NDW), total number of T-units (LENGTH), mean length of T-units in words (MLT-W), total number of T-units that contain two or more clauses (COMPLEX), and the proportion of complex T-units (PROCOMPLEX) (Justice, Bowles, et al., 2006). These values are presented in Table 8.7. Be cautioned that these data are from a pilot study, albeit a well-done one, and that there is wide variability among TD children, as seen in the standard deviation (SD). Within one standard deviation is where the normal population is considered to be.

TABLE 8.6 Types of Elaboration Found in Narratives by Age 9

Evaluations—Most frequent; increase with age		
Modifiers	Adjective, adverbs, and adverbial phrases*	*mighty, angry, shy, slowly, in between*
Expressions	Multiword modifiers	*as quietly as she could, wrong side of the tracks, all of a sudden*
Repetition	Repetition of a word for emphasis	*He ran and ran to get way, They were very, very happy*
Internal States	Words reflect intentions, thoughts, feelings, emotions, motivations, and reactions	*thought, sad, angry, tired, decided, planned*
Dialogue	Portions of narrative in which characters speak	*She shouted, "Stop that!"*
Orientations—Increase with age		
Names	Characters identified specifically on first mention	*King Juan, Jack, Monica*
Relations	Relationships of jobs defined	*Monica's sister, teacher, pet*
Personality	Personal attributes that endure throughout the story	*always late, too young to, grumpy old woman*
Appendages—Least frequent; increase with age		
Introducer	Beginning of narrative marked	*Once upon a time, One night, Yesterday*
Abstract	Summary prior to narrative or story title	*This is a story about why you you shouldn't run away, This is called "My Best Day"*
Theme	Summary within narrative	*And this is why he was so scared*
Coda	Effect of narrative or lesson learned	*So they decided never to ride their bikes in the woods again*
Ender	Formal indication narrative is over	*That's it, The end, And they lived happily . . .*

*Some occur so frequently that they should not be noted. These include *some, other, another, one, little, big, bad, on top, outside, behind,* and *after.*
Source: Information from Ukrainetz, Justice, Kaderavek, Eisenberg, Gillam, & Harm (2005).

TABLE 8.7 Narrative Microstructure

Age	TNW		NDW		LENGTH		MLT-W		COMPLEX		PROCOMPLEX	
	M	SD	M	SD	M	SD	M	SD	M	SD	M	SD
Oral Narratives												
5	68	(± 47)	39	(± 20)	8.5	(± 5.4)	6.8	(± 1.7)	3.1	(± 3.2)	.33	(± .2)
6	77	(± 54)	43	(± 22)	9.6	(± 6)	7.5	(± 1.6)	3.5	(± 2.8)	.37	(± .2)
7	96	(± 74)	52	(± 28)	11.3	(± 9.1)	8.5	(± 3.8)	4.6	(± 4.3)	.38	(± .2)
8	137	(± 77)	69	(± 27)	15.8	(± 8.9)	8.1	(± 1.4)	7.6	(± 5.2)	.45	(± .2)
9	162	(± 96)	79	(± 30)	17.3	(± 9.6)	8.4	(± 1.4)	8.9	(± 6.1)	.51	(± .2)
10	237	(± 196)	101	(± 49)	21.5	(± 14.5)	8.9	(± 2.1)	12.2	(± 9.8)	.55	(± .2)
Written Narratives												
11							9.14	(± 2.2)				
14							11.19	(± 3.9)				
17							11.27	(± 2.1)				

Note: Columns include total number of words (TNW), number of different words (NDW), total number of *T*-units (LENGTH), mean length of T-units in words (MLT-W), total number of T-units that contain two or more clauses (COMPLEX), and the proportion of complex T-units (PROCOMPLEX).
Source: Information from Justice, Bowles, Kaderavek, Ukrainetz, Eisenberg, & Gillam (2006); Sun & Nippold (2012).

In the narratives of teens, we find that both mean length as measured in T-units and clausal density increases with age. In addition, throughout adolescence the use of abstract nouns, such as *accomplishment, loneliness,* and *mystery,* and metacognitive verbs, such as *assume, discover,* and *realize,* in narratives also increases (Sun & Nippold, 2012).

Episodic or episode structure and syntactic accuracy are good measures of language in children from CLD backgrounds (Muñoz et al., 2003). More semantically based quantitative measures, such as the number of different words, seem to vary with the method of elicitation (Uccelli & Páez, 2007).

Cohesive Devices

Cohesion is the use of various linguistic means to link narrative utterances together into a unitary text (Hickmann & Schneider, 2000). To tell an effective story, narrators must use cohesive devices that carry concepts across utterances. Three major categories of cohesive devices are

- referential cohesion, which maintains appropriate reference to the characters, objects, and locations.
- conjunctive cohesion, which sustains concepts across phrases and utterances.
- lexical cohesion, which effectively uses vocabulary to link concepts across utterances.

Refential cohesion across utterances is controlled using noun phrases and pronouns and articles. As the name implies, conjunctive cohesion uses conjunctive words and phrases (*and, but, because, besides, in addition, finally, in contrast*). As noted previously, children with LI have more difficulty with correct use of cohesive devices.

Children with LI and those with poor reading abilities exhibit some difficulty communicating well-organized, coherent narratives. In general, they produce event and essential relationships more poorly than do their age-matched TD peers. The most common cohesive errors among children with LI are an *incomplete tie,* in which the child references an entity or event not introduced previously, and an *ambiguous reference,* in which the child does not identify to which of two or more referents she or he is referring.

Of interest in the text are cohesive devices that linguistically connect the components. In short, any sentence element that sends the listener outside of the sentence for a referent is a cohesive device. For example, a pronoun may require referral to the previous sentence in order to determine the referent. The five types of cohesive relations are reference, substitution, ellipsis, conjunction, and lexical items. Of these, lexical cohesion may be the most difficult to assess reliably.

Because there is little normative data on the development of these relations, descriptive analysis is the best diagnostic approach. In general, mature story grammar develops prior to mature use of cohesive devices. It is possible, therefore, to have good episodes but poor cohesion. The two are related but not dependent. The cohesion within and between episodes becomes important as children develop complex and interactive episodes. There is a metalinguistic quality about cohesion in that the speaker must pay attention to the text apart from the story itself. Cohesive relations are discussed in Chapter 7 and are reviewed only briefly in this section.

Reference

Reference devices, which refer to something else in the text for their interpretation, consist of pronouns, definite articles, demonstratives, (*this, that*) and comparatives (*bigger shown*). The link with the referent should be clear and unambiguous. Referring expressions are adequate if they are appropriate for the listener's knowledge, shared physical context, and preceding linguistic context (Schneider & Hayward, 2010). Clarity is often a problem when a child changes the story narrator frequently, uses dialogue, or includes several characters.

Adequate first or initial mention includes the use of an indefinite article and a noun, as in "*A boy* was eating *a cookie*." In contrast, subsequent mention makes use of definite articles and pronouns, as in "*He* dropped *it*." There are exceptions, of course. For example, if two people are looking at a picture, a pointing gesture or glance can serve as the initial mention and one speaker, referring to the picture, might say, "Look, *he* dropped *it*." The references are understood because the listener can refer to the context and relate the referring expressions to the pronouns.

Children's ability to introduce and maintain referents in narratives develops gradually during the early school years. Younger children frequently introduce referents in a confusing way, possibly assuming that the listener understands the referent. On initial mention, they often use pronouns and definite articles. Although these children can use indefinite articles and nouns in other contexts, they seem to be unsure of the appropriate choice of these forms in the context of an extended discourse, such as a narrative, in which the knowledge state of the listener needs to be constantly monitored. It takes some linguistic skill to bring a listener along as a narrative progresses.

Kindergartners correctly introduce referents more often when they are retelling a recently heard fictional story than when they are formulating the story themselves from pictures unseen by a listener. This would suggest that when kindergartners must choose referents based on listener knowledge, they tend to be less adept at doing so. Even young school-age children have some difficulty with initial mention, although after age 9 or so, in simple stories, children introduce characters similarly to adults. The ability to introduce referents in narratives continues to develop for some time after age 9 (Schneider, 2008).

Although children have some inadequate referring in subsequent mention, preschool and young school-age children have more difficulty with first mentions of referents. Difficulty in subsequent mentions seems most related to story complexity. This is because in simple, short narratives it may only be necessary to refer to characters once or twice after initial mention. Multiple characters, especially of the same gender, can also complicate subsequent reference.

Semantic elaboration can be used to assess the language differences of children, especially those with FASD (Thorne, Coggins, Carmichael Olson, & Astley, 2007). Semantic elaboration is measured by the use of nouns and pronouns to reduce ambiguity in the narrative, the specificity of the nouns and verbs used to introduce an entity (*thing* vs. *hammer*) or action (*went* vs. *drove*), and noun and verb elaborators (***large angry*** *dog* and *ran* ***quickly***, respectively). The Semantic Elaboration Coding System (Thorne, 2004) offers a convenient way to analyze this data.

Demonstratives locate referents on a continuum of proximity. Nominals, such as *this, that, these,* and *those,* refer to a person or a thing; adverbs, such as *here, there, now,* and *then,* refer to a place or a time. Use of *now* and *then* usually is restricted to referring to the time just mentioned. In addition, *now* and *then* can serve as conjunctions.

Finally, comparatives are both general and specific. General comparatives include such words as *another, same, different(ly), equal(ly), unequal, identical, similar(ly),* and *else.* Specific quantity words include *more, less, so many, as few as, second, further,* and *fewer than.* Quality words and terms consist of *worse than, as good as, equally bad, better, better than, happier than,* and *most happy/happiest.*

Substitution and Ellipsis

Substitution and ellipsis both refer to information within the narrative that supposedly is shared by the listener and the speaker. In substitution, another word is used in place of the shared information. The words *one(s)* and *same* can be substituted for nouns, as in "Make mine the *same*" or "I'll take *one*, too." Such words as *do* can be substituted for main verbs, as when we emphasize, "I *did* already." Finally, such words as *that, so,* and *not* can be substituted for whole phrases or clauses, as in "I think *not*" or "Mother won't like *that.*"

Ellipsis differs from substitution in that shared information simply is omitted. Whole phrases and clauses may experience ellipsis.

Conjunction

The four types of conjunctive relations, mentioned in Chapter 7, are additive, temporal, causal, and adversative. Whereas additive relationships usually are represented by *and,* temporal ones may be signaled with a variety of words, such as *then, next, after, before, at the same time, finally, first, second,* and *an hour later.* Causal conjunctive relationships may be expressed with a variety of terms, such as *because, as a result of, in that case, for, and so.* Finally, adversative conjunctions include *but* and others, such as *however, although, on the other hand, on the contrary, except,* and *nevertheless.*

Conjunction use may be independent of the specific clausal structures linked. In other words, conjunctions link the underlying semantic concepts and thus represent the relationship of these units, which may be expressed by various syntactic units. The way episode parts are linked may reflect a child's underlying episodic organization. We would expect, therefore, that conjunctive relationships between episodic elements would be more complex and difficult than those between sentences. This increase seems to be true for both children with LI and those without. This may account for the fewer conjunctions found in the narratives of children with LI (Greenhalgh & Strong, 2001).

Lexical Items

Words themselves express relationships by the morphological endings used. The following example demonstrates a clear understanding of the relationship of the process to the product:

> He *had been writing* for several months. After the book was finally *written,* he celebrated for days. He swore never *to write* another novel.

Categorical relationships can be expressed and demonstrate convergent and divergent organizational patterns. Convergent thought goes from the members to the category, as in "She had *petunias, dahlias, roses, and pansies* in her garden, but she could never have enough *flowers.*" Divergent thought goes from the category to the members, as in "She liked several kinds of *sports* but was best at *soccer, rugby, and lacrosse.*"

Finally, words can express relationships, such as opposition or part-to-whole. In a narrative, the SLP can look for antonyms, synonyms, ordered series, and part-whole or part-part relationships. Ordered series include memorized sequences, such as the days of the week, or hierarchies, such as instructor, assistant professor, associate professor, and full professor. Part-whole relationships are expressed by entities that form a portion of the whole, as in rudder-boat, pedal-bike, and January-year. Finally, part-part relations contain parts of the same whole, as in nose-chin, finger-thumb, and rudder-sail.

Summary

Assessing children's use of cohesive ties has been attempted in several ways (Schneider & Hayward, 2010). These range from frequency counts and distributions to judgments of correctness or adequacy (Girolametto, Wiigs, Smyth, Weitzman, & Pearce, 2001). Normative data is difficult to obtain given the influence of story complexity on these measures. In addition, not all cohesive ties are equal in the degree to which they contribute to cohesion. For example, consider the relationships conveyed by various conjunctions. In contrast, focusing solely on certain linguistic forms may miss the overall cohesive abilities of a child. Referential cohesion may be best considered in terms of function rather than particular linguistic forms. While related, the ability to introduce and maintain referents differs from mastery of individual linguistic forms.

Other researchers have suggested calculating referential adequacy or RA by dividing the number of adequate referring expressions by the total number of referring expressions (Norbury & Bishop, 2003). Again, this methodology overlooks different types of cohesion and degrees of inadequacy. Nonetheless, RA measures have the advantage of focusing on the function of referring expressions in context.

Unfortunately, for all these reasons, we are still searching for a normed narrative instrument of referential cohesion. The likely reason is the difficulty in specifying the rules for determining adequacy of subsequent mention, which depends on both the length of a story and the number and order of referents mentioned.

It might be more appropriate to focus, at least in part, on initial mention, which is more straightforward than subsequent mention (Schneider & Hayward, 2010). In addition, it's possible with initial mention to restrict analysis to same set of referents by controlling for the number and type of referents. This can be accomplished using picture cues. Scaled scoring on the degree of adequacy of the initial mention can also be helpful in distinguishing children's responses. A total score for all referents could be divided by the number of referents mentioned initially. This would permit comparisons across children. If you're interested in such a procedure, please refer to the article by Schneider and Hayward (2010) who used this methodology with the Edmonton Narrative Norms Instrument (ENNI; Schneider, Dubé, & Hayward, 2009). The authors were able to describe developmental changes with age and to distinguish between TD children and those with LI. The ENNI is available free of charge at www.rehabmed.ualberta.ca/spa/enni. A similar procedure could be used to establish local norms.

Reliability and Validity

Narrative analysis is not without its detractors. Naturally, reliability and validity will vary with the aspects of narratives measured.

Establishing developmental level by the number of story grammar components present appears to have very high inter- and intrajudge reliability. This developmental level and other quantitative measures, such as words per T-unit and words per clause, also correlate strongly with language test scores, suggesting that narrative analysis has strong construct validity.

One promising narrative assessment tool is the Narrative Scoring Scheme (NSS; Heilmann, Miller, Nockerts, & Dunaway, 2010). NSS rates a range of microstructural and macrostructural narrative skills required for school-age children to effectively tell a narrative. To do this, the NSS incorporates multiple aspects of the narrative process into a single scoring system, combining both the basic components of story grammar approaches and higher inter-utterance text-level narrative skills.

The hybrid approach enables the SLP to examine each component of the narrative process while reflecting on a child's overall narrative skill. The NSS is broken into seven skill areas:

- Introduction, a key element in story grammars
- Character development of both main and supporting characters and the use of voice
- Mental states expressed through metacognitive verbs
- Referencing through the use of nouns and pronouns
- Conflict resolution
- Cohesion, including the relationship between and the logical order of events
- Conclusion, in which the elements of the narrative are wrapped up

Each component is rated as proficient, emerging, or minimal/immature and contributes to a score of overall quality.

As an assessment tool, the NSS appears to be both an efficient and informative way to measure development of narrative macrostructure. The NSS is significantly correlated with age and with each of the microstructural measures. In addition, there is a unique relationship between vocabulary and narrative macrostructure.

Children with CLD Backgrounds

Narrative performance among various cultural, ethnic, and linguistic groups may differ greatly. These differences reflect both cultural and individual differences in storytelling. Storytelling is never context or culture free. Rather, it is the product of the contextual interaction of the narrator and the audience and of the sociocultural norms of each, which shape each person's presuppositions and expectations. Even the purpose and context for narratives varies across cultures.

Telling narratives is a social event governed by cultural norms and values. Not every culture expects the narrative monologues seen in American English. Among some Latinos, Native Americans, African Americans, Jewish Americans, and Hawaiian Americans, stories are produced conversationally with audience cooperation. The story is built by the storyteller acting out the parts as the audience challenges and contradicts.

Although there do not appear to be any significant differences between ethnic groups in narrative organizational style or use of paralinguistic devices, there are some differences of which SLPs should be aware (Gorman, Fiestas, Peña, & Reynolds Clark, 2011). In the narratives of first and second graders, African American children include more fantasy, Latino children named the characters more often, and Caucasian children make more references to the nature of character relationships. While these changes do not significantly change the character of the stories, they give us added insight when soliciting narratives from these children.

SLPs must be alert to possible bias in interpretation of children's narratives. For example, with little guidance in the professional literature, SLPs may have their own preference for what constitutes a good narrative. Current literature focuses almost exclusively on the story structure over the performative aspects of storytelling, although there are potential sociocultural influences on children's use of stylistic and creative features in their narratives.

Planning ecologically valid narrative intervention requires an SLP to be mindful of the many functions narratives can serve in various cultures, such as informing and entertaining. An SLP should attempt to foster narrative skills valued by children's culture (Bliss, McCabe, & Mahecha, 2001).

Narrative Collection and Analysis

The cultural variability of narratives requires an SLP to assess narrative development in a wide variety of culturally relevant contexts approaching the natural environment of the child. If the child does not consider the task "worthy," he or she may give less than an optimum or even typical performance.

A dynamic assessment of narrations consists of a collection and analysis, mediated instruction, and a second collection and analysis (Peña, 2002). With school-age children, the SLP first can collect narratives in response to wordless picture books and analyzes each for the number of words, C-units, clauses, clauses/C-unit, episodic structure, story components, and story idea and language. Possible wordless picture books include *Bird and His Ring* (Miller, 1999b), *Frog, Where Are You?* (Mayer, 1969), *One Frog Too Many* (Mayer & Mayer, 1975), and *Two Friends* (Miller, 1999a).

In the second step, the SLP can choose one or two areas of the narrative for a mediated language experience (MLE). The SLP helps the child explore the goals of a story, the importance of these goals, the consequences of omitting these goals, plans for using this information, and developing strategies.

The second collection and analysis is similar to the first but attempts to answer five questions (Peña, 2002):

Was the child able to form a more complete and coherent narrative?

How difficult was it for the SLP to achieve positive change?

Did the child pay attention and include more elements in the second narrative?

Was the child able to transfer the learning without SLP support?

Was learning quick and efficient?

Children developing typically usually make rapid changes and are very responsive.

For more-mature children and adolescents, several narratives can be collected in various contexts and analyzed as above and for the "rules" appropriate for each type of narration. The characteristics of each type of narration based on temporal, referential, causal, and spatial coherence are included in Table 8.8. The SLP must remember that the "rules" for certain types of narration may be unfamiliar to some children and may be a difference, rather than a deficit. The types of cohesion used by the child should reveal his or her narrative style.

TABLE 8.8 Types of Narration and Cohesion

Temporal Coherence
Is there a temporal order of events?
Are temporal connectives necessary? If so, are they used?
Are shifts in time marked?
Causal Coherence
Are physical and mental states used to interconnect actions? (He was very tired, so he went to sleep.)
If not, can connectives be inferred easily?
Are causal connectives necessary? If so, are they used?
Referential Coherence
Participants
Is adequate reference to the participants made?
Are new characters introduced clearly? If not, are they referred to as if introduced elsewhere in the text?
Are characters reintroduced in an unambiguous manner?
Can the referent be inferred from general world knowledge?
Props
Is identification of specific objects necessary? If so, are props mentioned adequately? If not, are props introduced by gestures or deictics, such as "that thing"?
Can the identity of props be inferred from descriptions or functions?
Spatial Coherence
Is information about location necessary? If so, are locations identified?
Are shifts in location clearly marked?

Source: Information from Gutierrez-Clellan & Quinn (1993).

In the second step, the different types of narratives are explained to the child by using cues, such as "Talk like a book in school" or "Talk like you would to a friend," and examples. Within the training, the child is given different types of narratives to produce. Feedback is used by the SLP to seek clarification, additional information, relevant comments, and reference. After some intervention, the SLP attempts to determine whether the child can learn different types of narration, can transfer the types of cohesion across contexts, and can tell narratives without cuing and feedback.

Two measures that seem particularly important are the length of causal sequences and the number of unrelated statements. Among children speaking Spanish, an increase in the length of causal sequences and a decrease in the number of unrelated statements are indicators of greater causal cohesion.

Dynamic procedures work well with children from different sociocultural backgrounds. The procedures require that the task be explained, that the reasons for certain responses be stated adequately, and that the child respond differentially to the SLP's cues.

Conclusion

The near universal use of some form of narrative suggests its importance in communication. As in dialogue analysis, it is important to analyze narratives simultaneously at several levels. Although there are few normative data on narrative development against which to compare a child's or adolescent's performance in any culture, an SLP can use the model described in this chapter as a basis for analysis and description of a child's narrative performance.

In general, the more mature the narrative, the more complete the structure and the story grammar. In addition to causal chains, more-mature narratives contain greater cohesion to aid the listener in interpretation. Mature narratives are structurally cohesive and proceed from one event to another in a logical fashion that demonstrates the narrator's attempt to guide the listener.

More-mature narratives also include more insight into the thoughts and feelings of the central characters and greater use of devices for expressing time and place. There are fewer extraneous details and loose ends.

An SLP should be cautious when evaluating children from cultures whose narratives do not closely follow the pattern described in this chapter. Children from some Spanish-speaking and some Native American cultures may have less experience with story narratives. To varying degrees, these cultures make extensive use of more descriptive narratives. The use of pictures and elicitation techniques, such as "Tell me a story about this picture," may evoke a very different narrative from what is sought.

Chapter 9

A Functional Intervention Model

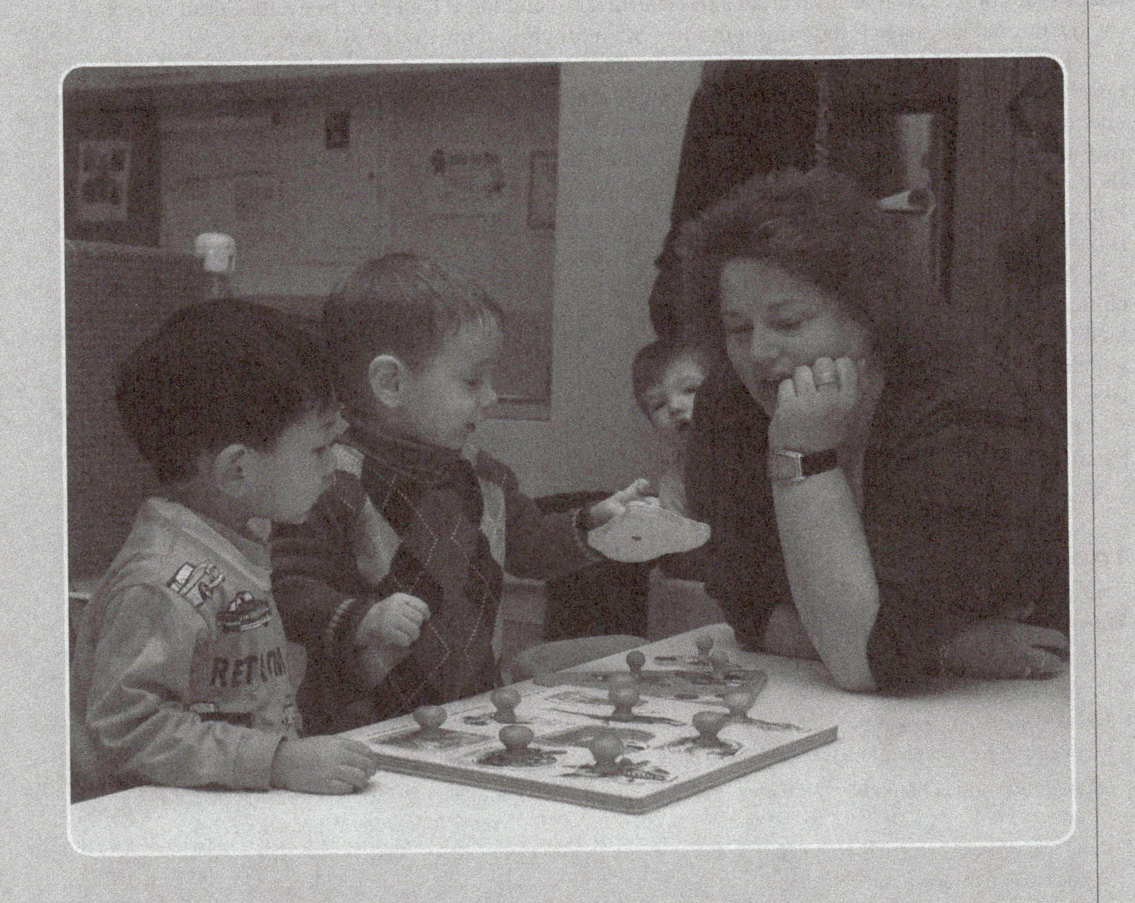

Traditional language intervention does not consider either the integrated nature of language or the context of language use. Language is viewed as a hierarchically organized set of rules, rather than as a holistic set of variable context-sensitive rules. Although the focus may include form, content, and use, the overall design is usually additive, rather than integrative. Often, the stated goal is to learn specific language units, not to enhance overall communication. Language methods that emphasize very specific skills seem to have very specific effects. There is little evidence that newly acquired forms generalize to everyday conversational use.

Clinical intervention should be a well-integrated whole in which the various aspects of language combine to enhance communication. The purposes of intervention should be (a) to teach a generative repertoire of linguistic features that can be used to communicate in socially appropriate ways in various contexts and (b) to stimulate overall language development (Duchan, 1997a).

A functional language intervention model discussed throughout this text attempts to target language features that a child uses in the everyday context, such as the home or the classroom, and to adapt that context so that it facilitates the learning of language. Table 9.1 presents a comparison of the traditional language intervention model with a functional integrated approach.

The functional approach recognizes a need to orient language training toward the inclusion of family members and teachers as language facilitators and toward the use of everyday activities for encouraging functional communication. Therefore, routines within the home, school, and community are used with an array of language facilitators. In this way, aspects of language can be trained as they relate to one another within the context of a meaningful experience. As a result, the intervention experience more closely approximates patterns of nonimpaired language development. Content is based on common experiences.

A functional approach, with its integrative and interactive aspects, changes the nature of the clinical interaction and the role of the SLP. The SLP becomes a consultant for the other language facilitators, who interact more frequently with the child, training them to modify the contexts within which language can occur and to elicit and modify the child's language. The SLP and caregivers collaborate in the child's language intervention.

Concern for generalization is foremost and governs the overall intervention approach. Planning by an SLP, along with the language facilitators, is essential. Implementation and generalization may

TABLE 9.1 Comparison of Traditional and Functional Intervention Models

Traditional Model	Functional Model
Individual or small group setting using artificial situations.	Individual or small or large group setting within contextually appropriate setting.
Isolated linguistic constructs with little attention to the interrelationship of linguistic skills.	Relationship of aspects of communication stressed through spontaneous conversational paradigm.
Intervention stresses modeling imitation, practice, and drill.	Conversational techniques stress message transmission and communication.
Little attention to the use of language as a social tool during intervention sessions.	The use of language to communicate is optimized during intervention sessions.
Little chance or opportunity to develop linguistic constructs not targeted for intervention.	Increased opportunity to develop a wide range of language structures and communication skills through spontaneous conversation and social interaction.
Little opportunity to interact verbally with others during intervention.	Increased opportunity to develop communication skills by interacting with a wide variety of partners.

Source: Information from Gullo & Gullo (1984).

be hampered or impeded by any number of factors, such as the targets selected, the intervention setting, the training methods used, and caseload and scheduling considerations.

Intervention should begin with a generalization plan that identifies features of a child's communication environment relevant to generalization. All too often, generalization is the last step in the intervention planning process, rather than the overall organizing aspect.

Once the appropriate generalization variables have been identified, an SLP can begin to design intervention strategies. The relevant features of the communication environment that have been identified can now be enlisted. Ideally, such intervention enables an SLP to (a) develop linguistic constructs at a child's developmental functioning level, taking into account the strategies children normally use when acquiring language, (b) integrate all linguistic areas within the communication framework, and (c) provide meaningful and age-appropriate contexts.

In this chapter we discuss principles of intervention in a functional approach and an overall model for intervention, focusing on the variables that affect generalization.

Principles

Use of a functional approach to language intervention requires an SLP to change some methods and to be mindful of certain principles that aid communication with and learning for a child. It is important to engage a child in meaningful dialogue or in some other communication event, and this event becomes the vehicle for learning and generalization.

The following section includes some of the most important principles of the functional approach. Undoubtedly, some important ones have been omitted that the reader will want to include in her or his repertoire.

The Language Facilitator as Reinforcer

As communicators, we continue to interact with those individuals who provide positive feedback and reinforcement. As much as possible, you avoid communicating with certain individuals who are nonresponsive, caustic, or overly critical. Children avoid certain potential conversational partners for many of the same reasons. If you want children to communicate with you, then you must be someone with whom children want to communicate.

Children respond most readily to adults who convey genuine caring and respect for them. These attitudes are conveyed by meeting a child halfway. Adults who desire to be effective conversational partners must appreciate the world from a child's perspective. It may help to recall that for children the world is full of wonder and delight, full of things that cannot be explained, and full of magic.

Adults demonstrate concern for children and adolescents when they are willing to attend to children, to listen, and to accept their topics. As much as possible, intervention should be nonintrusive, with facilitators providing supportive, evaluative feedback to a child. By reducing your authority-figure persona, demonstrating an attentiveness and a willingness to adopt a child's topics, and remaining accepting while providing evaluative feedback, you, as an SLP, can send a message of acceptance of the child as a partner.

Few child linguistic responses are totally wrong. Even seemingly incorrect utterances can demonstrate the child's understanding of the situation and of the underlying relationships. Acceptance of a child includes acceptance of these utterances. Usually, some portion of the utterance can be reinforced.

Child: I need ear-gloves.
SLP: That's right, they are like little gloves for your ears. We call them *earmuffs*. Here, let me help you put on your earmuffs.

The partner has accepted the child's utterance, recognized the child's understanding of the situation, corrected the utterance, and left the child's ego intact.

The intervention setting itself should "create and sustain an atmosphere containing fun, surprise, interest, ease, invitation, laughter, and spontaneity" (Cochrane, 1983, p. 160). In such an atmosphere, children will be eager to participate. One of my best lessons on verbal sequencing used mime, complete with whiteface. The children enacted familiar everyday event sequences, such as making breakfast, while other students tried to guess the name of the sequence. After the correct guess was given, the actor stated each event in the sequence while performing it. Finally, each actor attempted to reconstruct the sequence verbally. The lesson was messy, fun, enjoyable, and thoroughly successful.

Children also respond favorably if the facilitator occasionally plays the clown or buffoon. I may wear a cooking pot on my head in order to evoke a response. On other occasions, I purposely may make incorrect verbalizations or actions. I've even dressed as a chicken. These behaviors add to the magic of the communication situation and encourage children to communicate in an accepting atmosphere.

Close Approximation of Natural Learning

Language intervention strategies should approximate closely the natural process of language acquisition. The strategy should be communicative in nature and should use language as it naturally occurs. Teaching language devoid of its communicative function deprives a child of intrinsic motivation and of one essential element of generalization.

Natural language models—parents, teachers, aides, and others—should be the principal resources for implementation of language intervention. These individuals serve as language models with or without the SLP's input. Their potential as language facilitators can be exploited best, however, when they are guided in content selection and trained in facilitative techniques. When using these language facilitators within the child's everyday situations, the role of the SLP changes to that of collaborator.

Following Developmental Guidelines

The language development of typical children can guide the selection of training targets. As a group, these children develop language in a similar, albeit individualistic, manner. Generally, language form is preceded by function, with easier, less complex structures being learned first. Children use the language they possess to accomplish their language goals. These uses are the framework within which new forms develop. The overall result is a hierarchy that suggests steps for training language.

Of course, no SLP would ever adopt a language intervention hierarchy without adaptations for a child and the contexts in which he or she functions. Slavish adherence to a developmental hierarchy is inappropriate. Good teaching may suggest alternative hierarchical teaching patterns.

An SLP should be aware of the prerequisites for successful communicative behaviors at the functioning level of a child. The child learning plurals need not be able to count but must have a notion of one and more than one. Likewise, successful use of *why* questions and answers requires an ability to reconstruct events in reverse. These cognitive skills may need to be taught prior to attempting the linguistic manner for noting this knowledge.

Similarly, the child needs to understand the requirements and demands of different communication situations to communicate effectively within them. For example, the requirements of classroom give-and-take are very different from having a face-to-face conversation or from talking on the telephone.

As with much learning, simple rules are combined and modified or enlarged to form higher-order rules. By carefully analyzing each new training target and monitoring progress, an SLP can ensure that a child possesses the appropriate skills for new learning.

Language development and impairment can be very individualistic and may not follow the dictates of a developmental hierarchy. Aspects of language will develop at rates influenced by perception and cognition, opportunity, needs, and training. Of more importance for intervention is the designation of training targets that help the child function more effectively within the everyday environment.

The language rules of most children are valid for those children at that time. For example, young children say such things as "Mommy eat" and "More juice," which demonstrate adherence to simple word sequencing rules. The rules are appropriate to the child's level of linguistic competence. At various levels of intervention, it is appropriate to target child rules rather than the correct but more difficult adult ones that will eventually be learned. To require children with LI to use adult sentence forms seems unfair, especially when we do not require such behavior from young children developing typically.

Even the expectation that a child will use a new or adultlike language rule or feature following brief periods of intervention may be unrealistic. Children developing typically learn and extend or retract their language rules gradually after many encounters and trials. Over time, these rules come to resemble those of adults. Therefore, it is inappropriate to expect near perfect performance from children with LI shortly after a target is introduced. Rule learning is complicated and time-consuming. As a child progresses, the language training should be modified accordingly.

Following the Child's Lead

Often, the expectation that a child will not communicate effectively becomes self-fulfilling. If facilitators expect a child to communicate and plan for it, the child will.

It is important, therefore, that the SLP or other facilitator attend to the content and intent of each child utterance and respond appropriately. In this way, teaching occurs when a child is paying attention and because using the language being taught has positive consequences.

Language facilitators can choose either to direct and maintain a child's attention or attend to what interests the child (Kovarsky & Duchan, 1997). Although the former is a trainer-oriented approach (or adult-centered) that gives the trainer virtual control of the entire interaction, it may not be the most effective approach. Children with ID are less likely to follow such trainer attempts to redirect attention. In contrast, these children learn some things more easily when the trainer follows their attentional lead and builds on the focus of their attention.

A more child-centered approach guarantees joint or shared reference, enhances semantic contingency, and reduces noncompliance by a child. With semantic contingency, an adult comments on a child's topic or previous utterance, thus facilitating processing by the child. Children appear to attend most to and be best able to comprehend speech during joint-attention activities.

Responses to child actions or utterances provide contextual support. Such support aids the processing of children with ID who have memory storage and retrieval problems that complicate encoding and decoding.

A child's verbal behavior should be interpreted by others in terms of its possible intention, rather than viewed as inappropriate or incorrect. In other words, a request is still a request even though the form may be wrong, the item desired misnamed, and so on.

Children signal those things in which they are most interested by their actions or through verbalizations. This gauge can be used to keep child interest and motivation high in the intervention setting. Often, I will say to a child, "What toy do you want to play with?" Although the topic is open-ended, the technique is very specific—as we see later—permitting a flexible choice of topic.

When a child initiates an interaction and is responded to accordingly, the value for learning is greater than when a child's initiation is ignored or penalized. Ignoring or penalizing a child will result in a decrease in future initiations.

While observing a lesson in a training apartment in preparation for an older teen's move to his own apartment, I overheard the following exchange:

SLP: What are you doing?
Client: (Matter-of-factly) Dusting furniture.
SLP: Good. What else are you dusting?
Client: You live in apartment?
SLP: You didn't answer my question. What else are you doing?

The client obviously was interested in living arrangements and would have joined such a conversation willingly if the SLP had followed his lead. The SLP can follow the client's lead and manipulate the conversation to encourage the desired language features. Continued use of directive responses by this SLP will diminish the client's initiating behavior. Who wants to talk about dusting anyway?

Active Involvement of the Child

Language acquisition occurs with the active participation of the learner. Language learning is not a passive process. In like fashion, more rapid learning occurs when a child with LI is participating actively in some event. In general, the more actively involved the child, the greater and more stable the generalization. Ideally, intervention should consist of motivating participatory activities with the potential for a variety of language use contexts.

Heavy Influence of Context on Language

Context can be a big determiner of what is said and how it is said. Language is a socially based cultural form whose use reflects an individual's linguistic, interpersonal, and cultural competence within a given contextual situation. An individual's knowledge of the event or situation influences the way he or she uses language in that situation.

Language intervention should occur within the contexts of everyday events and within the context of conversational give-and-take or of other communication events. The language facilitator needs to create a rich context in which a child with LI can experience a variety of linguistic and nonlinguistic stimuli and be supported in his or her linguistic attempts.

The content for these dialogues is the common experience of the intervention setting. The skillful SLP or other language facilitator can manipulate both the linguistic and nonlinguistic context to attain desired targets from the child. So can you!

Familiar Events Providing Scripts

A *script* is an internalized set of expectations about routine or repeated events organized in a temporal-causal sequence. As such, scripts contain shared event knowledge based on common experiences that aid and enhance memory, comprehension, and participation.

Routinized events for which children have scripts provide specific situations in which children can learn appropriate language. Familiar activities of high interest, such as making popcorn, pudding, or cake, can be used as the contexts for language intervention. The event sequences contained in scripts can be used to teach language expression and comprehension and can aid recall.

Naturally, scripts will differ with a child's maturational level and, to some extent, with the individual, although even very young preschoolers remember events in an organized manner similar to adults in general structure and content. As children mature, their scripts become longer, more detailed, and contain more options ("Sometimes . . ."), alternatives ("You either . . . or . . .), and conditions ("If . . ., then you . . .").

TABLE 9.2 Possible Generalization Plan Format

Training targets:

Identify settings, situations, and persons across which training can occur.

		Settings:								
		Situation:	Situation:	Situation:	Situation:	Situation:	Situation:	Situation:	Situation:	Situation:
P										
e										
r										
s										
o										
n										
s										

Cues:

Consequences:

Designing a Generalization Plan First

Considerations of generalization are essential to treatment program design and should be identified prior to beginning training. Table 9.2 is a suggested generalization plan format. In designing such a plan, an SLP considers the individual needs of the child and environment and the relevant variables that will affect generalization.

Generalization Variables

To ensure generalization to the everyday environment of a child, the SLP must manipulate the generalization variables most likely to result in that outcome. As you may recall from Chapter 1, the variables that affect generalization can be grouped by content and context (Table 1.2). Content variables include the training targets and training items. Context variables include the method of training, language facilitators, cues, contingencies, and location of training. Each of these variables and considerations for intervention within a functional model will be discussed, expanding on the brief presentation in Chapter 1.

Training Targets

As mentioned previously, teaching the complex process of language as discrete bits of language actually can slow growth. Language intervention needs to be relevant to the child's communication within the environment and to target the language process, rather than language products or units. Therefore, intervention must answer two questions:

1. What will be the function of the forms and content we are teaching?
2. Are the forms and content being trained in the context of communication events in which the intended function can actually be accomplished?

In general, more frequently used or attempted targets are more relevant to a child's world and, therefore, are more likely to generalize. Communicative utterances observed to occur in the home, albeit incorrectly, can be introduced in therapy as natural outcomes of the context. Once introduced, they can be modified by the adult.

Language targets need to increase the effectiveness of a child as a communicative partner. The first goal of intervention should be successful communication by a child at the present level of functioning.

As mentioned, developmental guidelines can aid target selection. Goals approximating a developmental sequence are more successful than those that do not. Earlier emerging forms can be learned in fewer trials and prior to later emerging forms. In addition, earlier emerging forms seem to generalize more readily into a child's use system and at a higher level of use.

A functional model would suggest teaching forms useful in the natural setting while attending to the developmental order of these forms. The overriding criterion for target selection should be to aid the child in communicating what is necessary in the contexts in which she or he most frequently communicates. This practical approach is especially important for children who experience pragmatic difficulties, such as those seen in children with TBI and some psychiatric disorders.

The best way to determine need is through environmental observation. If, for example, a child frequently requests items in the environment but is generally ineffective, then requesting might be chosen as a target. When there is very little opportunity for a possible training target to occur, it might be best to identify other content for training.

Infrequent opportunity for possible training targets to occur may be the result of low environmental expectations or few requirements for a child to produce these forms or functions. For example, there may be few opportunities for a child to ask questions when there is little expectation that she or he will do so. In such cases, low expectations can become self-fulfilling. The communication environment may need to be restructured to facilitate use of newly acquired communication skills.

An SLP can identify both targets and everyday situations in which each target is likely to occur and in which its use will be affected by and, in turn, affect the context. For example, questions should be trained in situations in which they make sense and in which they perform their intended function of gaining information. SLP instructions such as "I'm coloring a picture. Ask me what I'm doing" violate the function of questions. Usually, we do not ask questions for which we already have the answer. Similarly, an SLP's attempt to elicit an answer with the instruction "What am I doing?" also violates the function of questions and answers. Although we might wonder about the mental capacity of SLPs who do not know what they are doing, we can modify both the situation and the cue to elicit an answer more appropriately. For example, the SLP might sit behind a screen, give clues, and ask the child, "Can you guess what I'm doing?"

Training Items

An SLP should plan to train enough examples of the feature being targeted to enable a child to generalize to untrained members. For example, it is neither desirable nor possible to train all noun-verb combinations. The goal should be to train enough examples from the noun class in combination with examples of the verb class so that the child will generalize the rule *noun + verb* to all members of these two classes. Obviously, this process is being simplified in this discussion, and more planning and thought are required.

In addition, a sufficient number of items must be trained so that a child can determine both the relevant and irrelevant aspects of the communication context. For example, words or phrases such as *yesterday, last week*, and *in the past* are relevant to use of the past tense. The child forms a hypothesis that states, "In the presence of *yesterday, last week*, or *in the past*, use the past tense." Other aspects may be irrelevant, such as the specific nouns, pronouns, or verbs used. For example, the pronoun I is irrelevant and can be used with any tense. If the child is trained to use the form *Yesterday, I . . ., Last week, I . . .,* and *In the past, I . . .,* the resultant incorrect hypothesis might be "In the presence of I, use the past tense." Knowledge of both the relevant and irrelevant aspects of the context are essential for learning. A child needs to learn those cases in which the target is required and those in which it is not.

Initially, training should limit irrelevant dimensions. For example, the child first may learn to use regular past tense with *yesterday*. Such words as *today* do not signal the tense as clearly and should be introduced later. Gradually, more irrelevant dimensions, such as longer sentences, are introduced.

When a particular syntactic form or function is being targeted, it is especially important to select content words or utterances already in the child's repertoire. With the targeting and introduction of new words, an SLP selects familiar structural frames. New structures should be trained with familiar words. This principle is called "new forms–old content/old forms–new content."

Processing constraints are the limited capacity of the brain to process information. When these boundaries are reached, tradeoffs occur. For example, children omit more grammatical markers in longer, more complex sentences than in shorter, less complex ones. Children with LI are particularly susceptible to these constraints because the linguistic processing uses more capacity than among TD children. Training items that exceed the information-processing constraints of these children may result in inadequate learning and poor generalization.

Often a language feature fails to generalize because a child has not learned the conditions that govern its use. For example, if a child learns only by imitation, he or she internalizes the variables that affect imitation, not the variables found in conversation. In order for a behavior to generalize to another context, such as conversation, the behavior must be taught with the variables found in that context.

Because a child with LI often lacks metalinguistic awareness, rule explanation is not a viable clinical tool. An SLP must structure the environment so that linguistic regularities are obvious.

Contrast training is one method of overcoming generalization problems. In contrast training, a child learns those structures and situations that obligate use from those that do not. For example, use of the third-person *-s* marker is required with singular nouns and third-person singular pronouns. A child must recognize also that plural nouns and other pronouns do not require this marker.

Conversational use requires recognition of contexts within which the target does or does not appear. Using several different contexts, both linguistic and non-linguistic, ensures that a child does not misidentify linguistic variables nor assume that the SLP and the therapy setting are the only contexts in which the target is to be used. Ideally, functional training uses multiple examples, such as the several categories of linguistic response classes or training items, several facilitators, and several settings. This feature is essential for generalization.

Method of Training

Language is a set of rules that allow a person to use language features in communication contexts to express intentions. A rule is an abstraction that describes similarities. If language is rule governed, then the goal of intervention should be to learn the rules.

The most effective intervention approach for older school-age children and adolescents with deficits in grammar is an integrated one in which naturalistic stimulation approaches are supplemented by deductive teaching procedures. In a deductive method, children are presented with a rule guiding the use of a morphological inflection along with models of the inflection (Finestack & Fey, 2009). While this statement would seem to fly in the face of functional approaches outlined in this text, this is not the case. Strict stimulation-only approaches occur in natural context, but the child is usually unaware of the teaching target and not required to respond. This approach is much more open-ended than the functional intervention we'll be discussing in which an SLP can engage a school-age child's metacognitive abilities in the learning process by helping the child to become conscious of the intervention target and informing her or him of the principles and patterns underlying the target. Rules can then be deduced from the SLP's specific examples and from actual use by the child.

It is not practical with most children with LI and most intervention targets simply to explain the language rule being trained. Instead, training consists of the rule being applied within situations that contrast the critical conditions that apply to the rule. For example, can you imagine trying to teach regular past tense to a child as follows:

> When a verb is used in the past tense, an *-ed* is added to it to produce a past tense verb, as in *walk/walked.*

Instead, we might teach regular past tense in the following manner:

Every day *I walk*, yesterday I *walked*.
Every day we *talk*, yesterday we *talked*.

The word *yesterday* tells us to add the /t/ sound. Now you try it. I'll start.

Every day I walk, yesterday I _____.
Every day they rake, yesterday they _____.

An SLP's role is to provide organized language data to a child as an illustration of rule use. Thus, the child would be presented with paired minimally different situations that do and do not invoke the rule. For example, pronoun use might be contrasted with noun use.

SLP: We're going to play imagination. I'll tell you about something in my mind and you try to find the picture. I'm thinking about a *ghost*. Which ghost? *He* has a big nose. Wow, you found that really fast. Okay, you think of something else.
Child: It has blue eyes.
SLP: I don't know what you're talking about. What's the name of it?
Child: A doll.
SLP: Um-hm. What about the doll?
Child: It has blue eyes.
SLP: I found the doll with blue eyes. It's easy when I know what you're talking about. Try another. I'm thinking . . . .
Child: Thinking of a dinosaur. He's got sharp teeth.
SLP: Oh, I know which dinosaur has the sharp teeth. This one.

By presenting these contrasting situations and encouraging the child to practice, the SLP helps the child amass the data necessary to identify the critical elements of the rule. Once the child is aware of the critical elements, the SLP has the flexibility to present these elements in any communication situation.

The strength of the rule-teaching approach is in the way it simplifies the learning task by condensing relevant input and highlighting critical conditions. Abstract grammatical rules are difficult for children with LI to learn directly.

Functional techniques are more effective than stimulation alone because they incorporate behavioral principles and also use the context of naturally occurring conversations that can be modified systematically by the language facilitator. For example, the following exchange might occur with a child for whom we have targeted future tense.

SLP: That sounds like fun. What about tomorrow?
Child: Zoo?
SLP: What about the zoo?
Child: Go zoo.
SLP: Now?
Child: Go zoo tomorrow?
SLP: You *will*? John *will* go too, right. Tomorrow you both. . . .
Child: Will go zoo.
SLP: Yes. Tomorrow John and you ***will*** go to the zoo. I love the zoo. I wonder what *will* happen there.

Generalization is more likely than with more structured drill-like approaches because the cues used resemble the varied ones found in communication events. In addition, the child's attention is focused on a topic while receiving linguistic input about that topic.

A functional model provides a dynamic context for teaching language. Language training that works for a child in communication events should generalize to those events. The focus should not be merely the correctness of a child's language, but its communicative potential.

In general, functional intervention in combination with more structured remediation facilitates both acquisition and generalization of language targets to usage within natural environment situations. The functional approach involves

- selecting appropriate language targets for a child and environment.
- arranging the environment to increase the likelihood that a child will initiate.
- responding to a child's initiations with requests for elaboration of the target forms.
- reinforcing a child's attempts with attention and access to objects in which the child has expressed interest.

Interactions between adults and children arise naturally in unstructured situations, such as play, and can be used systematically by the adult to give the child practice in communication.

A child signals a potential topic by demonstrating interest or requesting assistance. Thus, the child provides the topic and the opportunity for the language-facilitating adult to teach the language form. The child is more likely to talk and be more interested in the content of this talk if the topic has been established by the child.

Within these communication contexts, an SLP models the responses that fulfill a child's communication goals. Because the purpose of language already is established in the natural environment, form and content may be learned more easily. In short, the child is taught a more effective way to communicate within a particular context. The SLP also models behaviors for the caregivers in order to facilitate training and increase the likelihood that natural situations will occur in which the child is successful.

When the desired interactions do not occur, the SLP can manipulate the environment to enhance its language-training potential. Both linguistic and nonlinguist aspects of the context can be altered to elicit the desired communication.

Activities can be planned around communication contexts that are highly likely to occur for the child. Training outside the normal environment should be as close to that environment in materials, situations, and persons as possible. Activities should include a child's usual reasons for talking and typical topics, rely on previous experiences and introduce new ones, use familiar focuses of communication, and include the child's normal communication partners.

Each child's individual learning or cognitive style also must be considered by the SLP. Children are most comfortable with new experiences and information presented in a manner consistent with that style.

By considering why and how children use words and gestures, you can increase your ability to provide the most natural and optimal situations for eliciting and teaching communication. The combination of appropriate context and specifically targeted language features facilitates maximum carryover and generalization outside the clinical environment.

Language Facilitators

If the goal is language use within a child's everyday context, then a lone SLP working only in a clinical setting is limited as to what he or she can accomplish. The brevity of child–SLP contact necessitates the use of a wider variety of social contexts, including various communication partners. These partners supply a strong social base for intervention, providing a reason for language use.

The appropriate partners to be used in training will vary with the age and circumstance of the child. Whereas parents may be appropriate for preschool children, they may have more limited interaction with their school-age children for whom teachers and peers may be more effectual. Successful use of the language taught in intervention programs depends, in part, on the expectations of these significant others in the child's environment.

Parents have been successful language facilitators with their children. Most success has been reported for children in early stages of language and cognitive development. For example, parents of children with ASD have been taught to provide intervention services within the daily routines of their preschool children at home (Kashinath, Woods, & Goldstein, 2006).

Without intervention, it is often difficult for toddlers with LI and their parents to establish mutually rewarding interactional patterns. Such children are less likely to succeed in a preschool setting. Their experience level and their success in communicative interaction are often minimal, and they may exhibit poor listening skills. Children who are not successful in communication often become resistant or negative and develop attention-getting behaviors.

A child must have the opportunity to communicate; thus, a facilitator must be attentive and responsive. A facilitator must consistently recognize a child's attempts to communicate and provide appropriate responses. Parents need to be taught more than just modeling language and their progress as trainers must be monitored.

Communication partners, such as teachers and parents, can be an effective part of an intervention team if they are trained and monitored thoroughly. A facilitator must be trained in both (a) the *how*, or the best teaching techniques, and (b) the *what*, or the goals and materials for intervention. Training of facilitators can be accomplished in a combination of ways, including direct training and modeling, in-service training, and the use of telephoned and written/illustrated instructions. To provide effective intervention services at home, parents need realistic input. For example, training might include user-friendly written handouts explaining the teaching strategy and/or target, video-recorded and live demonstrations, practice and critique, and discussion.

Caregiver Conversational Style

The difficulties experienced by children with LI reflect their everyday contexts as much as their so-called disorder. If this is so, then conversational partners must assume some of the responsibility for the communication of these children. For example, although adult interaction-promoting strategies, such as extended conversations and questions to promote turn taking, are positively related to language productivity in preschool children, adults in childcare centers are more responsive to the context of interactions than to the language abilities of preschool children (Girolametto & Weitzman, 2002). If we want change to occur, we need to change these adult behaviors. The quality and quantity of spontaneous conversational behavior of children with LI are negatively related to the number of verbal initiations and directives by their adult conversational partners.

Partially in response to these children's language deficits, adults modify their own language. Mothers of children with LI repeat more than do mothers of TD children. Most of these maternal repetitions are imperatives (demands) or directives (commands). The frequency of these parental directions and of self-imitations is negatively correlated with the rate of a child's language growth. In a highly directive interaction style there is often no connection between the directive and any utterance of the child.

Adult verbal control of interactions also seems to affect adversely the verbal output of children with LI. For example, although the question-answer style of adult communication may help children to maintain a conversational topic, it can discourage children from commenting outside the topics initiated by the adults and is counterproductive to the goal of spontaneous conversational behavior.

An adult directive style includes verbal conversational behaviors that

- control and initiate conversational topics.
- lead the conversation.
- structure the nature of the child's contribution.

These behaviors ensure a cohesive and fluent conversation at the expense of the child's spontaneous initiations.

In contrast, the use of an adult facilitative style of conversation can increase the use of topic initiations, questions, and topic comments by children with LI. An adult facilitative style

- allows a child to control and initiate conversational topics.
- follows a child's conversational lead.
- encourages a child to participate in various ways.

A facilitative adult is less interested in conversational flow than in providing an opportunity for a child to participate and to assume control of the conversation. Specific behaviors that define each style are given in Table 9.3.

We know that a parental directive style is not as effective as a conversational style in helping children develop language. For example, with children with ASD, parental utterances that follow a child's current focus of attention or respond to child verbal communication acts facilitate the process of vocabulary acquisition by mitigating the need for children with ASD to use attention-following of others as a word-learning strategy (McDuffie & Yoder, 2010). As has been mentioned several times throughout this text, following the child's attentional and conversational lead is an effective clinical tool.

Mothers who receive facilitative training are more responsive to and less directive of their children's behavior than are untrained mothers. These changes in parental behavior are related to such child language changes as increased MLU, increased number of utterances, increased lexicon, and improved standardized test scores. Children whose parents receive training initiate more topics, are more responsive, use more verbal turns, and have a more diverse vocabulary. These results suggest that the effect of parental conversational strategies may be greater on semantics and pragmatics than on linguistic form.

An increase in the percentage of semantically related or contingent utterances can, in turn, provide greater opportunity for topic maintenance and turn taking. With more opportunity to participate, the child gains more control over both the adult's behavior and the exchange process.

Children's spontaneous verbalizations can be enhanced when adult facilitators provide a high level of verbal feedback coupled with little verbal directing. Examples are given in Table 9.4. Data from several studies suggest that children's conversational abilities can be increased by adult behaviors that are highly responsive to a children's spontaneous communicative behaviors. Best results seem to occur when facilitators receive frequent, regular, structured training, including role-playing and critiques.

TABLE 9.3 Characteristics of the Directive and Facilitative Styles

Directive	Facilitative
Initiate at least half of the topics of conversation.	Initiate fewer than half of the topics of conversation.
Use direct questions to initiate most topics.	Use indirect questions or embedded imperatives to initiate most topics.
Use primarily direct questions and occasional imitations or expansions to maintain topics.	Use primarily direct statements, encouragements, imitations, expansions, or expansion questions and occasional direct questions to maintain topics.
Do not ask for clarification directly, relying instead on encouragement, imitation, and expansion strategies.	Use direct clarification questions or statements when necessary and appropriate.
Do not allow lapses in turn taking to occur, but use direct questions to require the child to respond.	Allow lapses between turns to occur and after a short wait, initiate topics as noted above.

TABLE 9.4 Examples of Minimally Directive Verbal Feedback to Children

Child: I went to the zoo, yesterday. *Partner:* Oh, that's one of my favorite spots. I love the monkeys best.
Child: I have a birthday party, tomorrow. *Partner:* Oh, that should be fun. What do you want for your birthday?
Child: We went whale watching on vacation. *Partner:* I've always wanted to do that. Bet it was exciting. Tell me about it.
Child: My picture is a cowboy. *Partner:* A big cowboy on a spotted horse.
Child: I'm gonna be a ghost for Halloween. *Partner:* Don't come to my house; I'm afraid of ghosts. I think I'll be a witch and scare your ghost.

Note: In each of these five exchanges, the adult followed the child's lead by commenting on the child's topic and then cueing the child to provide more information or waiting for a reply.

It is feasible even for parents in dire economic situations to participate in and benefit from language-based group intervention with their children while residing in family homeless shelters. Despite the many demands made on and restrictions faced by mothers and children who are homeless, homeless parents, even those with limited language skills, can be taught to use facilitating language strategies during interactions with their preschool children in shelters (O'Neil-Pirozzi, 2009). The time families reside in homeless shelters offers an opportunity to provide language-based interventions for children in need.

In one study, children living in shelters showed positive language growth when parents received as little as four 90-minute small-group program sessions, held weekly over the course of four weeks (O'Neil-Pirozzi, 2009). Attendance by parents can be increased if training sessions are offered at a convenient time and place and by providing childcare and light refreshments.

Intervention may empower homeless parents' sense of self-worth and foster strong, positive parent–child bonds during a time of family instability. Given the temporary nature of shelter living, intervention should be as brief and convenient as possible, while maximizing effectiveness by training across multiple contexts (Dickinson & Tabors, 2001; Tabors, Roach, & Snow, 2001).

The results of a meta-analysis of eighteen studies of parent-implemented language interventions with preschool children found such approaches to be effective (Roberts & Kaiser, 2011). Parent-implemented language interventions have a significant, positive impact on both receptive language and expressive syntactic skills. Parent training has a positive effect on parent–child interaction style in terms of responsiveness, use of language models, and rate of communication. Parents receiving parent training are significantly more responsive than those who do not. However, we must be somewhat circumspect in generalizing results. Many studies do not adequately describe the parent training procedures or long-term results. Without specifics of the parent training and its actual implementation, it is difficult to determine what specific parent training works best.

Families and Children from CLD Backgrounds

Cultural identity is not a stereotype. Families within the same culture differ. Recognition of cultural contributions by an SLP, however, increase the likelihood of appropriate and effective intervention. Table 9.5 presents guidelines for SLPs to follow when interacting with culturally diverse families.

SLPs should be mindful of the differing expectations and perceptions of various ethnic and racial minorities. The role of parents, the expectations for children, and the attitudes toward disability, medicine, healing, self-help, and professional intervention within a minority population should be understood thoroughly prior to intervention. For example, mothers from Puerto Rico who live on the mainland seem to hold beliefs about early education and literacy that reflect both

TABLE 9.5 Guidelines for Interacting with Culturally Diverse Families

Do not make assumptions based on cultural stereotypes.
Cultural rules govern each encounter for both the family/child and the speech-language pathologist. Be aware that responses to stimuli, such as a clinic room, may be very different across cultures.
Learn about the cultures of the families and the children you serve.
Use cultural mediators or interpreters when necessary.
Learn to use words, phrases, and greetings from the culture of the family/child.
Be patient; allow more time for interactions. Use as few written instructions as possible, unless a family member has good English reading comprehension. Allow time for questions.
Recognize that the family may not be prepared for the amount of professional-family collaboration found in functional approaches.
Encourage family input without embarrassing family members. Involve the family to the extent that they wish to be involved.
Ensure that goals and objectives of the professionals and the family match.
Involve the cultural community when possible.

Source: Information from Lynch & Hanson (2004); Wayman, Lynch, & Hanson (1990).

their original culture and more North American notions (Hammer, Rodriguez, Lawrence, & Miccio, 2007). Children and professional intervention services are viewed quite differently across Asian, Latino, and African American cultures. Likewise, an SLP's conversational style may have a great effect on future involvement with members of that community. Successful SLP–family collaboration should be characterized by mutual respect, trust, and open communication.

Although I have tried to make the teaching techniques mentioned in the next chapter culture-free, the model of intervention proposed in this text is based primarily on North American psycholinguistic research of white, middle-class families and, therefore, contains an implicit, if unintended, cultural bias. When we ask mothers to use these techniques at home, we need to be very sensitive to cultural differences that define how parent–child interactions occur (Johnston & Wong, 2002).

An SLP must determine these cultural belief systems and modify intervention techniques accordingly. Otherwise, intervention may be less effective, or worse, parents may actively resist intervention efforts. Information can be gleaned from reading research studies, talking with community representatives, and working closely with parents. Nothing beats getting involved with the cultural community, attending religious services, clubs, and festivals, and talking with and listening to parents and community members.

Once we enter someone else's culture, many of our assumptions must be set aside. Even when things seem similar, they may not be. Let's use Chinese culture as an example and explore the implications for intervention (Johnston & Wong, 2002). Based on research literature, we can make the following broad characterizations of Chinese cultural beliefs:

- The ideal self is embedded in interdependent social relations, requiring obedience and respect of others over self-fulfillment and independence.
- Human behavior is very malleable rather than biologically based.
- When a child goes to school, he or she passes from a period of nonunderstanding to one of understanding in which the child can be expected to succeed.

As a result, parents are less likely to join preschool children in play or to engage them in social communication. Instead, parents are more directive, focusing or refocusing a child's attention.

These beliefs impact intervention in myriad ways. For example, a parent may not understand our insistence on the importance of early intervention. Any discussion of this topic must include the importance of early intervention for later success in school, a Chinese cultural value. Similarly, the notion of following a child's lead does not flow naturally from beliefs in interdependence and respect for elders. It might be better to help Chinese mothers construct more formal teaching lessons to be used several times each day within the home (Johnston & Wong, 2002). Note that the use of the home environment still retains the basic functional nature of intervention.

Given differences in cultural beliefs, there are likely to be occasions when well-intentioned intervention recommendations run counter to cultural expectations of the family you serve. To be successful, an SLP must find "functional equivalents" that achieve the same ends (Johnston & Wong, 2002). For example, parents of young children with LI are often encouraged to engage in book-sharing activities. The goal is social communication, not book reading *per se*. Other methods can be found that attain the same goal while being more culturally appropriate to the child and family, such as oral storytelling.

Language is one of the primary modes of socialization and acculturation for children. When a child learns a second language, such as English, in an English-intensive educational program, he or she is in danger of losing the first language. This may be especially true for children with LI who receive remedial intervention for English but no help with their initial language in which they are most likely also impaired. Given the interdependence of emotional, cognitive, and communication development in young children and the needs these children have for family support, it is important that SLPs also support the home language of these children (Kohnert et al., 2005). This does not necessitate intervention in both languages.

Potentially, well-trained parents can be as effective as SLPs in administering intervention in the first language (Law, Garrett, & Nye, 2004). As mentioned, an SLP can directly train a parent to become the primary intervention agent for the child. Successful parent training requires the following:

- Specific language facilitation strategies vs. general stimulation
- Use of multiple sessions and instructional methods with parents
- Systematic progression of skills
- Activities tailored for the individual child

Rather than suggest that parents cease using one language at home—a huge imposition, especially for families that freely mix languages—it seems best to target activities, such a book reading, in which one language would be used exclusively. Where necessary, it may be helpful to use paraprofessionals from the language community or siblings as in-home trainers.

Preschool Teachers

High-quality preschool language experiences are especially important for children from disadvantaged backgrounds and those at risk for language impairments (Dickinson & Tabors, 2001; Hubbs-Tait et al., 2002). Sadly, many preschool classrooms, especially those serving children from low socioeconomic status (SES) backgrounds, do not provide an optimum environment for facilitating children's language skills (Dickinson, Darrow, & Tinubu, 2008; Justice, Mashburn, Hamre, & Pianta, 2008). Teachers may provide little explicit facilitation of children's language skills through use of questioning, modeling, and recasting. In turn, young children may have limited opportunity for multi-turn conversations with their teachers (Justice et al., 2008).

Unfortunately, evidence-based practice (EBP) provides little guidance on how to achieve higher quality language instruction in preschools short of intensity-sustained levels of interaction that may lack feasibility for real-world settings. One promising approach, training preschool educators to be more conversationally responsive to children within the classroom setting, benefits children's language, especially vocabulary, and literacy development, especially print-concept knowledge, but requires further study (Cabell et al., 2011). It is not surprising, given their better overall language skills, that children of high and high-average language ability seem to benefit most.

Responsivity education attempts to increase adults capacity to be conversationally responsive partners with children and to promote "reciprocal interactions" that support children's active participation in an exchange. Adults promote reciprocity by smiling and maintaining eye contact, consistently responding to children's communication efforts and recasting or expanding a child's productions, cuing a child to take another turn, using a slow pace so as to not dominate, and asking open-ended questions (Girolametto & Weitzman, 2002; Yoder & Warren, 2002).

Training Cues

If one accepts the premise that pragmatics is the governing aspect of language, then an SLP must be concerned with the context within which training occurs. Certain linguistic and nonlinguistic contexts require or provide an expectation of certain linguistic units.

In part, the problem of lack of success in generalization is due to response *programs* in which children are taught specific responses to specific cues. A child's everyday world lacks this careful control. The everyday context contains many irrelevant stimuli that do not and cannot elicit trained communication behaviors.

At the same time, parents and teachers may be presenting cues and prompts in such a diverse manner as to inhibit learning. They can be trained to focus their attention and to manipulate the environment to elicit the behaviors desired.

Too often, the traditional approaches rely on very narrow and somewhat stilted cues unlike those found in conversation. The use of these traditional cues, such as "Tell me the whole thing," may result in training characterized as "apragmatic pseudoconversational drills" (Cochrane, 1983). Pragmatically, the cues may not make sense. As a result, the conversations within which training occurs are little more than drill with a conversational veneer.

Verbal and nonverbal cues can be varied to ensure that the child does not become dependent on one stereotypic stimulus. A *system of least prompts* can be used, in which an SLP rates each type of prompt from least to most intrusive and supportive (Timler, Vogler-Elias, & McGill, 2007). Through the course of intervention, the SLP works to minimize prompting whenever possible and to allow the context to prompt the targeted language features. For example, children with ASD can be taught to initiate requests and to make comments through a system of decreasing prompts, moving from sentence completion (*Can I . . .*) through answering (*What could you ask your friend?*) (Thiemann & Goldstein, 2004).

Relevant, common stimuli within the everyday communication context can serve to elicit a child's new language targets if these stimuli are included in the training. Targets can be trained across several behaviors, facilitators, and settings to ensure generalization. The overall goals are for the newly trained behavior to be emitted in response to a variety of stimuli and for a single stimuli to result in a variety of responses. These goals can be achieved by using contrast training, response variations, and linguistic and nonlinguistic cue variations. In contrast training, mentioned previously, relevant and irrelevant stimuli are presented together so that a child learns which ones affect the newly learned behavior.

Response variation teaches a child that several responses can be used to achieve the same communication goal. For example, a drink can be attained by saying, "Want drink," "Drink please," "May I have a drink?" "I'm thirsty," and, "Are you as thirsty as I am?"

Use of a functional conversational approach requires an SLP to assess thoroughly the effects of certain cues and to explore the possibilities of eliciting language with a variety of linguistic and nonlinguistic cues. Those SLPs who rely on traditional cues are unaware of the rich variety of cues available for creating contexts in which language targets can occur.

Contingencies

Once a child has produced language, the adult facilitator can begin to modify that language if necessary. In short, the child's utterance is the stimulus to which the facilitator responds. These responses or contingencies help form the context for the child's utterance.

Natural maintaining consequences should be identified prior to beginning training. As much as possible, these consequences should be related directly to the response. Such consequences as "Very good" and "Good talking" should be avoided. When a child message ("I saw monkeys") and the consequence ("Good talking") are unrelated, the child's language fails to retain its communicative value. Communication behaviors can be maintained by conversational responses ("Oh, I think monkeys are funny. What did they do?"). Often, simply attending to a child is sufficient to maintain the child's participation.

As much as possible, conversational consequences should be semantically and pragmatically contingent and should serve to acknowledge a child's utterance. *Semantic contingency*, the relatedness of a parent's or facilitator's response to the content or topic of a child's previous utterance, has a positive effect on the rate of language development. In the above example, "I think monkeys are funny," the adult response is semantically contingent.

Adult speech that is semantically contingent decreases the amount of processing a child has to do to understand and analyze the structure and meaning of an adult's utterances. The sharing of a conversational topic and common vocabulary decreases a child's memory load. The facilitator's utterance provides a prop or scaffolding for the child's own analysis and subsequent production. For children with expressive vocabulary delays, the semantic contingency of adult responses has more effect on a child's language than does the structure of the adult response. In contrast, frequent topic changing or refocusing of a child's attention by an adult impedes the child's language acquisition.

It is not enough, however, just to comment on a child's topic. In the following example, the facilitator's response is semantically contingent but lacks *pragmatic contingency*.

Child: I want cookie, please.
Facilitator: Johnny wants a cookie.

The facilitator's response should make pragmatic sense within the conversational framework. In this example, more appropriate responses might be, "What kind of cookie do you want?" "Okay, but just one," "Help yourself," and, "No cookies until after lunch." This example shows why contingencies such as "Good talking" violate pragmatic contingency and do not help continue the interchange. A child's language is reinforced more naturally when its purpose and intention are met.

The SLP can recast a sentence containing the target structure or can recast a sentence that does not contain the structure so that the recast will do so. In the first instance, the child says "Boy eating cookie" and the adult recasts "He *is* eating." In the second example, the child says "Boy cookie" and the adult recasts, "The boy *is eating* the cookie." As we've noted in this chapter, you can manipulate the environment to increase the likelihood of the child's original utterance containing the target structure. Children with SLI and low MLUs benefit more from recasts following utterances in which the child is prompted to attempt the structure prior to the adult's recast (Yoder, Molfese, & Gardner, 2011).

In brief, behaviors that attempt to increase a child's participation in the interaction, that is, a child-centered interactional style, enhance a child's language skills. By relinquishing some control and adopting the child's topics, language facilitators can ensure more child participation and interest.

Overall, in the clinical setting it is important that facilitators accept a child's utterance as representative of the child's understanding of the world and of the requirements being asked. Answers considered wrong by the adult may, in fact, represent a child's somewhat different perspective. A child's meaning can be negotiated by the facilitator and the child as the conversation continues. Such child-centered language interventions are correlated with greater generalization gains in grammar for children with SLI than are therapist-directed methods (Yoder & McDuffie, 2002).

Location

As noted in Chapter 1, location of training includes both the physical location in which training occurs and the conversational context formed by a child and a facilitator. In many ways, the conversational context is more important for generalization because it does not depend on physical setting and transcends the clinic, classroom, and home. In the light of the flexibility of these natural communication sequences, training is more a matter of *how* than *where.*

Physical Location

When possible, training should occur wherever a child is likely to use the newly trained language skill. Most communication takes place within familiar events that influence the way the participants communicate. Storytelling at home, conversation in the ear, and classroom interactions all have different rules for participation. Therefore, language intervention should take place within these types of discourse events and others as they occur in a child's everyday physical locations. The everyday environment provides natural and familiar stimuli for intervention and for generalization. Children with lingering pragmatic deficits, such as those with TBI, are particularly in need of environmentally based intervention.

Obviously, parents and teachers will need to be trained for their new roles as language facilitators. Parents may come to a clinic or school to be trained. If this is not possible, evening group sessions or written guidelines can be used. Even if parents only modify their expectations for the child, this will help with the generalization of language training.

Conversational Context

Language should be evaluated and trained within some dynamic context in order to make sense to the child. Language and communication are influenced heavily by the context of what precedes and follows (linguistically and nonlinguistically) and by the expectations for participation with that specific context. Ordering at a fast-food restaurant presents different expectations from chatting with a friend on the phone. Each event follows certain scripts.

Sentences trained out of context are, therefore, more difficult for a child to learn. Ideally, SLPs are not training static forms but a generative, versatile system. The contextual expectations and scripts must be examined prior to beginning intervention within each context. Teaching approaches can be adapted to this setting to approximate more closely conversational exchange.

Conclusion

By carefully considering the variables that affect generalization, an SLP can modify training to maximize this effect. Targets and design decisions can be made on the basis of the likely effect on generalization and on ultimate use within the events and situations of a child's everyday environment. Language can be elicited and modified by using techniques that mirror the conversational style used by a child's usual partners within these contexts. Motivation is provided by a child's desire to participate in enjoyable activities with responsive and attentive adults.

Facilitators should adhere to the following guidelines:

1. Expect the child to communicate.
2. Respond to the child's topics and initiations.
3. Respond conversationally and build the child's utterances into longer, more acceptable ones.
4. Facilitate communication within the everyday activities of the child.
5. Cue the child in a conversational manner to elicit the language desired.

All of these principles are discussed in Chapter 10.

Chapter

10

Manipulating Context

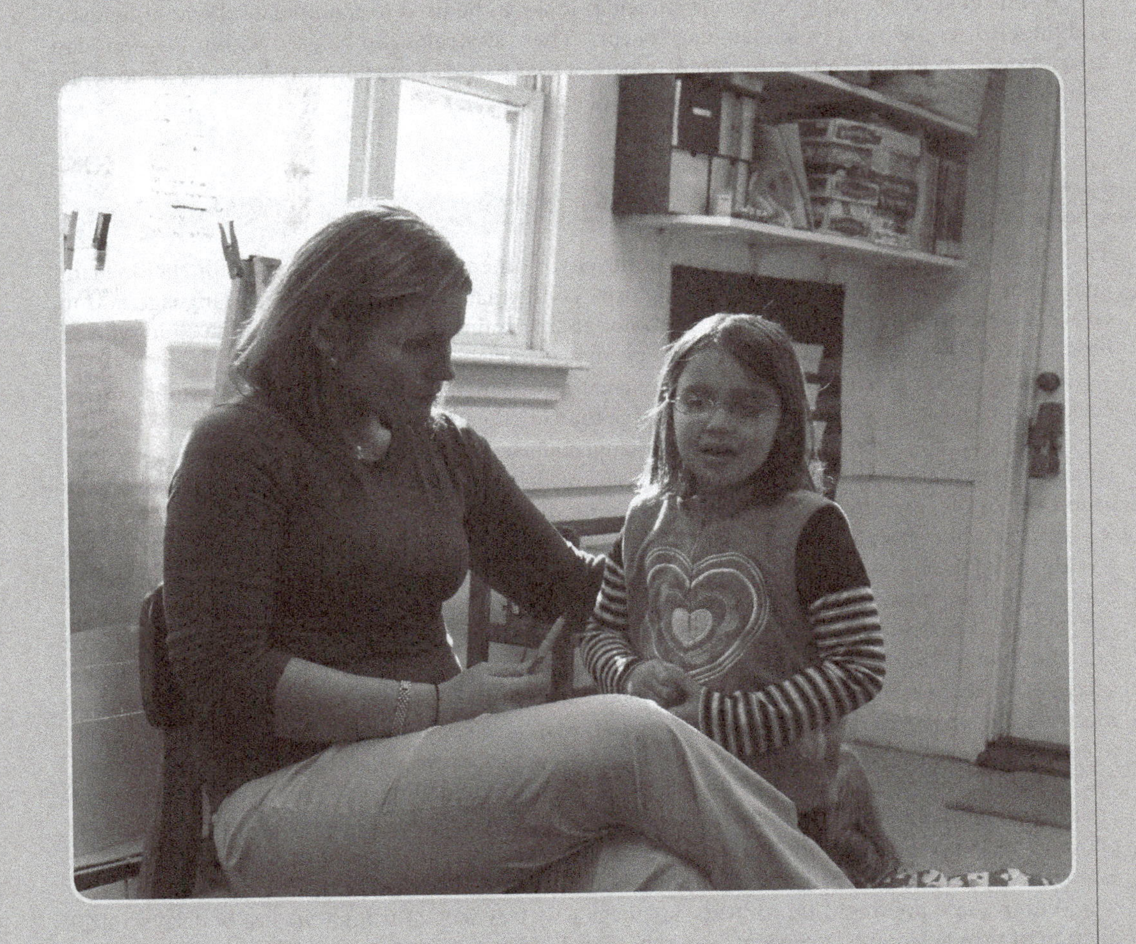

Language is pragmatically based. The demands of the nonlinguistic and linguistic context give rise to both the form and content of the language expressed. Therefore, a primary goal of language intervention should be for a child to learn the appropriate language skills to function effectively within everyday communication contexts or environments.

Within each activity, a language facilitator strives to provide an active experience with language use. It seems appropriate, then, that the SLP and other language facilitators learn to manipulate these contexts to provide a child the maximum learning possible. A facilitator's role is "to accept the child's spontaneously occurring verbal or nonverbal behavior as meaningful communication, interpret it in a manner that is contextually appropriate, and become a collaborator with the child in communicating the message more effectively" (J. Norris & Hoffman, 1990b, p. 78).

When language can be used to achieve goals within everyday communication contexts, the chances of generalization to these contexts increase. Language acquires a purpose or function, and thus, training becomes functional in nature.

In this chapter we explore various strategies that can be used to manipulate the nonlinguistic and linguistic contexts in which language occurs. These strategies can be used within the everyday activities of a child and, thus, can become a part of that natural environment. As much as possible, natural and conversational strategies are recommended.

Nonlinguistic Contexts

The nonlinguistic context—what happens in the environment—offers a rich source for eliciting language. An SLP can manipulate the nonlinguistic contextual cues to elicit desired language and to ensure that a child initiates language. All too often, the training paradigm allows the child with LI little control. Therefore, the child assumes a passive, responsive role.

Certain nonlinguistic contexts naturally elicit more language than do others. For most adults, cocktail parties are more likely to elicit language than are theater engagements.

Some situations also dictate the type of language used. Most adults do not question and challenge sermons—at least not while the sermon is being delivered. In contrast, learning situations, such as in a classroom, are supposed to encourage questioning.

If targets have been selected to help a child communicate better, then, hopefully, the SLP already has identified the contexts in which the child attempts these targets. In other words, the nonlinguistic contexts that are highly likely to elicit the target are known.

Ideally, the nonlinguistic context serves to elicit the target language behavior: The SLP then can help the child modify the target into a correct form for that situation. In theory—and this is key to our success—a child who makes a meaningful response in context will be interested in that response and motivated to change it in the desired manner. This corrected response should generalize more easily to everyday use because it is being trained within the context of everyday events and conversations.

Table 10.1 contains a sample of nonlinguistic contexts and the type of language each may elicit. Small group projects or tasks usually elicit lots of language from children. For younger children, role-play and dress-up are good contexts for language. Routines also can either be previously identified or established within the home or the classroom.

Within these nonlinguistic contexts, language may be elicited through the use of delays, introduction of novel elements, oversight, and sabotage. Delaying or waiting for a child to initiate communication is often a very effective nonlinguistic strategy, especially after a child has demonstrated use, however incorrect, of a desired behavior. Too frequently, adults do not expect a child to communicate, and this expectation becomes self-fulfilling when the adult communicates for the child.

Let's assume that the language facilitator is waiting for a child to initiate the interaction. The facilitator may sit near the child and look questioningly or display some interesting item while looking at the child. When the child looks at the adult, the adult does not speak for a specified period of

TABLE 10.1 Nonlinguistic Contexts and Language Elicitation

Turn taking and requesting objects:

Provide only one plastic knife for children to share as they make a fruit salad.
Provide one highly desirable outfit in the dress-up corner of the class.
Provide only enough art supplies for half of the children and request that children share equipment.

Following directions and directing others:

While working in a group, re-create the teacher's construction-paper collage. The teacher should be careful not to supply precut paper or to help children with the color tints. The goal is to get the children to ask for help and to direct others and themselves.
In groups of two, duplicate a cake decoration previously completed by the teacher.
As a group, plant seeds in cups as the teacher has done previously. A more involved project might involve planting a garden, keeping the different crops straight, and making signs.
Bake while following a written or pictured recipe.
Put together a model by following written or oral directions.
Play dumb. By making lots of mistakes, the teacher can have children direct or correct the behavior.
Have a child explain how to do something known by only that child.
Have children direct each other through activities blindfolded.
Have the child be the teacher.

Requesting information:

Give only partial directions for completing a task.
Put objects that the children need for a task in an unusual location so that they will need to ask for the location.
Introduce visually interesting items but do not name them or explain their function to the children.

Giving information:

Have children explain class projects to children from another class.
Have children explain class projects to parents at a special event or Parents' Night.
Have children tell about events they experienced: for example, summer vacation, a weekend trip, a birthday party. This task and explaining how something is accomplished are excellent vehicles for sequencing.
Have children request information from children who need to improve their ability to give information.
Have children tell make-believe stories.

Reasoning:

Have children try to float or submerge objects in water. Include objects that float and those that do not so that the children must find various combinations.
Build a suspension bridge from straws, string, toothpicks, and tongue depressors.
Design a city with transportation, schools, recreation facilities, and residential, industrial, and business areas.
Play initiative games in which groups of children must solve a common problem.
Make large projects in connection with class projects. For example, children might design the "perfect" world, make montages that demonstrate male and female roles, or design a board game, such as On the Way to Your Birthday, that illustrates stages of fetal development.

Requesting help:

Pose problems that children cannot solve themselves.
Sabotage activities, such as holes in paper cups, dried markers and paints, glue bottles glued shut, not enough chairs, missing gloves and hats, and so on. The list is endless.

Imagining and projecting:

Set up a drama or dress-up center. Set up a puppet stage with a variety of characters.
Set up simulated shops and stores or a housekeeping center.
Role-play. (Role-play can elicit a variety of intentions.)

(*Continued*)

TABLE 10.1 (*Continued*)

Protesting:
Play dumb, as in forgetting to give children peanut butter and jelly with which to make sandwiches.
Miss a child's turn or withhold needed objects.
Violate a routine or an object function by using objects in novel or nonsensical ways.
Give a child too much of something or more than is needed.
Put away objects before the child is finished using them.
Ask a child to do something that is not physically possible (but safe).
Initiations:
Pose problems and wait for children to initiate communication.
Ask children to talk to lonely animals for you.

time unless the child does. If the child does not verbalize, the adult may use a linguistic model or prompt to get the desired verbalization.

Novel or unexpected events can be introduced into a situation to evoke communication. Most individuals will notice and remark on such events. For example, a kitten, guinea pig, or bright toy might be found in an unexpected spot. Even children functioning at the single-word level will comment on elements in a situation that are novel, different, or changing.

Oversight or forgetting by a facilitator will elicit language from a child who's eager to become the teacher. I often play dumb, forgetting object locations or children's turns. Needed objects, such as glue or scissors, can be omitted or used by the facilitor in unusual ways to prompt a reaction by the child.

Finally, sabotage of activities or routines involves taking actions or introducing elements that will not permit the activity to continue or to be completed. My favorite example is the classroom teacher and aide who would buckle the children's boots together and turn their coats inside out sometime during the day. One can imagine the chaos at the end of the day and all of the language elicited as children requested assistance.

Linguistic Contexts

The goal of language use within a conversational context necessitates a thorough evaluation of the linguistic cues used with children in the training situation. Cues such as "What do we say?" and "Now, tell me the whole thing" are examples of pseudoconversational cues mentioned previously. Both cues have their place but tend to be overused in intervention while rarely occurring in the real world.

Eliciting language through constant prodding or interrogation can be unpleasant and actually result in less talking by the child. Such communication is one-sided, with the child assuming the role of passive receiver or occasional reluctant speaker.

Linguistic contexts can be divided into those that model language with or without a child's response and those that directly and indirectly cue certain responses. Contingencies are strategies used following a child's utterance that attempt to confirm the utterance, or, if necessary, modify it in some way.

Modeling

The efficacy of the modeling approach has been demonstrated repeatedly. *Modeling* is a procedure in which an SLP produces a rule-governed utterance at appropriate junctures in conversation or activities but initially does not ask the child to imitate. The technique compares favorably with more active techniques, such as question-answer, that require responses by a child.

Modeling can be used in any of the following ways:

- As a high-frequency response in very structured situations
- As a specific language stimulation technique
- As an element in comprehension training

In general, modeling closely approximates the language-learning environment of TD children and is an effective language-learning strategy for a child with LI.

It is expected that the child will acquire some aspect of the language behavior of the facilitator and use it in a similar context later. Interactive modeling considers the child to be an active learner who abstracts the rules used in forming utterances and associates these utterances with events and stimuli in the environment.

It is best to model the training target for a child prior to attempting to elicit the target. Within such *focused stimulation*, an SLP produces a high density of the targets in meaningful contexts without requiring the child to respond. Two varieties of this stimulation are *self-talk* and *parallel talk*. In self-talk, an SLP talks about what he or she is doing, whereas in parallel talk, discussion centers on the child's actions. Obviously, activities must be chosen carefully to provide sufficient opportunities for the target to occur.

Focused stimulation should be semantically and pragmatically appropriate. The target feature is presented frequently while, at the same time, placing little pressure on the child. The following is an example of focused stimulation within a conversational context:

Child: Mommy made hamburgers. Mommy made 'tator salad.
SLP: *She* must be a good cook. What else did *she* make?
Child: A cake.
SLP: *She* did? *She* made a cake. Yummy. Did *she* cook any hotdogs?
Child: Uh-huh.
SLP: *She* made a very nice picnic for the family. Did *she* get to play any games or did *she* just work?

The language feature being targeted—the pronoun *she*—appears in the initial part of the sentence or in elliptical utterances in which shared information is omitted. Such frequent modeling plus recasts of the child's utterances, explained later, have been effective in facilitating use of several language structures.

Although a grammatical feature can be made more salient or conspicuous by emphasizing it, this can change the basic meaning of a sentence. Say the following sentences out loud, emphasizing the boldfaced word:

I'll see you next week.
I **will** see you next week

While the first is probable, the second is definite. Or the following:

I do my homework every day.
I **do** my homework every day.

We have a statement of fact followed by an argumentative accusation or defensive response. An SLP must be careful, therefore, that added emphasis does not change the meaning of the utterance.

Targets can also be placed at the end of a sentence to aid working memory and enhance learning (Fey et al., 2003). This can occur in syntax (*The girl is running to school. She really is.*), morphology

(*He rides to work. He doesn't walk; he rides.*), or semantics (*Don't put the block on the box. Put it in.*) Here's an example of how it might work (Fey et al., 2003):

Child: I do it.
Adult: What about me?
Child: You too.
Adult: Great. You won't do it alone. We will. We **will** do it.
Child: We will.
Adult: Yes. We will do it together. We **will!**

Once a target has been modeled thoroughly, the SLP can ask the child to respond in a manner similar to the model. Note this change. Children who are young, low-functioning, or delayed may need imitation training, with a complete model presented immediately before their response. *Imitation* is a procedure in which the child repeats the language behavior of a facilitator, with the expectation that the child will acquire some aspect of the facilitator's language. Imitation by a child enables him or her to become accustomed to the language feature being taught and its phonological patterns. This is especially important if the feature is difficult to produce.

Imitation can be used as a first step in programs to teach specific language targets or as a correction procedure when the child fails to respond or responds incorrectly. The procedure has been used successfully with several types of LI. By monitoring a child's progress, an SLP can provide varied cues, including partial models and/or delayed imitation.

This methodology, called **priming**, occurs when the utterance of one person influences the structure, vocabulary selection, or sounds used by a second speaker. For example, semantic priming occurs when the second speaker uses words previously used infrequently or not currently in the child's vocabulary. Phonological priming is seen when the sounds (*st*op) of the first speaker influence the sounds of the second (*st*art). It should be easy to see that priming can have uses in language intervention.

Structural priming occurs when a sentence produced by one speaker influences the structure of the sentences of a second speaker. This influence occurs even when the second speaker's productions do not contain the same words or thematic relations as the preceding sentence. For example, after hearing *The woman sent presents to her friends*, a speaker is more likely to produce a sentence such as *The girl gave cookies to her parents*. The sentence heard by the second speaker is referred to as the *prime sentence*, and the sentence produced by this speaker is the *target sentence*.

The effects of priming are not fleeting or limited to the effects on the next sentence. Priming effects persist even when there is intervening information or sentences (Bock & Griffin, 2000; Hartsuiker, Bernolet, Schoonbaert, Speybroeck, & Vanderelst, 2008; Konopka & Bock, 2005). Although our discussion will of necessity be short, I suggest that you read the excellent tutorial by Leonard (2011) from which much of this discussion is taken.

Priming is sometimes used in **parallel sentence production** in which the SLP provides a model of the *type* of utterance desired. The child is not expected to imitate the model but to provide a similar type of sentence. For example, I might describe a picture with "The girl is throwing the ball" and then ask the child to describe a second picture of a boy *catching a ball*.

Structural priming has it limits and appears to work best at the phrase level (Pickering & Ferreira, 2008). In other words, priming for the present progressive (*is catching*) would work best if the child already has the structure of the basic sentence into which it fits (*subject + verb + object*).

As you might imagine, the effects of priming on a child varies with the child's age. In general, parallel sentence production occurs with 3-year-olds only when

- there is considerable lexical overlap between the priming sentence and the child's target sentence (Bencini & Valian, 2008).
- the child is able to repeat or imitate the priming sentences.

In contrast, 4-year-olds showed the effects of priming effects after only hearing the priming sentences (Savage, Lieven, Theakston, & Tomasello, 2003; Shimpi, Gámez, Huttenlocher, & Vasilyeva, 2007). Newer studies are finding much more parallel sentence production among TD 3-year-olds and children with SLI (Leonard et al., 2000; Miller & Deevy, 2006; Thothathiri & Snedeker, 2008).

Both strategies that require a child response, such as questions, imitation, parallel sentence production, and those that do not, such as stimulation, result in improved language but not for all children. Given that priming works best at the phrase or the less-than-a-sentence level, we can target elaborated noun and verb phrases and other phrasal structures such as prepositional phrases.

A child may be asked to respond to questions for which an SLP has modeled the answers. Initially, the modeled answer may follow the question, but this format can be altered so that the answer precedes the question, is given partially, models a similar answer, or precedes the question by increasingly longer periods of time.

Although the modeling procedure seems stilted in writing, it can be applied very flexibly and works well with groups of children. In small groups, children who have acquired a certain target can serve as models for those who have not. By varying turns, an SLP can ensure that sufficient models are provided for different children. In a reversal of roles, the SLP can serve as a model for a child, while the child cues the SLP.

Modeling alone may be less effective than other, more structured methods. Although modeling is effective in changing the behavior of TD children, it is less effective than imitation with children with LI who may benefit more from other approaches.

Direct Linguistic Cues

Linguistic cues for certain targets can be direct or indirect. Direct elicitation techniques might include the following target questions:

To elicit . . .	Use . . .
Verbs	"What is he doing (are you doing)?" Use any tense. A benefit is that the question contains the target tense.
Noun subjects	"Who/what is verbing?" Again, the tense can be altered for the situation.
Noun objects	"What is he/she verbing?" Tense can be altered for the situation. Obviously, verbs that do not take objects should not be used.
Adverbs or adverbial phrases	"When/where/how is he/she verbing?" Tense can be altered. "How" questions can be used also to elicit process answers, as in "How did you make the airplane?"
Adjectives or adjectival phrases	"Which one . . . . ?" Tense can be altered. There should be an obvious contrast between choices for the response, such as *big* and *little*. These differences might be noted prior to questioning. Responses of a particular type can be modeled, as in "Which one ate the cookie, the littlest bear, the middle-size bear, or the biggest bear?" To keep the child from responding, "That one," the SLP may want to cover the child's eyes or use some barrier.
Specific words	Completion sentences, as in "She is playing in the ______." Rising intonation after the last spoken word will signal the child to respond. If the SLP plays dumb or acts forgetful, the child's behavior makes more sense conversationally.

Substitution requests also can be used. For example, pronouns can be substituted for old information. The facilitator might make a statement, such as giving one descriptor ("The dog is little"), and then ask the child to make a comment ("What can you tell me about the dog?"). This procedure also can take the form of a guessing game, as in "Is the dog little? Well, if the dog isn't little, what can we say?" Of course, our goal is "He is . . ."

Although these linguistic cues are conversational in nature, they will seem very nonconversational if used in nonlinguistic contexts in which they make no sense pragmatically. Questions should be used when the facilitator really desires the answer and when the child is interested in the topic of discussion.

An SLP can model a response prior to asking the child a question, as mentioned previously. For example, "I think I want the yellow one. What about you?" This type of cue is more likely to elicit a longer utterance and is more conversational in tone. The goal is a sentence of similar construction. If you ask, "which do you want?" you may get "Red" in reply.

One variation of the direct linguistic cue is a *mand model*. This technique has been used effectively with preschoolers and with children with SLI. This procedure follows a routine that is established prior to beginning any activity. The routine serves as a chain in which one stimulus cues the next. The mand-model approach typically is used for teaching new language features.

In this approach, access to desired items is through an adult, who determines the criterion for acceptability. In this way, the adult, not the object, becomes the stimulus for talking.

In the four-step mand-model training sequence, an adult first attracts a child's attention by providing a variety of attractive materials. This inducement may not be necessary if the child already displays an interest. Thus, the adult establishes joint attention with the child. In the second step, after the child has expressed interest, the adult (de)mands, "Tell me about this," or, "Tell me what you want," requesting a behavior trained previously. If there is no response, the adult moves to step three and prompts a response or provides a model to be imitated. In step four, the adult praises the child for an appropriate response and gives the child the desired item.

Even preschool peers can be trained to use the mand-model technique effectively. In these situations, production by children with LI generalizes to unprompted productions.

Indirect Linguistic Cues

Indirect linguistic cues are more conversational and situational in nature. For example, when attempting to elicit questions, the SLP might use unfamiliar objects hidden in boxes to set the nonlinguistic context. Beginning with "Boy, is this neat," the SLP peeks into the box. An exchange might continue as follows:

Child: What's in there?
Facilitator: This. (Takes the object out. Waits.)
Child: What is it?
Facilitator: A flibbity-jibbit. It does everything.
Child: What it do?

Notice the elicitation of questions. It is easy to see the interplay of nonlinguistic and linguistic cuing.

Another indirect linguistic technique requires the SLP or language facilitator to make purposefully wrong statements. A child's clothing can serve as the focus of this conversation, a technique I have dubbed "the emperor's new clothes."

Facilitator: (Touching child's red sweater) What a nice blue blouse.
Child: This no blue blouse.

In both examples, the child has given a final response that may be something less than what is desired. The SLP now can respond and begin to shape the child's previous utterance into an acceptable form, as in *This isn't a blue blouse.* We'll use contingencies to correct the utterance.

These examples are only a very few of many indirect techniques. Others examples are listed in Appendix D. Take a look. The possibilities are only limited by your imagination.

Contingencies

Conversational consequences can be divided roughly into those that do not require a child's response and those that do. Each type provides some feedback to the child, and each differs with the functioning level and degree of learning exhibited by the child.

Contingencies Requiring No Response

Contingencies that require no response from a child are nonevaluative or accepting in nature and can be used to increase correct production or highlight incorrect production for self-correction. When a child initiates or responds to some cue, the facilitator focuses full attention on the child, creating joint focus on the child's topic. Because the child has established the topic, it now acts as a motivator for the child and can be used to modify the child's language. Modifying techniques that do not require the child's response include *fulfilling the intention, use of a continuant, imitation, expansion, extension* and *expiation, breakdowns* and *buildups*, and *recast sentences*.

By *fulfilling the intention* of a child's utterance, such as handing the child a requested item, the facilitator signals the child that the message was acceptable as received. No verbal response is required.

A *continuant* is a signal that a message has been received and acknowledged. These signals usually consist of head nods or verbalizations, such as "uh-huh" and "okay." Continuants fill a speaker's turn by agreeing with the previous utterance.

In *imitation*, the facilitator repeats a child's utterance in whole or in part but makes no evaluative remarks. Rising intonation, signifying a question, is not present. Again, this behavior primarily acknowledges the child's previous utterance. Imitation is especially helpful to the child when correctly produced features of interest are emphasized ("She **is** riding the bike"). Imitations might be preceded also by phrases such as **That's right** ("That's right, she **is** riding the bike").

In contrast to imitation, expansion or recast/expansion is a more mature, or more correct, version of the child's utterance that maintains the child's word order, for example:

Child: It got stolen by the crook.
Facilitator: Uh-huh, it *was* stolen by the crook.

The use of expansion as a teaching tool is very limited for children functioning above about 30 months of age. In a variation of expansion, the SLP can prompt the child to imitate the expansion, although such requests disrupt the flow of conversation. A more appropriate variety of expansion for older children is a reformulation in which two or more child utterances are combined into one utterance that includes the concepts of each, as in the following:

Child: The dog bit the man. The man ran away.
Facilitator: Oh, the dog bit the man, who then ran away.

The use of expansion and of a cloze, or fill-in-the-blank, procedure by adults produces more responses, more interpretations, and more syntactically complex utterances by children than does a question-and-answer procedure (Bradshaw, Hoffman, & Norris, 1998).

For older children, extension is a more appropriate response. *Extension* is a reply to the content of the child's utterance that provides additional information on the topic, as in the following:

Child: It got stolen by the crook.
Facilitator: Oh, I wonder if the crook stole anything else.

Much of our behavior in conversations consists of replies to the content of the other speaker, and these comments can be used effectively regardless of the age or functioning level of the child. Extensions signal the child that the facilitator is attentive and interested.

Breakdowns and buildups consist of dividing the child's utterances into shorter units and then combining them and expanding on the child's original utterance. The purpose is to help the child understand intrasentential relationships. I use this strategy as my great-great-uncle used to do to aid the processing of information, mulling it over before commenting.

Child: It got stolen by the crook.
Facilitator: (Emotional, disbelieving) It was? (Hmmm) It was stolen. Stolen by the crook. (Disgusted) By the crook. (Finally) It was stolen by the crook.

This strategy works well, especially if the SLP or facilitator plays dumb or uses a silly puppet who just does not seem to get things right. The child may shake his head or say, "Uh-huh," in agreement between the facilitator's utterances.

Finally, *recast sentences* maintain the child's meaning or the relations while modifying the structure, and they immediately follow the child's utterance. Recasts repeat at least one of the major lexical elements while modifying other parts of the utterance. For example,

Child: He not eat.
Adult: The dog is not eating his food. Is he hungry?
Child: Not hungry.
Adult: The dog is not eating his food. He is not hungry. Is the cat eating?
Child: Uh-huh.
Adult: The cat is eating his food. The dog is not eating his food.

We may be splitting hairs in this example because these types of recast are very close to expansions. Sentences can also be recast in another form:

Child: It got stolen by the crook.
Facilitator: Was it stolen by the crook?
OR
It was stolen by the crook?
OR
The crook stole it.
OR
Did the crook steal it?

These sentences can be recast in whatever form the SLP has targeted, although adult comments are easier for children to process than question forms. Note that even though the form is changed, the relations are not: *crook-steal-it*. Although children with SLI can benefit from the use of recasts, this consequence must be produced in much greater quantity than found in typical conversation to be of value (Proctor-Williams, Fey, & Frome Loeb, 2001).

Input effects are especially strong when the adult utterance builds on a preceding child utterance, providing new grammatical information. Theoretically, given that the child initiated the interaction, the adult's semantically related reply or recast will be regarded as conversationally responsive and will thus hold the child's attention. The immediacy of the adult's recast will enable the child to more easily process the difference between his or her utterance and that of the adult. In a conversational recasting, the SLP selected a grammatical target ahead of time and looks for opportunities to produce this target as part of a conversationally appropriate response to a preceding child utterance.

Children with language impairments vary in the degree to which they benefit from this treatment approach. In addition, good clinical practice would suggest that the form of the recast should change as the child's language and facility with the target form change.

Although the nature of learning that takes place following conversational recasting varies according to the relationship between child and clinician utterances during the recasting process, additional research is needed to assess the many variables that affect treatment outcomes (Hassink & Leonard, 2010). For example, it seems that even noncorrective recasts can have some positive effect (Hassink & Leonard, 2010). Noncorrective recasts continue the child's topic, occur immediately after the child's utterance, and contain a new grammatical form. Providing a new grammatical form in a recast may set in motion a different learning process from that which may occur when children view a recast as providing a correction of their preceding utterance.

If the child says little, the SLP can recast his or her own utterances. If the child will not stop talking, the SLP can interrupt with "yeah" or "uh-huh" and insert a recast sentence.

The effectiveness of recasts is based on four assumptions (Fey et al., 2003):

- It is easy for the child to attend, because the recast sentence is based on the child's utterance.
- It is easy for the child to comprehend, because the recast sentence is similar to the child's sentence.
- It is easy for the child to notice the change, because the recast sentence differs from the child's sentence primarily in the use of the targeted feature.
- It is easy for the child to understand underlying relationships, because the recast sentence occurs in context.

Conversational Contingencies Requiring a Response

Conversational contingencies that require a response are used when a child is able to produce the target reliably but has failed to do so in conversation or has produced the target inaccurately in conversation. A skilled use of both nonlinguistic and linguistic contextual cues should set the stage for production of the target in a situation in which it makes good pragmatic sense. As a fully participating conversational partner, the child has an interest in the conversation and in his or her own utterance. Thus, the child is motivated to modify production in order to maintain the conversation and receive the adult's attention.

Most of these contingencies note the child's error or require the child to find the error and request that the child produce the target more correctly. A second contingency type requests repetition or a correct or expanded utterance to strengthen correct production. A hierarchy of both types, ranging from contingencies that provide maximum input to the child to those that provide the minimal, would be *correction model/request, incomplete correction model/request, reduced error repetition/request, error repetition/request, self-correction request, contingent query, repetition request, expansion request*, and *turnabouts*.

In a *correction model/request*, the facilitator repeats the child's entire utterance, adding or correcting the target that was omitted or produced incorrectly, for example:

Child: I *builded* a big tower out of blocks.
Facilitator: I *built* a big tower out of blocks. Now you say it. (or "Tell me that again.")

The child is requested gently to repeat the facilitator's model. Note that the error has been corrected for the child.

Initially, the target may be emphasized to aid the child in locating the corrected unit. Later training might restate the child's utterance as a question, as in, "You *built* a big tower out of blocks?"

Because the entire utterance is desired in the child's response, the facilitator can act confused to maintain the conversational nature of the interaction rather than saying "Tell me the whole thing."

Facilitator: You *built* a tower out of big blocks? No, you *built* a big tower out of blocks? Oh, I'm confused, tell me again.

In a correction model/request, the child is provided with a complete or only slightly altered model of the correct utterance.

The facilitator should require the child to produce correctly only those units that are currently targeted for intervention. It is difficult for some facilitators to reinforce utterances even when they contain errors, as in the following example:

Child: I *builted* the most biggest tower out of blocks.
Facilitator: You *built* the biggest tower out of blocks?
Child: Yeah, I *built* the most biggest tower out of blocks.
Facilitator: Uh-huh, how big was it?
OR
Yeah? What kind of blocks did you use?
OR
Oh! Where is the tower now?

Note that the facilitator ignored "most biggest."A conversational approach requires the language facilitator to remain focused on the target and on the hierarchy of teaching strategies being used.

In contrast to a correction model/request, an *incomplete correction model/request* provides only the corrected target. The child must provide the rest of the utterance, as follows:

Child: I *builded* a big tower with blocks.
Facilitator: Built.
Child: I *built* a big tower with blocks.

Initially, the child will need a cue to repeat the utterance with the corrected target.

As the child begins to exhibit some success at self-correcting, the facilitator can offer *choice-making*: "Is it *builded* or *built*?" The facilitator must be careful to use this form occasionally when the child's initial utterance is correct as well as when it is incorrect. Otherwise, the child will recognize that the question is only used when he makes an error. In addition, the location of the correct answer should vary so that the child does not develop a strategy of always picking the first or second of the pair choice.

Once the child has learned the target reliably within more structured situations, the language facilitator can use other techniques that require the child to supply the missing or correct target. With *reduced error repetition/request*, the facilitator repeats only the incorrect structure with rising intonation, thus forming a question. This contingency informs the child that the language unit in question is incorrect and must be corrected, for example:

Child: I *builded* a big tower with blocks.
Facilitator: Builded?
Child: Built.

The facilitator's question is more conversational than the cue found in correction model/requests and is less disruptive to the flow of conversation. If the child fails to recognize the error, the facilitator can provide a corrected model by using an incomplete correction model/request.

With *error repetition/request*, the facilitator repeats the entire utterance with rising intonation. The child must locate the error or omission and correct it, as in the following:

Child: I *builded* a big tower with blocks.
Facilitator: I *builded* a big tower with blocks?

The emphasis on the error can be increased or decreased as needed. For example, increased emphasis might be used to aid the child in finding the error. If this technique is unsuccessful, the facilitator might provide a reduced error repetition/request.

Once the child's target knowledge is reasonably stable, the facilitator can use the error repetition/request even when the child is correct. This procedure helps children scan their productions spontaneously and to self-correct.

A *self-correction request* does not provide the child with a repetition of the previous utterance. Instead, the facilitator asks the child to consider the correctness of that utterance from memory, for example, "Is/was that right/correct?" and "Did you say that correctly?" If the child is unsure, the facilitator can provide an error repetition/request.

In contrast to the somewhat stilted tone of the self-correction request, the *contingent query* is very conversational. It is concerned more with comprehension of the message being sent than with specific targets. Nonetheless, this technique can be used effectively to signal the child that something may be amiss with the production. The child is left to scan recent memory to determine where communication breakdown occurred.

Use of contingent queries should be limited because they can disrupt communication and frustrate the speaker who is continually asked to repeat. Young school-age children dislike having to repeat more than once or twice.

Contingent queries may be specific or general, depending on the abilities of the child. In response to the sentence "I *builded* a big tower with blocks," the facilitator might respond, "What did you do with blocks?" "What did you do?" or simply, "What?" If the child falsely assumes that his or her production was correct and merely repeats the error or omission, the facilitator might use a self-correction request.

Correct productions of the target can be strengthened by asking the child to repeat. With a *repetition request*, the facilitator simply says, "Tell me that again," or, "Could you say that again?" This technique also can be used conversationally, implying that the listener missed some portion of the transmission, not that the transmission was in error.

If the child produces the target correctly but in a smaller unit than desired, such as a one-word response following a reduced error repetition/request, the facilitator can use an *expansion request*. The typical cue "Tell me the whole thing" is not conversational in tone. It is better for the facilitator to fake confusion and ask for a total restatement, as in the following example:

Facilitator: Built? What was built? Who built it? I get so confused. You better tell me again.

The advantages of using this routine to elicit language from children were discussed previously.

Turnabouts may be more effective than repetition requests and are more conversational in nature. In a *turnabout*, the facilitator acknowledges the child's utterance or comments and then asks for more, as in "Uh-huh, and then what did you do?" or "Wow, what will you do next?" or "That sounds like fun; what happened then?"

The turnabout technique has been taught successfully to high school peers and parents and has been used effectively in conversation with children with LI. This partner-as-facilitator strategy reportedly can improve conversation skills significantly.

The *wh-* questions used in turnabouts should be of a topic-continuing nature and thus support the child's efforts to maintain the topic. This style of responding is especially helpful to preschool children and children with LI.

Several relational terms also may be used in open-ended utterances to aid the child in providing more information of a specific nature. For example, the facilitator might repeat the child's utterance with the addition of *but* to elicit contrary or adversative information, or *and* to elicit complementary information.

Child: We played games at the party.
Facilitator: What fun. You played games at the party *and . . .*
Child: And we had cake and ice cream.

Other types of relationships and terms are as follows:

Temporal	*and then, first, next, before, after, when, while*
Causal	*because, so, so that, in order to*
Adversative	*but, except, however, except that*
Conditional	*if, unless, or, in case*
Spatial	*in, on, next to, between, etc.*

The conversational contingencies just discussed can be arranged in a hierarchy similar to that in Table 10.2. This arrangement and the specific techniques will differ with the language unit being targeted. The facilitator who is familiar with this hierarchy can respond to the child's utterances in a top-down manner that enhances language stimulation and facilitates language learning.

Top-Down Teaching

The methods presented so far are helpful no matter what method of intervention used by an SLP. It is in the arrangement of these techniques that everything changes. A functional approach is one that uses conversation whenever possible as the milieu for instruction. Employing a top-down intervention model, an SLP helps a child repair conversational errors as they occur within context.

Initially, the SLP selects targets based on the child's needs and activities and topics of conversation based on the child's interests and experience. Placing intervention within everyday routines or play is ideal. By manipulating both the nonlinguistic and linguistic context, the SLP can elicit

TABLE 10.2 Hierarchy of Conversational Contingencies

For the examples, the child's utterance is "I sawed two puppies." The facilitator should use the contingency farthest down on the list that ensures the child's success with minimal input.

Facilitator Input	Conversational Contingency	Example
Maximum ↑	Correction model/Request	I saw two puppies. Can you tell me again? (The cue to say it again is optional, unless the child does not repeat spontaneously.)
	Incomplete correction model/ Request	*Saw.* Can you tell me again? (Again the cue is optional.)
	Choice-making	Is it *saw* or *sawed*?
	Reduced error repetition/ Request	*Sawed*?
	Error repetition/Request	I sawed two puppies?
	Self-correction/Request	Was that right?
	Contingent query	I didn't understand you. Say it again, please. (Other options include *Huh*? and What? or, in this example, *What did you do*?)
	Expansion request	Tell me the whole thing again.
↓	*Repetition request	Tell me again.
Minimum	*Turnabout	You did? I love puppies. What did they look like?

*Used with complete, correct responses.

the targeted language feature and then provide just enough input to aid the child's production. The amount of input needed by the child depends on the child's ability and will differ across children.

Let's assume that a child is working on irregular past tense and the SLP is inquiring about the past weekend, specifically what the child *saw, ate, drank*, and so on. In this case, built on the examples in Table 10.2, the child can self-repair but requires that the error be highlighted in order to do so. Note in the following example how the child needs more assistance than first assumed by the SLP. It is also important to note that the SLP does not correct the error for the child. Supplying the correct response builds dependence on this type of help and does not foster independence.

Example of hierarchy in use:

Child: I sawed two puppies.
Partner: Was that right? (Self-correction request)
Child: Uh-huh.
Partner: I sawed two puppies? (Error repetition/request)
Child: Yeah.
Partner: Sawed? (Reduced error repetition request)
Child: Saw. I saw two puppies.
Partner: Uh-huh, tell me again. (Repetition request to strengthen correct production)
Child: I saw two puppies.
Partner: I think I love puppies more than kittens. Where did you see them? (Turnabout)

When the child gives the correct response, the SLP does not respond with that tired old "Good talking!" Instead, he or she strengthens the correct response by asking for a repetition, then replies conversationally and uses a turnabout to elicit the next response. Let's eavesdrop some more.

Child: At the pet store.
Partner: I'm confused. What happened?
Child: I saw the puppies at the pet store?
Partner: Oh, you saw them at the pet store. Pet stores are fun. When did you go?
Child: I goed on Saturday.
Partner: Was that right?
Child: I went on Saturday.
Partner: Oh, you went to the pet store on Saturday and saw the two puppies. Did you go alone?

Each response by the SLP tries to elicit another that includes use of the target, the irregular past tense, but not just any irregular past tense verb. The specific verbs were chosen well in advance and taught using a variety of methods.

The functional approach to intervention can be challenging for an SLP at first. Once she or he begins to think in a new way, and with practice, functional teaching becomes second nature—just simply the way the SLP talks with children. The intervention approach can be used in almost any interaction with a child, thus giving an SLP ultimate flexibility.

Conclusion

As an SLP, you are a teacher. Not a classroom teacher, although you may do that on occasion, but a teacher nonetheless. What does that mean? One of the best explanations is provided by Melanie Schuele and Donna Boudreau (2008). In fact, it's so good, I'm quoting it for you:

> Teaching involves helping a child do something that he or she was not able to do previously, or helping a child do something better or more independently (Vigil & van Kleeck, 1996). Thus, a teacher . . . explains, models, highlights critical concepts, carefully sequences teaching, provides sufficient practice, and scaffolds, contingent on the child's current level

> of performance. At the outset of learning, the adult literally carries the child through the task. The adult controls the learning situation, provides ample input, and shows the child how to move from question to answer. . . . Over time, the adult gradually yields control; the adult guides the child to successfully complete the pieces of the task, providing support when needed. As the child gains skill and independence, the adult provides less and less support (Vigil & van Kleeck, 1996). Learning is best characterized . . . by moving a child from successful performance with maximal support to successful performance with little or no support. At each step along the way, the teacher or clinician must be proficient at providing the appropriate amount and type of support. . . . (pp. 10–11)

Commit this to memory!

Throwing out questions or cues and hoping for the right response or providing the answer when the child is incorrect is not teaching. Teaching is a systematic analysis of what the child is lacking that results in his or her non-success. It's essential for an SLP to break any learning task into the sequential steps required to move from where the child is now to where we want the child to be, which is successfully learning the task, whether it's using plural *-s* or initiating a topic. To be an effective teacher, the SLP must now plan how intervention will proceed within and between each step of the sequence.

Decisions on sequencing should be determined by the complexity of the task. It goes without saying that simple tasks are targeted before complex tasks. Success in earlier tasks should lead to success on later ones. Earlier tasks need to target emergence and initial establishment of a skill and provide enough support that there is a high probability of a child being successful.

To teach effectively, the SLP must plan how intervention will proceed at each step. This requires consideration of the task but also necessitates paying attention to the learning characteristics of the individual child and the cognitive and linguistic requirements of the task.

The SLP must consider the way in which he or she cues or prompts a child's response. Framing the question is essential to success in responding. As a child becomes more successful, the SLP can provide less scaffolding or structure. You can enhance teaching by anticipating the types of support that a child is likely to need and the types of error the child is likely to make. Both should be used to plan scaffolding strategies (Schuele & Boudreau, 2008).

In addition, effective intervention depends on ways in which the adult responds to the child's attempts. Both cuing and responding should be designed to facilitate growth toward more independent and more complex performance. The nature of the child's errors and successes, indicates the amount of scaffolding a child needs. Guidelines include the following precepts.

- Formulate a response based on the reason for a child's error.
- The manner of responding will depend on where the child is in the learning process.
- The SLP response should be designed to facilitate achievement of the teaching goal while still preserving the goal of maximum independence with minimal support.
- Responses to correct an inadequate response may be similar because they both highlight the problem-solving task for the child.

Both the nonlinguistic and linguistic contexts can be manipulated by an SLP and other language facilitators to teach language to a child and to encourage use of structures recently acquired. By using the various techniques described in this chapter, facilitators can maximize interactions with child with LI. Although it would be ideal if facilitators used the full range of techniques, even the adaptation of some would help make learning more conversational in nature.

Chapter 11

Specific Intervention Techniques

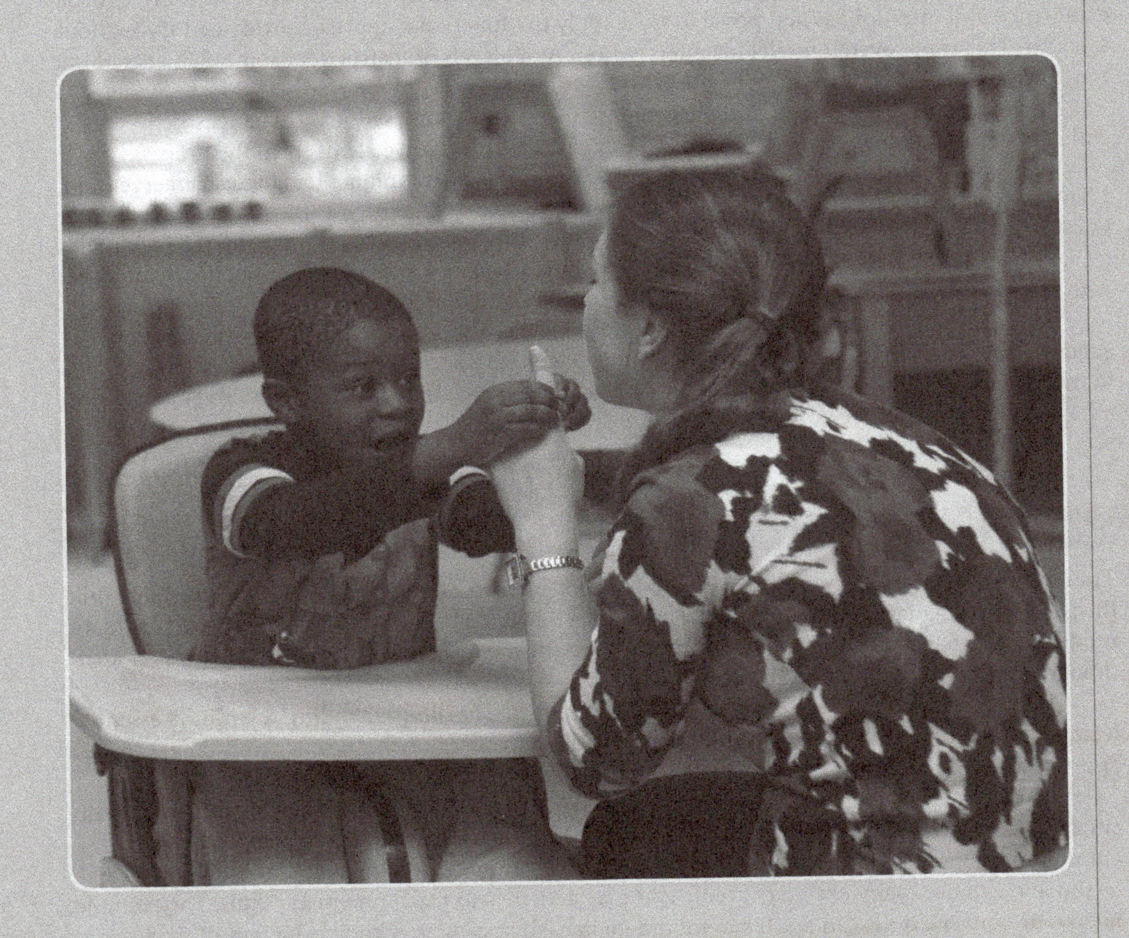

number of teaching techniques are effective. The success of intervention varies with the particular linguistic feature trained, the manner and duration of the training, and the characteristics of the individual child.

Prior to beginning intervention, an SLP should examine all deficit areas for a given child and apply a "so what?" criterion. In short, an SLP is concerned with the importance of individual deficits for a child's overall communication. Each deficit should be evaluated to the extent that it contributes to a child's communicative functioning. Those that do not affect overall communication may fail "so what?" test.

It is also important that you, as an SLP, consider generalization at the beginning of intervention and make crucial training decisions on the basis of generalization to the everyday environment. At least a portion of each lesson should involve use in a conversational context. Intervention that focuses solely on linguistic form can result in limited progress and lack of generalization.

In this chapter we will discuss a developmental hierarchy for intervention, modified where appropriate by sound teaching principles, research and evidence-based practice, and my clinical experience and intuition. When possible we'll apply the functional approach explained throughout this text. This is my overall model for intervention. At all levels of instruction, some elements of the functional intervention model can be used.

Intervention should be fun and challenging, using real conversational exchanges between the child and partners wherever possible. Thus, both partners are involved actively in the process.

In this chapter we explore some proven and some promising techniques for language intervention. I have attempted to include the best evidence-based practices. For clarity, I have divided the chapter into four aspects of language: pragmatics, semantics, syntax, and morphology. We discuss hierarchies for training and techniques that lend themselves well to each area. The final portions of the chapter deal with the special needs of children from CLD backgrounds and the clinical application of computers.

The best intervention addresses language holistically so that a child can experience newly acquired language as it is used in communication. Some SLPs accomplish this goal by targeting skills in more than one area of language or by using a stage approach in which a few training targets from a stage of development are targeted simultaneously. Suggested activities are presented in Appendix E.

Pragmatics

Traditional language intervention goals are product oriented. Language forms are targeted, while the process of language use is tangential. Although a theoretical shift has occurred toward pragmatic models of language, all too often communicative context is used only to create fun or as an afterthought relative to generalization.

Children can acquire very complex forms without totally comprehending them. It is essential, however, that they understand the functional qualities or uses of the forms being taught. When appropriate, linguistic forms can and should be targeted within a functional context.

Through role-playing and the use of videotaped interactions, an SLP can teach a child to identify situations in which the desired information, action, or material was requested inadequately, inaccurately, or inappropriately. An SLP may directly target a number of pragmatic skills within a single lesson and can use many everyday events and play activities to teach pragmatic skills. For example, telephone conversations can teach several pragmatic skills, such as acknowledgment of the interaction, conversational opening and closing, topic maintenance, and referential communication. The use of different situations can help a child adapt to differing scenarios. For example, by pretending that he or she is lost, an SLP can teach requesting and giving assistance and information, roles, and following directions.

Construction toys, such as Legos, can teach requesting assistance, referential communication, giving and following directions, and topic maintenance. More difficult tasks will require requesting assistance.

Several children's stories can be enacted to help a child learn roles. The use of puppets or dolls or different costumes also will aid the learning of role taking.

Finally, an SLP can use any number of activities for referential communication. Children can describe objects seen in books, on computers, or through toy periscopes. Such activities as I Spy and Twenty Questions also aid referential communication growth and foster requesting and giving information. In addition, object descriptions can be a part of requesting similar objects, as in "I want the fuzzy bear."

Effective intervention should enhance language and social skills while generalizing to authentic interactions (Timler et al., 2007). Although more structured clinician-centered intervention methods may be required for some children and targets, generalization to a child's everyday environment is key to success.

Intentions

Children select and acquire utterances that are communicatively most useful. As an SLP, you'll be concerned with the breadth of intentions that a child is able to express. The following section addresses the training of several intentions. In Chapter 12, some methods to be used in the classroom are discussed. Appendix D also provides several indirect linguistic cues useful for eliciting different functions.

Calling for Attention

Children seek attention from adults who provide it. Within the classroom, teachers might give a child an object and ask him or her to take it to an adult who, for the purpose of training, initially ignores the child. The child also might be asked to relay a message to someone else.

Facilitators should attend to a child as soon as the child requests attention. If the child continually demands attention or uses inappropriate behavior to get attention, the facilitator will have to set some limits, such as only responding in certain situations and never responding to inappropriate behavior.

The form of attention-requesting is usually a child calling a facilitator by name or gaining attention by some other means, such as tapping the listener's shoulder, moving into the visual field of the listener, leaning in the direction of the listener, or using eye contact. The child also may specify how the facilitator should respond by making a request. These sequences are easy to train within a variety of activities.

Requests for Action or Assistance

Requests for action can be trained at mealtime, within small group projects, or during almost any physically challenging task. A facilitator will need to design situations in which children require assistance to complete a task. To encourage requesting, a facilitator can use games in which children must solve problems. Tasks also may be sabotaged by a facilitator (see Table 10.1). In requests for actions or assistance attention is gained first, and the form of the utterance is interrogative or imperative.

SLPs can enhance the discriminability between two communicative forms by decreasing the reinforcement for the less desirable form in a given situation while providing reinforcement for a second, more acceptable approximation. It is important to establish well-generalized use of the acceptable communicative act in situations previously associated with the less conventional alternative.

Although young children with ASD can learn a new communicative behavior, they may fail to use that behavior conditionally (Sigafoos, O'Reilly, Drasgow, & Reichle, 2002). **Conditional use** means using the behavior that best matches a particular context. In some cases, individuals with significant DDs find a socially unacceptable response option more reinforcing than a more conventional one. Screams may get more attention than politely asking and may require less effort

(Sigafoos et al., 2002). It may also be that the child doesn't have sufficient teaching examples during initial training to know when to use and when not to use a particular option.

An SLP cannot assume that a child's obligatory use of a communicative behavior, such as requesting assistance, will result in correct conditional use. Conditional use of a requesting requires a child to use one communicative behavior when it is needed but refrain from using it when it is not. For example, when items are nearby or easy to manipulate, a child can be taught to help himself or herself, and when items were distant or difficult to manipulate, the child can be taught to produce a request. This can be accomplished in graduated steps in which a child attempts a desired task and is initially successful. As the task becomes increasingly more difficult, the child must request assistance. In this way, conditional use can be established even with children with ASD (Reichle, Dropik, Alden-Anderson, & Haley, 2008; Reichle & McComas, 2004).

Requests for Information

Children with LI often do not see other persons as sources of information and may produce few such requests of this type. Although the environment can be manipulated to encourage requests for objects and actions, it is not as easy to encourage or increase a child's need and desire to seek information.

Requests for information require that a facilitator omit essential information for some novel or unfamiliar task, such as an art project, a new game, or some challenging academic task. Objects unknown to a child may be introduced without being named or their purpose explained. A child can be prodded gently to ask questions if asking does not occur spontaneously.

A child must recognize both the need for this information and that another person possesses the knowledge. Recognition of need is often the most difficult aspect of this training. Confrontational naming tasks, such as pulling objects out of a bag, with objects known and unknown to a child, may encourage initial requesting for information. The form of requests for information is either a *wh-* or *yes/no* interrogative with rising intonation, as in "what's that?" or "Is that a marker?"

A facilitator also might encourage the child to ask questions by questioning him or her about other people's feelings or actions of which the child has little knowledge. The child then can be cued with "Why don't you ask (name)?" This tactic can be used with naming tasks as well, as in "See if Juan knows what this is."

A child should be expected to ask questions that reflect the forms he or she is capable of producing. The facilitator's verbal responses discussed in Chapter 10 can be used to help the child modify incorrect, inappropriate, or immature responses or learn new ones.

Requests for Objects

A facilitator can easily train requests for objects within art tasks, group projects, snacktime, job training, or daily living skills training, such as dressing and hygiene. It is essential that a child actually desire the object he or she is to request and that the facilitator can provide it.

A facilitator can change the environment to increase both the opportunities for requesting and the behaviors that direct a child's attention to these opportunities. Many situations, especially those with groups of children, provide an opportunity for overlooking a child's turn, thus encouraging requesting. Of particular importance is a coordinated program designed to teach requesting for use in the everyday environment by approximating that environment and by training those within that to model and elicit requests. Table 11.1 includes general guidelines for caregiver elicitation techniques.

Expression of this intention usually begins with eye contact or some attention-getting behavior, such as calling a name. The form, usually accompanied by a reaching gesture, is interrogative ("can I have . . . ?") or imperative ("give me . . . ") and specifies the desired object.

An SLP can elicit denials by giving the child something other than what he or she requested or by giving the child something undesirable. The child can reject either an action or proposal. The speaker uses emphatic stress, and the utterance is in a negative form.

TABLE 11.1 Guidelines for Caregiver Elicitation of Requests for Objects

Make statements throughout the day about objects that the child might prefer. Wait for a response.

Use elicitation behaviors to accompany high-interest activities and play. These behaviors include the following:

Modeling with an imitative prompt. Facilitator provides a model of a request and asks the child to imitate.

Direct questioning. Facilitator asks, "What do you want?" or "What do you need?"

Indirect modeling. Facilitator provides a partial model followed by an indirect elicitation request, such as, "If you want more *X*, let me know (or, "ask me for it") or, "Would you like to *X* or *Y*?"

Obstacle presentation. Facilitator requests that the child accomplish some task but provides an obstacle to accomplishment.

"Please get me the chalk over there." (There is no chalk.)
"Pour everyone some juice." (The container is empty.)

General statement. Facilitator makes a verbal comment about some activity or object that the child might want to request. The facilitator entices the child.

"We could play Candyland if you want to."

"I have some Play-Doh on that high shelf."

Set up specific situations to elicit requesting.

Provide direct and indirect models as often as possible without requiring the child to imitate.

Provide a model at appropriate times when the child appears to need assistance or is looking quizzical.

Have the child attempt difficult tasks in which help is occasionally needed.

Respond *immediately* and *naturally* to any verbal request.

Responding to Requests

Responses may take the form of an answer to a question or a reply to a remark. These forms are very different and require different skills and syntactic forms.

In responding to questions, children must recognize that they possess the answer and that they are required to reply. Initial training might disregard the correctness of the answer in favor of reinforcing answering in general. Responding with an incorrect answer is preferred over no answer at all.

Some children with LI have difficulty identifying the emotions of others and of themselves and placing these in a form of expression. We can teach awareness and expression through a three-step intervention model (Way, Yelsma, Van Meter, & Black-Pond, 2007):

1. Connecting physical experience and emotions
2. Increasing awareness of own emotional state
3. Connecting emotion to expression

Activities within each step are presented in Table 11.2.

Replies

Replying is more difficult to teach than answering because a response is expected from the child but not required. A child can be helped to recognize the need to reply by physical signs from the SLP, such as a head nod, or the passing of an object to signal "It's your turn."

A child's ability to reply may be hindered by an inability to determine the topic or to formulate a response. A facilitator may enhance linguistic processing by having the child repeat the previous speaker's comment. Over time, the facilitator can modify this procedure to teach the child to whisper the

TABLE 11.2 Teaching Emotional Awareness and Expression

Connecting Physical Experience and Emotions
• Bodywork, such as recognizing one's heartbeat, sweating, flushing, or a stomachache, can help a child turn his or her attention internally. • Connecting physical states to specific feelings and learning methods to calm oneself when feeling anxious or upset.
Increasing Awareness of Own Emotional State
• Drawing the child's attention to the important features of expression, then modeling language to express those feelings. SLPs might observe and comment on facial expressions, body expressions, vocal affect, and labels or words in affective experiences. • Role-playing various feelings. • Identifying feelings of characters in stories, videos, or photos; or using art therapy. • Using *feelings strips* on which is the unfinished sentence, "I feel . . . " into which children can insert feelings faces to describe their feelings. In this way, children are taught physical cues for different feelings at the same time as they learn to become aware of their own. • Identify single feelings and then learn to recognize multiple feelings at a particular moment. Begin with *primary* emotions such as joy, sadness, anger, fear, disgust, and interest, and then progress to more sophisticated *complex* emotions that require self-reflection, such as empathy, sympathy, guilt, envy, shame, regret, and pride.
Connecting Emotion to Expression
• Drawing pictures to express feelings nonverbally in preparation for addressing them verbally. • Expressing emotion through role playing, pretend play, and acting out dramas. • Creating a skit from an index card listing multiple feelings, and then having other children guess the feelings being portrayed. • Acting out stories from books, TV shows, and movies. • Reading and listening to narratives and making sense of character perspectives in the context of story events. SLPs can use questions that probe linguistic and socioemotional awareness, questions that guide students to reflect on feelings and organize these ideas using language to describe, report, predict, and interpret feelings and motivations. • Oral and written storytelling to share personal narratives while developing integrated language skills and expressiveness.

Source: Information from Denham & Burton (1996), Hyter, Atchison, & Blashill (2006).

speaker's comment, mouth it, and silently repeat until the process is internalized by the child. In this way, children can be helped to identify important information in comments and in formulating replies.

Statements

Show-and-tell, discussions, and current-event activities help children state information. During discussions of high-interest topics, such as, holidays, pets, and family events for children or dating, friends, and competitive games for adolescents, a facilitator can encourage offering of opinions. A facilitator also can use mock radio and television broadcasts. With a little cutting and some paint, he or she can convert a large appliance box into a television from within which children can deliver daily newscasts of information.

A conversational partner may or may not know the information being shared. In the first instance, the child might recall a shared event; in the latter, the child presents new information and can assume that the facilitator has very limited knowledge. Each situation has different informational needs and requires some presuppositional skill to determine the necessary amount of information to convey. Children can be taught how much information to include (see under Presupposition heading on page 288).

Initially, the child must secure the listener's attention and state the discussion topic. Statements can be expanded into narratives whose purpose is also to convey information.

Conversational Abilities

More than other areas of language intervention, the training of conversational abilities requires the use of actual conversational situations. Ritualized communication that interferes with interpersonal communication, such as echolalia, can be modified gradually into acceptable and conventional routines, such as greetings, conversational initiations, and requests for repair (Magill, 1986). For children with Asperger's syndrome, high-functioning autism, or other social interactional difficulties, the following conversational goals seem appropriate (Kline & Volkmar, 2000):

- Conventions of verbal and nonverbal communication, including initiating a conversation and selecting appropriate topics.
- Social awareness and social problem solving, including perceiving verbal and nonverbal cues and making inferences.
- Self-evaluation and management, including ability to participate in diverse communication activities and to control one's own behavior.

Social routines can be memorized and practiced in different situations that help a child become more flexible in their use. Variations can be taught through different facilitators and situations. For example, one does not offer to shake hands when the potential partner has her or his arms full.

In a study of TD adolescents, several behaviors that may or may not be present in teens with LI occur frequently (Turkstra, Ciccia, & Seaton, 2003). These include

- looking at a conversational partner, especially when listening.
- nodding and showing neutral and positive facial expression.
- responding verbally to acknowledge understanding (*Uh-huh, Yeah*).
- giving contingent responses.

These four behaviors suggest targets for helping children with LI interact more appropriately. You may recall that contingent responses may be semantically contingent (on-topic) and/or pragmatically contingent (appropriate).

While only limited research data exist, they suggest intervention methods that may work for some teens (Brinton, Robinson, & Fujiki, 2004). A two-step intervention program could target

- helping youth with LI think of conversation as a reciprocal endeavor that requires adjustment for one's partner.
- providing interactive strategies to solicit and act on conversational contributions by others.

Intervention can occur within structured, conversation-focused, small-group activities (Nippold, 2000). The atmosphere should be positive with plenty of opportunity for success. Within this context, the SLP models appropriate responses, and this modeling is followed by teen practice, then peer analysis and feedback with the use of video recordings and small-group discussion. Scripted sequences and role-play can be very helpful.

Video clips and guided observation and comment can be used to aid an adolescent to comment on the nature of exchanges, feelings and thoughts of participants, and interpretation of reactions. The bulk of the time, however, should focus on interactive strategies, moving from highly structured situations in which turns and topics are controlled to more free-flowing conversations. Clients can be trained in variations of comment-question, in which they make a contingent comment on their partner's utterance and then ask a related question, as in turnabouts. Listening and comprehension skills can also be enhanced. From here, additional interactional techniques, such as how to ask someone's opinion or how to draw listeners into the conversation, can be taught.

Entering a Conversation

Although entering an interaction can be a formidable challenge to children with LI, children can be taught play-entry strategies through modeling and prompting by an adult (Selber Beilinson & Olswang, 2003). Four nonverbal "low-risk" strategies can be taught initially through modeling and visual picture prompts:

- Walk over to your friend.
- Watch your friend.
- Get a toy like the one your friend is using.
- Do the same thing as your friend.

A fifth, "high-risk" strategy includes verbal initiation.

In modeling verbal initiation, the classroom teacher, aide, or SLP helps a child select a toy similar to that of another child and says to the second child, "We're building with blocks just like you." This can be an opening for the other child to respond by asking the child to join. A more direct model might include telling a child what to say. When a child can successfully imitate the opening behavior, the adult gradually reduces the model and tries to prompt it through toys and picture and verbal prompts. These are also reduced until a child can initiate spontaneously. Other strategies might include interpreting (*I think Mohammed wants you to play with him*), giving suggestions (*Maybe Kwanzi would like to see what you made*), referring to a peer (*Maybe Alex can help you hold the paper while you glue it*), and commenting on similarities (*Jin is making a costume too. Tell him about yours.*) (Weitzman & Greenberg, 2002).

Presupposition

A speaker's semantic decisions are based on her or his knowledge of the referents (the thing to which words refer) and the situation and on *presuppositions*, or social knowledge of a listener's needs. A speaker needs to provide information that is as unambiguous as possible. In other words, the speaker and the listener need to share the same linguistic context. Often, children with LI are unaware of their audience's needs.

Two aspects of training might be (a) what information to relay and (b) how much. The first can be trained with descriptive or directive tasks in which a child is the speaker. A listener tries to guess or draw the described object or to follow the directions. The facilitator can use barrier games, in which he or she places an opaque barrier between the speaker and the listener. Because the speaker and the listener do not share the same nonlinguistic context, the bulk of the information must be carried by the linguistic element in an unambiguous manner if the listener is to comprehend. The list of fun activities in which a child directs an adult in how to do something is endless.

When the child is the listener, the SLP can send ambiguous or incomplete messages or directions to give the child an opportunity to identify the missing semantic elements. Obstacle courses are a good vehicle through which the child can be directed or direct others.

Training the correct amount of information to transmit may be more difficult. Of course, giving insufficient information in the tasks previously mentioned would make the directions difficult to follow. The SLP can train children to give more, as well as more accurate, information. For a child who gives too much information, these tasks may be trained initially one descriptor or one step at a time. These tasks then can be grouped into multidescriptor or command steps so that the child experiences offering more information. The relating of very discrete or limited events, such as combing your hair or washing your face, also can control the amount of information to be relayed.

The SLP can help the child monitor his or her own production to know when redundancy occurs. This is accomplished by gently remainding the child that certain information was relayed previously. In subsequent training, the SLP can quiz the child about the novelty or the lack of information presented. This will help the child identify the correct amount of information.

Referential Skills

Referential skills include identifying novel content and describing this content for a listener. Children with LD have been trained successfully to use referential skills through the use of barrier games. The description of physical attributes ("It's big and white and furry.") is somewhat easier to teach than are relational terms, such as location ("He's in front of the computer."). Guessing games can be lots of fun and very instructive.

Topic

Topic offers an encompassing framework for considering other language skills. Unlike greetings, which vary only slightly across situations, topics and methods of topic introduction and identification are context-dependent.

Topic Initiation. *Initiation* is the verbal introduction of a topic not currently being discussed. Children with LI often do not understand the purpose of conversations or are reluctant to introduce topics for discussion. Topic initiation implies an active conversational strategy. A child with LI may not be adept at introducing topics clearly or may have very limited topics to discuss. Children with ASD or TBI may introduce unusual or inappropriate topics.

Adolescents with moderate-to-severe ID have been taught to initiate a topic through the use of SLP or facilitator waiting and through training in the purpose of conversation. In the first step of training, a facilitator maintains eye contact for 10 seconds but does not speak. Planned delay can be an effective strategy for prompting clients to initiate.

If the child does not initiate the conversation during this wait, the facilitator can explain the purpose of conversation and the enjoyment that can result. He or she also can describe the roles of speaker and listener. Then the facilitator returns to the waiting strategy. If the child still does not respond, the facilitator can suggest that the child find something of interest to discuss by looking through a magazine or pictures from the child's life. The facilitator then returns to the waiting strategy. If the child fails to initiate again, the facilitator can model a topic initiation.

It is important that the facilitator focus fully on the child when he or she initiates and follow the child's lead. The facilitator should try not to interrupt the child.

The SLP might first teach the child to gain a listener's attention. When the child inadequately introduces a topic, the facilitator can request further information to identify the topic.

The SLP initially can tolerate inappropriate topics to give the child some success. Gradually, the SLP can discuss the inappropriateness of these topics and gently steer the conversation to more appropriate ground. He or she can suggest topics ("Maybe you'll tell me about . . . ") and leave it for the child to initiate. The SLP also can train the child to ask other people about their likes and dislikes, favorite foods, sports, TV shows, or exciting trips or vacations in order to include other- oriented topics in the child's repertoire.

To increase the frequency of memory-related topics, the facilitator can encourage the child to talk about feelings or activities engaged in prior to the conversation. Elicitation can be direct ("What did you do yesterday?") or indirect ("I wonder what you did yesterday"). The SLP can encourage the child to ask the same information in turn. In addition, she or he can engage the child in activities and then ask the child to discuss what was done. The SLP can provide feedback. Future-related topic initiations are similar, such as discussing what the child will do next. The use of such conversationally based strategies can increase nonimmediate topic initiations, as well as the general level of syntactic performance.

Topic Maintenance. An SLP can continue the conversation by commenting on the topic a child initiates and by cuing the child to respond. The SLP can use turnabouts—usually a comment followed by a cue for the child to respond, such as a question—to keep the conversation flowing and on-topic. Questions should make pragmatic sense; that is, the facilitator should not know the answer prior to asking. Table 11.3 is a list of various turnabouts.

TABLE 11.3 Variety of Turnabouts

Type	Example
Tag	*Child:* Baby's panties. *Mother:* It's the baby's diaper, *isn't it?*
Clarification (contingent query)	*Huh?* *What?*
Specific request	*What's that?*
Confirmation	*Horse?* *Is that a hippopotamus?* (Hand object to partner and give quizzical glance)
Expansions	
Suggestions	*I want one.*
Corrections	*No, it's a zebra!* (Expectant tone)
Behavior comment	*You can't sit on that.*
Expansive question for sustaining conversation	*What would the police officer do then?*

Off-topic responding may indicate that a child is inattentive or cannot identify the referent or topic presented. Children who are inattentive may be distracted easily and need help determining how to focus their attention.

A facilitator can help a child who cannot sort through the information to identify the referent or topic through the use of questions and prompts that highlight those semantic cues of importance to the child. Practice conversations with various partners and topics can provide an opportunity to learn and generalize. The facilitator can keep the child on-topic with such cues as "Anything else you can tell me about (topic)?" and "Tell me more about (topic)."

When a facilitator and a child have shared the same experience, the facilitator can act as a guide to keep the child on-topic. The facilitator also can help the child sequence events through the use of questions ("Then what happened?") or probes ("Are you sure that happened next?").

The facilitator should avoid dead-end conversational bids. Dead-end bids result in a short response, such as "yes" or "no," that ends the interaction.

Duration of Topic. An SLP or a facilitator can help an incessant talker by using very limited topics with definite boundaries, such as "What animals did you see at the zoo?" If the child strays beyond the topic, the facilitator should interrupt. He or she then can remind the child of the topic and gently bring him or her back to it.

The facilitator also should alert the child when he or she has provided enough information or is redundant. Such phrases as "You've already told me about *X*" or "I'll only answer that question one more time" help the child establish boundaries.

Children who provide too little information can be encouraged to provide more with "Tell me more." An SLP also can play dumb with such utterances as "Well, I guess it was pretty boring if that's all that happened." In general, children remain on-topic longer when they are enacting scenarios, describing, or problem solving.

Turn Taking

It is important not to initiate turn-taking training while also attempting to train topic maintenance. Too many new training targets may confuse the child. A facilitator may have to tolerate off-topic comments initially to correct inappropriate turn taking.

Turn taking can begin at a nonverbal, physical level. An SLP and a child can pass items back and forth as they use them. The item then can become the symbol for talking when you hold it. Many structured games also require turn taking. The SLP also can provide a turn-taking model by imitating the child's spontaneous speech or using verbal games and motion songs with groups of children. Later, the SLP can use turnabouts or a question-answer technique to help a child take verbal turns. Nonlinguistic cues, such as eye contact and nodding, can also signal the child to take a turn. The SLP can decrease questioning gradually in favor of these nonlinguistic cues and wait for the child to take a turn. Children can be taught attention-getting devices, such as increased speaking volume, to gain a turn. Games in which the child directs other people are highly motivating.

Turn taking is appropriate if it does not interrupt others. A child who is overly assertive and who continually interrupts may need to be reminded not to do so. The SLP might focus instruction on identifying when speakers have completed their turns. He or she also should explain appropriate interruptions, as in emergencies. Structured exchanges through use of an intercom or mock police radio may help children understand the importance of turn allocation through play. Structured games, such as Twenty Questions, also foster turn-allocation learning. In fact, there are many games that require turn-taking skills and can be adapted for conversational training.

Conversational Repair

Children with LI often seem unaware of the distinction between understanding and failure to understand and rarely act when they do not.

An SLP may modify comprehension monitoring through the use of audiotaped language samples in the following training sequence:

1. Identification, labeling, and demonstration of active listening.
2. Detection of and reaction to inadequate signals.
3. Detection of and reaction to inadequate content.
4. Identification of and reaction to comprehension breakdown.

Although this sequence can be trained easily in an audio-recorded mode, generalization to actual conversational use should not be neglected. The introduction of puppets, dolls, or role-playing at each step can facilitate this generalization. Written scripts may be used with older children, targeting frequent conversational contexts.

Comprehension monitoring can be facilitated when a child takes an active role in the process. The child is taught first to identify, label, and demonstrate active orientation to listening behaviors, such as sitting, looking at the speaker, and thinking about what the speaker says. After learning to distinguish successful and unsuccessful performance of the three active listening behaviors, the child labels and demonstrates each. The child also might repeat the previous speaker's utterance or reply to such questions as "What did (name) just say?" This can be worked into many play situations, such as playing store or restaurant.

Next, the child is taught to detect and react to *signal inadequacies*, such as insufficient loudness, excessive rate, or competing noise. These concrete obstructions that prevent representation of the message are relatively easy to identify and enable a child to learn the difference between understanding and not understanding.

Within everyday activities, the facilitator can encourage clarification requests from the child by mumbling or talking too fast. This technique works especially well when giving directions needed to complete some fun task. The SLP or facilitator occasionally can ask the child, "What did I say? How can we find out?"

Once able to identify signal inadequacies, a child can be taught a variety of responses for requesting clarification. Requests may include general appeals, such as "Pardon?" (or "What?"), "I can't hear you," and "Wait . . . Now say it again" (or "Again please"), or more specific requests, such as, "Talk louder please" (or "Louder"), "Could you talk more slowly?" (or "Slow down"), and "Did you say *X*?" It is best to begin with more general requests and then move to more specific ones. The request form should reflect the child's overall syntactic level.

Next, a child can be taught to detect and react to *content inadequacies*, such as inexplicit, ambiguous, and physically impossible commands. For example, because inadequate content may not always be obvious, the SLP can ask the child to repeat the message to himself or herself and/or to the speaker and to attempt the task demanded. Again, the child is taught various methods for requesting clarification of inadequate content.

This part of the training can be great fun, with the facilitator making outrageous statements and ridiculous demands of the child as in a game of "Simon says." I still remember the expression on the face of a child with Down syndrome whom I had asked to get into his lunch box. The SLP can insert intentional content inadequacies into any number of daily activities.

Finally, the SLP can teach the child to identify and react to messages that exceed his or her comprehension capacity by the presence of unfamiliar words, excessive length, and excessive syntactic complexity. This level of comprehension breakdown may be the most difficult to detect.

A child can practice identification and reaction in the form of clarification requests in real-life situations in which these difficulties are likely to occur. Most novel activities include unusual jargon that the facilitator can use to confuse the message. For example, cooking offers such words as *ladle*, *simmer*, and *skillet*.

As training progresses, the child should learn to identify the point of actual breakdown for the speaker. The child can be aided in identifying where the breakdown occurred through questions from the SLP.

Narration

Language intervention with narratives may focus on the organization of, cohesion within, or comprehension of the narrative. The length and complexity of narratives is positively related to the amount of exposure to narratives in intervention. Modeling and practice are especially important. Specific targets will vary with the maturity of the child.

Whether the training target is comprehension or narrative retelling, or story production, it is important to control for the many variables that can affect a child's performance, including (Boudreau & Larsen, 2004):

- Number of characters
- Plot line clarity
- Number of episodes
- Number and complexity of utterances
- Clear resolution
- Age appropriateness
- Interest level

It is also important to manage the external prompts needed by a child, such as the use of sequential pictures and verbal prompts, which can range from those needed to craft the narrative, such as "In the beginning . . . " and "How did the story end?" to more open-ended prompts, such as "What happended next?"

Narrative Structure

Young children use a script-based knowledge organization system. *Scripts* are sequences of events that form unified wholes. When this event sequence is placed in linguistic form, it is called a text, the basis of narratives.

Knowledge of episode structure forms a narrative framework within which the child can interpret complex events and unfamiliar content. An SLP can facilitate development of internalized narrative organization through

- involving children in organized activities, such as daily routines, to help them organize their own real-life scripts. Go over each event in a routine with children.
- using scripted play in which children enact everyday activities that gradually become more variable and less bound to the immediate context.
- reading and telling real-life stories with clear scripts. The narratives can be based on the child's experience.
- helping children transfer from event-based to linguistic organization by telling them narratives with clearly structured story grammars and then having them dramatize the stories.

These exercises may be performed orally with young children or in writing with older.

Scripted play is especially useful with preschool and early school-age children and will be discussed in detail in Chapter 12. Initially, it is very important that the scripts describe familiar motivating events, such as going to the market or getting ready for school. The script should be introduced and discussed prior to play. The script is played and discussed afterward.

With each replaying, the children change roles, modify the events, and use fewer concrete objects. As children become more adept at recounting the script, the SLP encourages telling of the narrative without an enactment. Again, familiar roles and situations are used.

The SLP or teacher can facilitate production of event descriptions by having children describe familiar events as they occur or as recalled from slides, pictures, or videotapes. Children can role-play and describe familiar events as they occur.

Familiar events depicted in child drawings can be used for sequencing. An SLP can help the child identify the setting and characters by asking him or her to describe the picture; for example:

Facilitator: Well, what do we have here?
Child: This is me in the kitchen, and I'm making breakfast.
Facilitator: So, we might say, "This morning, I was in the kitchen making breakfast." What did you do first? (or Then what happened? or What's this next picture?)

After completing a step-by-step description, the child can be encouraged to tell the entire narrative.

As an SLP, you can teach a child with LI to structure personal narratives and to use narratives in different contexts. Initially, the SLP elicits and models a simple chronological sequence of a limited number of past events using temporal words such as *first, next,* and *last* to focus on the chronological ordering of events. Once a simple structure is mastered, additional details and events can be added to elaborate the narrative. These might include descriptions, causal factors, emotions, and dialogue. Teachers and parents can be enlisted to elaborate a child's personal narratives (Boland, Haden, & Ornstein, 2003). Intervention might target the use of narrative organizational knowledge and skills in other contexts, such as learning to speak to different listeners and about different experiences.

Training fictional narratives does not result in increased functional communication (Cannizzaro & Coelho, 2002). Most likely this is because there is only a minimal to nonexistent relationship between use of the two genres (Shiro, 2003). Personal narratives are used in a variety of natural contexts. In contrast, fictional stories have a more focused use. Another aspect of generalization is the frequency of target's use, and personal narratives occur more frequently than fictional ones.

Episode knowledge can be taught through the use of children's books. Book selection should be based on the following criteria (Naremore, 2001):

- Familiar event scripts
- Pictures that support the episodes
- Clearly sequenced episodes

- Appropriate length and language level
- Stories "pretested" for retelling by the SLP

The actual story is not of prime interest. The SLP should select stories that contain all episodic elements. Intervention can begin with a mediated approach by discussing with the child the importance of stories for communication.

After reading a book together, the SLP can help the child analyze the story following a "problem-solution-result" format. Learning structure is the goal. Terminology is not. The SLP helps the child break the story into pieces, identify the parts, and recombine them again into a cohesive narrative. For children who can't relate to books, the SLP can construct one-episode narratives of experiences familiar to the child. Pictures and real objects may aid the child's participation.

Preliminary data suggests that we can improve some young school-age children's functional use of both the macrostructure (story grammar) and microstructure (causality) in their narratives through literate narrative intervention (Petersen, Laing Gillam, Spencer, & Gillam, 2010). More sophisticated oral narratives share a variety of microstructural features with written language, including the use of causal and temporal subordinating conjunctions, coordinating conjunctions, adverbs, elaborated noun phrases, mental and linguistic verbs, and specific nouns with clearly referenced pronouns (R. B. Gillam & Ukrainetz, 2006; Greenhalgh & Strong, 2001; Nippold, Ward-Lonergan, & Fanning, 2005). Steps in literate narrative intervention are presented in Table 11.4.

Narratives can be retold repeatedly, although retelling is not the overall goal. Ideally, the child will internalized knowledge to use composing and comprehending conversational and book-based narratives (Naremore, 2001). Both narrative length and structure can be improved if children have a model on which to base their narrative and a structure inherent in the model, such as story retelling using pictures (Tönsing & Tesner, 1999).

TABLE 11.4 Possible Steps for Narration Training

1.	The SLP models storytelling from pictures in a book.
2.	The SLP and child co-tell the story in the same format with story grammar icons as prompts.
3.	The child retells the narrative with SLP verbal prompts and pictures in a book but no story grammar icons prompts.
4.	The SLP and child co-tell a story from a single complex scene picture and story grammar icon prompts.
5.	The child retells the story from a single complex-scene picture while the SLP uses verbal prompts but no story grammar icons prompts.
6.	The SLP and child listen to the child's recorded narrative while looking at the single complex-scene picture. The SLP places an icon on table when each story grammar element is heard. After listening, SLP and child identify missing story grammar elements and co-tell the story using the same single simple-scene picture and story grammar icon and verbal prompts.
7.	The child retells the story from a single simple-scene picture while the SLP only uses verbal prompts as needed.
8.	The child tells an oiginal narrative using story grammar icons prompts and SLP verbal prompts as needed. Simultaneously, the SLP draws pictures illustrating the narrative.
9.	The child retells the story using these pictures but without story grammar icons prompts and only minimal verbal prompts.
10.	The child retells the narrative without using any visual prompts and only minimal SLP verbal prompts as needed.

Source: Information from Peterson et al. (2010).

Retelling can begin with short stories of a few minutes' length. If the story is longer, the SLP may choose only a segment for retelling. Generalization can be enhanced if the narrative is related to classroom content or to events in the child's life. Pictures can be used to depict elements of the story grammar. With older children, an SLP can explicitly teach the elements of story grammar and use graphic story organizers to help children produce complete episodes. Stories retold many times can be modified by one element that will change the outcome. Commercially available resources include *The Magic of Stories* (Strong & North, 1996), *Narrative Tool Box* (Hutson-Nechkash, 2001), and *Storybuilding: A Guide to Structuring Oral Narratives* (Hutson-Nechkash, 1990).

Narrative telling can be extended in both speech and in writing. If a child is able to retell a story with two or three complete episodes, she or he is probably ready to begin composing original narratives (Naremore, 2001). This can be accomplished within a story context with the SLP supplying the supporting structure initially. Gradually, the SLP supplies fewer episode portions. In each narrative, the child completes the story by supplying the final elements until he or she can compose an entire narrative. The teaching of longer written narratives will be discussed in Chapter 13.

Children then can progress to fictional narratives or their own original stories. The facilitator can use questions to move children to more sophisticated ways of organizing and expressing concepts and relationships. Chapter 12 includes a discussion of replica play and narratives in the classroom.

Narrative discourse is the next logical step. Children should have the opportunity to practice forms of narration within a variety of role-playing situations.

Cohesion

Cohesion comes in many forms *Conjunctive* cohesion is the easiest form to teach. Children's oral narratives can be collected and transcribed into a "book." Use of conjunctions and the relationships expressed can be analyzed. Simple stories containing various clausal relationships also can be read to children. In a retelling, a child usually will not express relationships and conjunctions that he or she does not use in everyday speech.

Once a child's narrative relationships and conjunctions have been analyzed, the SLP can begin to introduce other conjunctions. A developmental order of introduction may be helpful, although the first priority should be conjunctions omitted or used incorrectly in the relationships expressed. For example, in ". . . stoled all his money. He robbed a bank. He was starving . . . ," cause and effect are suggested but without the use of *because*.

The SLP can introduce narrative relationships with or without a conjunction and then, using a question-answer technique, prompt a child to produce the desired conjunction. If the child responds incorrectly, the SLP can reread or retell the relevant portion of the narrative, model a response including the conjunction, discuss the meaning, and prompt the child to respond again. The important aspect of the training is an understanding of the relationship expressed, not a regurgitation of the correct conjunction. The final stages of training would include original narratives produced by the child.

Referential cohesion uses nouns, pronouns, and articles to designate old and new information in the narrative. Questions and answers can be used to direct the child as a narrative is told. Retellings by the SLP might use a fill-in-the-blank technique, in which the child provides the appropriate word. Gradually, less narrative-structured and more expository materials can be introduced. It is more difficult to comprehend and produce cohesion without the narrative frame.

Comprehension

Narrative comprehension can be improved by beginning with predictable narratives concerning everyday events or routines familiar to a child. The child's internalized event script aids both comprehension and recall. As in scripted play, variations in the narrative are introduced gradually, and the text moves to more unfamiliar and fictionalized events and stories. Comprehension and recall can be facilitated by having children draw or write common event sequences.

Before beginning a narrative, an SLP should review it with the child. Help the child bring his or her knowledge to the task. This prenarration task is discussed in detail in Chapter 12.

Data suggest that the use of subjectivity or the character's thoughts and feelings can enhance comprehension of fictional narratives. Children can be taught to focus on a character's reactions as a way of making sense of the events in the narrative. Thus, the child focuses more on the reasons for and outcomes or results of events within the narrative. There are no right or wrong answers; rather, the child's responses explain events in a manner comprehensible to the child.

Semantics

Semantic intervention consists of several different but related levels of intervention involving a variety of interrelated intervention strategies that are much more complex than simply training vocabulary words. At its core, word meaning consists of concepts or knowledge of the world. Semantic training must recognize the importance of these underlying concepts and include cognitive aspects of concept formation.

Inadequate Vocabulary

Meaning is the relationship of a sign or word to the underlying concept. Different strategies are used by different children and by the same child at different developmental times to construct meanings. meanings. Knowing a word's meaning is not the same as being able to construct a definition.

Children with LI often use one strategy exclusively or predominantly. For example, the meanings expressed by some children with ASD seem to be unanalyzed, situationally related "chunks." Children with ID are often deficient in their ability to form complex concepts.

An SLP may assist with the building and extending of individual reference systems by providing situations in which children encounter the physical and social world. Dynamic events seem to encourage early concept development better than do static ones. Therefore, feature learning can be enhanced by focus on movement, contrast, and change. The most successful strategy is to

- build on an experiential or prior knowledge base and establish links to new words.
- teach in meaningful contexts.
- provide multiple exposures.

The experiential base is important, especially for the child below age 7. The child should have the opportunity to have meaningful, real experiences. For example, play in the snow could be followed by a lesson on the words used in the activity. As mentioned previously, repeated input and practice retrieval are beneficial for vocabulary teaching with children, especially those with Down syndrome (Chapman et al., 2006).

World knowledge, or what the child knows about her or his world, is very important for vocabulary growth. Early word meanings are acquired within event-related experiences, especially predictable, everyday routines and their accompanying scripts. Groups of children on a field trip can experience the world by touching, smelling, and even tasting an old log and describing the sensation. Language facilitators can encode features of events and entities to which children attend. Older elementary school children can learn from the experiences of others, much as adults do.

Exposure to storybook reading has been shown to be an effective way for kindergarten children to learn new words, especially those children with poor vocabularies (Justice, Meier, & Walpole, 2005). To be effective, reading should be paired with other word-teaching strategies, such as explaining an unfamiliar word when it occurs in the story, offering synonyms, acting out the word, and pointing to the referent.

Children and adolescents with LI need to learn how to use the context to establish word meaning. Contexts provide a number of cues that can be classified as temporal (time), spatial (location), value (relative worth), stative descriptive (physical description), functional descriptive (use), causal (cause and effect), class membership (type), and equivalence (similarity/difference). Class membership and functional descriptive are the easiest for children, whereas stative descriptive seems to be the most difficult.

Context should be established for the child prior to introducing the word numerous times. A child will need help in determining what he or she knows from the context and repeated exposures in a variety of play or interactive contexts. Novel word learning is enhanced when words receive emphatic stress while being presented within stimulus sentences (Ellis Weismer & Hesketh, 1998). Stress is important given the difficulty children with SLI have in using syntax to acquire vocabulary (Rice, Cleave, & Oetting, 2000). Narratives also may provide a context for introducing a novel word.

In vocabulary training with children with SLI, a mand-elicited imitation (MEI) model is reportedly a better teaching method than focused stimulation alone (Kouri, 2005). In the MEI method, nonverbal cues, such as the presence of toys, and verbal cues, such as "What do you want?" are used to elicit requests from children. If a child does not request an item by name, the SLP can give an imitative prompt.

For children with SLI, different teaching cues seem to affect learning in differing ways (Gray, 2005). For example, semantic cues (*It's made of wood*) foster comprehension, while phonological cues (*It begins with /s/*) aid expression. Because children with poor vocabularies can have difficulty with both the phonological and semantic aspects of words, intervention with both should be explored (Nash & Donaldson, 2005). Overlearning of new words in both expressive and receptive mode seems warranted, especially for children with SLI (Gray, 2003).

Several factors may influence new word learning. For example, children acquire new words more readily if they consist of frequently occurring phonemes in common word locations, if the attached morphology, such as plural *-s*, is not modified between the learning and testing phases, and if the novel word is presented before the referent is shown (Bedore & Leonard, 2000; Storkel, 2001; Storkel & Morrisette, 2002). In general, access paths to words for both TD children and those with LI become strengthened with successful use.

Other factors that can affect word learning include lexical similarity, which seems to speed learning, and semantic similarity, which slows it (Storkel & Adlof, 2009). One measure of lexical similarity is *neighborhood density*, which is the number of words that differ by one phoneme from a given word. TD preschool children tend to learn high-probability/high-density novel words more rapidly than low-probability/low-density novel words (Storkel, 2001, 2003, 2004; Storkel & Maekawa, 2005; Storkel & Rogers, 2000).

Semantic similarity involves the closeness of semantic representations or meanings. Known words that are similar to many semantic representations compete with those similar representations. Among adults, this can lead to poorer performance in recognition or recall of known words with a large set of semantically similar ones (D.L. Nelson & Zhang, 2000).

Many academic terms—the ones children need to succeed in school—such as *evolution* and *triangle*, have low probability and low neighborhood density but few semantic similarities. While we cannot change the word in order to increase neighborhood density, morphological approaches could strengthen understanding of word formation. It is also helpful to teach morphological variations, such as *evolution, evolve*, and *evolving*.

Expressive use and retrieval among 7- to 12-year-olds is positively influenced by a child's greater familiarity with the word. Other factors include greater familiarity with the word's lexical neighbors and surprisingly, given the beneficial learning effects of high density, lower neighborhood density (R.S. Newman & German, 2002).

Four different methods of vocabulary teaching are recommended (Alderete et al., 2004):

- Engaging in interactive book reading
- Direct vocabulary instruction
- Teaching word-learning strategies for using morphological knowledge
- Fostering word consciousness through "playing with language"

In interactive reading, children can be encouraged to immediately talk about objects, characters, and events and also to expand to more nonimmediate talk that goes beyond the text. The child can be taught via levels of abstraction to progress away from the immediate text. Immediate prompts ask children to point to, name, and describe by physical traits. Reordering their perceptual skills, children are asked the meanings of words used in the text, identifying characters and events by less perceptually based descriptions. Finally, children reason in response to questions about why events occurred or why emotions developed. After-reading activities can focus on discussion of words from the text and their meaning in context.

Direct vocabulary instruction should focus on high-frequency words, especially those used in the classroom and essential for academic success. Words can be taught through a variety of methods and across several situations, relating them to other words and building on the initial knowledge a child may possess. Multisensory approaches in which the child both listens to and produces the word will help to form a phonological representation. SLPs should provide examples from other contexts and encourage the child to do likewise.

Word-learning strategies should focus on morphology, teaching root words and various morphological affixes. This intervention can be combined with spelling instruction; etymology, or dividing words to discover their meaning; and sorting words by morphological affixes.

Perhaps the most fun comes in fostering word consciousness, the last of the four strategies. This involves word play, matching synonyms, riddles, art, drama, and poetry. Try this using figurative words and phrases. Children also enjoy creating words that do not exist in the dictionary or giving existing words new definitions. Such original words can be used along with real words to try to encourage children to make educated guesses about the meaning. In a recent conversation, ELL students used the word *skinship*, which they defined as the relationship between family members who touched frequently.

No one likes to give verbatim definitions. It is important to remember that the child may not need a full adult definition when the word is first introduced. The facilitator should not expect dictionary definitions from children below age 12. By that age, however, a TD child should be able to define words, draw conclusions, and make inferences.

The SLP should expose a child to multiple examples of events and things in familiar contexts in order to help the child perceive features of words being used. In class and at home language facilitators can act as mediators, framing, focusing, and providing salient features of experiences for the child.

Within activities, children can be encouraged to describe features. Descriptors then can be used to determine similarities and differences and to label the world. Instead of naming unfamiliar entities such as types of leaves, children can be encouraged to stretch their existing language and give descriptive names, such as *five-pointed leaf tree.*

Facilitators also can target words used frequently at home and school in everyday activities and events. In general, it is easier to learn words for known concepts than to learn both words and concepts at the same time. The choice of which words to teach should be based on the likely frequency of use, typical development, need within the classroom and use in textbooks, and likelihood of the child learning the word from context alone. Even slang expressions might be taught to aid socialization, especially among adolescents.

Training should include words that mean the same (synonyms), sound the same (homonyms), or are opposites (antonyms). This training will help the child organize language for easy storage and retrieval. Common prefixes and suffixes are also important, as is syllabication. A child's existing meanings can be consolidated by building on the child's current vocabulary while correcting errors and misconceptions of meaning.

Training also should proceed from more contextual meanings, as in "hit the ball," to less contextual, more figurative meanings, such as "hit the roof," and multiple meanings, such as "a hit musical."

The facilitator can help the child understand that meaning varies with context. Varying contexts provide for maximum usage and exposure. Storytelling in which a novel word must be used is also a good strategy and uses context to facilitate use.

The semantic features of words can be analyzed to expand the characteristics associated with words and to aid categorization. Words can be classified according to their semantic features, as in

	Transportation	Four-Wheel	Two-Wheel	Engine-Powered	Pedal-Powered	Runs on Rails
Motorcycle	X		X	X		
Bicycle	X		X		X	
Car	X	X		X		
Bus	X	X		X		
Train	X			X		X

	Animals	Bird	On Farm	Wild or Zoo Animal	Gives Milk	Four-Legged
Chicken		X	X			
Duck		X	X			
Cow	X		X		X	X
Elephant	X			X	X	X
Goat	X		X		X	X

FIGURE 11.1 Analyzing semantic feature similarities.

Figure 11.1. Sorting tasks perform a similar function, and children can be encouraged to make their own associations.

A root-word strategy can be used with school-age children to help them discover meanings and their modifications. Suffixes are easier to learn than prefixes and should be introduced first (see Morphology section of this chapter). Prefix training should begin with concrete, easy-to-define prefixes, such as *un-*, and proceed to more abstract ones. The most frequently used prefixes in American English are *un-*, *in-*, *dis-*, and *non-*.

Many commercially available games can be used as is or modified for vocabulary training, including *Boggle*, *Pictionary*, and *Scrabble*. Semantic organizers, such as spidergrams, can be used to build associations. Children can use semantic organizers to "brainstorm" or to tell all they know about a word. Figure 11.2 is a typical spidergram.

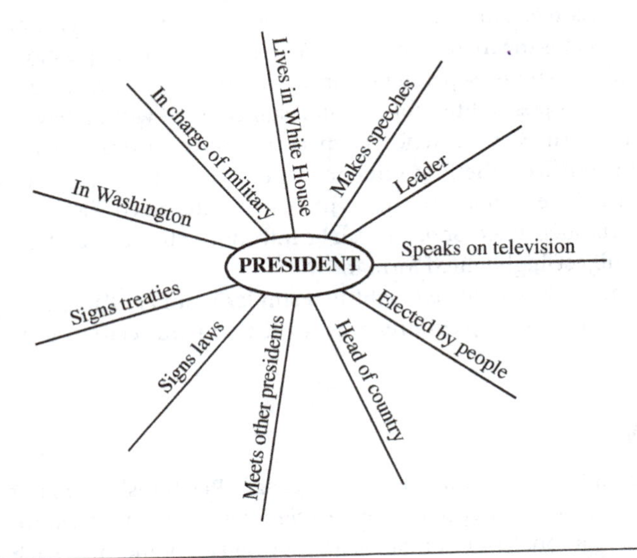

FIGURE 11.2 Spidergram of word meanings and associations.

Semantic Categories and Relational Words

Meanings extend beyond the word level. Words fulfill different semantic roles, such as agent and action, that specify the relationships among those referents. Thus, a child forming a sentence must keep in mind both the referent and the semantic role.

Words and phrases also modify the meaning of basic sentence elements by indicating qualities, such as perceptual attributes (*big, old*), manner (*quickly*), temporal aspects (*first, later*), and relationships between larger sentential units, such as additive (*and*) or causal (*because*). As a listener, the child can only comprehend other people to the extent that she or he understands the various relationships underlying their utterances.

Semantic Classes

An SLP can teach words to children while placing the words in different semantic classes that govern word use. A portion of word definition is the semantic class into which a word can be placed. The best way to teach is through actual use. That's functional! Let's just use one class as an example.

The *agent* is usually found in the subject position of a sentence. English is a subject-prominent language in which a large number of elements are associated with the subject of the sentence. These elements include subject-verb agreement, as with variations of the verb *to be* (*am, is, are*) and the third-person singular, present tense *-s* ending; pronouns; and auxiliary verb-subject inversions in questions. These elements, while important syntactically, are not critical to the content of a sentence, and they can be omitted without greatly affecting the understanding of the sentence. For example, "Mommy eat soup?" gets the general meaning across.

An SLP can teach the concept of *subjecthood* using a functional approach in which he or she teaches the child the purpose of a subject. The function of a sentence's subject, represented by a noun or a noun phrase, is to designate the perspective used in the sentence. If the sentence contains action, the agent designates the actor. Subjects can also be identified by the pronouns used with them.

The SLP can train children to identify the subject by using the following forms:

- Subjective: ***He*** *is running*
- Objective: ***Him****, he is running*

The first is taught in conversational response to a "Which one is . . . ?" type of question, and the second in response to a "What is the man doing?" or "Who is . . . ?" type of question. Children can deduce the function of the subject and its separateness from the topic by the varying contexts in which they are used. There are endless possibilities for teaching subjecthood within play and conversation.

Children can learn each sentence form in response to questions within ongoing activities. Training should begin with the first sentence type because it is included within the second. Once children have learned the formats, the questions can be alternated. Later, the habitual or simple present form of the verb, such as *eat* or *drink*, can be introduced to teach children subject-verb agreement within the same subject-highlighted format.

Other semantic classes may be taught in a similar manner. Table 11.5 presents suggestions for training. Question cues can help children identity the semantic class of different words within a variety of activities.

Relational Words

Relational words fulfill many functions in language. Relationships may be based on quantity or quality and may be general or specific. Other relational words are used to mark location and time. Conjunctions are relational words that relate one clause to another. Each type of relational word requires specific intervention considerations.

TABLE 11.5 Suggestions for Training Semantic Classes

Instrument
Initially, this class can be trained in the final position of the sentence, preceded by the word *by*, as in "The wood was split *by his axe*." Position and the preposition *by* act as signals for this class. This class can also be signaled by the verb use, as in "John *used the rake* to gather the leaves." This sentence type can be prompted by questions such as "How did. . . ?" and "What did John use to. . . ?"
Patient/Object
This class may be taught initially by using the final position in the sentence as a direct object to transitive verbs. Question prompts such as "What did Carol throw?" may be used to elicit this class. It is somewhat more difficult to teach this class in the subject position because that position is usually occupied by an agent. If agents are taught in response to a *who* type of question, patients might use *what*, as in "What grew in the park?"
Dative
The dative class is most frequently and obviously used as an indirect object. This function can be clearly signaled initially by use of the prepositions *to* and *for*. Question prompts can include these cues and the word *whom*, as in "For whom did Mary buy the flowers?"
Temporal, Locative, and Manner
These classes are relatively easy to teach because each has specific questions that prompt usage. Prepositions, such as *in, on,* and *at*, are used with these functions, as are *to, with,* and *by*, which are used to mark other semantic class use.
Accompaniment
The final position in the sentence and the preposition *with* should be used in training to signal this class. A *with whom* question prompt can be used to elicit response.

In general, relational terms can be acquired through descriptive tasks, in which a child must differentiate between one entity and another, or through narrative tasks, in which a child must aid the listener to differentiate characters. An SLP can help the child initially by keeping the task context-bound and by controlling the number of items or characters. By playing dumb or acting confused, the facilitator can help the child provide additional or essential information. Narratives are also effective vehicles for acquiring conjunctions, especially when the facilitator synthesizes larger, more conceptually complex sentences based on those of the child.

Quantitative Terms. A child does not need to be able to count to learn quantitative terms. Initial training can begin with the concepts of *one* and *more than one*. The second concept can be marked variously by *many, much, some*, and *more*. Such terms as *these* and *those* should be introduced with some caution because of deixis, or interpretation from the perspective of the speaker.

The distinction between *many* and *much* is complex and should not be introduced with children functioning at a preschool level. In general, *many* is used with regular and irregular plural nouns, such as *cats, shoes*, and *women*. In contrast, *much* is used with mass nouns—nouns that refer to homogeneous, nonindividual substances, such as *water, sand*, and *sugar*.

Later quantifiers can include words such as *few* and *couple*. These can be followed by other quantifiers, such as *nearly, almost as much as*, and *half*. Table 11.6 presents common quantitative words. The ordering of these words in the noun phrase is very important and is discussed in the syntax section of this chapter. The use of numerical terms and fractions and percentages must wait until school-age and requires some mathematical skill.

Quantitative terms can be taught within many naturally occurring situations, using anything from counting blocks and Legos to candy and treats. Books and many fingerplays also contain counting.

TABLE 11.6 Common Quantitative and Qualitative Terms

Quantitative	Qualitative
One, two, three, four . . .	Big, little, long, short
Many, much, lots of	Large, small, fat, thin
Some, few, couple	Soft, hard, heavy, light
More, another	Same, different, alike
Nearly, almost all	Old, young, pretty, ugly
As much/little as	Blue, green, red. . . .
Plenty	Hot, cold, warm, chilly
Half, one-fourth, two-fifths	Wide, narrow
10%, 75%	Sweet, sour
Units of measure: inch, foot, mile, cup, pint, quart, gallon, centimeter, meter, kilometer, liter, ounce, pound, gram, kilogram, acre	Nice, mean, funny, sad
	Fast, slow
	Smooth, rough
	Clean, dirty
	Empty, full
	Angry, afraid
	Comparative and superlative relationships: *-er*, *-est*, as *x* as, *x-er* than

Narratives can contain several characters or objects that can be grouped in various ways throughout the story, using words such as *both, only one,* and *all three.* It is also easy to create situations in which children request a number of objects, as in response to "How many do you want?" Quantitative terms also naturally occur within any play that replicates commerce, such as a fast food restaurant or market.

Qualitative Terms. Qualitative terms include such words as *big* and *tall,* plus *bigger* and *tallest,* which use the *-er* and *-est* morphological markers, and such phrases as *as big as, not as wet as, smaller than,* and the like. Table 11.6 presents common qualitative terms. In general, children learn to use the comparative *-er* before the superlative *-est,* and training should follow that pattern. It is best to begin with the regular use of these two markers before introducing exceptions, such as *better* and *best.* Words can be expanded into phrases, for example, from *bigger* to *bigger than.*

Children seem to acquire concepts one semantic feature at a time. A corollary to this hypothesis is that broad, nonspecific concepts (e.g., *big*) are learned before more specific concepts (e.g., *long*). In this example, *big* refers to overall size, whereas *long* refers to size only in the horizontal plane.

The SLP should introduce terms and relationships in the order in which comparative terms develop. Table 11.7 includes common pairs of comparative terms and the approximate age at which most children can use them correctly.

In general, conceptual word pairs are acquired asymmetrically. Children ages 3 to 7 appear to learn the positive member of conceptual pairs, the one that represents more of the dimension characterized by the pair, prior to learning the negative member (Bracken, 1988). For example, *big* and *little* are opposite poles of the dimension *size. Big* represents more size and is, therefore, the positive member. These data suggest that positive members should be taught first to children with LI.

Many play situations and narratives include qualitative terms. It is also easy to devise conversations in which children must contrast one thing with another. By acting confused and asking "Which one?" a facilitator can elicit responses such as "The big one" or "The green fuzzy one." Within several situations, such as play or snack, children can be offered choices based on some contrasting feature, such as size or color.

TABLE 11.7 Common Comparative Word-Pairs

Positive-Negative (age)	Positive-Negative (age)	Positive-Negative (age)
same-different (36–60 months)	inside-outside	high-low (42–60 months)
in front of-behind (48–54 months)	over-under (42–48 months)	forward-backward
into-out of	front-back (48–52 months)	happy-sad
top-bottom (48–54 months)	above-below (66–72 months)	old-young
rising-falling	right-wrong	large-small (78–84 months)
healthy-sick	heavy-light (30–48 months)	long-short (horizontal) (54–60 months)
big-little (30–48 months)	tall-short (30–84 months)	hot-cold
deep-shallow	loud-quiet	dark-light
thick-thin	sharp-dull	tight-loose
hard-soft (30–42 months)	solid-liquid	a lot-a little
smooth-rough	full-empty (36–48 months)	fast-slow
more-less (42–72 months)	with-without (48–54 months)	early-late
all-none	arriving-leaving	always-never
old-new	first-last (60–66 months)	
before-after (66–72 months)	on-off (24–36 months)	
open-close	up-down (36–60 months)	

Note: The order represents when each member is learned respectively, i.e., *high* at 42 months and *low* at 60 months.
Source: Information from Bracken (1988); Edmonston & Thane (1990); Wiig & Semel (1984).

Spatial and Temporal Terms. Several words are used to mark both space or location and time and, thus, are potentially confusing. Among the most commonly used words in English are prepositions, such as *in, on, at,* and *by*. In the Syntax section of this chapter I discuss prepositional phrase training. Other terms, such as *first* and *last*, also note place and time.

Spatial concepts are best taught first in relation to the child; then with "featured" or fronted objects, such as a video screen, and finally with nonfeatured objects, such as a wastebasket or a ball. The latter is more difficult to learn because it involves deixis, or interpretation based on the speaker. In general, vertical dimensions (*on top*) are learned before horizontal. Horizontal front and back terms, such as *in front of* and *behind*, are learned before horizontal side-to-side terms, such as *beside* and *next to*. The order reflects the underlying concepts. Terms that denote order, such as *before, after, first*, and *last*, usually are learned before terms for simultaneity, such *as at the same time, during*, and *when*. Duration terms, such as *a long time*, generally are acquired last.

In general, it is better to begin with concrete definitions and progress to more abstract ones. For example, with *first, last, before*, and *after*, training can begin with objects in a line or with a train. The facilitator can have the child touch individual train cars ("which car is first?") then a short sequence of objects (*first, last*) and finally a reverse sequence. Sequenced objects should be used before sequenced events and the concept of time sequencing.

The greater the number of contexts, the more learning and generalization that will occur. Language can be used to help a child organize the environment by marking experiences of space and time. Table 11.8 includes common spatial and temporal terms.

The SLP can use direction-following games and activities to train children about space and time. It might be best to begin with routines that the child knows, such as those that occur at home or in the classroom, and then move into less familiar activities, such as using an ATM, in which the child must rely more on linguistic input rather than physical memory. Activities involving making or cooking are excellent sequential tasks.

Later, the SLP can use sequenced pictures or storytelling in the training. Children can identify what happened first, next, and last.

TABLE 11.8 Common Spatial and Temporal Terms

Spatial			Temporal		
next to	under	in front of	next	today	days
before	over	behind	before	tomorrow	weeks
after	below	beside	after	calendar dates	hours
on, on top	corner	right	in, to	months	minutes
in, into	bottom	left	soon	seasons	through
in between	inside	through	later	numerals for years	away from
between	outside	high, tall	now	morning	toward
middle	side	upside down	above	afternoon	sometimes
above	end	together	yesterday	evening	

Deixis and the use of deictic terms are very difficult concepts to teach. The facilitator who takes both the role of speaker and prompter for a child violates the roles in a conversation. The simple example of *here* and *there* is illustrative. The request "Put the ball *here*" is said from the speaker's perspective. To the listener, the speaker's *here* is most likely *there*. If the speaker then shifts to the listener's (the child's) perspective and says, "Yes, put it *there*," it may confuse the child further. How can it be both here and there for the speaker?

When training the child about deictic terms, it is best to sit next to the child so that you both can share a perspective. From this shared perspective, deictic terms for location would be similar. Another facilitator, puppet, or prerecorded tape may act as the other conversational partner. The teaching of deixis is discussed also under the topic of pronouns in the Syntax section of this chapter.

Conjunctions. An SLP can teach conjunctions by noting the relationships expressed in each. For example, *because* represents cause and effect and may not be fully acquired until about age 12. Table 11.9 presents the general order of conjunction acquisition. The conjunction *and* can first be taught to combine entities, as in "cats *and* dogs." In a cooking activity, the facilitator might say, "Which two types of cookies do you like best?" or, "Tell me your two favorite types of cookies." In similar fashion, *but* can be used for like/dislike distinctions ("I like cookies, *but not beets.*").

A *clause + conjunction + clause* format can be employed initially to help the child acquire the underlying relationship. For example, sentences might be presented as follows:

We wear a coat *because* it is cold.
We wear a coat *if* it is cold.
We wear a coat *when* it is cold.

Once a child understands these relationships, the order of the clauses can be reversed, as in "Because it is cold, we wear a coat." These specific sentences can accompany dress-up play.

Next, the SLP can present clauses for the child to combine. The breakdown and buildup technique, described in Chapter 10, may be used to help the child identify clauses and conjunctions and then reconstruct the sentence. This can be accomplished conversationally.

TABLE 11.9 A Rough Acquisition Order for English Conjunctions

and, and then	but, or, because, so, if when	until, before, after	although, while, as	unless, therefore, however

Conjoining clauses with conjunctions is a natural occurrence within narratives and can be prompted through storybook retelling or with pictures. The SLP can reply to a child's utterance by supplying the desired conjunction and then asking for a restatement as in the following:

Child: And the whole bridge fell down.
Adult: Why? Because . . .
Child: 'Cause the water was going so fast.
Adult: That sounds very exciting, but I'm not sure I understand the whole thing. The bridge . . .
Child: The bridge fell down because the water was going fast.
Adult: The bridge fell down because the water was going fast. That's really scary. What happened next?

Word Retrieval and Categorization

Word-finding difficulties can result from two possible sources. The first is lack of elaboration or lack of a well-established, thorough representation of the word within the child's internal dictionary, or lexicon. Children who exhibit difficulties often have less extensive vocabularies and poor word knowledge.

The second source of problems is in retrieval. Although many elaboration difficulties occur alone, retrieval problems usually do not and may be an additional difficulty found in some children with elaborative problems.

Children with word retrieval problems appear to benefit from both elaboration and retrieval activities. Word-finding activities can be incorporated easily into a number of everyday activities and conversations about these activities.

Prior to beginning intervention, it is important to determine the source of the problem. An SLP should derive naming data from a variety of activities to be certain of the cause of the problem. In general, children name real objects and colored pictures with a higher accuracy than black-and-white pictures (Barrow, Holbert, & Rastatter, 2000). Naming words in a meaningful context is also performance enhancing.

Children with storage problems have difficulty understanding and retrieving words that are not stable in their memory. Inadequate storage is the result of shallow meanings, reference-shifting problems, and poor analytical and synthesizing skills. The goal of intervention for storage difficulties is to improve word knowledge and storage.

Those with retrieval-only problems have difficulty with search and recovery. Somewhere in the process of discriminating the desired word from among competing words and constructing the phonological specifications for production, the process breaks down. The goal of intervention for retrieval is improved access.

Memory storage seems to be affected by the depth or level of processing. In general, recall is best for words processed at the deepest levels. Acoustic processing, such as rhyming, is surface processing; categorical is mid-level; and semantic/syntactic is deep.

Words are remembered in relation to other words and form meaning networks. When one member of the meaning family is accessed, it activates others. In other words, *ride* might elicit ***drive*** or ***pedal*** but not elicit ***stride***, a phonological variation. Likewise, *cad* might elicit *villain* but not ***cadet***.

Networks of semantic-related morphemes are also part of each individual's memory system. Thus, *stain, stained glass*, and *stainless steel* are perceived to be related.

Elaboration training focuses on organization of the child's lexicon and generalization of word meanings to everyday use. In elaboration training, an SLP can use semantic focus strategies, such as nonidentical examples and word comparison tasks. Nonidentical examples of the word in several linguistic contexts enrich a child's definition and word associations. Examples for *house* might include *dollhouse, housefly*, and *greenhouse*. In comparative tasks, the SLP expects the child to identify similarities and differences between two words with related meanings, such as *house* and *hotel*.

A mnemonic or "key word" strategy also might be used to aid elaboration and recall of new vocabulary. New words are linked with acoustically or visually similar words with which the child is familiar. For example, *dogged* might be linked with *dog*. This initial linkage is gradually modified by the child through use to a semantic strategy with deeper processing.

Pictures and written descriptions may be used to link two words. A known word is used to aid learning and storage of an unknown one. In the above example, a *dog* would be portrayed being stubborn or determined (dogged). Under the picture, it might read *The* ***dog*** was ***dogged*** *and would not give up*. Note also that the definition of *dogged* has been included. Other examples are given in Figure 11.3. The key word now becomes the retrieval cue.

Children using this approach reportedly are able to recall 50 percent more definitions than those taught vocabulary by a more traditional method. In addition, the combined picture and sentence format appears to be more effective than either used separately.

Children seem naturally to enjoy word games and word play, and these teaching strategies can be incorporated into many types of activities. As a communication partner, I like to get very "confused" and use words in silly ways. Children laugh and freely correct their somewhat slow-witted communication partner.

Data from TD children suggests that taxonomic or categorical relations, such as things to write with (crayon, marker, pencil), and thematic or event relations, such as the act of writing (paper, pencil), develop differently and can affect word recall (Hashimoto, McGregor, & Graham, 2007). In addition, taxonomic relationships are originally based by children on observable perceptual features (shape, size). For preschool and kindergarten children thematic cues might assist word recall. Taxonomic cues with school-age children should begin with obvious perceptual similarities.

Retrieval training may include categorization tasks, such as naming members of a category or identifying the category when given the members. Categories include animals, clothing, grocery items, and the like that can easily be introduced into functional methods. For example, "I heard you were going on a class trip. What will you put (clothing) in your suitcase?"

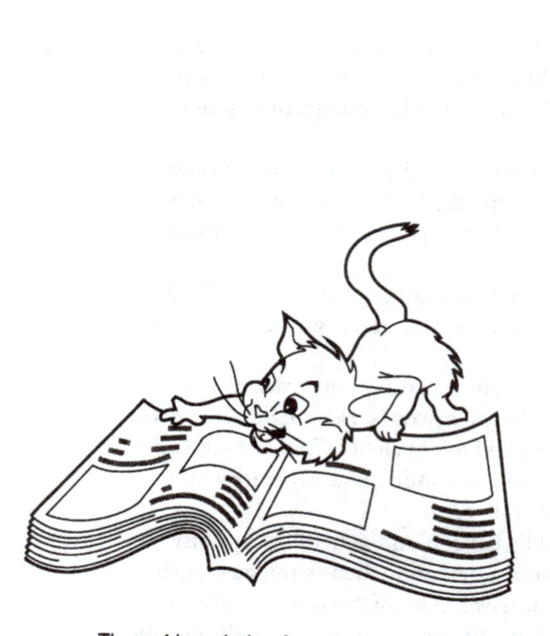

The **cat** is ordering from the **catalog.**

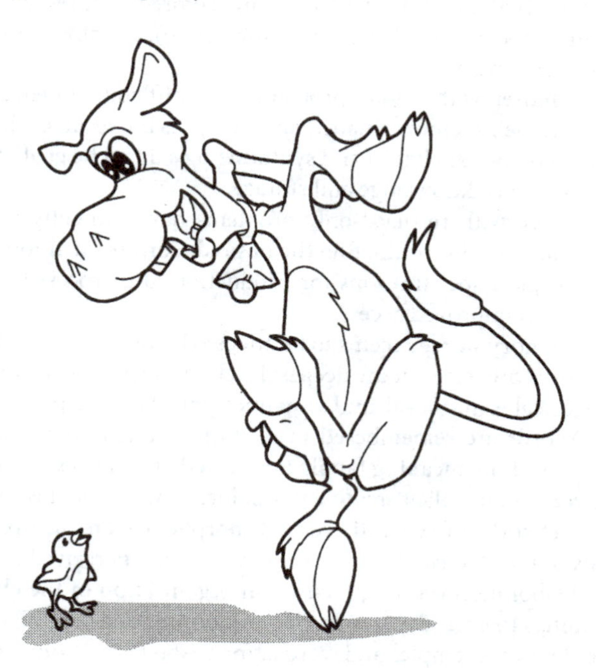

The **cow** is a frightened **coward.**

FIGURE 11.3 Examples of mnemonic strategies.

As a group, children with LI are less likely than children developing typically to discover semantic organization strategies on their own and usually require more examples to determine a basis for organization and for generalization of organizational skill. Word-substitution errors should demonstrate the predominant organizational framework of the child and alert the SLP to the patterns that need strengthening.

Categorization tasks, especially such familiar ones as Saturday morning cartoon shows, in which the child names members of the category, facilitate recall by building associational and categorical linkages between words. Of course, the possibility still exists that a child will access the right category but retrieve the wrong member.

Categorization tasks can be elaborative in nature when members of more than one category are presented together. For example, the items *chair, bed,* and *table* can be classified as furniture; *chair, swing,* and *bicycle* are things on which you sit; and *bicycle, car,* and *bus* are vehicles. The facilitator could present these items together and ask the child to classify them in as many ways as possible.

Training might begin with actual objects and children making piles of objects that go together (Parente & Hermann, 1996). As a child, I sorted my comic books by main character and my baseball cards by team. Similar tasks are found in several everyday activities. After objects and pictures, then words can be used. Entities might be classified by description (e.g., cold) or by function (e.g., things that you ride on). The facilitator should encourage the child to use as many different sensory descriptions as possible.

After a sorting task, a child can be asked to recall the categories. Once the child has recalled categories, he or she can be asked to recall members. Everyday tasks such as preparing grocery lists, organizing chores, or planning items to take on vacation or items that go in your backpack or your room have more relevance than arbitrary groupings.

Verbal training should begin with common words for everyday concrete objects. Familiar everyday objects and events should be used. I am reminded of a teacher who tried to teach zoo and farm animal categories but found the children very unresponsive. Both categories were outside their realm of everyday experience. When one child suggested the category of animals seen "squashed" on the highway, every child became a participant. Although the example is somewhat gruesome, the lesson for SLPs is very practical. Everyday natural environments, the ones functional intervention tries to use, provide specific cues that aid memory.

Word-retrieval difficulties can be helped by (a) naming/descriptive tasks ("It's a bicycle; you ride on it by peddling"), (b) associational activities ("Red, white, and ______"), and (c) sentential elaboration tasks based on syntactic characteristics of two words drawn at random ("The *trailer* was parked near the *restaurant* while the driver ate") and open-ended fill-ins and completions ("We eat with a ______") that involve deeper levels of processing. Word-sorting tasks can aid in the development of categorization and recall skills. Taxonomy charts, especially for newly introduced classroom content, also can help children develop categorization strategies.

With some children, a combination of phonological and perceptual strategies may also be effective, although semantic elaboration and retrieval activities produce better results than phonological strategies alone. In phonological training, the child participates in segmentation exercises such as rhyming, initial sound matching, and counting syllables and phonemes. The rationale for this method is that, in part, breakdown is the result of poor phonological representation of the word. Phonologically based treatment that focuses on words that begin with the same phoneme and words that sound alike can reduce semantic substitutions. Perceptual strategies involve imagery activities, such as simultaneous picture and auditory exposure, visualization with eyes closed, and silent name repetition.

The SLP can help a child note features and attributes that determine how members are categorized. One mediational strategy might be to teach the child to ask a set of questions to establish an association between a new item and something familiar. Questions might include the following (Parente & Hermann, 1996, p. 50):

What does it look (sound, smell, taste) like?

What does it mean the same thing as?

What groups does it belong to?

Who is it commonly associated with?

It is important that children note a similar attribute on more than one object. Otherwise, children may begin to associate certain attributes with specific items. For example, several very different objects may be described as *wet*. This kind of task naturally leads to categorization. Attributes should appear also in many different linguistic forms, rather than just "It's . . . " in order to enhance storage and memory.

Categorical identification seems to be the best cue for recall when a child is stuck or blocks on a word. By naming the category, the facilitator can help the child locate the desired word more easily. Other strategies include partial word cues, sentence completion, and nonverbal, gestural cues. Additional retrieval strategies are listed in Table 11.10. In intervention, retrieval units should move from single words to longer units.

The relationship between responses to drill-like naming exercises and word finding in conversation is unknown. At a minimum, therefore, it is essential that training include a strong conversational element to ensure generalization of word-finding skills.

Comprehension

Language comprehension consists of a complex set of processes, including (Linderholm et al., 2000)

- encoding of facts.
- activation of knowledge.
- generation of inferences.

Inferencing connects information in ways that make that information understandable and memorable. Comprehension difficulties occur when children have difficulty remembering what they

TABLE 11.10 Word-Retrieval Strategies

Retrieval Strategy	Description
Attribute cue	Attribute of the word or meaning is presented. Types: Phonemic: Initial phoneme, vowel nucleus or syllable is presented, as in *It begins with /b/.* Semantic: Category name or function is presented, *boat* for *canoe* or *mixes* for *blender.* Visual: Picture or revisualization is presented. Gestural: Motor scheme is presented as in miming shoveling.
Associated cue	A word typically associated with the word is presented, such as *hiking* for *boot* or *orange* for *juice.*
Semantic alternative	Another word with a similar meaning is presented. Types: Synonym or category substitution: A synonym other category members are presented, such as *afraid* to elicit *frightened* or *goats, cows, and horses* to elicit *pigs* Multiword substitution or description is presented as in *It lives on a farm* or *You cut your hair with them*
Reflective pause	Child is reminded to pause and think in order to reduce competitive responses

Source: Information from German (1992).

have heard or read, applying their world knowledge to what they heard or read, or focusing on the important ideas and concepts presented (Kibby, Marks, Morgan, & Long, 2004).

The goal of intervention is to teach the child to retrieve relevant word and world knowledge as a comprehension aid and to help the child decide how and what to remember from what he or she hears or reads. Comprehension and memory are aided by familiar, meaningful contexts. The degree and type of experience the child has with events strongly shapes his or her expectations and, thus, comprehension. Language within familiar play and role-play of everyday events can enhance comprehension.

The level of involvement also affects memory and comprehension. The more involved a child is, the more he or she comprehends and recalls. Song lyrics, nursery rhymes, and finger play occur regularly in school classrooms and can be used to help a child make active associations between words and the nonlinguistic context. Repetitions aid comprehension.

Finally, comprehension intervention should be pleasurable. Fun activities keep children engaged, a necessity for comprehension and comprehension training.

Initial comprehension training may need to be very concrete and highly contextual. Preschool children benefit more from activities with more immediate recall versus narrative recall. The use of gestures and a slower rate of talking by the SLP also enhances comprehension by young children and children with SLI (Montgomery, 2005). As children approach school age, training should become more decontextualized, similar to many of the literate activities found in school.

Comprehension training might begin with recall from pictures or objects and progress to literal recall of one or more details from verbal sources. Gradually, an SLP can require a child to recall more details. Later, the child can detail these in sequence, possibly using sequential pictures, photographs of past events, or comic books as aids. Daily events can provide a script to aid comprehension. Next, the SLP can require the child to relate cause and effect from familiar or recently read narratives. Once able to reconstruct these relationships, the child can begin to make inferences, to draw conclusions, and to predict outcomes from stories, riddles, and jokes. Finally, the child can learn to synthesize information and create subjective summaries of the meanings of narratives, TV shows, or movies.

To assist comprehension, you can shape question-response strategies by manipulating the semantic content, question complexity, context, and function. The therapy process moves from simple, context-embedded yes/no questions to the use of questions in more abstract contexts, while controlling the length of the questions to highlight semantic content.

In the second stage, early-developing *wh-* question forms might become the targets, with yes/no questions used to highlight the semantic content desired. Take, for example, the question, "What is the girl wearing on her head?" A nonresponse, an inappropriate response, or an inaccurate response might be followed by "Is she wearing a shoe on her head?" If the child responds negatively, the prompt would be "That's right, what is she wearing on her head?" Print, pictures, or signs can be used to highlight the *wh-* words and, thus, emphasize the information desired. These prompts can be faded gradually.

In the third stage, new *wh-* forms are added systematically. Developmental data suggests a logical order for teaching *wh-* words and question types based on concept learning. Initial *wh-* words, concerned with things (objects), persons (agents), possession, and locations, include *what, who, whose*, and *where* respectively. Soon children learn distinctions between things, as expressed in the word *which*. Around age 4, they become aware of sequence, time, and causality, or the *wh-* words and questions *how, when*, and *why* respectively. In stimulus content is shifted gradually from concrete, predictable, factually based academic topics to more abstract, less predictable conversational ones.

School-age children might manipulate objects or pictures and match them with the sentences heard. Similarly, the child might select a picture described by the facilitator from among a set of pictures. Written cues also could be used.

Figurative Language

Figurative language consists of idioms, metaphors, similes, and proverbs. Idioms are a form of figurative language that is particularly troublesome to comprehend for school-age children with LI and for children from CLD backgrounds. The most common error is literal interpretation. Children with

LI may lack a strategy for determining meaning. Some common high- and low-familiarity idioms are listed in Table 11.11.

Intervention should begin with comprehension of transparent or easily decipherable idioms. Narratives may be the best teaching milieu because of the contextual support. The child can be instructed prior to the narrative that it will contain a certain idiom and that he or she will be able to

TABLE 11.11 Common American English Idioms

Animals		
A bull in a china shop	Playing possum	Clinging like a leech
As stubborn as a mule	Go into one's shell	Grinning like a Cheshire cat
Going to the dogs	A fly in the ointment	Thrown to the wolves
Body Parts		
On the tip of my tongue	Put their heads together*	Put your best foot forward
Raise eyebrows	Vote with one's feet	Turn heads
Turn the other cheek	Breathe down one's neck*	Put one's foot down*
		Lead with one's chin
Clothing		
Dressed to kill	Wear the pants in the family	Strait-laced
Hot under the collar	Fit like a glove	Talk through one's hat
Colors		
Grey area	Tickled pink	Red letter day
Once in a blue moon	Has a yellow streak	True blue
Foods		
Eat crow	That takes the cake	In a jam
Humble pie	A finger in every pie	Put all your eggs in one basket
Games and Sports		
Ace up my sleeve	Paddle your own canoe	Get to first base
Cards are stacked against me	Rise to the bait	Keep the ball rolling
Got lost in the shuffle	Skate on thin ice*	On the rebound
Keep your head above water	Ballpark figure	Go around in circles*
		Cross swords
Plants		
Heard it through the grapevine	Beat around the bush*	Shaking like a leaf
Resting on his laurels	No bed of roses	Withered on the vine
		Hoe one's own row
Vehicles		
Fix your wagon	On the wagon	Missed the boat
Like ships passing in the night	Don't rock the boat	Take a back seat
Tools, Work, and School		
Bury the hatchet	Throw a monkey wrench into it	Hit the roof
Has an axe to grind	Read between the lines*	Nursing his wounds
Hit the nail on the head	Doctor the books	Sober as a judge
Jockey for position	Has a screw loose	
Weather		
Calm before the storm	Steal her thunder	Right as rain
Haven't the foggiest	Come rain or shine	Throw caution to the wind

*Highly familiar

figure out the meaning from the story. Questions can be used throughout the narrative to help the child attend to important information. After repeated exposure and the child's correct interpretation, he or she can be encouraged to invent his or her own narratives that illustrate use of the idiom. Finally, conversationally appropriate use can be discussed and role-played.

Proverbs depend on context. The context in which the proverb is used facilitates understanding. In general, concrete proverbs are easier to interpret than abstract, and familiar easier than unfamiliar.

The ability to interpret and use proverbs develops during late elementary school and continues into adulthood and is related to reading and metalinguistic abilities. With this in mind, an SLP is advised to teach proverb interpretation within the context of reading (Nippold, 2000). Working in small groups, adolescents can discuss interpretations. The SLP can use contextual cues, questions, and analysis, to help teens become independent learners. Through both asking and answering factual and inferential questions, adolescents learn to interpret the context. Analysis of the main characters' motivations, goals, actions, and feelings further aid interpretation. Finally, adolescents need help determining the relationship between the proverb and their own lives.

Verbal Working Memory

Although the depth and breadth of this topic is beyond the scope of this text and the topic fits only loosely—if at all—under semantics and comprehension, I would be remiss were I not to mention verbal working memory given the deficits mentioned in Chapter 2, especially for children with SLI.

Unfortunately, there is not a great deal of research on effective methods for teaching working memory (WM) skills with children with LI. That said, a critical component of successful intervention is placing significant storage and processing demands on WM and then systematically increasing or decreasing demands based on a child's performance (Boudreau & Costanza-Smith, 2011).

Given the academic difficulties of children with WM deficits, it seems wise to intervene with children in two ways. First, the SLP can train WM abilities directly. Second, the SLP in collaboration with classroom teachers can identify WM demands in the classroom that impact a child's academic performance and then modify the classroom environment to support each child. Let's discuss intervention in that order. See both Montgomery and colleagues (2010) and Boudreau and Costanza-Smith (2011) for more specifics than we have space to discuss here.

The focus of intervention for children with SLI and WM deficits should focus on remediating weak cognitive processing and promoting stronger language abilities and should be grounded in the principles of evidence-based practice (EBP). Inclusion of intervention for cognitive processes is warranted for several reasons (Montgomery et al., 2010).

- The response of children with SLI to language-only intervention is inconsistent (Bishop, Adams, & Rosen, 2006; Ebbels, 2007; Law et al., 2004).
- The psychological literature supports the use of memory training with students with SLI (S. Gillam & Gillam, 2006).
- The suggestion by some SLI researchers that failure to consider cognitive processing in students with SLI leads to poor language intervention outcomes (Bishop et al., 2006; Gathercole & Alloway, 2006).

SLPs can address child-specific variables that will allow a child to manage his or her WM skills and available resources more effectively.

SLPs and teachers can support children with poor WM skills by first helping them develop awareness of their WM limitations. A child who is aware of his or her difficulties can reflect on the demands inherent in a situation, the skills he or she brings to a task, and the strategies needed to ensure success.

A child also needs the metacognitive skills to compensate or make adjustments for WM limitations. Studies with TD children suggest that as they mature and WM demands increase, children become more efficient at selection and use of processing strategies. For a child with WM deficits, this requires teaching a child, especially as he or she gets older and education tasks increase in complexity, to analyze a learning situation and then select appropriate strategies for successful task completion. Although children with LI are less likely than their TD peers to use memory strategies, they can be taught to manage these limited resources more efficiently (Minear & Shah, 2006; Swanson, Kehler, & Jerman, 2010). Table 11.12 presents some strategies to improve the academic success of children with SLI and/or WM difficulties (Boudreau & Costanza-Smith, 2011).

In the following section, we'll quickly discuss intervention in three areas: phonological short-term memory (PSTM), working memory capacity, and automaticity and rate.

PSTM. Interestingly, improving phonological memory seems to improve WM abilities overall as well as language. Rehearsal of repeating phonological forms that are unfamiliar may assist a child in perceiving the essentials of the phonological structure of language. Enhancing the efficiency of phonological encoding may improve the retention and the quality of phonological information in WM, as well as potentially improving reading ability (Maridaki-Kassotaki, 2002; Minear & Shah, 2006).

Phonological memory may also be improved through training of other phonological processes as well (O'Shaughnessy & Swanson, 2000). For example, intervention focused on rhyme and phoneme awareness improves phonological awareness skills as well as fostering significant improvement on new word recognition tasks.

Direct intervention with reading and writing interventions can also improve phonological memory skills. For example, phonological spelling intervention, explained in Chapter 13, including specific training with syllable and phoneme segmentation of unfamiliar words as well as phoneme-grapheme relationships, can result in children's improved ability to spell, repeat, and read pseudowords (Berninger, Winn, et al., 2008).

WM Capacity. There is emerging evidence that training can lead to increases in WM capacity and in fluid intelligence in adults and children. In addition, WM capacity training can also increase reading comprehension accuracy, nonverbal reasoning, attention, and reading speed in young elementary

TABLE 11.12 Techniques to Use for Working Memory Intervention

Technique	Explanation
Rehearsal	Explicit training and rehearsal training can enhance the STM storage and recall of children with SLI and other language impairments (Gill, Klecan-Aker, Roberts, & Fredenburg, 2003; Loomes, Rasmussen, Pei, Manji, & Andrew, 2008). Older children and adolescents with SLI and/or WM deficits can be taught to rehearse information that is critical to a task. This, in turn, reduces WM demands. Memory strategies, such as systematically chunking words or information together, also make the information easier to remember (Minear & Shah, 2006).
Task analysis	Children can be taught to identify the current goal of a task and helped to systematically identify appropriate strategies.
Visualization	Using key words to organize verbal information into a visual representation can improve our ability to follow instructions and to remember complex information (Gill et al., 2003; Hood & Rankin, 2005). Visual representations constrain the amount and complexity of the information, reducing the amount of cognitive resources required (Alloway et al., 2009).
Study and organizational	Children with WM difficulties often struggle with organizing information. Organization and study skills might include visual or key word cues to represent steps in a process or instructions to follow.

Source: Information from Boudreau and Costanza-Smith (2011).

school children, although none of these studies have directly targeted children with SLI (Klingberg et al., 2005; Loosli, Buschkuehl, Perrig, & Jaeggi, 2008; Thorell, Lindqvist, Nutley, Bohlin, & Klingberg, 2009).

The purpose of WM capacity intervention is not just to help children with SLI enhance their WM capacity but also to allow them to better manage the dual demands of information processing and storage during language-related activities. It may be best to begin intervention with visuospatial WM training, given that children with SLI seem to struggle with verbal storage more than visuospatial storage (Archibald & Gathercole, 2006c, 2007). Visual stimuli might enable a child to learn to manage WM resources under more storage-friendly conditions (Montgomery et al., 2010). Once a child demonstrates good responses under these conditions, intervention could switch to auditory stimuli.

Several computerized training programs, such as *Cogmed Working Memory Training* (www.neurodevelopmentcenter.com/index.php?id=128), *Fast ForWord Language* (Scientific Learning Corporation, 1998), and *Soak Your Brain* (www.soakyourhead.com), are available. In general, these programs require a child to complete a task while remembering rules, such as responding whenever a certain letter appears. Even at the verbal level, an SLP might find it advantageous to combine verbal and visual input to help a child manage the demands of cross-modal information processing and storage common to academic learning.

Although computerized programs are effective in producing gains in general language abilities and WM, traditional interventions seem equally effective, indicating that lower tech, lower-priced interventions can yield comparable gains (Cohen et al., 2005; R. Gillam, Frome Loeb, et al., 2008). Computerized programs alone, without direct SLP input, are less effective than a combination of both methods.

Automaticity and Rate. The SLP can help a child decrease WM demands by making some components of a learning situation more automatic. By analyzing learning situations in the classroom, the SLP and teacher can identify the knowledge and skills important for its completion. Through repeated practice, overlearning, and overrehearsal of this knowledge and skills, the task becomes automatic for the child. For example, the SLP might focus on language abilities that are critical for assignments in reading and writing and also help to support WM limitations. The SLP might also target vocabulary and syntax that are closely tied to a task, thus reducing the demands on available WM resources. For example, if a child has a store of vocabulary terms on a certain topic, writing a paper on this topic is less demanding. Intervention might also focus writing routinely used sentence frames for particular classroom activities, such as compare and contrast essays.

For young children with WM deficits, it is especially important to ensure that they can understand and follow directions. This may include learning sentence frames with causal or conditional clauses (e.g., *if/then, because*), temporal terms (e.g., *before, after, first, last*), or specific terms (e.g., *describe, explain, compare*).

Learning situations that require accessing prior knowledge place great demand on a child's WM abilities. By collaborating with the classroom teacher, the SLP can ensure that background knowledge is readily available to a child. This will result in greater resources dedicated to the task.

Many students with SLI have significantly slower processing than age-matched TD peers. The *Fast ForWord Language*, a popular computerized intervention program, is designed to improve the processing speed and language processing abilities of children with SLI. The program provides practice with acoustically and temporally modified syllable, word, and sentence material. As stimulus recognition and comprehension improve, the properties of the stimuli are modified to more closely approximate normal speech rate. Computerized training has also been used to improve both verbal and visuospatial WM skills in preschool and school-age children with ADHD (Klingberg et al., 2005; Thorell, Lindqvist, Nutley, Bohlin, & Klingberg, 2009). The use of computers will be discussed at the end of the chapter.

Processing within actual use contexts is the goal of intervention. Each session should provide real conversational and academic activities within which the SLP can functional monitor each child's behavior and aid participation.

Syntax and Morphology

Although language use improves syntax, the reverse is not true. It is important, therefore, that syntactic training be as conversational as possible. When language forms or constructions are taught outside a communication context, the forms may be mastered without the knowledge of how to express ideas within and across these forms. In addition, utterances produced in a context such as conversation strengthen cohesion and relationships across linguistic units.

The linguistic techniques discussed in Chapter 10 are particularly applicable to syntactic and morphologic training. Methods requiring response by the child are reported to be superior to those presenting only a model, although focused stimulation can be very effective in the initial stage of intervention. Evaluative feedback is also very important.

During training, it is important that the SLP control for vocabulary and/or sentence length, especially when teaching new structures. If the facilitator changes too many variables at one time, it may confuse a child or make the task too complex for successful completion.

The SLP also should be careful not to require metalinguistic skills beyond a child's abilities. Although recognition and comprehension usually precede production, judgments of correct usage do not. Judging a sentence to be grammatically correct is a metalinguistic skill that develops in the middle elementary school years. Asking children to form sentences with selected words or to unscramble words to form a sentence (*coat john a yesterday new bought*) also requires metalinguistic skill and WM. In short, any task that requires the child to manipulate language abstractly takes some degree of metalinguistic skill.

The development of syntactic and morphologic forms is well documented and provides a guide for intervention. In the following section, hierarchies for intervention with several different forms are discussed. The purpose is to offer general guidelines for the ordering of structures to be taught.

Just as development is a gradual process, especially for older children and adolescents, so too is intervention. It may be unrealistic to expect error-free production following teaching. Some low-frequency forms are difficult even for adults.

Morphology

Inflectional suffixes develop early and lend themselves well to teaching within a conversational milieu. Other morphemes may best be taught in a more explicit manner first, beginning with derivational suffixes, followed by prefixes. Explicit rule learning is not recommended for preschool children. The unique learning style of children with SLI also may make explicit rule learning less effective. Common bound morphemes are listed in Appendix C. Because derivational relationships are complex and irregular, memorization is of little value as a learning tool. It is essential that the child understand the underlying changes in meaning.

Although data for school-age morphological development are scarce, some suggestions for teaching do exist. These are presented in Table 11.13. Training should begin with the most common, early developing morphemes and proceed toward those that are more complex and cause phonological and orthographic or spelling changes.

Increasing syntactic difficulty decreases use of morphology for all children. In other words, processing demands influence morphological accuracy. With greater MLU, children are less affected by sentence complexity. Although children with SLI have similar performance to TD children on morphological tasks, they are less accurate (Owen, 2010).

Specially constructed "syntax stories" that provide numerous examples of forms, such as *be*, can be used to increase language input of these forms. Stories tailored to the child and intervention target, can serve as models for parents of how to provide intensive positive input for their child. Books can be part of an integrated intervention approach, resulting in significant improvements in young children's grammar. A list of children's books for this purpose is included in Appendix F. Westby

TABLE 11.13 Suggested Order for Teaching Morphemes

1. Establish awareness of syllables and sounds. Practice counting both.
2. Identify roots and affixes. Practice pronouncing and defining roots and affixes in contrasting words that are similar in sound or appearance, such as *happy-sunny,* and *include-conclude.*
3. Generate a formal definition in the form "A/An *X* is a (superordinate category) that (restrictive attributes)."
4. Discuss relationships with other words.
5. Use words in meaningful contexts and in analogies and cloze activities.
6. Use words in reading activities if appropriate.
7. Introduce spelling and spelling rules if appropriate.

(2005) provides several titles that can help clinicians and parents enhance the intensity of input for target forms.

The school-age child should be taught to analyze from derived words (theorize) to word stems (theory) and to synthesize from word stems to derived words. Meaning relationships should be emphasized. The metalinguistic skill of awareness of word structure is essential to the analysis of complex structures. These skills can be taught and used in conversation.

Middle-school children can be taught complex derivational morphology. Training can occur in both the oral and written modes. Training for middle-school children also should include root words that frequently occur in science, math, and social studies.

Verb Tensing

Verb learning takes several years and is very difficult for children with LI, partly because of the many ways verbs are treated syntactically and morphologically. Studies with TD preschoolers suggest that verb learning is enhanced when specific movements are associated with different verbs as opposed to general verbs, such as *do* (Brackenbury & Fey, 2003).

The teaching of verb tensing can be adapted easily to everyday activities in which children discuss what they are doing at present, did previously, or will do in the future. Art projects and building toys such as Legos are especially useful. Appendix E offers a number of activities for targeting verb tensing.

Training with very young children can begin with protoverbs, such as *up, in, off, down, no, there, bye-bye,* and *night-night.* These verb-like words usually are used in relation to some familiar action sequence.

More specific action verbs should be introduced in their uninflected or unmarked form. The language facilitator can cue by asking what a child is doing or by directing the child, "Tell *X* to (verb)." To facilitate learning, action word meanings might be taught with specific actions or objects. While playing, the facilitator can hide his or her eyes or turn away from the child and ask, "What are you doing?" Although the cue requires an *-ing* ending on the verb in the response ("Eating"), this form need not be required of the child at this very low level of training.

Familiar event sequences, such as play or routines, facilitate action verb usage because of the mental representations of the scripts of these sequences that children possess. These event sequences enable the child to focus on the communication, rather than on the extralinguistic elements of the event.

In verb learning, children with SLI benefit from multiple and well-spaced presentation of labels (Riches, Tomasello, & Conti-Ramsden, 2005). Massed training in which several words are presented in a single session requires a greater number of presentations of each word before learning occurs.

Once a child is able to form simple two- and three-word utterances with an action word, as in "Doggie eat meat," the present progressive verb form can be introduced without the auxiliary verb.

The SLP can model this form through self-talk and parallel talk. The SLP can cue the child to use this form with "What's doggie doing?" or "What's he doing?" Pronouns, such as *he*, must be used with caution at this level because many children with LI use very few.

At this level of training, a child only needs to deal with the immediate context. A sense of time beyond the present, however, is essential for further verb training.

The SLP can use a few high-usage irregular past tense verbs, such as *ate, drank, ran, fell, sat, came,* and *went*, to introduce the past rather quickly and to forestall overgeneralization of the regular past *-ed*, the next target form. With both past tense forms, storytelling, show-and-tell, and recounting past events are good vehicles for training and use. Initially, the facilitator can ask the child a question like "What did you eat (or other action verb)?" to teach the child the form. When the child responds with "Cookie" or another entity, the facilitator can reply, "What did you do with the cookie?" Later, the sequence can begin with the question, "What did you do?" The child responds, "Ate cookie," or, "I ate a cookie." It is important that question cues not violate pragmatic contingency, which requires that questions make sense. When possible, facilitators should not ask questions to which they know the answers. This strategy is achieved easily by asking about unobserved actions or having a puppet ask questions.

Before training additional verb forms, the SLP should introduce singular and plural nouns and subjective pronouns because the child will need these for the third-person singular present tense *-s* marker and for present tense forms of the verb *to be*.

The SLP can introduce the third-person marker with singular nouns, contrasting "The dog eats" with "The dogs eat." Subjective pronouns can be introduced gradually with such cues as "What does he do every day (all of the time)?" or such fill-ins as "Every day, she (verbs)," or "All of the time, he (verbs)."

Two-year-olds produce the third person singular *–s* markers more accurately (Sundara, Demuth, & Kuhl, 2011; Theodore, Demuth, & Shattuck-Hufnagel, 2011)

- on verbs in sentence-final position (*He walks*) as compared with verbs in sentence-medial position (*She sleeps in a bed*).
- in simple phonological vowel-ending words versus cluster-ending one (*sees* vs. *jumps*).

The sentence final position seems to be most influential.

Although children hear the third-person singular *–s* in sentence-medial position in conversation five times more frequently, they still selectively attend to the third-person marker in sentence-final position. This would suggest that the final position is more salient and should be where we place the third-person marker when teaching. Perceptual factors also play an important role (Sundara et al., 2011). This has relevance for children, such as those with SLI, who have perceptual difficulties. SLPs need to do everything possible to help these children perceive the third-person marker.

Targeting of third-person -s or the auxiliary verbs *is/are/was* in a focused stimulation story followed by a play period in which the SLP recasts the child's sentences containing the target result in significant gains in target learning (Leonard, Camarata, Brown, & Camarata, 2004; Leonard, Camarata, Pawlowska, Brown, & Camarata, 2006). In a variation, the SLP acts out the story with toys as she tells it. Children demonstrate learning of nontargeted forms that also demonstrate verb-tense and noun–verb agreement. In other words, learning of the third-person *-s* marker generalizes to *is/are/was*, and vice versa.

The SLP should not target the phonological variations of the *-ed* marker (/d/, /t/, and /Id/) and those of the third-person *-s* (/s/, /z/, and /Iz/) in initial training. When the marker is first being emphasized in training, the SLP should use one form exclusively, such as the /d/ or the /s/. As the emphasis on the marker becomes more natural or lessens, its cognate can be introduced without any fanfare. Be careful when talking with a child about morphological change. It's not the "D" or "S" sound being added but /d/ and /s/. Saying that "we add a 'D'. . ." may help spelling but is incorrect for speech.

The SLP should not expect a child to understand the phonological rules relative to ending sounds and added markers. Usually, deemphasis of the marker's sound will allow the child to produce naturally either two voiced or two unvoiced sounds at the end of each word. The /Id/ and /Iz/

markers should be avoided until later. Children developing typically usually employ the cognates by late preschool. It takes them a few more years to acquire the */Id/* and */Iz/* forms.

It's easier for children with LI and those developing typically to use the past-tense *-ed* on verbs of short duration and a definite end, such as *drop* (Leonard, Deevy, et al., 2007). Other verbs with less distinct end points, such as *play*, are more difficult. Lists of both types of verbs are presented in Table 11.14.

Use of pronouns enables the child to begin training on forms of the verb to be used both as an auxiliary verb and as the copula or main verb. This does not preclude earlier targetting of *is*, the most common form, with singular nouns. Because the form is *noun (or pronoun) + be + X*, in which the *X* can be a noun, adjective, adverb, or verb with *-ing*, these two forms of *be* as auxiliary and copula can be trained together, thus facilitating carryover. As a rule, the uncontracted form is taught first, and the contracted next.

The verb *to be* has different forms for various persons and tenses. These different forms should be introduced slowly. Children developing typically generally learn the *is* form first.

Other auxiliary verbs, such as *do*, also can be introduced to facilitate the development of more mature negatives and interrogatives. For example, the negative form of *do* can be elicited with "Let's play school. Remember to tell me (some other person) not to (*verb*)."

Using the present progressive form *be + going*, the child can begin to form early future tense forms. Facilitators should be willing to accept this form because it marks the concept even though less mature than *will*.

Training should begin with *going to noun*, as in "going to the zoo," before *going to verb*, as in "going to eat." The former is more concrete and does not require use of an infinitive phrase, such as *to eat*. The more mature *will* form of the future tense can be introduced later.

Guidelines for training *can, do*, and *will/would* include the following:

- Allow some delay between mastery of one form and introduction of another in order to avoid confusion.
- Use self-reference in the form of either first-person pronouns or the child's name initially because this is the first referent associated with these forms.
- Link these forms with actions because this is the first association of children developing normally.
- Initially, use short utterances with the word at the end in order to increase saliency ("Can you jump?" "Yes, I *can*."). Use the popular Bob the Builder refrain "Can we do it?" "Yes, we *can*."
- Provide meaningful situations in which the concepts and forms serve some purpose.

TABLE 11.14 Easy and Difficult Words to use with Past-Tense *-ed*

Actions with a Definite End	Actions of Longer Duration
Close	Brush
Cover	Carry
Drop	Chase
Dump	Crawl
Jump over	Dance
Kick	Hop
Knock	Play
Open	Pull
Pop	Push
Scare	Rake

Source: Information from Leonard et al. (2007).

Children with SLI have particular difficulty with verbs, verb endings, tenses, and verb phrases. These children are more likely to use an auxiliary verb if it is included in the preceding sentence, but both the form and location must be considered (Leonard, Miller, Deevy, Rauf, Gerber, et al., 2002). Although the exact form of the verb does not need to be in the preceding sentence, some forms do facilitate others. For example, use of *are* facilitates *is*. The sentence-final position (Yes, we *can*) also facilitates learning, but the sentence-initial position as in questions (*Can* we do it?) does not (Fey & Frome Loeb, 2002).

With the addition of the future tense, a child now can discuss the past, present (progressive), and future. Language activities, such as baking cookies, can now include planning (*will mix*), execution (*am mixing*), and review (*mixed*).

After teaching other auxiliary verbs, the SLP can introduce *modal auxiliaries*. These are helping verbs that express mood or feeling, such as *could, would, should, might*, and *may*. The shades of meaning across the various modal auxiliaries are often very subtle, and the facilitator should not expect mature usage for some time.

Finally, the SLP may wish to target verb particles, multiword units, such as *pick up* and *come over*, that function as verbs. Although verb particles emerge in early preschool years, they are not fully acquired and differentiated from prepositions until age 5.

The particle—*up, down, in, on, off*—may either precede or follow a noun phrase, as in *kick over the pumpkin* **or** *kick the pumpkin* ***over***. The same words used as prepositions, always precede noun phrases. The acquisition of verb particles is especially difficult for children with LI, possibly because they are unstressed units and may appear in either position vis-à-vis the noun phrase.

Particles should be introduced with a limited set of verbs used regularly by the child. It might be helpful to use position cues to teach the distinction between particles and prepositions. Particles could be taught following the noun phrase and prepositions preceding. Particles preceding the noun phrase could be introduced later.

Procedures for teaching verb tensing should make sense both semantically and pragmatically. Examples are asking the child to perform various tasks ("Will you please . . . ?"), problem solving ("What will happen if . . . ?" "What might happen if . . . ?"), and role-playing ("What should we do if . . . ?"). Many children's books—discussed in the next chapter—lend themselves to predicting tasks as well.

Pronouns

Pronouns are extremely difficult to learn because the user must have syntactic, semantic, and pragmatic knowledge. In general, an SLP should teach the underlying concept first and should model appropriate use for the child. Use of pronouns requires an understanding of the semantic distinctions of number, person, and case. The noun in the sentence generally determines use, but the conversational context is also a determinant.

Children often avoid making an overt pronominal error by overusing nouns. This mistake can be avoided somewhat in training by limiting the number of referents. For example, if the SLP uses too many characters in a story format, the child may overuse nouns in an attempt to remember who is being discussed. Using nouns can help children whose memory is somewhat limited.

In general, the first person *I* should be trained before the second person *you*, followed by the third-person *he/she*. This developmental order reflects increasing complexity with shifting reference and the number of possible referents.

Deictic terms, such as *I* and *you*, are difficult to teach. A second SLP, facilitator, or child can serve as a model to avoid confusing the child's frame of reference.

Development by typical children would suggest that facilitators target subjective pronouns (*I, you, he, she, it, we, you, they*) before objective pronouns (*me, you, him, her, it, us, you, them*). Possessive pronouns would follow (*my, your, his, her, its, our, your, their*), and, finally, reflexive pronouns (*myself, yourself, himself, herself, itself, ourselves, yourselves, themselves*). Although there are exceptions to this hierarchy, it approximates typical development. Subjective and objective case can be taught by location in the sentence.

This hierarchy and the error patterns of young children suggest that reflexives might be trained initially as possessives (*my self*). The exceptions (*himself* and *themselves*) can be introduced later.

One exception to the suggested hierarchy might be third-person singular pronouns. It appears easier for children to learn *her-hers-herself* than *him-his-himself*, probably because of the consistency in the feminine gender. The three feminine pronouns might be trained as a unit before the masculine.

Conversational training with so many varied forms can be very confusing. Initially, the facilitator must target carefully the desired pronouns and practice cues to elicit these forms.

Pronouns can be taught in any context where an object, toy, doll, action figure, character, or the child does something repeatedly, as in play or a narrative. After something or someone has been introduced, we use pronouns on repeat mention. For example, while telling a story from a book, a child might point and say, "He's running," or "They want to eat." While directing play, a child may say, "You be the boy and I be the girl. And this bes your fairy. He jump and he follow you everywhere. Now you both go sleep." When pronouns are not used, they can be prompted or modeled for the child. For example, if the child said, "And this bes your fairy. Fairy jump and fairy follow you everywhere," the SLP might reply, "He does. He jumps and he follows me everywhere. What else?"

Plurals

To learn plurals, the child must have the concepts of *one* and *more than one*. Numbers or words such as *many* and *more* may serve as initial aids. Begin with comparisions of one item versus many. Cue with "Show me (touch block) more," then respond, "Yes, more blocks!"

As with the past-tense *-ed* and third-person *-s* markers, the facilitator should not expect mastery of the phonological rules until later. Again, training should begin with either the /*s*/ or the /*z*/, gradually introduce the other, and wait some time before introducing /*Iz*/.

The SLP may wish to introduce a few common irregular plurals to forestall overgeneralization. As mentioned in the Semantics section of this chapter, words such as *water* and *sand* are not irregular plurals and present a special case, especially with the modifiers *any* and *much*.

Because so many toys have parts, play is almost a natural for teaching plurals. Use a key word such *as many* or *more* to signal the child to use the plural marker. Once a child is responding correctly with *many* or *more*, expand into more quantity words or counting. Use replica play of a birthday party or grocery shopping to elicit plurals. At birthday parties, there can be balloons, favors, treats, cookies, presents, cards, and games. Teaching of plurals lends itself nicely to a top-down approach.

Articles

Articles are extremely difficult for children to learn because of the two different operations they perform. Articles may mark definite (*the*) and indefinite (*a*) reference and also new (*a*) and old (*the*) information. When in doubt, preschool and early elementary school children tend to overuse *the*.

Articles and adjectives are acquired gradually along with development of the noun phrase (Kemp, Lieven, & Tomasello, 2005). Pragmatic reference (new/old) may be more difficult than the definite/indefinite distinction. Late preschool and early school-age children tend to use both articles with specific words, suggesting that individual words may influence use. For example, a child may use *the white kittie* but not *the white snow*. This suggests going slowly at first.

An SLP can use objects and pictures in play or books and instruct the child to describe what is seen ("A puppy"). Next, the SLP and the child can describe each object or picture, as in the following exchange:

Facilitator: Tell me what you see.
Child: A duck.

Facilitator: A duck? Let's see. I can tell you that *the duck is yellow. What* can you tell me?
Child: The duck is swimming.

The article *an* should not be introduced until a child is functioning at the early elementary school level.

Once pronouns have been introduced, the facilitator can switch back and forth between pronouns and articles, as in the following:

Facilitator: Here's *a* puppy. What can you tell me about *him*?
Child: *He* has a cold nose.
Facilitator: Who does?
Child: *The* puppy.

The possibilities are endless within a conversational paradigm. Remember that many Asian languages don't have articles, so this feature may be especially difficult for some ELL Asian children.

Prepositions

Although nine prepositions (*at, by, for, from, in, of, on, to,* and *with*) account for 90 percent of preposition use, these nine have a combined total of approximately 250 meanings! No wonder some children with LI have difficulty with this class of words. ELLs will find prepositions especially difficult. Prepositions were discussed briefly in the Semantics section under relational terms. Here's more.

Development of prepositions suggests the following hierarchy of training:

in, on, inside, out of

under, next to

between, around, beside, in front of

in back of, behind

In general, children will learn more easily when real objects are used in training. Spatial and directional aspects should be trained with a number of objects and/or examples so that a child understands the concept separately from any specific referent. Variety may preclude the child's focusing on the objects and referents rather than on the relationship. Large muscle activities also can be used as children go *in* and *out* of boxes or closets, *on* and *off* tables and chairs, and the like. Thus, the child's body becomes a referent and it's fun. Spatial terms may be taught in a naturalistic context of play with puppets, dolls, action figures, or the child's body. In one lesson, I played the tiger who pursued a preschool child *in* the cage, *out* of the cage, and so on.

Word Order and Sentence Types

Word order and different sentence types are best trained within conversational give-and-take, although school-age children and adolescents also may benefit from both oral and written training. Miniature linguistic systems have been used in initial training to teach word combinations. In these systems, a matrix is developed with one class of words on each axis. A child need not learn all possible combinations to acquire the rule. Good generalization to untrained combinations has been reported. Figure 11.4 presents some sample matrices and the teaching models that have been effective. A matrix can be used to tell a narrative or to direct play.

Noun phrases initially can be expanded in isolation. A question-answer paradigm will enable an SLP to target specific aspects of the noun phrase (How many . . . , Where . . . , Can you tell me . . .?).

	Cookie	Cake	Pudding	Pie	Bread
Eat	X	X	X	X	X
Bake	X				
Mix	X				
Want	X				
Give	X				

	Pet	Dog	Cat	Horse	Ferret
Feed	X	X			
Bathe		X	X		
Groom			X	X	
Walk				X	X
Brush	X				X

Verbs on one axis are combined with nouns on the other to form short phrases. Each combination taught is marked with an X. Rule learning will generalize to the untrained combinations.

FIGURE 11.4 Miniature linguistic systems.

Once placed within short sentences, the noun phrase can be expanded in the object position, followed by the subject position. Early expansion rarely goes beyond two elements, as in *a kittie* or *big horse*. The order of noun modifiers is discussed in Chapter 7 under analysis of the noun phrase (Table 7.17).

It's worth recalling from the discussion of articles that children initially use both articles and adjectives with specific words, suggesting that individual words may influence use. To me this means three things:

- Acquisition is gradual and intervention should be also.
- Contrastive training makes sense, e.g., the ***white*** *kittie, the* ***brown*** *doggie*.
- Generalization won't just happen; it must be planned for.

Adjectives can be taught in contrastive situations in which the child must distinguish between two objects that differ along one parameter, as in *big ball* and *little ball*. Incorrect or inadequate adjective use in conversation would result in misunderstanding and the misinterpretation of the child's message leading to some fun possibilities. In a similar fashion, post-noun modifiers can be used with objects in different locations, as in *the ball in the box* and *the ball on the table*.

Verb phrases and accompanying clause types should be chosen carefully. Specific verbs that clearly illustrate transitive and intransitive clauses might be chosen. Equitive verb phrases and the use of *be* can be trained in elliptical answers to questions, as in *He is* and *We are* responses to questions such as "Who is at the zoo?" A similar method of teaching transitive and intransitive verbs can be used to teach auxiliary verbs, as in "Who should eat?" and "Who can jump?". The response "We should" or "He can" place the auxiliary verb in the very salient final position in the sentence.

Infinitive phrases can be taught within play situations with dolls, puppets, or action figures or within storybook reading (Eisenberg, 2005). Of the two types of infinitives, noun–verb–to-verb (*Oscar wants to eat*) and noun–verb–noun–to-verb (*Oscar wants Ernie to eat*), the former is easier to learn and develops first. Early-developing and frequently used verbs that take an infinitive complement in the N–V–to-V form include *want, like,* and *try*. A possible format for training is presented in Table 11.15.

Using both oral and written techniques, an SLP can aid later-school-age children and adolescents to form longer sentences and more concise sentences and to use more low-frequency structures and intersentential cohesion. Compound and complex sentences can be formed from a child's own

TABLE 11.15 Top-down Model of Intervention with Infinitives

Target Response	Adult Cues	Verbal Prompts in Order of Increasing Input*
N–V–to-V		
Want to	Nonverbal: Playing house. Ernie stumbles around.	Verbal: *Ernie says to Elmo, "I'm very tired. Can I sit?" You finish the story. Ernie wants . . . ?* *Ernie wants* ***to*** *. . .* *Does Ernie want* ***to eat****? No. What does Ernie want?* *Ernie doesn't want* ***to eat****. Ernie wants . . . ?* *Ernie doesn't want* to eat. *Ernie wants to . . . ?* *Ernie wants* ***to sit****. What does Ernie want?*
Like to	Nonverbal: Playing with tools. Elmo wants the hammer.*	Verbal: *Elmo says to Oscar, "I will hammer. That is my favorite thing to do. Elmo likes . . .?* *Elmo likes* ***to*** *. . .* *Does Elmo like* ***to saw****? No. What does Elmo like?* *Elmo doesn't like* ***to saw****. Elmo likes . . . ?* *Elmo doesn't like* ***to saw****. Elmo likes to . . . ?* *Elmo likes* ***to hammer****. What does Elmo like?*
Try to	Nonverbal: Playing eating. Cookie Monster wants to jump over the table.	Verbal: *Cookie Monster says, "I will jump over the table." Cookie tries . . . ?* *Cookie tries* ***to*** *. . .* *Does Cookie try* ***to run****? No. What does Cookie try?* *Cookie doesn't try* ***to run****. Cookie tries . . . ?* *Cookie doesn't try* ***to run****. Cookie tries to . . . ?* *Cookie tries* ***to jump****. What does Cookie try?*
N–V–N–to-V		
Want N to	Nonverbal: Play eating. Elmo won't eat.	Verbal: *Ernie says to Elmo, "Eat your food." You finish the story. Ernie wants Elmo . . . ?* *Ernie wants Elmo* ***to****. . . ?* *Does Ernie want Elmo* ***to jump****? No. What does Ernie want?* *Ernie doesn't want Elmo* ***to jump****. Ernie wants Elmo . . . ?* *Ernie doesn't want Elmo* ***to jump****. Ernie wants Elmo to . . . ?* *Ernie wants Elmo* ***to eat****. What does Ernie want?*

(*Continued*)

TABLE 11.15 *(Continued)*

Target Response	Adult Cues	Verbal Prompts in Order of Increasing Input*
Tell N to	Nonverbal: Ernie is frightened by a big dog.	Verbal: *Bert says to Ernie, "Let's run!"* *You finish the story.* *Bert tells Ernie . . . ?* *Bert tells Ernie* ***to*** *. . . ?* *Does Bert tell Ernie* ***to sleep****?* *No. What does Bert tell Ernie?* *Bert doesn't tell Ernie* ***to sleep****.* *Bert tells Ernie . . . ?* *Bert doesn't tell Ernie* ***to sleep****.* *Bert tells Ernie to . . . ?* *Bert tells Ernie* ***to eat****. What does Bert tell Ernie?* *Bert tells Ernie****to run****. What does Bert tell Ernie?*

*The SLP provides more input only if needed by the child to be successful.

Source: Information from Eisenberg (2005).

simpler sentences. Subordinate clauses, such as *who is driving the red car*, can be transformed later into more concise ***phrases***, such as *The girl* ***driving the red car*** *is from Iowa*. Low-frequency structures, such as apposition (*Mary* ***my sister*** *. . . or John* ***the psychologist*** *will . . .*), complex noun phrases (*the large red dog with the bushy tail* or *teachers such as Ms. Meeker* or *Ms. Lilius*), perfect aspect (*has been verbing*), and passive voice (*The cat was chased by the dog*) can be targeted later. Finally, intersentential cohesion can be attempted by using adverbial conjuncts such as *therefore* and *however*. Acquisition is often very gradual. Less common types, such as *conversely* and *moreover*, should be introduced to mature language users.

Several strategies discussed in Chapter 10 can be used very effectively to strengthen word order. For example, expansion can provide a more mature model than a child's utterance, and recasts can help the child analyze relationships.

Table 7.16 presents some guidelines on the acquisitional order of certain sentence types. By the time most TD children begin school, they are using adultlike declaratives, imperatives, and *wh-* and yes/no interrogatives in both the positive and negative forms.

Summary

Although an SLP cannot always use all elements of the functional model simultaneously, he or she usually can employ several elements within any given teaching situation. Facilitators within the environment, everyday activities, and conversational give-and-take usually can be adapted to the individual child and language target(s). Some training may necessitate the initial use of structured approaches. Generalization to conversational use, however, will require incorporating everyday settings and activities into the training.

Children with CLD Backgrounds

Contrary to the popular belief, children with LI are capable, with appropriate support, of learning two languages (Paradis, Crago, Genesee, & Rice, 2003). Of course, the process will be less efficient than for TD bilingual children. In addition, there is every reason to believe that young L_1 speakers with LI are at greater risk for rapid regression or loss of L_1 if it is not supported (Restrepo & Kruth 2000; Salameh, Håkansson, & Nettelbladt, 2004).

Although bilingual approaches have been found to be as effective as English-only approaches in regular education (Rolstad, Mahoney, & Glass, 2005), there is a lingering fear among some professionals that intervention using a child's L_1 contributes to confusion or delays in development of L_2.

Although bilingual language intervention would seem appropriate for many reasons, less than 6 percent of SLPs in the United States are proficient in other languages (ASHA, 2009). In addition, very few SLPs speak many of the languages present in the United States, such as Hmong, Somali, and Vietnamese. Thus, the vast majority of bilingual U.S. children with LI receive services solely in English (ASHA, 2009, 2010; Kohnert, Kennedy, Glaze, Kan, & Carney, 2003).

It is crucial that English-only SLPs collaborate with bilingual SLPs and colleagues, interpreters, and families to design and implement intervention programs that promote development of a child's L_1 alongside English. Collaboration might include

- team approaches.
- use of interpreters and family members.
- use of bilingual classroom teachers.
- incorporation of technology or computer software.

The SLP could use a computer interface and prerecorded audio files in both L_1 and English to teach vocabulary (Pham, Kohnert, & Mann, 2011). Such a bilingual approach has the advantage of being just as effective as English-only approaches for English while having the additional benefit of promoting continued growth in a child's L_1.

As little as 30 minutes of instruction in Spanish daily is enough to promote L_1 learning among prekindergarten children in Spanish sentence length in words and clausal subordination (Restrepo et al., 2010). Effective programming might target five to ten vocabulary words a week, dialogic book reading, phonemic awareness, and letter knowledge.

English vocabulary learning of 4- to 6-year-old Spanish-English speakers is promoted by English vocabulary instruction enhanced with Spanish expansions when compared to English-only vocabulary instruction (Lugo-Neris, Wood Jackson, & Goldstein, 2010). Children can make significant improvement in naming, receptive knowledge, and expressive definitions. Their initial proficiency in both languages is important, and children with limited skills in both languages show significantly less vocabulary growth. Spanish expansions of novel vocabulary words during English storybook reading might include providing synonyms of words, using role-playing, and providng meanings or explanations. Over time, a bilingual child's vocabulary knowledge in both languages grows with multiple exposures and contexts. Children can associate additional semantic features with words and begin to recognize how words in English relate to the corresponding words in Spanish and vice versa.

Similarly, intervention with children speaking AAE can be bidialectal (Stockman, 2010). African American children are likely to come to therapy with varying levels of competence in both AAE and the majority dialect. Therapy should focus on a child's level of dialect use.

Dialectal issues should influence the SLP's judgments of correctness and appropriate teaching contexts. For example, because the use of the plural marker (*-s*) is context sensitive in AAE, an SLP should be alert to the absence of a plural marker on nouns preceded by a quantifier, as in *two shoe*. It's best to first target *noncontrastive* or non-differing AAE and majority dialect patterns instead of *contrastive* or dissimilar patterns. Such a strategy recognizes that African American children with and without LI will use contrastive patterns typical of AAE. LI should be most apparent on the noncontrastive patterns.

Trust is especially important if faculty, staff, and parents from CLD backgrounds are going to act as language facilitators. If, as an SLP, you know little of the local culture, you need to be proactive in seeking this information. It is not the child or parent's responsibility to educate you.

Use of Microcomputers

Microcomputers can enhance language instruction when well integrated into an overall language program in a cohesive manner. The computer can complement—but should never replace—face-to-face learning situations.

Children enjoy using computers. Preschoolers prefer computer-based training to traditional therapy drills and desktop activities. Most interventive programs are user friendly, lowering the threat to children with LI.

The goals of intervention and the methodology should be established prior to determining the role of the computer and integrating it into the overall plan. It is all too easy to fall into the trap of allowing the computer program to determine intervention goals. This *train-for-the-program* approach is not individualized for each child.

Children with LI are best served by computers when both the child and the SLP actively participate, when computer use is individualized, and when software specific to the intervention goal is used. The most effective integration occurs when the SLP or other facilitator and the child interact around the program being used, commenting and discussing choices offered and the child's selections. In this way, computer programs can be tuned more to the needs of each child. Similarly, software designed to address specific language problems is better than generic, mass-market software. Computers seem especially useful for writing training and will be discussed in Chapter 13. Possible intervention activities are presented in Table 11.16.

Computer programs should be used with caution. Prior to using any program, the SLP should ask fundamental questions about its theoretical underpinnings, the design of studies reporting success, and the clients who will seem to benefit most from program use. Of special concern for functional communication are the naturalness of the approach, its effect on overall communication, and generalization to real-life situations.

We have mentioned *Fast ForWord-Language* (FFW-L, Scientific Learning Corporation, 2009), a computer-based program, a few times in various contexts. *FFW-L* targets children's ability to process information from the speech stream by increasing the ability to rapidly process information. The program consists of seven computerized listening games with acoustically modified nonspeech and speech stimuli. Unfortunately, although some children make substantial gains in language performance, there is little to demonstrate enhanced learning ability (Tallal, 2000). In addition, more recent studies have found either no treatment-related effects on language test performance or

TABLE 11.16 Examples of Integrating Computer Activities into Language Intervention

Language Objective	Computer Activity
Giving directions	Write directions for making or baking something.
Sequencing events	Explain how to accomplish a common task such as making a peanut butter and jelly sandwich.
Future tense	Write an announcement explaining what will happen at the Fourth of July celebration or the class party.
Past tense	Write a "news" story about the class trip. Write a narrative about some past event.
Questions	Plan an interview with questions for your favorite musical performer or actor.
Negatives	Compile a list of dos and don'ts for the cafeteria or the school bus.
Syntax	Write a letter inviting someone to your class and in it explain why you want him or her to come.
Summarizing/syntax	Write a synopsis of your favorite movie, TV show, or book.

clinically significant gains not related to FFW-L (Cohen et al., 2005; Gillam et al., 2008; Pokorni, Worthington, & Jamison, 2004; Rouse & Krueger, 2004). In its defense, FFW-L does seem to improve attention, but the effects on subsequent language learning are not known (Stevens, Fanning, Coch, Sanders, & Neville, 2008).

In a study using FFW-L and narrative-based language intervention, FFW-L did not significantly improve language nor did it enhance learning of subsequent language material (Fey, Finestack, Gajewski, Popescu, & Lewine, 2010). When the results of intervention using FFW-L, nonspecific academic enrichment, computer-assisted language intervention, and individualized language intervention are compared, FFW-L was not more effective at improving general language skills or temporal processing skills than the others that did not contain modified speech stimuli (Gillam et al., 2008). This would suggest the benefits of using a more broad-based approach to intervention.

Conclusion

Even though you may feel overwhelmed by all the recommendations in this chapter, we have discussed only a small percentage of the available intervention techniques. Limited space necessitates a rather cursory examination of these procedures. SLPs can seek further information in source materials or in published clinical materials. In addition, they will conceive their own creative and innovative methods for intervening with children with LI. It is hoped that these methods will be adapted to fit the conversational model presented in Chapters 9 and 10.

Not all specific language problems are treated easily with a functional approach, but the entire model does not have to be discarded. Caregivers, for example, are a valuable resource and can be used in various ways, whatever the specific language problem being targeted. Likewise, training can occur in meaningful contexts within everyday events.

Chapter 12

Classroom Functional Intervention

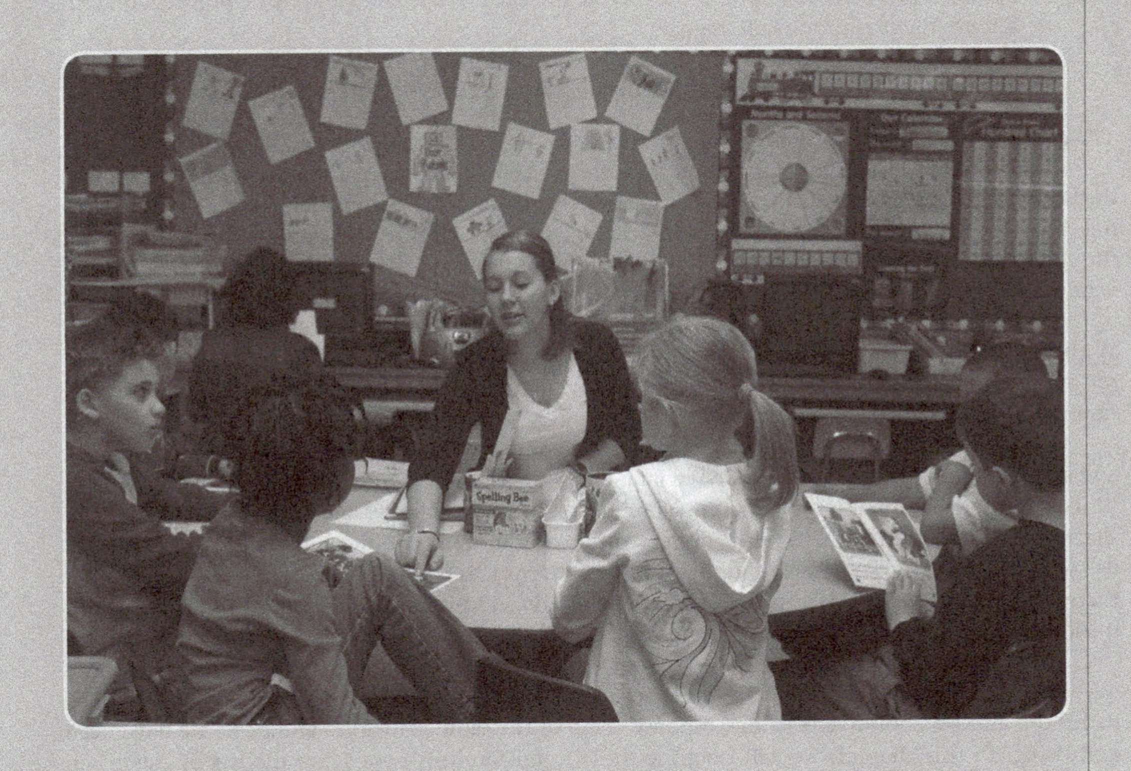

In school, children encounter the language of instruction, which is very different from the child's previous conversational interactions. Language is treated in the abstract as children learn to talk about it and to manipulate it. Metalinguistic skills are very important. The child with inadequate language skills or inadequate strategies for making sense of different situations is apt to become lost.

On an oral-to-literate continuum, school tasks are at the extreme literate end, requiring the child to understand and express information displaced from her or his own experiential base. Language itself creates the context within which information is conveyed.

An SLP can support a child's communication efforts in the following ways:

- Socially, by modifying his or her role and modeling appropriate roles for the child and by creating contexts in which the child can take varying roles.
- Emotionally, by preventing ostracism and by aiding the child to resolve conflict and to be tuned to the needs of others.
- Functionally, by redesigning contexts when needed by the child and by helping all children achieve their communication goals.
- Physically, by arranging the environment for maximum participation.
- Communicatively, by providing scripts for participation.

The goal is for each child to be successful in the classroom with diminishing adult support.

A functional approach to intervention shifts the focus from the child as the source and solution of the language problem to a holistic view that includes the child and the child's language uses and learning strategies, the contextual demands, the expectations and beliefs of other people within that context, the child's interaction, the context, and the child's communication partners. Thus, the focuses of intervention become the contexts that surround a child with LI and the manipulation of these contexts.

The classroom's cognitive activities are an excellent context for stimulating language growth. Within the classroom's constructive activities, children create, change, relate, and compare entities; set goals; encounter and try to overcome problems; make errors; reflect on success or failure; and note problem-solving procedures.

Context, especially in the school, has a significant effect on children's classroom discourse skills, and several contexts should be included in language assessment and intervention with children with LI. For example, within a journal-writing conference, a small-group lesson, a peer play session, and sharing time, children with LI perform very differently in language productivity and complexity, use of self-monitoring strategies, and turn-taking patterns (Peets, 2009). More specifically, although there is a wide range, children produce the most words and utterances during peer play but speak most rapidly, take longer turns, and have higher type-token ratios during sharing time.

The functional model discussed throughout this text can be adapted to these differing classroom needs. In fact, some of the recent changes in education, such as Response to Intervention (RTI), inclusion, and collaborative teaching, espouse some of the same principles and goals we have been discussing. In this chapter, we will examine these trends and propose some models of classroom intervention. Following that, we will describe the new role of the public school SLP and elements of a classroom intervention model, including specific intervention targets for preschool and school-age children. Finally, we will discuss implementation of classroom intervention.

Background and Rationale: Recent Educational Changes

Language training within the school classroom offers a special challenge for an SLP and a classroom teacher. School systems throughout the United States and Canada are adopting and modifying many models of intervention to provide more appropriate and effective intervention. These new models reflect recent educational changes in inclusion and collaborative teaching.

Response to Intervention (RTI)

Response to intervention (RTI) is a multitiered, problem-solving approach to education that addresses the learning difficulties of all children not just those with LI or other special needs conditions, incorporating both prevention and intervention. As such, RTI provides a structure within which educational teams can identify areas of concern and the need to provide appropriate levels of support for struggling children. Jackson, Pretti-Frontczak, Harjusola-Webb, Grishám-Brown, and Romani (2009) offer an excellent overview of RTI and its implications for early childhood professionals that is worth consulting.

The number of children with LI in the schools highlights the need for SLPs to understand the principles of RTI and ways to ensure their successful application. Within the RTI model, SLPs have expanded opportunities to collaborate with teachers and other education professionals.

From its beginning in early childhood education, RTI was envisioned as a interdisciplinary team approach within a comprehensive curriculum framework. Although the concept has been around since the 1970s, the term "response to intervention" first appeared within educational literature with the reauthorization of the Individuals With Disabilities Education Act (IDEA) in 2004. Principles originally devised within special education to embed service delivery within the general education setting began to be adapted to support the learning of all students, not just those at risk of academic failure. The goal of RTI is the academic success of all children.

So far, this discussion seems rather vague, so let's examine RTI principles and how they affect the responsibilities of SLPs. Common principles of RTI include (Jackson et al., 2009):

- Many tiers of support for each child exist in RTI, incorporating different levels of instruction.
- High-quality instruction from knowledgeable team members who use of a variety of instructional approaches, ongoing assessment procedures, and experiences that match the needs of each child, and collaboration among professionals.
- An evidence-based core curriculum that is evaluated for effectiveness.
- A data collection system, including both formative and summative, multiple informational sources, used to evaluate children's performance.
- Evidence-based intervention, which uses validated practices across multiple environments to support individualized learning.
- Family and professional procedures for identifying, selecting, and revising instructional practices based on child data and the learning context.
- Measures to monitor ensure effective and accurate implementation of instructional strategies and interventions.

These characteristics of RTI offer SLPs new dynamics and standards for providing services and supports.

Ensuring progress for all children has to be a collective effort involving families, educational professionals, related services providers, researchers, and legislators. SLPs play a crucial role in collaborating with other professionals and family members in the provision of language- and literacy-based services.

If we assume that the school, district, and/or state curriculum sets our goals for education, then those goals can serve as a comprehensive guide for day-to-day instruction. By operating within the curriculum, SLPs can promote active engagement and learning, individualize and adapt practices for individual children, provide opportunities for learning within daily routines, and ensure collaboration and shared responsibilities (Grisham-Brown, Hemmeter, & Pretti-Frontczak, 2005).

A possible curriculum framework might be composed of (Jackson et al., 2009)

- assessment.
- scope and sequence.

- activities and instruction.
- progress monitoring.

Within the last three, there are instructional tiers or levels of instruction that vary based on the size of the instructional group, location, intensity of instruction, and service providers. For example, as a child progresses through language intervention, SLP services may move from intensive one-on-one instruction to a small-group less-frequent model.

Operating within a curriculum framework enables various childhood professionals and disciplines to work together and move away from traditional service delivery models. Implementing a curriculum framework provides a series of challenges; in particular, challenges in reconceptualizing

- how to gather information on children's abilities.
- what to teach whom and in what order.
- how and when to teach.
- where children are making progress.

This leads to four expanded and redefined professional roles for the SLP as collaborator, problem solver, interventionist, and coach. Let's discuss each element of the curriculum framework.

Assessment

Within RTI, assessment is an ongoing process of observation and documentation of a child's performance, interests, and preferences and her or his family's priorities and needs (Grisham-Brown et al., 2005; Neisworth & Bagnato, 2004). Implementation begins by establishing each child's present level of performance. This assessment is for "program planning" purposes, requiring identification of all individual children's strengths, interests, and areas of concerns relative to common curricular outcomes.

In other words, SLPs are expected to administer, summarize, and interpret findings to better understand how all children are accessing, participating, and making progress across daily activities. Such as assessment requires multiple sources of information, multiple assessment approaches, and collection in multiple settings and across time (Neisworth & Bagnato, 2004). A key here is the use of **authentic assessment practices** that encourage children to show what they know and can do in the ways in which they would typically do so, something we have stressed throughout this text. The focus of assessment shifts, therefore, from more traditional norm-referenced assessment approaches to authentic, transdisciplinary collaborative assessment practices that focus on all areas of child development.

Scope and Sequence

The link between assessment and instruction is both the scope (concepts, skills, academic learning) and sequence or order of instruction. Individual children may need additional practice and support to gain independence with components of a curricular standard. This may even entail the teaching of underlying or prerequisite skills. For example, classroom reading instruction is based on the acquisition of phonological awareness, which, as we'll see in the next chapter, is a deficit for many children with LI.

SLPs bring specific expertise to the problem-solving task of determining which tier or level of instruction is appropriate for a child's needs. Within the curriculum framework, the SLP is expected to know how to support each child's language and communication development within the instructional tiers. By tailoring the type of instruction to the needs of these children, professionals are able to prevent children from falling behind and to do so without resorting to individual intervention.

In collaboration with teachers, the SLP can share communication development information, scientifically based literature, and pedagogical sequences that the classroom teacher can embed into classroom routines to provide increased learning opportunities in the child's natural environment. As a result, services responsive to a child's needs can be provided within daily routines to increase the amount of time that a child spends in quality instruction and intervention (Pretti-Frontczak & Bricker, 2004).

Activities and Instruction

Activities are the context in which important concepts and skills are addressed. Daily activities are designed to integrate concepts and skills from across developmental and content areas (Pretti-Frontczak & Bricker, 2004). For example, language skills are used in a variety of contexts throughout the school day. The SLP can consult with other team members to ensure that sufficient communication learning opportunities are created. By demonstrating ways to incorporate evidence-based instructional strategies into daily activities, SLPs can act as coaches for teachers addressing language and literacy development.

Instruction refers to the practices, actions, and methods used to deliver the content. Based on the assessment data for each individual child, quality instruction is developmentally responsive, enabling each child to create his or her own knowledge through interactions with the social and physical environment (Pretti-Frontczak & Bricker, 2004). Thus, quality instruction is responsive to the child and changes as the child's needs and personal preferences change.

Within activities and instructional tiers, SLPs need to embrace both direct and indirect interventionist roles. A direct interventionist role is the more traditional model of providing services directly to children and families. Less directly, as we have suggested throughout this text, an SLP may provide models and prompts for other professionals to use with children with LI to foster growth and development of communication abilities.

Progress Monitoring

Information gained from monitoring children's performance is used for

- evaluating the degree to which outcomes or goals are being met.
- serving as the foundation of decision making.
- identifying children in need of additional or more intensive support or instruction.

In these ways, progress monitoring efforts produce both formative and summative data that can be used to inform day-to-day practices and guide program-level decisions.

Data are gathered periodically to assess a child's progress. Quarterly or annually, data are used for setting direction for what to teach, comparing individual or group progress toward common outcomes, meeting accountability mandates, and evaluating program effectiveness. The SLP will collaborate with other team members to gather data, interpret findings, and problem-solve.

Inclusion

The Individuals with Disabilities Education Improvement Act mandates that all students with disabilities have access to the general education curriculum. Inclusion is based on sound research documenting the benefits to both children with special needs and their typically developing peers (Odom, 2000). There is a growing consensus that children with disabilities should be educated alongside their TD peers whenever possible within the context of daily routines and activities.

Beginning in the 1980s and continuing today, a movement has developed to raise education standards for all children. These changes have led to inclusive schooling and to the Regular Education Initiative (REI). **Inclusive schooling** is an educational philosophy that proposes one integrated educational system based on each classroom becoming a supportive environment much as we saw with RTI. Instead of separate systems of education, inclusive schooling proposes a unitary system of education adaptive enough to meet individual children's needs in a flexible manner. The result is (a) a shift in focus from the deficits to the abilities of children with special needs, (b) collaborative learning, (c) curriculum-based intervention, and (d) placement of all children in regular-education classrooms, with special services as needed.

REI is the movement toward an educational continuum that extends from regular-education classrooms for most children through regular-education classrooms with special services to adaptive environments for a small majority of the children most severely involved. At the latter end of the continuum, children will require services from trained professionals and curriculum-based intervention services to enhance their classroom participation. For example, in reading readiness training, children with LD need explicit, systematic, and intense instruction in areas such as phonological awareness and letter-sound relationships (Silliman, Bahr, Beasman, & Wilkinson, 2000).

The notion of inclusion is predicated on the assumption that children can learn and thrive in general education settings. It is not inclusive education when children with special needs are simply placed in a general education classroom without making sure they have full access to the curriculum. Inclusive education only occurs when all children have the supports and assistance they need to be able to engage in meaningful learning opportunities throughout the day (Grisham-Brown et al., 2005). That's where RTI comes in.

Despite widespread support for inclusion, there is concern that preschool-age children with disabilities are not provided specialized instruction by general education teachers (Markowitz et al., 2006). In fact, only a small fraction of these children receive specialized instruction embedded in common classroom activities. In general, teachers' lack of knowledge, specialized training, and confidence are barriers to providing inclusive care or early education that supports children's access to the general education curriculum (Chang, Early, & Winton, 2005; Knoche, Peterson, Edwards, & Jeon, 2006).

Collaborative Teaching

The possible negative effects of pulling children out of class to receive speech and language services are not found when these services occur in the classroom. Ongoing classroom activities can serve as the basis for intervention, with content coming from a child's assignments and projects and the interactions of the classroom. Thus, intervention is relevant for the environment in which it is being used. In addition, a child can benefit from the social dynamics of the classroom.

The variety of formats for classroom intervention includes the following:

1. An SLP team-teaches with a regular classroom teacher and other specialists.
2. An SLP provides small group or one-on-one classroom-based intervention with selected students in the classroom by using course materials.
3. An SLP acts as a consultant for a classroom teacher and other specialists, assisting primary caregivers with intervention strategies. Within a therapeutic partnership, the SLP helps the teacher set objectives, reinforce and modify behavior, and assess progress (Ehren, 2000).

The model for discussion in this chapter incorporates some elements of each of these, although primary emphasis is on the collaborative format.

Collaborative teaching is a combination of consultation, team teaching, direct individual intervention where needed, and side-by-side teaching in which a teacher and an SLP share the same goals for individual children. In partnership, an SLP and classroom teacher combine their efforts to serve children with LI. Parents are also members of the intervention team. The approach is a problem-solving one in which all participants share the responsibilities of decision making, planning, and implementation. All aspects of speech and language services are built around the skills a specific child needs to function better in the classroom environment. That's functional language intervention!

This model includes, but is not limited to, the following elements:

- An SLP provides in-service training for staff and parents.
- A classroom teacher helps identify potential children with LI through observation of classroom behavior. An SLP evaluates the speech and language skills of these children and others who fail speech and language screenings.
- An SLP, classroom teacher, and aide provide individual and small- and large-group intervention services within the classroom and the curriculum. In addition, the SLP continues to provide individual or small group therapy outside the classroom to children in need.
- A classroom teacher, aide, and parents interact daily with the children in ways that facilitate the development of language skills.

Classroom training has been shown to be effective in increasing both elicited and spontaneous language production. For example, with very young children, a classroom intervention model is superior to individual intervention methods in generalization of learned words. Providing language intervention in the classroom also has been shown to be effective in teaching some language concepts, such as key vocabulary, to elementary school children (Throneburg, Calvert, Sturm, Paramboukas, & Paul, 2000).

By working closely with classroom teachers, the SLP can become well-informed of the language demands of the curriculum. The SLP can gain this information by

- meeting with teachers to discuss classroom activities.
- listening to classroom instruction.
- observing classroom demonstrations.
- reviewing materials and upcoming assignments.
- analyzing tasks to determine the skills needed to participate effectively.

Through this process, the SLP can gain insight into the lexical, syntactic, and discourse development required for students to succeed (Nippold, 2011). As teachers share their knowledge of the curriculum, the SLP can share his or her expertise in language development, language disorders, and language intervention techniques. Inclusion of classroom content and vocabulary in intervention increases the relevance of language intervention. Ideally, the classroom provides an interactive model in which language features are modeled and embedded in familiar, ongoing activities. Real conversations and meaningful activities provide motivation and experiences that are usually not available in isolated individual intervention. Activities are meaningful and experience based.

Summary

Educational trends have combined to change the teaching and remediation of language. In many schools, an SLP is working with children and their language impairments within a naturalistic language curriculum in regular education classrooms. The principles we have been discussing in this book are a near perfect match to the demands of this intervention situation.

Role of the Speech-Language Pathologist

Any classroom intervention model raises questions about the SLP's role and about others' expectations of the intervention team. There are no quick answers. The model of intervention that evolves is a blend of the child's needs and the desires of the school, the individual teacher, and the SLP. Ideally, the SLP will assume the roles of co-teacher, consultant, and direct service provider and will be integrated fully into the classroom.

The SLP is the school's language expert. As such, he or she advises administrators, teachers, and special needs committees about children and language impairment. The SLP is also responsible for speech and language assessment, for the planning and implementation of all speech and language programming, for record keeping, and for training personnel who will work with the children with LI. Although evidence-based data are very few, they tentatively suggest that highly trained language facilitators can provide effective services for children with LI under very specific conditions (Cirrin et al., 2010).

Relating to Others

Functional intervention in the classroom necessitates coordination of intervention goals and schedules. This coordination requires that an SLP interact daily with a variety of individuals.

Classroom Teachers

The SLP is uniquely qualified to assist a classroom teacher in assessing each child's level of functioning, analyzing the language requirements of various activities and materials, and developing intervention strategies in conjunction with the classroom teacher. This is an ongoing process, accomplished through in-service training and individual consultation and training, as well as with co-teaching within the classroom. Both teachers and SLPs rank team teaching and one teach/one drift as the most appropriate model for collaborative teaching. Team teaching is supplemental teaching in which one team member adapts the material for children with LI. In a one teach/one drift model, one member teaches and the other moves around the classroom assisting students as needed.

The SLP and the classroom teacher have unique skills that they can use to help each other and a child with LI. The SLP understands language development and the remediation of speech and LI. The classroom teacher knows each child and understands the use of large and small group interactions for teaching.

It is imperative that the SLP avoid the "tutor trap" in which she or he becomes a glorified classroom aide. Classroom requirements should not dictate clinical content. In addition, the SLP should work to enhance the classroom environment as well as to change the child's language. It is important to retain a therapeutic focus. This requires the interrelated steps of planning and implementation (Ehren, 2000). Planning requires intervention services for children that target skills underlying the curriculum. In implementing intervention, the SLP should focus on the goals for children on the caseload and not on general educational activities. Examples of classroom *dos and don'ts* are presented in Table 12.1. The role of the SLP is not to provide specific curriculum teaching or tutoring nor to relieve the teacher of the responsibility to teach all students in the class.

TABLE 12.1 Examples of *Dos and Don'ts* of Classroom Speech and Language Services

Do . . .	Don't . . .
Help child to identify the important information on a math worksheet and decide on a way to perform the operation.	Help the child complete the math problems.
Teach relevant vocabulary by focusing on the words and figurative language of the science text that may be difficult for the child with LI, and encourage the teacher to establish a language learning center.	Preteach the science vocabulary next chapter.
Co-teach a social studies lesson by guiding the students with LI to practice the language strategies learned in therapy. Simple note cards containing reminders can be given to each child.	Co-teach a social studies lesson for all students without addressing the IEP goals of the children with LI.

Source: Information from Ehren (2000).

The SLP and the classroom teacher are part of the intervention team and should contribute in that fashion. Each has special expertise to impart.

Parents

Not all parents can or wish to participate in their children's speech-language intervention. Parents tend to fall into three identifiable groups, the largest being those who desire participation. Next are those who desire no participation, and the smallest group is composed of parents who only want more information. The first group of parents can be involved in planning and implementation of intervention, and parents who want information can be served through parent meetings and in-service training.

School Administrators

Administrators may not understand generalization and the need to provide language remediation within the classroom. Caseload dictates and contact hour requirements may have to be modified to accommodate the classroom model. Both teachers and SLPs agree that finding enough consultative time is a big problem (Beck & Dennis, 1997). Discussion should center on how best to serve the children and how to use professional time commitments most efficiently.

Language Intervention and Language Arts

Classroom teachers and administrators are sometimes confused about the difference between language arts and language remediation. Unless this distinction is clear, the SLP's role also may be misunderstood, especially as it relates to classroom intervention. *Language arts* accomplishes several things:

- Provides children with labels for the language units they have been using in their speech.
- Requires children to stretch their language abilities into new areas, such as fictional and expository writing.
- Enables children to have language growth experiences, such as performances.
- Helps children reason and problem solve by using linguistic units.

All of these valuable accomplishments presuppose that each child has a well-formed language system. Children with LI are at risk of failure.

In language intervention, a child is taught language features that are not present or are in error. These problems can have a huge impact on a child's success within the curriculum.

Elements of a Classroom Model

As mentioned, the classroom model consists of identification (assessment), intervention, and facilitation. In each phase, the classroom teacher and the SLP, although a team, have individual inputs that affect the delivery of quality services for a child.

Identification of Children at Risk

Teachers play a vital role in identifying children with LI. Most teachers are not trained in language development or impairment, and the SLP must alert them to the behaviors that signal a possible impairment.

Teacher training can be accomplished through in-service sessions. Teachers also can be given aids to use in identifying a potential language problem. Table 12.2 presents a list of some signs for

TABLE 12.2 Recognizing Children with Language Impairment in the Classroom

The child may have some or all of the following:
Seems to fail to understand and follow instructions.
Is unable to use language to meet daily living needs.
Violates rules of social interaction, including politeness.
Lacks ability to read signs or other symbols and to perform written tasks.
Has problems using speech to communicate effectively.
Demonstrates a lack of appropriate organization and sequence in verbal and written efforts.
Does not remember significant information presented orally and/or in written form.
May not recognize humor or indirect comments.
Seems unable to interpret the emotions or predict the intentions of others.
Responds inappropriately for the situation.

Source: Information from N. Nelson (1992).

recognizing children having difficulties in the classroom. Table 12.3 or its adaptation might be used by teachers for referral to the SLP.

Teachers should be trained to observe and describe classroom behaviors as precisely as possible. The SLP's complaint that teachers refer children who have rather nonspecific vocabulary problems or are inattentive reflects poorly on the SLP's training of teachers to recognize LI and its manifestations. Teachers are a valuable source of raw data on classroom performance when they know what to observe and measure.

In addition, the SLP and the classroom teacher can identify the individual classroom's or grade level's special communication requirements as a gauge against which each child can be measured to assess achievement. Called *curriculum-based assessment*, this method uses a child's progress within the school curriculum as a measure of her or his educational success. Children are assessed against the curriculum within which they are expected to perform. Thus, intervention focuses on changes in the child's behavior that are relevant to the educational setting.

From preschool through high school, the curriculum changes in the types of demands made on each student. These changes are as follows:

Preschool: Learning focuses on sensorimotor, language, and socioemotional growth with materials that are manipulative, three-dimensional, and concrete.

Early grades (K–2): Learning focuses on perceptual-cognitive strategies with materials that are one-dimensional, abstract, and symbolic.

Middle grades (3–4): Learning places higher demands on linguistic and symbolic skills with less direct instruction. The child is expected to make inferences, analyze data, and synthesize information.

Upper grades (5–6): Learning focuses on content areas, with the child expected to recall past learning and display fluency with basic academic skills.

Middle and high school: Learning emphasizes lectures in content areas, with students expected to reorganize material as they listen and to gain the main or important points. From 75 percent to 90 percent of the day may be spent receiving information.

Some school districts have identified skills that children need to succeed in each grade. Table 12.4 (on p. 338) presents some of the skills needed in the first three grades.

In addition to the school's official curriculum, children encounter several other curricula. These include the *de facto curriculum* that is actually taught and the cultural and school curricula needed to

TABLE 12.3 Teacher Referral of Children with Possible Language Impairment

The following behaviors may indicate that a child in your classroom has a language impairment that is in need of clinical intervention. Please check the appropriate items.

____ Child mispronounces sounds and words.

____ Child omits word endings, such as plural *-s* and past-tense *-ed*.

____ Child omits small unemphasized words, such as auxiliary verbs or prepositions.

____ Child uses an immature vocabulary, overuses empty words, such as *one* and *thing*, or seems to have difficulty recalling or finding the right word.

____ Child has difficulty comprehending new words and concepts.

____ Child's sentence structure seems immature or overreliant on forms, such as subject-verb-object. It's unoriginal, dull.

____ Child's question and/or negative sentence style is immature.

____ Child has difficulty with one of the following:

____ Verb tensing	____ Articles	____ Auxiliary verbs
____ Pronouns	____ Irregular verbs	____ Prepositions
____ Word order	____ Irregular plurals	____ Conjunctions

____ Child has difficulty relating sequential events.

____ Child has difficulty following directions.

____ Child's questions often inaccurate or vague.

____ Child's questions often poorly formed.

____ Child has difficulty answering questions.

____ Child's comments often off-topic or inappropriate for the conversation.

____ There are long pauses between a remark and the child's reply or between successive remarks by the child. It's as if the child is searching for a response or is confused.

____ Child appears to be attending to communication but remembers little of what is said.

____ Child has difficulty using language socially for the following purposes:

____ Request needs	____ Pretend/imagine	____ Protest
____ Greet	____ Request information	____ Gain attention
____ Respond/reply	____ Share ideas, feelings	____ Clarify
____ Relate events	____ Entertain	____ Reason

____ Child has difficulty interpreting the following:

____ Figurative language	____ Humor	____ Gestures
____ Emotions	____ Body language	

____ Child does not alter production for different audiences and locations.

____ Child does not seem to consider the effect of language on the listener.

____ Child often has verbal misunderstandings with others.

____ Child has difficulty with reading and writing.

____ Child's language skills seem to be much lower than other areas, such as mechanical, artistic, or social skills.

succeed within each context. The expectations of the latter are often very confusing for the child with language-processing problems. The implicit expectations of individual teachers and other children form a fourth curriculum.

The SLP first must become familiar with the curricula that affect the individual child with LI. He or she can assess the child through a combination of interview and observation of the child's ability to

TABLE 12.4 Some Possible Language Skills Needed in the First Three Grades

First Grade. The child will be able to:

Recognize correct word order auditorily.
Identify singular and plural common nouns and proper nouns.
Identify regular and irregular past and present verbs.
Identify descriptive and comparative adjectives.
Use nouns and pronouns, adjectives, and verbs correctly in sentences, including verb-noun agreement.
Give and write full sentences.
Categorize words by opposites, by sequence, by category, and as real/nonreal.
Retell a story.
Identify the main idea in a paragraph.
Classify narrative and descriptive writing.
Rhyme words and identify words that begin with the same sound.
Identify declarative and interrogative sentences and use correct ending punctuation for each.
Capitalize the first word in a sentence, days, months, people's names, and the pronoun I.
Alphabetize.
Give directions and explanations and follow two-step directions.
Read aloud.
Listen attentively and courteously to others.

Second Grade. In addition to the skills needed for first grade, the child will be able to:

Use correct word order.
Identify incomplete sentences.
Recognize singular and compound subjects of a sentence.
Identify possessive and plural nouns, contracted verbs, and superlative adjectives and use correctly.
Capitalize holidays, titles of people, books, stories, and places.
Identify correct comma use.
Use an apostrophe in contractions.
Identify the topic sentence and sentences that do not relate in a paragraph.
Write an explanation or set of directions.
Address an envelope.
Write rhyming words to complete a poem.
Identify figurative language and synonyms.
Recognize characters, plot, setting, and the major divisions in a story or play, and the difference between fiction and nonfiction.
Tell and write a clear, original story.
Use the title page and table of contents in a book.
Use the dictionary for spelling and meaning.
Read critically for sequence, main idea, and supporting details.
Use tables and graphs as sources of information.
Recognize types of poetry.
Listen discriminately for rhyming, sequences, and details.

Third Grade. In addition to the skills needed for first and second grade, the child will be able to:

Identify imperative and exclamatory sentences, simple and compound sentences, and run-on sentences.
Recognize compound predicates in a sentence.
Recognize articles and conjunctions in sentences.
Use an exclamation point.
Use an apostrophe in possessive nouns.
Define a paragraph and identify the main idea and supporting sentences.
Write a paragraph, a book report, and a letter with correct capitalization and punctuation.
Write a clear, original story with title, beginning, middle, and end.
Recognize the difference between biography and autobiography.
Use a dictionary for pronunciation.

(*Continued*)

TABLE 12.4 *(Continued)*

Use an encyclopedia, telephone book, newspapers, and magazines as references.
Identify compound words, homophones, and homographs.
Use prefixes and suffixes.
Read critically for sequence, main idea, and supporting details.
Organize information by category and sequence.
Recognize real and make-believe, relevant and irrelevant, and factual and opinionated statements.
Identify characteristics of different types of narratives.

meet the language demands of the curricula. The interview phase can provide information on the curricular expectations, and observation can focus on the specific linguistic demands made of the child.

An analysis of the linguistic demands must consider all aspects of language and the many reception and production modes. Such an analysis also should note metalinguistic skills demanded in the classroom.

An educational language assessment focuses on a child's oral and written abilities and capacity to learn, rather than on his or her deficits. Data are gathered by direct testing, dynamic assessment, and real-life observation within the classroom. The level of support necessary for learning is determined, including evaluation of the effectiveness of various instructional and intervention strategies. Most standardized tests are too global, and more specific measures should be used to measure the child. The parents and the teacher, as well as the child and the SLP, should participate.

The SLP follows up these reports and collects her or his own data within the classroom setting. These data can be corroborated by further testing and sampling.

Assessment with Preschool Children

With preschool children, an SLP is interested in pragmatic abilities, semantics, especially the child's lexicon or "personal dictionary"; language structure; and narrative forms. Additional areas of importance for literacy education include role-play and representational play, decontextualization, and adaptations for non-oral responding.

Play is particularly important for preschool children, especially as a context within which to experiment with language. Of particular importance in play are the level of decontextualization, thematic content, organization, and self/other relations. Play can be very context-bound, using only real objects, or relatively decontextualized, using imaginary or symbolic objects. The familiar versus unfamiliar themes of play are also important for later intervention. The organization of play can demonstrate cohesion, logical connections with the theme, and planning. Finally, the roles a child takes and assigns may be important for later training and may tell an SLP something about the child's ability to take the perspective of others and to style switch.

Decontextualization in a child's language is important for later reading and is demonstrated by reference to nonpresent entities and to past and future tense. Reading is very decontextualized because all meaning comes from print and little from the physical context.

Even though a child cannot read, pre-literacy skills are important for further development. An SLP is interested in a child's comprehension of text, knowledge and awareness of print, and sound-symbol associations and decoding abilities.

Finally, non-oral methods of communicating are also important. These include gestures, facial expression, and body posture, but also drawing and preschool "writing."

Assessment with School-Age Children and Adolescents

In addition to considering the language features mentioned in Chapters 6 through 8, the SLP is interested in the child's language as it relates to the specific requirements of the classroom. An authentic, or real, assessment should include a dynamic be a *train-test-train* procedure, with both the SLP and the classroom teacher determining the best instructional strategies for individual children. An evaluation also consists of systematic observation of real teaching and learning in the classroom.

Systematic observation might include rating scales and checklists, narrative records, and descriptive tools by the teacher, SLP, and student. Possible rating scales for use with school-age children and adolescents are listed in Table 12.5. Teacher logs, notes, journal entries, and student assignments and self-evaluations should be gathered to ascertain the child's oral and written language skills. Of interest is the amount of scaffolding or structure and assistance needed by a child for success.

Interviews with the student are also helpful. Students can be asked to describe their most difficult and easiest subjects and their strengths and weaknesses, to relate recent classroom events that made them feel bad and to prioritize changes they would like to make in themselves and in the classroom and manner of instruction.

The SLP may gain additional information by informally sampling the child's performance. For example, the SLP might compare a secondary school child's notes with those of a higher-performing student in the same class. Audio recordings of classroom instructions can be analyzed to determine the level of complexity that each child must be able to process. The SLP may want to collect samples of the child's oral reading or help the child complete assignments, noting the child's language-related work skills.

Within the classroom, children use language for self-monitoring, directing, reporting, reasoning, predicting, imagining, and projecting thoughts and feelings. Using a "speak-aloud" technique, a child can verbalize as she or he tackles classroom tasks. Also of interest is the breadth of functions demonstrated in conversation and narration.

School semantic features include abstract terms, refinement and decontextualization of word meanings, the ability to define words, multiple word meanings and figurative language, organization of a semantic network, and use of metalinguistic and metacognitive terms. Semantic networking, or relating ideas to a theme, is another important skill for children to acquire. Those with better-formed, more-extensive networks are better able to comprehend and follow a topic or theme.

TABLE 12.5 Tools for Assessment of Classroom Skills

Observation/Interviews
Clinical Discourse Analysis (Damico, 1991a)
Environmental Communication Profile (Calvert & Murray, 1985)
An Interview for Assessing Students' Perceptions of Classroom Reading Tasks (Wixson, Bosky, Yochum, & Alvermann, 1984)
Pragmatic Protocol (Prutting & Kirchner, 1983, 1987)
Self-Attribution of Students (SAS) (Marsh, Cairns, Relich, Barnes, & Debus, 1984)
Social Interactive Coding System (SICS) (Rice, Snell, & Hadley, 1990)
Spanish Language Assessment Procedures: A Communication Skills Inventory 3rd edition (Mattes, 1995)
Spotting Language Problems (Damico & Oller, 1985)
Systematic Observation of Communication Interaction (SOCI) (Damico, 1992)
Testing
Classroom Communication Screening Procedure for Early Adolescence (CCSPF-A) (Simon, 1989)
Curriculum Analysis Form (Larson & McKinley, 2003)
Interactive Reading Assessment System–Revised (Calfee, Norman, & Wilson, 1999)
Lindamood Auditory Conceptualization Test, 3rd edition (Lindamood & Lindamood, 2004)
Pre-Literacy Skills Screening (Crumrine & Lonegan, 1998)
Test of Awareness of Language Segments (Sawyer, 1987)

TABLE 12.6 Common Metacognitive and Metalinguistic Terms

afraid	assert	assume	believe	concede	conclude
confirm	disgusted	doubt	embarrass	feel	forget
guess	happy	hypothesize	imply	infer	interpret
know	mad	predict	propose	proud	remember
sad	surprised	talk	think	understand	

Networks can be evaluated by having the child name everything he or she can related to a given topic or category or place pictures and words into categories. Picture tasks can be made more challenging by the use of pictures with differing perspectives.

Success in the classroom requires that a child be able to explain decision making, to discuss mental processes, and to reflect on mental processes of others and him- or herself. Related metalinguistic and metacognitive terms are listed in Table 12.6. Some terms are acquired prior to school age, but many are not mastered until adolescence.

Syntax and morphology gradually change throughout the school years. Initially, structure is more complex in oral language rather than in written, but this reverses. Therefore, the SLP is interested in the structure of both. Analysis would include clause and T-unit length and elements of the noun phrase and verb phrase. Cohesive elements such as pronouns and conjunctions are especially important.

Narrative and expository writing and speaking also should be analyzed. Difficulty at these levels may signal underlying problems. Pictures can be used in an assessment to elicit both oral and written samples. Of interest are the clarity of cohesion and the types employed.

For children with word-finding difficulties, the SLP can analyze reading and writing errors to determine the strategies used by the child. Word substitutions may highlight the type of storage and retrieval being used by the child. Categorization strategies may also be revealed. A curriculum-based assessment should attempt to identify the discrepancy between the child's knowledge of classroom content and his or her ability to retrieve it.

Finally, auditory discrimination and articulation skills are important for spelling and should also be assessed. Similarly, phonemic awareness is important for writing and reading.

As language becomes more complex in school-age and adolescent years, the assessment and intervention tasks also become more challenging. Add to this the deficits found in reading and writing and the task becomes even more formidable. Reading and writing assessment and intervention will be discussed in Chapter 13.

Curriculum-Based Intervention

Children with LI may need assistance transitioning from preschool to kindergarten and elementary school (Prendeville & Ross-Allen, 2002). Not only is the child-to-adult ratio increased, but children are also expected to work increasingly in small groups and to negotiate using language. In addition, there is also increased expectation for a child to work independently while receiving less individualized support. The curriculum is different and language based, as is the manner of instruction. Children need instruction and activities that help them "bridge" to the curriculum (Masterson & Perrey, 1999). Planning for each child's transition should be systematic, individualized, timely, and collaborative involving both the family, classroom teacher, and SLP. Through collaborative intervention, the SLP can model interactive teaching styles and help the teacher to combine listening, speaking, reading, and writing activities into each lesson but structured in such a way as to ensure success for children with LI.

Within the classroom, an SLP can work with individuals or small groups of children and adolescents while the teacher works with the rest of the class. Group projects can provide the context for intervention by using the techniques discussed in Chapter 10. Other children can serve as models. Small group instruction is efficient and effective and increases generalization and interaction.

Children's individual needs can be addressed if the SLP or teacher carefully interacts with each child in ways that foster the targeted aspects of language. With planning, adults can accomplish such training individually even in groups of children.

The goals of classroom intervention are for a child to learn new ways of communicating and to have ample opportunity to practice newly acquired skills. The environment should be responsive so that a child learns that language can have some effect on that environment. The language of effective classroom communicators is characterized by fluency of word-finding skill, coherence or content organization, and effectiveness and control.

A child's learning within the classroom is a function of individual learning style and the environment. Both must be considered when assessing or attempting to intervene with learning. The language of a child's classroom and materials can provide the context and content for intervention.

Classroom Demands

With advancing grades, the emphasis shifts increasingly to independent work and to listening and note-taking abilities. Rules become implicit and children are expected to work independently (Westby, 1997). Each of these tasks is extremely complex. Intervention helps students learn strategies for analyzing various tasks and for determining the steps to take to accomplish them. The SLP might teach language-impaired students time management skills, study skills, critical thinking, and language use. He or she might develop a book of listening activities for teacher use within the classroom. Other innovations that might help children with LI organize their day and make sense of the classroom include encouraging use of a daily planner, helping teachers add graphic input to lectures, defining concepts and vocabulary, cuing to guide reading comprehension, developing guided questions to help children make inferences, discussing how to answer questions, and helping children to identify main ideas for note taking.

Study skills training might include text analysis, study strategies, note taking, test-taking strategies, and reference skills. Through text analysis, a child can be helped to understand the organization of texts and their more efficient use.

Study strategies might include active processes for reading, such as identifying the main ideas and reviewing periodically to organize the material. Children also can learn associative and other memory strategies.

Critical thinking is the collection, manipulation, and application of information to problem solving. Language is an integral part of this process. Therefore, a child with LI may experience difficulties with organizing information and with decision making. Likewise, sophisticated metalinguistic judgments also would be difficult. Critical thinking training might target the three components of general thinking, problem solving, and higher-level thinking.

General thinking includes observation and description, development of concepts, comparisons and contrasts, hypotheses, generalization, prediction of outcomes, explanations, and alternatives. Problem-solving skills include analyzing the problem into smaller parts, developing options, predicting outcomes, and critiquing the decision. Higher-level thinking includes deductive and inductive reasoning, solving analogies, and understanding relationships. These tasks become increasingly more abstract and require greater reliance on linguistic input.

Analogies (A is to B as C is to ______) are particularly difficult for children with LD. Analogical reasoning can be taught through a two-phase model in which steps for solving analogies are taught in Phase I and bridging activities to specific academic areas are taught in Phase II. Phase I targets the following skills:

Encoding. Translating each term into an internal representation of its attributes.

Inferring. Establishing the relationship of the first pair.

Mapping. Using the first relationship to identify a similar one in the second pair.

Applying. Picking the answer that has the same relationship as the first pair.

With increased emphasis on lectures at the secondary level, listening skills become even more important. In general, good listening skills are highly correlated with good overall language performance. Students can be taught to tune in to what they hear and to listen actively. Subsequent training can focus on recognition and understanding of lecture material. The child's semantic, syntactic, and morphological repertoire can be expanded as a base for comparison with new information from lectures. Such training might include word meanings, relationships and categories, sentence transformations, active and passive voice, embedding and conjoining clauses, and segmentation. Through critical listening training, a child learns to supply missing information, complete stories, find important information, and recognize absurdities in spoken information. Children who have difficulty attending will need special help in listening to what they hear.

In oral language production, the child can sharpen word-retrieval and figurative language skills. The SLP can teach children to verbalize important critical reasoning skills, such as questioning, comparing, and analyzing, and to discuss a task or topic and to give examples. Elementary school children and adolescents can also be taught metapragmatic awareness in order to judge inconsistencies, inadequacies, and communication failures. The SLP can help students with LI understand response requirements for relevancy and thoroughness.

An SLP can enhance written-language training by using computers and topics of interest to the child. Computer intervention can have a positive effect on language, especially vocabulary, and even can improve some social-interactive skills if the SLP mediates. Organizational skills gained in critical thinking training can be used in expressive writing training.

Finally, an SLP can enhance conversational skills by role-playing and practice. The child with LI can be helped to identify different communication contexts and their requirements.

Written information can be used to train oral language skills. Within a conversational or small group framework, written scripts can be used for practice in communicating between speaker and listener. Written material can be controlled systematically to ensure that it is well organized and cohesive and that it offers a variety of topics, roles, and situations. The use of social interactions enables the child to learn language as an integrated social-cognitive-linguistic experience.

Adolescents can offer a special challenge. The structure of an adolescent's day highlights the need for some stability in the teen's language input. These students need more time than short classes allow. In addition, each teacher's contact with individual students is limited to class periods. No one teacher is responsible for the teen's overall language functioning and success.

Essential to any successful adolescent program is destigmatization and the awarding of academic credit. Rooms selected for language group classes should be mixed with other classes. Classes should have names similar to other classes, such as "oral communication skills," rather than "speech therapy." The giving of credit aids motivation and gives the SLP clout and credibility.

Instructional Approaches

The overall intervention model might incorporate elements of two instructional approaches called strategy-based and systems models. The **strategy-based intervention** model assumes that learning problem-solving strategies is more powerful than learning factual content and will generalize more readily. Teaching includes strategies for verbal mediation and for the organization and retrieval of linguistic information. Verbal mediation is verbalizing the steps being used to accomplish a task. This model is highly appealing because of its potential for generalization outside the intervention setting.

In contrast, a **systems model** assumes that the source of the language impairment lies in the interactions of the child, the primary caregivers, and the content to be learned. Intervention strategies reflect the child's varying learning needs across several learning contexts.

Although classroom group intervention may suffice for some children with mild language problems, others will need individual services. This service can be accomplished in the classroom, through the more traditional pull-out model, or both. The functional conversational model is still very appropriate, as noted in Chapter 9.

Linguistic Awareness Intervention within the Classroom

In addition to providing individual or group services within the curriculum and the classroom setting, an SLP can increase linguistic awareness itself for all children. Within such activities, an SLP can be especially mindful of the needs of those children with LI. Each child should be encouraged to participate at her or his ability level.

Preschool

Nearly 60 percent of 3- to 5-year-old children in the United States attend center-based childcare and education programs (U.S. Department of Education, National Center for Education Statistics, 2006). Participation in high-quality preschool programs has the potential to equalize some early gaps in academic, social, cognitive, and language development for children who are at risk.

While a language-intense preschool curriculum may provide some added benefit for children with LI in accelerating their expressive language growth, such programs alone do not address the deficits associated with LI (Justice, Mashburn, Pence, & Wiggins, 2008). In other words, they are no substitute for intervention. Child language outcomes can be more readily improved through targeted intervention that is delivered within the preschool classroom setting's language-rich curriculum (van Kleeck, Vander Woude, & Hammett, 2006; Wasik, Bond, & Hindman, 2006)

Classroom teachers are a critical "first line" of intervention as they interact in an ongoing fashion with children. Preschool SLPs can provide professional development to teachers in the form of language-stimulating strategies for use within their classrooms (Girolametto, Weitzman, & Greenberg, 2003). Two contexts for intervention are classroom activities and instructional processes. Classroom activities include activities structures by teachers across the school day through a combination of materials, props, and physical classroom organization. These may include art, dramatic play, storybook reading, large- and small-group activities, music, and free-choice centers, such as a computer or discovery area.

Instructional processes complement the teachers' use of the specified activity contexts, especially the interactions that take place between adults and children, and might include use of strategies presented in Table 12.7. Some of these strategies have been discussed before in a more general context in Chapter 10.

Language-focused curricula are designed to improve at-risk preschool children's language outcomes through targeted improvements to both classroom activity contexts and instructional processes. Within these preschool classrooms, teachers find it easier to adhere to methods in activity contexts than to modify their behavior in instructional processes (Pence, Justice, & Wiggins, 2008).

To help adult language facilitators acquire, refine, or enhance their intervention skills or strategies, the SLP coaches them through the use of modeling, demonstration, and feedback techniques mentioned elsewhere in this text. In general, **coaching** is a process of observing, demonstrating, and providing feedback that can result in the acquisition and use of the skills necessary to provide effective intervention. Coaching offers the opportunity for individualized instruction and assistance, and its positive outcomes are well documented in early childhood intervention (Hanft, Rush, & Shelden, 2004). By training teachers and other adults, the SLP increases the chances that training will occur throughout the day in a variety of daily activities. In other words, embedded learning opportunities (ELOs) will occur in sufficient number and across sufficient numbers of activities to aid learning and generalization. The challenge is for the SLP and adult to create varied and multiple ELOs designed and implemented in a way that leads to improved outcomes for each child (Dinnebeil, Pretti-Frontczak, & McInemey, 2009).

To be maximally effective, the teacher and SLP must create a classroom environment that is warm, inviting, and instructive, and one in which positive and productive social interactions between adults and children occur on a regular basis while actively engaged in multiple learning opportunities (Petersen, 2003; Pianta et al., 2005). In addition, adults with whom children with disabilities spend

TABLE 12.7 Strategies for Classroom Use

Strategy	Explanation	Example
Event casts	Adult provides an running description of an activity or event	*Now we're pouring the dough into the pan.*
Expansions	Adult repeats child's utterance in a more mature form, providing additional semantic information	Child: *I had birthday.* Adult: *Yes, you had a birthday party last week.*
Focused contrasts	Adult highlights contrasts between language targets	*Yes, I am eating cookies and you are eating a cupcake.*
Modeling	Adult emphasizes language targets not used independently by the child.	*You rolled the ball and knocked over the dinosaurs.*
Open-ended questions	Adult asks questions with a variety of possible answers	*What should we do next?*
Recasts	Adult repeats the child's utterance with varied syntax	Child: *Sing song.* Adult: *That's right, yesterday we sang songs together.*
Redirects/prompted initiations	Adult prompts child to initiate interaction with a peer	*Juan is playing with the cars and you want to play. Ask Juan, "Can I play?"*
Scripted play	Adult provides appropriate verbalizations within familiar events	*Thank you. Here's your change. Drive to the next window* (Playing fast food drive-thru)

Source: Information from Pence, Justice, & Wiggins (2008).

the majority of their time must have the knowledge and skills and access to the resources necessary to support children's learning appropriately (Dinnebeil et al., 2009).

In order for SLPs and teachers to work effectively, they must have

- clear or consistent expectations of roles and responsibilities.
- sufficient uninterrupted time to consult.

For their part, SLPs must be confident and comfortable in their role and able to (Dinnebeil et al., 2009)

- work well with other people.
- share and gather information appropriately.
- use active listening strategies and respond appropriately to their partners.
- accurately assess and respond to the needs of others.

In addition, effective SLPs assume that teachers come together with them in a collaborative spirit that seeks to do the best they can for children.

Let's focus our discussion on preliterate activities as an illustration. Whole class, preschool, preliterate activities may include replica and role-play, narrative development, and the use of children's books. Each contributes to the general notion of narration and narrative form and is an important later development for literacy.

Replica and Role-Play. Play and narrative development are very similar. For children developing normally, the language of social make-believe play and the language of literacy have similar functions.

Language must be modified for the audience or participants, meaning must be conveyed, language is elaborated, and there are cohesive ties and integrated themes.

The imaginative function of language is acquired during preschool through social interactional play. The language is very explicit in order to convey meaning crucial to directing such play ("You be the baby now"). Language is used to refer to objects within the situation ("*This is* my horse") and to negotiate and compromise ("Okay, you can talk like that if you're the baby"). Integrated themes are evident in the beginnings and ends of play episodes, in the temporal organization, and in the enactment of everyday events or previously heard or seen narratives.

Imaginative language is heavily influenced by context. Both preschool boys and girls prefer replica toys, such as dolls, a simulated store, dress-up, and boys also prefer blocks. Replica toys reflect the real word. Toys generally are used as props for their intended purposes.

Unfortunately, many children with disabling conditions do not play like children developing typically. Sometimes, they do not have the experiential base for play. As a result, children with LI often are isolated in the regular preschool class, engaging in solitary play. Given the importance of play for later narrative development, it is essential that these children have normalizing play interactions.

Prior to beginning social play training, an SLP must plan the event carefully. First, he or she must create a play script. Theme selection should be based on a child's familiarity with the theme or script and the child's level of play. It is best to begin with everyday events. Table 12.8 presents events based on familiarity. For a child unfamiliar with replica play, the SLP might select getting ready for school or going to the market. By providing a supportive context, familiar routines provide natural events within which language can occur.

Some events emphasize roles; others emphasize sequences. For example, riding on the school bus is more role-dependent, while making a cake is sequential. Different types of events should be chosen over time to aid generalization.

A note of caution is in order. Event representations vary with cultures. A child in a preschool classroom from a different culture may not readily adapt to the event chosen.

Next, the SLP determines each child's involvement and develops the script. Children unfamiliar with play should be involved in planning so that the play can be explained and to provide some contextual reference. The script should begin with one sequence and progress to multischeme events. More detail should be added gradually, along with more story grammar components.

Once children have progressed through this type of replica play, they can reenact selected texts from children's books. Appendix F includes a list of children's books for reading and enactment. The use of literature is discussed in following sections.

TABLE 12.8 Themes for Training Replica Play

Every Day	Once in a While	Very Seldom	Fantasy*
Getting ready for school	Baking a cake	Going to the zoo	Being the teacher (police, grocer, mommy, etc.)
Getting dressed	Having a birthday party	Going to the circus	Being a dinosaur
Eating lunch	Going to a birthday party	Seeing a parade	Going to Mars
Riding on the school bus	Getting a haircut	Going on a boat ride	Piloting a plane
Going in the car	Going to the doctor	Going on an airplane	Being a caveman hunting animals
Getting a bath	Going to the market	Visiting ____	Painting a picture
	Celebrating (holiday)	Going to an amusement park	Flying with wings
	Going to church or temple	Going to a show/ concert	
	Eating at McDonald's		

*To preschool children.

Decisions will need to be made about roles, props, repetitive elements in the narrative, and elaboration. In general, children with LI should be assigned initially to more familiar roles. Props should be real objects, such as empty product containers and clothing. Gradually, roles can be modified and reassigned, and prop use can become more decontextualized and symbolic.

Table 12.9 presents a possible format for the training of play. The script is presented first in such a way as to provide a context for play. General play and the specific theme of this particular play are discussed with children, the adult models the appropriate roles, and children re-create the event. This step is replayed many times with varying roles and elaboration of the basic theme.

At each juncture, children are encouraged to describe and discuss the event enacted. The language of such group discussion and decision making is important for school success and helps more firmly stabilize learning.

Narrative Development. Training for narrative development and production is similar in many ways to that for play and may occur at the same time or following more elaborate forms of replica play. Gradually, the events in play become more decontextualized through the use of puppets or cutouts and imaginary or substituted objects. Children can take turns narrating the story as it continues.

After decontextualized enactment, the narrative might be repeated by the adult and retold by the children. With retelling, sequences can become even more elaborated so that a familiar event such as getting ready for school is modified with late arising, no clean socks, burnt toast, no toothpaste, a flat tire, and so on. Preschoolers may need to be cautioned to stay within the story frame. You do not get attacked by giants at the market nor rescued by the Transformers on the school bus.

Gradually, the SLP can introduce stories with familiar event sequences that have not been enacted by the children. These, too, can be retold and modified by the children. Finally, children's literature can be used and these narratives retold by the children.

Children's Literature. Significant differences exist in the activities and interactions with print for children with LI and those developing typically. These differences are reflected in the poorer letter

TABLE 12.9 Sequence of Sociodramatic Script Training

Step 1: Present script.
Step 2: Model roles including spoken parts.
Step 3: Have children re-present event and script. If needed, teacher prompts children for turn changes and for what to say and do. Prompting decreases over time.
Prompts for motor-gestural response.
Tell child what to do and give full physical prompt.
Gradually decrease the prompt to a partial one and then to a physical assist.
Tell child what to do and gesture or point.
Tell child what to do.
Point or gesture.
Ask child, "What do you do next?"
Prompts for verbal response.
Ask child to imitate and present child with model ("You say, 'I want a hamburger' ").
Ask child to imitate and present a partial model ("You say. 'I want ...' ").
Tell child it's his/her turn and gesture or point.
Point or gesture.
Repeat prior child's behavior and ask, "What do you say?"
Ask, "What do you say to X (other child's role)?"
Step 4: When children are familiar with roles, reassign.
Offer fewer prompts.
Step 5: Modify roles and script.

knowledge, interactive reading skills, story-listening abilities, and discussion of reading skills of children with LI. The normalizing benefits of interactive reading with these children are very important.

Sharing children's literature with preschoolers is not just reading to them. Prereading, reading, and postreading activities can enhance the experience and make it more meaningful, while bonding the class together.

Children's literature must be presented to children within a framework that makes sense for each child. Books should be introduced by their title and related to world knowledge that children already possess. The following is an introduction to *Brown Bear, Brown Bear, What Do You See?*:

> I'm going to read a book today called *Brown Bear, Brown Bear, What Do You See*? This is the cover. First, what is a bear? It's like a ... That's right, Angel. Angel said a bear is like a big dog. Where does he live? Does he live in your house? No, he *doesn't* live in your house. Does he live in your neighborhood? Good, Antonio shook his head "No." He doesn't live in your neighborhood. I wonder if he lives in the woods. Yes, he lives in the woods. And in the zoo, good, Shawna.
>
> Now, this bear is brown; he has brown hair. Who has brown hair? John, point to someone with brown hair. That's your hair, John. Point to ... yes, Billie Sue has brown hair. Put up your hand if you have brown hair. Good, Maria ... and Katie ... and Michel. And my hair is ... That's right, Angel, black hair just like yours.
>
> Well, our bear has brown hair. Here's a tough one: Do bears have any other color hair? ...

As is obvious, the children can bring a lot of information to the task. When the story is read subsequently, each child can use her or his personal knowledge to interpret the story.

Notice in my example that some children were allowed to respond by pointing. The SLP can ensure that every child has an opportunity to participate and facilitates their success by structuring their participation.

Often, children with LI do not understand books, temporal and causal sequences, story grammars, or logical consequences. The SLP can guide them in constructing their narrative representation.

Within the classroom, books might be used for chanting, rhyming, or predicting activities or for specific language targets. Art activities, sequential memory, and consequential language (*if ... then*) can follow reading. These activities and several resource books are listed in Appendix F. Books can be discussed with children at several levels of discourse and semantic complexity. These levels are presented in Table 12.10.

School-Age and Adolescent

Schools require extensive language skills from their students. Reading and writing are an essential part of the educational system. SLPs can encourage language use and aid development for those experiencing difficulties by actively engaging in classroom intervention. Skills targeted in intervention sessions can be enhanced in classroom application. Classroom linguistic awareness activities might include structuring classroom activities for success and metapragmatics. When asked to identify language targets that would facilitate successful communication interactions in high school, teachers highlighted the following as most important: relating narratives, presenting differing points of view or thoughts logically, employing conversation clarification and repair strategies, taking a conversational partner's perspective, and taking turns appropriately (Reed & Spicer, 2003).

To be successful, adolescents must have the ability to use and understand spoken and written language at an advanced level. Throughout the school day and beyond, adolescents are expected to use and understand language in a sophisticated manner. So it is not surprising that teens with LI frequently have poor academic performance and limited vocational options (Conti-Ramsden & Durkin, 2008; Nippold, 2007; Snowling, Bishop, & Stothard, 2000).

TABLE 12.10 Levels of Discourse and Semantic Complexity

Discourse levels of book discussion	
Collection:	Relatively unorganized list
Descriptive list:	Utterances coordinated through a central topic
Ordered sequence	Organized by temporal order
Reactive sequence:	Organized causally
Abbreviated structure:	Includes psychological intent and planning
Semantic complexity of book discussion	
Indication:	Nonlinguistic signals, such as pointing
Label:	Naming concrete, observable objects and agents
Description:	Characteristics and relationships
Interpretation:	Observable characteristics used to refer to internal states, motivations, and underlying qualities
Inference:	Own background used to go beyond observable characteristics in a situation
Evaluation:	Likes/dislikes, justifications, summarizations
Metalanguage:	Language applied to reflect on the way language is organized and used

Structuring Classroom Activities. When children find school too frustrating, success too elusive, they give up. Different learning contexts within the classroom can reduce feelings of failure. For example, a noncompetitive environment can keep students task-involved, rather than ego-involved. Motivation is the key. Motivated students are more persistent.

An SLP can make all students aware of the metacognitive and metalinguistic aspects of learning and employ strategies that enhance their application. He or she can explicitly teach learning strategies and provide guided practice and feedback. Each student can be guided and encouraged to participate at his or her functioning level.

Students can be aided in recognizing the features that influence comprehension and recall and the processing and retrieval demands of a task. General comprehension strategies to be taught include self-monitoring, drawing inferences, and resolving ambiguities. Study strategies that might be targeted include paraphrasing, summarizing, and note taking.

Metapragmatics. Children with LI are often unpopular and may seem odd or out of place in the day-to-day communication so common in the classroom. Among teenagers, perspective taking, comprehension of tonal changes signaling emotion, and nonverbal communication are considered important communication skills. Everyday communication is important for classroom success and can be improved by intervention focusing on metapragmatics.

Metapragmatic awareness is a conscious awareness of the ways to use language effectively and appropriately. More precisely, it is the knowledge of common ways of communicating, the ability to detect and judge inconsistencies, inadequacies, and failures, and the flexibility to change communication behaviors in order to increase efficiency. An SLP can improve metapragmatic awareness by presenting examples of good and poor communication, discussing the differences with students, and role-playing appropriate communication. Video-recorded examples of communication may also be employed. Gentle critiques and self-evaluation are essential.

With the entire class, an SLP helps students identify their communication goal and produce fluent, flexible, and efficient speech and language to reach that goal. The mature speaker is able to take and express another person's perspective and simultaneously formulate and test several communication hypotheses for effective language use. Within intervention, students can be taught to recognize patterns of social communication, to develop options and evaluate their effectiveness, and to organize communication behaviors to integrate communication goals, strategies, and perspectives.

Using scripted social drama as the vehicle for holistic training, an SLP can guide students through the following four steps of training (Wiig, 1995):

1. Awareness of pragmatic features and underlying plans, scripts, and schemes. For example, topic initiations can be signaled by phrases such as *That reminds me . . . , Speaking of . . . , You know . . . , Well . . . , and By the way.*
2. Extending pragmatic awareness to real-life situations.
3. Generalization training across different media, contexts, and partners.
4. Self-directed training to foster independence.

At each level and following each scripted drama, the SLP and students discuss feelings and reactions, identify alternative strategies, and apply the lessons learned to communication situations within their own lives. The SLP acts as coach while providing scaffolding and support.

Conversational narratives may be taught in a similar manner by first identifying the purpose of a narrative and then constructing the appropriate form to fulfill that function. Children can be helped to identify the cohesive ties, such as sequencing, word substitutions, conjunctions, and topic-comment relationships.

Syntactic structures also can be taught within verbal interactions. Awareness activities might begin with modeling. The SLP can "think out loud" and discuss his or her options in a given conversation. Embedded within highly interesting conversations, other activities might include sentence combining and detection and correction of errors.

Summary

An SLP can provide classroom language instruction that addresses the needs of the entire class while enabling every child to participate. The SLP can provide the linguistic scaffolding that teachers often neglect, thus helping children become meaning makers and be successful. In addition, he or she can provide preteaching for the child with LI, helping that child be successful.

Language Facilitation

Language facilitation includes (a) noting vocabulary of the classroom, (b) identifying the needs of certain contexts and giving children the opportunity to experience this context successfully, and (c) talking to children in ways that facilitate growth and highlight production. The classroom is a special context with its own demands. Facilitative techniques can be used there and in conversational interactions between children and their teachers, parents, and peers.

Vocabulary of the Classroom

Early word learning is highly related to frequency of input. Therefore, children growing up with varying input will develop different vocabularies (deVilliers, 2004). As a consequence, children from socially, culturally, and linguistically diverse backgrounds often struggle in mainstream school settings because of exposure to different vocabulary and to different emphasis on which words are central to their life experiences and ways of understanding.

Children with low socioeconomic backgrounds often are limited in the experiences needed to build background knowledge for vocabulary growth because experiences provided to these children are more limited overall than for those with greater economic resources. Early differences in children's vocabulary knowledge grow into larger ones in school-age and may be difficult to modify without intervention (Biemiller, 2001; National Institute of Child Health and Human Development Early Child Care Research Network, 2005).

As individuals learn language they learn the meanings of their culture. Children's early word learning reflects the values, expectations, and rules of their microculture. The language patterns of the group will influence the communication patterns a child develops. This may place children from ethnically diverse backgrounds at risk of academic failure because their word meanings may differ from those of the school environment and hinder their ability to be successful in literacy activities.

Classroom Language Requirements

Often, the type of language used in the classroom is very different from what a child experiences at home. For example, the teacher's language consists of many indirect requests and statements. Questions or statements such as "Can you show us where the answer is written?" and "I can't hear Lori because others are being impolite" contain requests or demands. In the classroom, the teacher asks questions that require responses. Certain question forms are difficult for children with LI. Table 12.11 presents ten rules for classroom participation.

The skill of knowing how to get things done in the classroom is not usually taught to children, but rather is taken for granted by teachers. The lack of such knowledge can be problematic for a child with LI asked to work with others to accomplish some task.

A child must be able to request and give information, action, and materials and to make judgments on the correct language and communication behaviors in and out of context. Each child is expected to be able to identify the information needed by all involved to complete a task and also to judge the appropriateness of information that is given.

Classroom language functions include the following:

- Relating socially to others while stating personal needs.
- Directing others and self.
- Requesting and giving information.
- Reasoning, judging, and predicting.
- Imagining and projecting into nonclassroom situations.

Relating socially to others while stating one's own needs contains a number of behavior categories, such as referring to psychological or physical needs ("I want to leave now" or "I'm hungry"), protecting one's self and self-interest ("That's mine"), agreeing or disagreeing ("You're wrong"), and expressing an opinion ("I hated that dessert").

The "directing self and others" function includes the categories of directing one's own actions, directing the actions of others, collaborating in the actions of others ("You be the mommy, and I'll be the daddy"), and requesting direction ("How do you do this?"). The directing function can be elicited

TABLE 12.11 Rules for Classroom Participation

Rules for Classroom Participation
Teachers mostly talk and students mostly listen, except when teachers grant permission to talk.
Teachers give cues about when to listen closely.
Teachers convey content about things and procedures about how to do things.
Teachers' talk becomes more complex in the upper grades.
Teachers ask questions and expect specific responses.
Teachers give hints about what is correct and what is important to them.
Student talk is brief and to the point.
Students ask few questions and keep them short.
Students talk to teachers, not to other students.
Students make few unsolicited comments and only about the process or content of the lesson.

Source: Information from Sturm & Nelson (1997).

by requiring children to accomplish tasks of varying difficulty. There will also be a need to direct others and to follow others' directions.

The "giving information" function includes labeling ("That's a piñata"), referring to events ("Yesterday, we got a kitty"), referring to detail ("That kitty is black and white"), sequencing ("We went to the party, and then we went to the movies"), making comparisons ("Yours is bigger"), and extracting the general point ("We're making Hanukkah presents"). This function occurs when the child shares an experience with someone who did not originally experience it, as in show-and-tell. If the classroom discussion involves activities in which the entire class has participated, children do not feel the need for relayed information to be as precise or detailed.

Requests for information vary with the type of information sought. For example, adults and children tend to use more direct requests when there are few, if any, obstacles to receiving the answer, as in checking short answers to problems. In this situation, the request is very direct: "What's the answer to number 4?"

As children mature, they learn to identify the type of information needed to help a requester. In general, children become more aware of the importance of information specificity. Children are also more likely with maturity to provide information on the process of solving a certain problem, rather than just the answer requested. In responding to the previous question about problem number 4, the child might try to presuppose the difficulties of the requester and respond, "5/8; I converted to 8ths after solving the problem in 16ths." School-age children who provide specific information and process explanations are more likely to be high achievers.

The "reasoning, judging, and predicting" function includes explaining a process ("When you get lost, you should find a police officer"), recognizing causal relationships ("The bridge fell because it was weak"), recognizing problems and solutions ("This box is too small; get another one"), drawing conclusions ("We couldn't finish the project because there wasn't enough glue"), and anticipating results ("If we pull this cord, the bell should ring"). In general, problem-solving tasks, such as designing or building an object, will elicit this function. Problem solving includes predicting, testing hypotheses, and drawing conclusions.

Finally, the "imagining and projecting" function includes projecting feeling onto others ("I think Carlos is afraid of the ghost") and imagining events in real life or fantasy ("I'm captain of the spaceship *Izits*. All aboard"). This function can be elicited by fantasy play.

Many activities can be projected into imaginings by asking children to imagine that they are some character in a story or what they would do in a particular situation. With older children, different situations can be role-played.

To be successful, children must be able to use all of these language functions with some facility. As noted, activities can be designed to aid this growth.

Talking with Children

Adult interactions with children should facilitate language growth and learning. In a nonthreatening way, whenever possible, the SLP should observe and comment on the use of language by teachers and parents. Teachers are often unaware of the effect their language has on the processing of children with LI. For example, teachers' oral directions can contain a large proportion of figurative expressions and indirect requests that are difficult for children with L1.

Teachers tend to respond to children with LI below the optimal level. In general, teachers reply infrequently and, often, in a manner that terminates the interaction. The teacher's frequent use of directives also may limit child–teacher interactions.

The SLP can efficiently introduce teachers, aides, and parents to facilitative conversational techniques at in-service training sessions or parent meetings. The SLP should help teachers, aides, and parents understand the importance of adult modeling and responding to communicative behaviors. He or she should attempt to decrease a directive style in favor of a more conversational approach.

TABLE 12.12 Guide for Parents' and Teachers' Interactive Style

1.	Talk about things that the child is interested in.
2.	Follow the child's lead. Reply to the child's initiations and comments. Share his or her excitement.
3.	Don't ask too many questions. If you must, use questions such as *how did/do . . . , why did/do . . . ,* and *what happened . . .* that result in longer explanatory answers.
4.	Encourage the child to ask questions. Respond openly and honestly. If you don't want to answer a question, say so and explain why. (*I don't think I want to answer that question: It's very personal.*)
5.	Use a pleasant tone of voice. You need not be a comedian, but you can be light and humorous. Children love it when adults are a little silly.
6.	Don't be judgmental or make fun of a child's language. If you are overly critical of the child's language or try to "shotgun" all errors, the child will stop talking to you.
7.	Allow enough time for the child to respond.
8.	Treat the child with courtesy by not interrupting when he or she is talking.
9.	Include the child in family and classroom discussions. Encourage participation and listen to his or her ideas.
10.	Be accepting of the child and of the child's language. Hugs and acceptance can go a long way.
11.	Provide opportunities for the child to use language and to have that language work for him or her to accomplish goals.

The SLP can provide teachers, aides, and parents with examples of good interactive styles. A handout, such as that in Table 12.12, is often helpful. The SLP should stress the importance of different facilitator behaviors and the need to tailor techniques to the child's individual style and language level. Whenever possible, the SLP should model these techniques for teachers, aides, and parents.

Peers as Facilitators. Classmates developing typically can serve well as models and can be taught functional strategies that promote interaction. Sociodramatic or replica play can provide a basis for interaction for preschoolers. With school-age children, many alternative activities can foster interaction and carryover.

One small set of facilitative principles to use with preschool peers can be stated as *stay, play, talk* (Goldstein, English, Shafer, & Kaczmarek, 1997):

Stay close to your buddy

Play together, use the other child's name, and attend to the same objects

Talk while you stay and play

This phrase plus adult modeling, guided practice, and independent practice with feedback and discussion of what it means to be a buddy and of the unconventional communication of some children can provide a model for effective peer training.

School-age TD classmates can be taught to increase communication interaction using a few simple steps. Questions seem to facilitate naturally occurring communication more than directive prompts, although males with ID respond more to comments by peers. Although specific techniques for cuing and prompting can be taught to peers, these are relatively ineffective and time-consuming to teach. The fewer strategies taught, the better.

One effective method, presented in Table 12.13, is to teach interactive strategies rather than teaching techniques to the TD peer and then to prompt and reinforce these strategies. This approach can increase interactions and on-topic responses by children with LI. Several precautions seem relevant. Strategies should do all of the following:

- Include only behaviors observed in high-quality interactions.
- Have a high likelihood of inducing the subsequent behavior.
- Not place the child with LI in a subservient role.
- Not target language features that take a great deal of effort or time to teach.
- Have the potential to produce balanced and sustainable interactions.
- Optimize typical social interaction, not simplify it.

Peer strategies reportedly continue when teacher prompts decline. Peers can also serve as effective tutors in narrative learning (McGregor, 2000).

School-age peers can be encouraged to interact through cooperative learning, homework monitoring, and language contracts. Cooperative learning fosters interdependence and individual accountability while encouraging face-to-face interactions and interpersonal skills. Students with different language abilities are paired for classroom language projects and rewarded for group achievement.

In homework monitoring, a child who has the skills needed to accomplish the assignment helps a child with LI. The SLP works with both to help them complete their homework, uses role-play to teach the tutor and tutored roles to the tutoring peers, and critiques role-played interactions between the tutors. In addition, the SLP monitors the peers when actual tutoring begins.

Finally, language contracts can be used to decrease inappropriate language behavior. Both the child with LI and the classroom peers must be able to identify the behavior and understand the need to decrease its occurrence. For example, one child with mild ASD continually touched other children annoyingly. The contract with the class defines the behavior and specifies the cues to reduce the behavior and to elicit a more desirable behavior. It is helpful in eliciting peer cooperation that the class be solicited for suggestions for decreasing the behavior. The contract is reviewed periodically and peers reinforced for success.

Classroom Support for Working Memory in Children with SLI

A first step for the SLP in supporting a child in the classroom is observing and analyzing the working memory (WM) demands of both classroom discourse and assignments (Boudreau & Costanza-Smith, 2011). Most important is identifying learning contexts in which WM limitations are most

TABLE 12.13 Training Peers as Facilitators in Preschool Classrooms

Step 1: Teach peer to interact.
Introduction
Explain purpose: To help friend "talk" better.
Model with another adult.
Direct instruction.
Children rehearse and adults critique.
Adults take role of child with disabilities.
Posters provide reminders.
Step 2: Prompt and reinforce use of strategies taught. Gradual change with less adult input and fewer peer facilitators and more children with disabilities.
Teacher prompts ("Remember to have your friend look at you first," "Remember to point").
Adults should try not to interrupt too much–inhibits children.
Whisper or point to posters.

Source: Information from Goldstein & Strain (1988).

likely to influence performance. As mentioned previously, greater WM demands are placed on a child when he or she is asked to store a considerable amount of information while at the same time engaging in mental operations related to that information. A child is most likely to experience difficulties with classroom instruction that is lengthy and does not reflect a routine classroom activity, activities that require both storage and processing of information, and writing activities that involve generating sentences or writing to dictation (Gathercole, Alloway, Willis, & Adams, 2006). The SLP will want to pay particular attention to the language of classroom instruction, noting how which information is delivered, assignments communicated, and participation facilitated (Boudreau & Costanza-Smith, 2011). Although significant attention to the WM demands of the language arts curriculum is warranted, it is important to remember that WM demands are not limited to reading and writing activities.

The SLP will also want to consider the WM demands within classroom texts and other materials. For example, complex narratives place more demand on a child than simple narratives, resulting in poorer performance in both narrative production and comprehension (Boudreau, 2007). Narratives used in the curriculum can be analyzed for the difficulty of language, the number of episodes, and the intricacies of plot and interaction of characters. Texts can be especially problematic if they contain complex sentences that place greater demand on WM than simple sentences do (Montgomery & Evans, 2009; Thordardottir, 2008). If a child must commit a great deal of mental resources to the comprehension of words or syntactic structure, then it is likely that fewer resources will be available to integrate the content with previous information.

Analysis of classroom demands also includes identifying supports and strategies currently in place that reduce WM demands (Boudreau & Costanza-Smith, 2011). These include visual supports and teaching practices that can reduce memory load. In turn, the SLP can inform teachers of ways in which these supports facilitate learning for children with WM deficits.

Four ways that SLPs can support the learning of children with WM deficits are by addressing teacher discourse strategies, visual support, preteaching, and breaking learning tasks smaller steps (Boudreau & Costanza-Smith, 2011). Teachers can present material in a manner that directs a child's attention and reduces overload on WM. Possible strategies are presented in Table 12.14.

The use of visual supports can also reduce WM demands in some learning contexts. I should caution that research is unclear as to whether visuospatial WM skills are also compromised in children

TABLE 12.14 Strategies to Use for Working Memory in the Classroom

- Repeat key points to assist child in knowing what is most important from a story, lecture, or discussion and provide child an opportunity to store key information in memory.
- Chunk information, such as periodic summarization of key content, to help reduce WM demands.
- Set clear expectations of what is expected in a task or assignment or what a child will be asked to do with information being presented or discussed. The child with WM deficits may also benefit from an example of the expected outcome of an assignment.
- Check a child's perceived understanding of an assignment.
- Request that a child restate the directions in his or her own words or demonstrate what he or she believes are the directions.
- Provide checklists or written lists of key steps to be accomplished in a classroom assignment or task.
- Reduce the rate of instruction, especially when new concepts are introduced. Slower rate results in better word learning in children with LI.
- Modify discussion characteristics to allow child with WM deficits to be an early contributor or to recap key points before asking the child to contribute. Asking a student to contribute after several contributors requires a child to hold prior information while formulating a response.

Source: Information from Boudreau & Costanza-Smith (2011); Gathercole et al. (2006); Horohov & Oetting (2004); Rankin & Hood (2005).

with LI. Nevertheless, visual support, especially when providing information related to assignments and when teaching new information, may help reduce WM demands. Children with poor WM skills may be more successful if a teacher uses gesture, written instructions, keyword lists, check-off forms, and object manipulation (Quail, Williams, & Leitao, 2009). Interestingly, physical manipulation of objects that correspond with written text can enhance reading comprehension in elementary-age children (Glenberg, Brown, & Levin, 2007; Glenberg, Jaworksi, & Rischal, 2005).

Demands on WM can also be reduced by preteaching key concepts. This might include providing background and related knowledge, such as relevant vocabulary and literate language features of a text. By providing this information, the teacher is enabling a child to dedicate relatively more WM resources to learning new material (Klingner, Vaughn, & Boardman, 2007).

Finally, children with WM deficits are likely to do better if tasks can be broken into smaller steps. By reducing the amount of information a child must process or store, complex tasks can be accomplished one step at a time with each part being a small piece of the larger whole (Gathercole & Alloway, 2008).

Instituting a Classroom Model

The transition from pull-out service to classroom-based, or "push-in," service takes careful planning. Central to success is the resolution of the following issues:

- Training of the SLP
- Training of other professionals
- Establishment of a clear source of authority and responsibility for intervention
- Administrative support in the form of adequate space, scheduled time slots, and financial commitment
- Identification criteria for students to receive services based not on standardized test scores but on classroom language processing and use
- Responsibility for IEPs

It may take three to five years to fully implement a collaborative classroom intervention model. The process is one of evolution. It is essential to begin slowly and to prepare parents and other professionals for the change.

The final model will vary with student needs and teacher/SLP flexibility. The teacher and SLP will need to consult for general language activities and for specific language support of individual children.

First, the individual SLP must train him- or herself. This training includes education in the use of a functional conversational approach and in the school curriculum. This text provides one step in that education. Workshops, convention presentations, observation, and further professional reading are also essential. In addition, the SLP should role-play the use of various techniques because they differ considerably from the more traditional behavioral patterns.

Classroom teachers can help the SLP become familiar with small and large group instruction. Possibly, the SLP could spend an hour per week in some group activity within a classroom.

Second, the SLP will need to recruit teachers and enlist administrative support. Informational meetings, breakfasts, and parent meetings can be used with demonstrations and video-recorded presentations. Administrators can be approached individually. The SLP can present a rationale for collaborative teaching, share scheduling, send brief memos of very successful interventions, invite administrators to attend sessions, and request time for discussion at parent events.

Third, the SLP must train other people. The initial purpose of this training is to educate teachers and administrators about the need for classroom intervention. This is best accomplished with in-service training stressing (a) the importance of the environment for nonimpaired language learning,

(b) questions of generalization, (c) the verbal nature of the classroom, (d) the practicality and efficiency of classroom intervention strategies, and (e) the need for and desirability of team approaches. A possible in-service training model is presented in Table 12.15.

Administrators may be reluctant to change current one-on-one pull-out services. A more functional classroom model can be presented emphasizing both inclusion and RTI. It is also important to remember that some children still will require pull-out services for special-skills training. Collaborative teaching is better suited to training of general communication skills. Goals and objectives, probably modest at first, should be established prior to implementation. At each step in implementation, administrators need to be kept informed of progress.

Several alternative models for collaboration are available. Peer coaching and co-teaching seem especially promising. In peer coaching, the SLP and the classroom teacher work as a team, coaching each other through observation and feedback, commenting on effective teaching strategies. In co-teaching, each professional focuses on his or her component of instruction on the basis of the curriculum goals of the class. The teacher and the SLP jointly determine student needs, develop goals and objectives and activities to meet them, implement these plans, and evaluate progress.

Once convinced of the need for such a model of intervention, teachers can begin to learn specific intervention techniques. These techniques may be introduced through in-service training, with individual instruction to follow. Videotaped lessons including children with LI are excellent training vehicles to demonstrate the use of various techniques. Professionals conducting the training

TABLE 12.15 In-service Training Model for Collaboarating Teachers and SLPs

Sessions	Description
1	Normal communication development and communication disorders in the classroom Help teachers understand development and the ways in which a communication disorder affects every aspect of classroom participation.
2	Language of the classroom Explain the collaborative model and the roles of the teacher and SLP. Help teachers understand how a communication problem makes participation difficult.
3	Scripts and identifying and managing classroom language demands Differentiate language arts from language intervention. Emphasize school "curriculums" and role of scripts in aiding participation. Stress (a) the process of language versus the product and (b) the need for a process approach to language problems.
4	Collaborative approach to identifying communication problems in the classroom Explain a curriculum-based approach. Describe the roles the teacher and SLP play in identifying students with potential communication problems.
5	Strategies for managing language Help teachers recognize the complexity of classroom language. Learn to adapt the curriculum to individual student needs. Learn strategies for collaborating to enhance a child's preformance.
6	Literacy problems Explain the oral language–written language link. Learn to recognize literacy problems. Learn strategies for using literacy in the classroom with children with literacy problems.
7	Issues in collaboaration Discuss roles, barriers, and issues of collaboration.

Source: Information from Prelock, Miller, & Reed (1995).

should be credible, knowledgeable, and practical. Appropriate materials and hands-on experience are essential to teacher training.

Fourth, clear lines of authority for language intervention must be established. It is vital to the success of this model that roles and responsibilities, as well as authority, be clearly established. This step requires administrative support and a definite statement of policy. New roles and responsibilities should be written into the curriculum, budget, and job descriptions. Responsibility is shared and roles shift within the classroom.

Fifth, administrative support in the form of space, scheduled time, and necessary financial outlays must be established. It is all too easy for administrators to declare a change in procedures without giving adequate support to ensure success.

The biggest single impediment to implementation is the lack of time. The SLP and the classroom teacher must allow time each week to discuss each child's success and to review targets and techniques.

Frequently, administrators have difficulty seeing the need to lessen dependence on standardized measures of language. Language test scores offer a quantifiable measure of behavior that can be used for determinations of student needs and progress. Yet, similar measurement can be made against the curriculum and from conversational samples. The implementation of this step requires the joint educational effort of the SLP and the classroom teacher.

Finally, IEPs will need to be written or modified to reflect the change in service delivery. Other members of the intervention team, including parents, will need to be educated on the rationale for such changes. Parents usually accept the classroom model when shown the increased service that their child will receive if the classroom teacher is also a language trainer. Many parents are also happy with the decreased amount of pull-out time.

The implementation phase should progress slowly and carefully because it is new to both the SLP and the classroom teacher. At first, one child in one classroom can be targeted. This can gradually be expanded to include several children in this classroom or one child in each of several classrooms.

The selection of the first classroom is critical. The SLP might begin with a best friend on the faculty, someone willing to learn, grow, and make mistakes. Teacher training should include SLP critiques of teacher use of training techniques. A checklist can ensure objectivity. It might be best for teachers to begin by attempting to integrate a child's newly acquired skills into the daily routine, rather than trying to teach new language skills.

The first class taught by the SLP should, likewise, begin cautiously. One goal per lesson is recommended. Later, individual IEP goals can be introduced through focused lessons with the whole class.

It's best to choose the initial child and classroom carefully to ensure some measure of success and to minimize friction with the classroom teacher. Once the SLP and the teacher begin to experience success, other teachers will be more willing to adopt the model.

There will always be administrators, classroom teachers, and/or parents who refuse to accept or cooperate with the implementation of the classroom model. Rather than become discouraged, the SLP should work with those individuals who accept the model and continue to try to educate those who do not. Usually, success with a few children is all that is needed to convince the foot-draggers. The key to success is your rapport with the educators involved.

Conclusion

Functional environmental approaches, as represented by the classroom model, are among the most progressive trends evidenced today. In many school districts throughout Canada and the United States, this model is a reality. Some districts are mandating the change from above, whereas others are experiencing a quiet revolution from below. No change as radical as this one can be accomplished without some difficulties.

The role of the SLP is changing. In many cases, SLPs are being asked to implement intervention models for which they have minimal training. Although such requests are expected in a professional field that is changing and growing as rapidly as speech-language pathology, it does highlight the need for continuing professional education.

Still, the SLP is the language expert responsible for identifying children with LI and for implementing intervention. In this new role of consultant, the SLP enhances this intervention process through others.

By itself, going into the classroom is only the most minimal of changes. In fact, data indicate that many SLPs engaged in a collaborative model are now modifying their intervention style to a more functional one. Although location, such as a classroom, was one of the variables of generalization addressed in the first chapter, it was not the only one. Functional intervention is conversational intervention. A truly functional approach uses language scaffolding techniques within real conversational contexts to accomplish communication goals.

Chapter 13

Literacy Impairments: Language in a Visual Mode

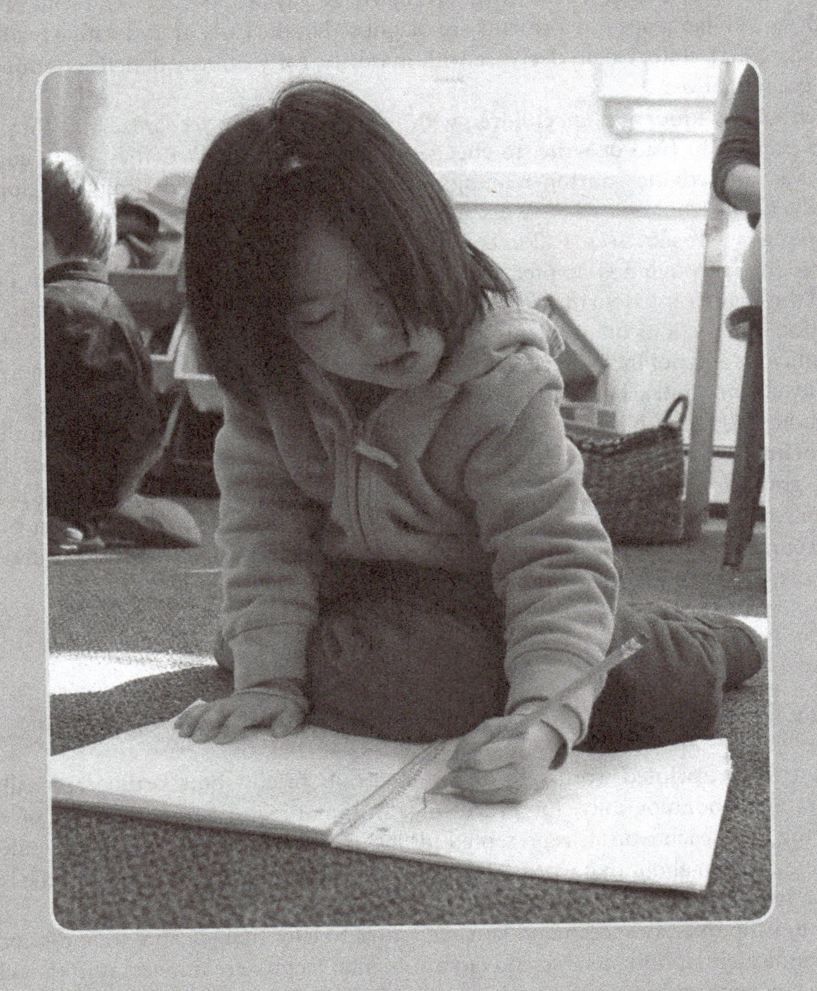

Children with LI are unprepared for literacy instruction because of a lack of preliteracy skills. Key indicators of this lack of skills can be found in their oral language and narrative ability, phonological awareness, alphabet knowledge, phoneme-grapheme (sound-letter) knowledge, spelling and orthographic knowledge, and word awareness (Justice, Invernizzi, & Meier, 2002).

Within a preschool or kindergarten setting, an SLP should (1) alert parents to the oral language-literacy relationship, (2) identify children at risk and notify parents, (3) refer parents to good literacy programs, and (4) recommend assessment and treatment in preliteracy skills, such as phonological awareness, letter knowledge, and literacy activities, when needed (Snow, Scarborough, & Burns, 1999). Within the school-age population, the SLP (1) continues to help children or adolescents develop a strong language base; (2) addresses difficulties in phonological awareness, memory, and retrieval; and (3) addresses difficulties individual children are encountering with both narrative and expository or curricular texts.

Children with language impairments are at greater risk for reading disability than TD children (Catts, Fey, Tomblin, & Zhang, 2002; Lewis Freebairn, & Taylor, 2000, 2002). From 40 to 65 percent of children with language impairments are diagnosed in the early grades with a reading disability (Catts et al., 2002). Rather than decrease with maturity, early literacy deficits continue to persist throughout the school years.

In preschool and kindergarten, children with LI are less able to recognize and copy letters and less likely to pretend to read or write, to engage in daily preliteracy activities, or to engage adults in question-answer activities during reading and writing than their typically developing peers. Unfortunately, many school-based SLPs are not providing any written language services to students with written language weaknesses (Fallon & Katz, 2011).

As we progress through this chapter, I shall address all the topics mentioned so far. For clarity, I have divided the chapter into two major sections, reading and writing. Within each, I have organized the information into sections on problems for children with LI, assessment, and intervention. I have tried to be judicious and not include regular reading and writing instruction, subjects more appropriately taught by classroom teachers and reading specialists.

Throughout this text, I have tried to take a top-down intervention approach. A similar strategy can be used in intervention with reading and writing. Obviously, some minimal phonics skills as well as phoneme–grapheme (sound–letter) knowledge are needed. Within guided reading practice, students can confront unknown words or grammatical structures and attempt to decipher the meaning from the surrounding text. They can be helped to read actively and to ask themselves questions about what they know, to summarize, predict, and interpret as they go.

Reading

For the skilled reader, printed words are represented only briefly, both orthographically through printed letters and phonologically, for processing. Automatic and below the level of consciousness most of the time, each word is represented for less than one-fourth of a second while the brain retrieves all information about that word. The process only becomes conscious when the reader tries to interpret an unfamiliar word based on the context.

The relationship of early speech and language skills to later literacy attainment is complicated. Twin studies indicate that both genetic and environmental factors are important in the relationship between early language skills and reading. In contrast, genetic factors alone seem to play a role in the relationship between early speech and reading (Hayiou-Thomas, Harlaar, Dale, & Plomin, 2010).

Reading ability is highly correlated with spelling ability. Poor readers tend to be poor spellers. Instruction and advances in one area help the other. Reading affects the memory for spelling, which in turn aids reading decoding.

Development of reading is a complex process based on the integration of its diverse components into a smooth and automatic foundation on which fluent reading and comprehension are based (Wolf, 2007). Phonological and orthographic processing are essential to word identification and linguistic and cognitive requirements are essential for fluent reading and comprehension of the text.

At another level of processing, language and world knowledge are used to derive an understanding of the text, much as one comprehends a spoken message. This comprehension process and the message being decoded are monitored automatically to ensure that the synthesized information makes sense.

Taken separately, neither word recognition nor comprehension is sufficient alone as an explanation of this developmental process. In order to fluently read and comprehend, multiple processes must be managed simultaneously (Bashir & Hook, 2009).

Fluency occurs as the rapid and accurate reading of a connected text is enabled by rapid retrieval of orthographic, phonological, and semantic processes, leading to an effective speed of reading to allow comprehension to occur (Wolf & Katzir-Cohen, 2001). The reallocation of attention from sub-word units, such as phonemes, to higher language and cognitive processes is essential for comprehension (Wolf & Katzir-Cohen, 2001). It would be simplistic to think of word identification abilities morphing automatically into text comprehension (Katzir et al., 2006; Torgesen, Rashotte, & Alexander, 2001; Wolf, 2007). The development of reading fluency depends on the interaction of multiple factors.

When something goes wrong in the reading process, it becomes less automatic and less fluent. Word decoding or understanding of language relationships expressed in the text may be impaired. Poor vocabulary may hinder understanding. Reading becomes labored and slow. The entire process may not make sense to some children, who may become frustrated and helpless.

Reading Problems

Good readers guide and control their behavior. It's purposeful and flexible. In contrast, poor readers lack such strategies. Many children who read poorly become passive, lacking persistence and accepting low self-esteem, and display apathy and resignation. Others will become aggressive or display acting-out behaviors. These affective problems interfere with subsequent learning and development.

Typically, children with SLI and LD who will later have written language impairment are slower in learning oral language during the preschool years. The oral language skills of children with ASD also parallel their reading development (Sénéchal, LeFevre, Smith-Chant, & Colton, 2001). Children with ASD may exhibit an uneven developmental profile predictive of reading behaviors. For example, a child may be able to decode words very effectively but not comprehend what is read.

Although children with ASD respond to phonological awareness and phonics instruction, they are likely to have persisting reading comprehension, spelling, and composition difficulties unless they receive instruction in morphological and syntactic awareness and comprehension strategy (Berninger, 2008). In contrast, children with a reading-based learning disorder usually have difficulty with phonological (sound) and orthographic (letter) coding in working memory, phonological decoding, and spelling, not with reading comprehension or syntax (Berninger, 2007a, 2007b, 2008).

Risk of difficulty with reading is greatest among children with a history of problems in both articulation and receptive and expressive language (Segebart DeThorne et al., 2006). In general, poor reading comprehenders have deficits in oral language comprehension but normal phonological abilities. On the other hand, children who are poor decoders have poor phonological abilities but little or no oral language comprehension difficulties (Catts, Adlof, & Ellis Weismer, 2006).

The relationship of early language difficulties and literacy problems may be more nuanced than a simple transference of problems to another modality. There seems to be an interaction between children's early reading abilities, their conversational language abilities, and their history of reported language difficulties (Segebart DeThorne, Petrill, Schatschneider, & Cutting, 2010). Conversational language skills contribute a small but significant amount to children's early reading.

Children with LI who have average or above-average intelligence may read initially by memorizing word shapes. However, without word attack or decoding skills, by second grade these children begin to fail. Serious reading comprehension problems may go unnoticed among beginning readers who have good phonological ability and appear to decode words well (Nation et al., 2004).

Children with LI tend to demonstrate a compensatory trajectory of reading development. This means children with LI have lower reading skills in preschool and overall reading growth that is faster than TD children as they try to compensate for their lower starting point. By fifth grade these children exhibit reading skills that are substantially lower than those of TD children.

Children with both speech and language difficulties, especially those who lack phoneme awareness at age 6, are at greater risk for literacy difficulties (Nathan, Stackhouse, Goulandris, & Snowling, 2004). Although children with LI in kindergarten are at greater risk for reading impairment, those whose spoken language abilities improve have better reading outcomes than those whose LI persists (Catts, Fey, Tomblin, & Zhang, 2002). As adolescents, poor readers also exhibit vocabulary, grammar, and verbal memory deficits in comparison with their TD peers (Rescorla, 2005).

Children with LI are at risk for reading impairment for several reasons (Hambly & Riddle, 2002; C. Miller et al., 2001):

- They begin with less language ability and have difficulty catching up.
- They have poor comprehension skills.
- Metalinguistic skills are not developing because of poor overall language skills.
- They have slower linguistic and overall information processing skills.

Most reading problems are related to deficient phonological processing. The errors of children with a reading-based learning disorder reflect the conventional English phonological system. Consonant clusters are especially difficult.

Phonological problems are often more severe in children with a reading-based learning disorder than in children with other forms of LI (Catts, Hogan, & Adlof, 2005). Although children with a reading-based learning disorder, LD, or SLI may have phonologically based spelling problems, only those with LD or SLI generally have impaired reading comprehension even in the absence of associated word reading problems (Catts, Adlof, & Weismer, 2006; Silliman & Scott, 2009). Those with SLI may have reading comprehension problems related to impaired working memory.

Children with SLI exhibit more graphophonemic (letter-sound), syntactic, semantic, and pragmatic miscues when reading than other children their age. Comprehension is less complete and more confused.

A number of types of linguistic awareness contribute to the acquisition of literacy, including phonological, orthographic, syntactic, semantic, and morphological.

- Phonological awareness: The ability to think about, reflect on, and manipulate the sound structures of a language.
- Orthographic awareness: The ability to translate spoken language into its written form based on the allowable spelling sequences of a language.
- Syntactic awareness: The ability to arrange words and morphemes in patterns that help a reader or listener to understand novel word meanings and larger concepts not encountered before.
- Semantic awareness: The understanding that words have meanings.
- Morphological awareness: The recognition that words can be divided into their component morphemes enabling listeners to identify families of words and their shared meanings.

Deficits in Phonological Awareness

Phonological awareness (PA), a metalinguistic skill, enables a child to analyze the sound structure of language. Metalinguistic ability allows us to think about language in the abstract and out of context. PA is a set of skills of varying complexity and depth, drawing on an underlying knowledge base (Anthony & Lonigan, 2004; Justice & Schuele, 2004). These skills include

- the ability to attend to and make judgments about the sound structure of language, such as dividing words into syllables, identifying and generating rhymes, and matching words with the same beginning sound.
- the ability to isolate and manipulate individual sounds or phonemes, called *phonemic awareness*, that is important in early word decoding.

Phonological awareness, often confused with phonics, is the ability to analyze the sound structure of *oral* language. In contrast, **phonics** involves *print* symbols or letters that represent the sounds of oral language. To be proficient in phonics a child needs PA. Alphabetic script makes little sense if a child does not appreciate that words are composed of sounds.

Children with expressive phonological delays have poorer phonemic perception and poorer phonological awareness skills than their TD peers (Rvachew, Ohberg, Grawburg, & Heyding, 2003). Difficulties seem to be related to failure to analyze words into syllables and these, in turn, into smaller phonological units.

Deficits in Orthographic Awareness

It's believed that orthographic awareness and knowledge plays an important role in literacy acquisition. **Orthographic awareness** is an individual's attention to orthographic knowledge. A metalinguistic skill, orthographic awareness is active and conscious thought and mindful consideration of this aspect of language. Late preschool and kindergarten children exposed to print obtain an implicit awareness of orthography, suggesting an early sensitivity to the regularities of print.

Orthographic knowledge is the information stored in our memory that tells us how to represent spoken language in a written form. I suggest reading the excellent tutorial by Apel (2011), but I'll try to explain orthographic knowledge as thoroughly as space allows. The term *mental graphemic representations* (MGRs) refers to the stored mental representations of specific written words or word parts (Apel, 2010; Wolter & Apel, 2010). This is similar to the stored phonological representations that underlie spoken words. MGRs contain specific allowable sequences of graphemes or letters representing written words.

Orthographic knowledge is an individual's knowledge of orthographic patterns, including

- how a letter or letters may represent speech sounds.
- how we represent sounds that go beyond one-to-one correspondence, such as spelling of long vowels and use of consonant doubling.
- how letters can and cannot be combined.
- positional and contextual constraints or orthotactic rules on the use of letters, such as not beginning a word with *tch*.

If we don't follow the patterns, we make spelling errors. An individual reads and spells either by accessing stored knowledge of specific words or by using knowledge of orthographic patterns. Figure 13.1 presents the manner in which the components of orthographic knowledge relate to one another.

Although phonological awareness skills are important for development of literacy, orthographic awareness and knowledge uniquely contribute to literacy development and are separate and important skills. In the earliest stages of literacy development, young children developed sensitivity to orthographic regularities.

Children with LI are less robust at developing initial MGRs than are their TD peers (Wolter & Apel, 2010). This poor ability likely places children with LI at risk for later literacy deficits. Childen, such as many of those with LD, who have little interest in print, may fail to extract recognizable patterns.

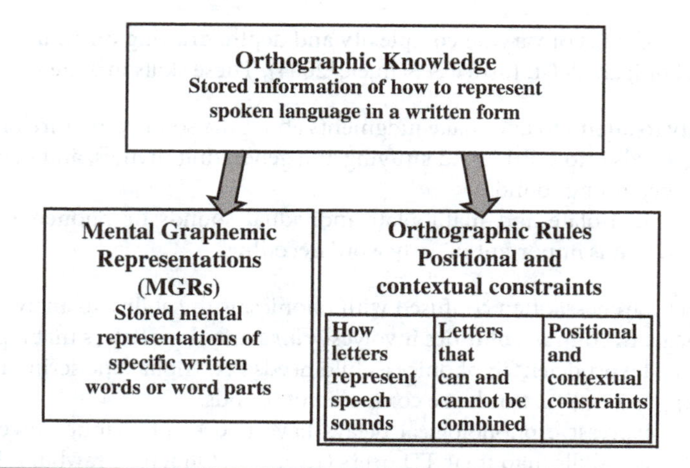

FIGURE 13.1 Components of Orthographic Knowledge.

Source: Information taken from Apel, K. (2001). What is orthographic knowledge? *Language, Speech, and Hearing Services in Schools*, 42, 592–603.

Deficits in Morphological Awareness

Although phonological awareness skills are essential for learning to read and write, recent findings suggest that by 10 years of age, if not earlier, awareness of and knowledge about the morphological structure of words is a better predictor of decoding ability (Mann & Singson, 2003). Children with speech sound disorders, and thus poorer phonological awareness, also have poor morphological awareness, suggesting a general insufficiency in linguistic awareness (Apel & Lawrence, 2011).

Children as young as first graders evidenced some morphological awareness, which influences their development of both reading and spelling (Wolter, Wood, & D'zatko, 2009). More specifically, first-grade children are capable of generating morphologically related words to fit a linguistic context, demonstrating some level of explicit awareness of both derivational and inflectional morphology. Interestingly, this metalinguistic task is generally too difficult for kindergartners. This has implications for early literacy instruction, which is often premised on the assumption that morphological awareness does not develop until middle elementary school.

As children progress through the elementary grades and into middle school, morphologically complex words make up an increasing proportion of the words they will encounter. If teachers and SLPs introduce children to awareness of morphemic structure from an early age, then they can provide children with additional strategies for use in spelling and reading morphologically complex words.

Contrary to what some professionals have assumed, the morphological awareness skills of African American children do not seem to be associated with the amount of AAE used by the children in their speech (Apel & Thomas-Tate, 2009). Students' performance on morphological awareness tasks is related to their performance on the word-level reading, spelling, and receptive vocabulary measures.

Deficits in Comprehension

Deficits in comprehension may not be evident in the early stages of reading acquisition when phonics is extremely important. Although phonics-based problems often decrease by third grade, comprehension problems persist for many children (Foster & Miller, 2007). Poor reading comprehension is associated not with phonics but with poor oral language (Nation & Frazier Norbury, 2005).

Many children and adults with ASD, even mildly affected or high-functioning individuals, have difficulty inferencing from reading and comprehending metaphoric expressions and ambiguity (Dennis, Lazenby, & Lockyer, 2001; Diehl, Ford, & Federico, 2005; Griswold, Barnhill, Smith-Myles, Hagiwara, & Simpson, 2002; Smith-Myles et al., 2002). Unfortunately, most children with ASD do not become skilled readers because of difficulties with interpretive language. Although children with high-functioning autism are able to understand words that convey an internal state, such as *know, remember, forget, think, believe,* they fail to infer what these same words mean in context (Dennis et al., 2001; Wahlberg & Magliano, 2004). Able to answer reading comprehension questions of a factual nature, they may be unable to inference, which is important for true reading comprehension.

The situation compounds itself as children mature (Stanovich, 2000). Students with poor reading comprehension are likely to read simpler texts, often below grade level, and to read less frequently. This lack of exposure to print containing more mature structure and content results in poor readers becoming poorer as they fall farther behind their TD peers.

Children with CLD Backgrounds

For many children from CLD backgrounds, especially those from impoverished home environments, school and family cultural notions of the value of literacy may differ greatly. This mismatch potentially places a child at risk of poor literacy development, especially if he or she is experiencing oral language difficulties with English.

Many children in publicly funded preschool and prekindergarten programs exhibit elevated risks for later reading problems because of poverty and its impact on precursors to reading achievement. The results of a survey of children in Head Start programs reveal that maternal education and the frequency of home literacy activities are strong factors in children's vocabulary and reading abilities (Scheffner Hammer, Farkas, & Maczuga, 2010). Findings regarding the benefits of current preschool language and literacy curricula are mixed and raise questions about the effectiveness of existing curricular tools (Preschool Curriculum Evaluation Research Consortium, 2008).

AAE-speaking students who learn to use Standard or majority American English (SAE) for literacy tasks, such as writing, outperform their dialect non-adapting peers in reading tasks (Craig, Zhang, Hensel, & Quinn, 2009). In fact, the rate of AAE use is inversely related to reading achievement scores. Dialectal variation alone cannot account for literacy differences. Socioeconomic status (SES) is also a large contributing factor, with lower SES negatively impacting literacy skills (Patton Terry, McDonald Connor, Thomas-Tate, & Love, 2010).

An SLP must be aware of ethnic and class parenting and shared book reading behaviors. For example, Mexican American mothers use a variety of communication behaviors during shared book reading, including interactive reading strategies, such as *wh-* and yes/no questions, directives/requests, labels, descriptions, positive feedback, and vocally directing their children's attention. Compared to white non-Latino mothers, the Mexican American moms rarely engage in interactive reading that supports comprehension, nor do they use literacy strategies, such as elaborating on their children's ideas as they share books. In general, middle-SES mothers use more positive feedback and yes/no questioning than do low-SES mothers (Rodríguez, Hines, & Montiel, 2009).

Kindergarten English vocabulary, phonological awareness, letter-word identification, and Spanish word-reading skills are significant predictors of English reading skills by first grade (Páez & Rinaldi, 2006). Although TD bilingual children from low-income backgrounds initially perform poorly in all three areas, they acquire these abilities quickly in kindergarten (Hammer & Miccio, 2006).

Although oral language skills in L_2 (English in this case) are a predictor of reading in L_2, oral language skills in L_1 are not (August et al., 2006). Rather, reading skills in L_1 are closely related to future ability in L_2. More specifically, children with high Spanish letter-name and sound knowledge tend to also show high levels of both in English (Cárdenas-Hagan, Carlson, & Pollard-Durodola, 2007). This may not be true for children with different first languages, especially those with different alphabets (Cyrillic, Arabic) or sound systems. Phonological awareness skills seem to transfer directly from Spanish to English. The good news is that all these skills—letter-name, sound knowledge, and phonological awareness—can be taught to these children easily.

Assessment of Reading

Language deficits associated with reading are often present during the preschool years. Prereading and reading assessment should be a portion of any thorough language evaluation.

Data Collection

Just as all children do not require an oral language assessment, neither do they all require a reading assessment. As mentioned in Chapter 3, Language assessments begin with an initial data-gathering step that may include use of questionnaires, interviews, referrals, and screening testing. Table 13.1 presents a checklist designed to identify kindergarten and first-grade school children at risk for language-based reading difficulties. No one item alone will indicate a possible problem.

Teacher reports are a moderately accurate predictor of children's literacy behaviors during assessment. In other words, teachers are moderately good predictors of those children who will experience reading difficulties in elementary school (Cabell, Justice, Zucker, & Kilday, 2009b).

On an early literacy parent questionnaire, parental reports of early literacy skills of their preschool children with LI compare favorably with professional assessments (Boudreau, 2005). Questions concern the frequency of book-reading behaviors, responses to print, language awareness, interest in letters, and early writing.

Early literacy can be screened using SLP-designed tasks such as those presented in Table 13.2 (Justice et al., 2002). For a wider view, data from these tasks can be combined with parental information on home literacy materials and activities.

Children who read poorly may exhibit learned helplessness or have negative attitudes toward the reading process. This information can be gathered from interviews with teachers, parents, and the child and by observation within the classroom. Interview questions should include the child's perceptions of the importance of reading and different types of reading and difficulties, along with self-perceptions. Scaled responses, such as a 0–5 disagree-agree scale, can be used with statements such as "Reading is difficult for me" or "My teacher helps me learn to read better."

Observation can confirm the child, teacher, and parent responses. Behavioral changes related to learned helplessness, such as nervousness, withdrawal, and aggression, may be noted. Lack of task persistence can be recorded as the amount of time or the number of attempts made in decoding a word or longer unit. A very high or very low number of requests for assistance also can be a good indicator. In addition, self-verbalizations blaming himself or herself ("I'm so dumb") or others ("This story is stupid" or "Why didn't you tell me I was next?") rather than stating alternative strategies for success ("Oh, this word is spelled like _____, so it's pronounced '_____' ") also may signal helplessness.

During more formal testing, either the SLP or the reading specialist might use one of the following standardized testing to determine if the child is functioning within normal limits:

- Test of Early Reading Ability (Reid, Hresko, & Hammill, 2001)
- Gray Oral Reading Test (Wiederholt & Bryant, 2001)
- Woodcock Reading Mastery Test–Revised (Woodcock, 1998)

The Test of Early Reading is designed for children ages 3 to 8 and assesses alphabet knowledge, phonological awareness, and ability to derive meaning from parts. A timed instrument, the Gray Oral

TABLE 13.1 Early Identification of Children with Language-Based Reading Impairment

The following checklist can be used by teachers to refer children to the SLP who exhibit possible language-based reading impairment.

The child has difficulty...

____ Counting and identifying syllables in words
____ Rhyming
____ Recognizing words that begin with the same sound
____ With sound-letter identification
____ Retrieving words and/or names
____ With specific words, preferring words such as *one* and *thing*
____ Recalling word sequences (alphabet, months of the year)
____ Recalling directions or instructions
____ Giving directions or instructions
____ Saying words
____ Confusing words that sound similar
____ Understanding questions and comments
____ Understanding simple stories
____ Telling stories, especially sequential events, clearly
____ With the give-and-take of conversations
____ Understanding the motivations and feelings of others
____ Initiating conversation

The child does not show an interest in...

____ Books ____ Play with others ____ Talking with others

The child's speech is characterized by frequent...

____ Word substitutions ____ Sound errors
____ Pauses and fillers, such as *you know* and *like*
____ Requests for repetition, such as *What?* And *Huh?*
____ Repetitions of words and phrases
____ Short sentences ____ Grammatical errors

Child has...

____ History of speech and language problems
____ Family history of speech and language problems
____ Limited home literacy

Source: Information from Catts (1997) among others.

Reading Test, is useful with slow readers. Finally, the Woodcock Reading Mastery Test assesses sight vocabulary, nonsense-word decoding, and comprehension.

Word-level working memory tasks may be appropriate for assessing word-level written language skills, such as reading and spelling. In contrast, sentence-level working memory tasks may be appropriate for assessing sentence- and text-level reading and writing skills, such as reading comprehension and composition or written expression of ideas (Berninger, Abbott, et al., 2010).

In a more functional task, a child might also be asked to read curricular materials in an attempt to assess her or his ability to function within the classroom (N. Nelson & Van Meter, 2002).

TABLE 13.2 Clinician-Designed Tasks of Early Literacy Screening

Areas	Tasks
Print Awareness	During shared book experience, differentiates written-language units, such as letter, word, and sentence, and identifies direction of print flow, location of cover, functions of books, etc. (Clay, 1979; Justice & Ezell, 2000; Lomax & McGee, 1987) Reads common environmental words (Gillam & Johnston, 1985)
Phonological Awareness	Finds one in three words that differs on the basis of an onset or rime or tells how two words differ on the same basis (Maclean, Bryant, & Bradley, 1987) Produces words that begin with a certain sound or rhyme (Chaney, 1992) Produces a "new" word after one sound has been deleted, as in "Say *cat* without the /k/ sound." (Lonigan, Burgess, Anthony, & Barker, 1998) Takes a word apart, then puts it together again Identifies the number of phonemes in a word
Letter Name Knowledge	Says the names of upper- and lowercase letters or points to letters named in two modes, at own pace or as fast as possible (RAN) (Blachman, 1984; Justice & Ezell, 2000)
Grapheme-phoneme Correspondence	Produces sound that goes with letter or names the letter that goes with a sound (Juel, 1988). Could also be accomplished with pointing to letter when sound is heard
Literacy motivation	Engages in a variety of literacy events and level of involvement is rated along a continuum from no engagement to high engagement (Kaderavek & Sulzby, 1998)
Home literacy	Parents complete checklist or questionnaire on home literacy activities and materials to determine child's access and participation (Allen & Mason, 1989; Dickinson & DeTemple, 1998)

Source: Information from Justice, Invernizzi, & Meier (2002). Readers are advised to read this article for a fuller explanation of the tasks mentioned.

The material should be new to the child to ensure that it has not been previously taught. Reading aloud gives the SLP information on decoding and can be audiotaped for later analysis. If curricular materials seem to be too difficult, the SLP or reading specialist could use graded passages, such as those found in the Qualitative Reading Inventory–III (Leslie & Caldwell, 2000). Regardless of the method of collection, some portion should be read aloud and audiotaped.

Comprehension can be assessed by using questions. Alternative forms include retelling or paraphrasing. Most standardized tests include a comprehension subtest.

The ability to paraphrase reading passages is closely related to measures of expository text comprehension (Laing Gillam, Fargo, & St. Clair Robertson, 2009). For this reason, data obtained during think-aloud sessions may be a useful supplement to traditional measures of comprehension. Think-aloud methods can reveal metacognitive processes that occur during thinking or reasoning. In think-alouds, children verbalize their thoughts or thought processes while reading, listening, or problem-solving (Braten & Stromso, 2003).

During a think-aloud task, the SLP periodically asks a child to report thoughts while problem-solving during tasks and to talk about why or how they arrived at particular solutions. A child's response might be classified as follows (Laing Gillam et al., 2009).

- *Exact repetition*: Utterance matches exactly or differs by only one word from the focal sentence.
- *Paraphrase*: A transformation of the focal sentence that preserves its meaning.

- *Explanation*: Utterance provides an answer to *why* questions.
- *Prediction*: Utterance provides answers to causal consequence questions. Predictive inferences may be produced in chains in which one prediction is necessary for and/or enables another one to occur.
- *Association*: Utterance in which content occurs concurrently with the event, state, or activity depicted in the focal sentence in the form of generalizations, specifications of procedures, and expressions of manner, features, and properties of characters or objects, as well as specification of temporal or spatial information.

While this list is not a strict hierarchy of comprehension, it does provide a systematic way to characterize a child's level of comprehension processing.

Data Analysis

Passages should be photocopied and used by the SLP to record discrepancies noted on the audiotaped reading samples. All attempts at word decoding, repetitions, corrections, omitted words and morphemes, extended pauses, and dialectal usages should be noted by the SLP and analyzed for possible strategies used by the child. There is little danger that children with SLI or LLD will inflate their performance by guessing words correctly, because a part of their reading difficulty is an inability to integrate syntactic, semantic, and textual information (N. Nelson & Van Meter, 2002).

The percentage of words correct on the first attempt should be calculated. Usually, children who experience less than 90 percent correct on their first attempt demonstrate frustration (Leslie & Caldwell, 2000).

Miscues can be analyzed by type at the word level (N. Nelson, 1994). These include reversals, in which word order is changed; semantic substitutions, in which an acceptable but different word is substituted; syntactic substitutions, in which a syntactically appropriate but semantically nonsensical word is substituted; insertions, in which a word is added; and deletions. The percentage of incorrect but linguistically acceptable words should be calculated as these indicate the use of linguistic cues to predict the correct word.

The SLP should note the way in which the child sounds out the words (N. Nelson & Van Meter, 2002). Good readers use several strategies. Common strategies include the following:

- Sound by sound.
- By consonant clusters including digraphs ("sh," "th," "on," "ch," "ay").
- Common rimes ("-ack," "-ent," "-ite," "-at").
- Morphemes ("un-," "dis-," "-ly").

Assessment of Phonological Awareness

Assessment for phonological awareness can be accomplished within an overall assessment of reading that includes measurement of reading, spelling, phonological awareness, verbal working memory, and rapid automatized naming (RAN). One caution: African American children from low-income families may score below expected norms on some phonological awareness measures, such as the Test of Phonological Awareness (Torgesen & Bryant, 1994), even though their reading performance is within normal limits (Thomas-Tate, Washington, & Edwards, 2004).

A thorough assessment of phonological awareness includes rhyming, sound isolation, segmentation, blending, deletion, and substitution. The rhyming portion is only predictive of reading with preschool and kindergarten children.

Formal testing can be accomplished using the Comprehensive Test of Phonological Processing (CTOPP; Wagner, Torgesen, & Rashotte, 1999) or the Phonological Awareness Test (PAT; Robertson & Salter, 1997). Designed for ages 5 through 21, the CTOPP includes subtests on deletion of sounds, sound and word blending, segmentation, and phoneme reversal, a difficult memory task. In addition, tasks on the CTOPP also assess verbal working memory and RAN. The PAT, designed for children ages 5 through 9, includes testing of rhyming, segmentation, phoneme isolation, deletion, substitution, blending, sound-symbol association, and word decoding.

Assessment of Morphological Awareness

Textbooks for adolescents and young adults contain a variety of morphologically complex words, such as *regeneration, reptilian,*and *strenuous.* Given the importance of derived words for academic success, morphological awareness should be assessed in older children (Nippold & Sun, 2008). At the very least, SLPs should examine adolescent students understanding of *–able* (*acceptable*), *–ar* (*molecular*), *–ic* (*genetic*) , *–ful* (*powerful*), *–less* (*speechless*), *–ment* (*concealment*), *–ship* (*citizenship*), *–tion* (*prediction*), *–ness* (*weariness*), and *–ity* (*diversity*). Additional suffixes might include *–ous, –like,* and *–ish* for adjectives and *–ian, –ster–,* and *–ology* for nominals. Actual word choice should be based on frequency of word use in curricular materials and in textbook glossaries.

Assessment of Comprehension

Assessment for comprehension is difficult because of the multifaceted character of the process. Kindergarten and first-grade screening tests focus on phonological awareness and phonics, thus identifying only children who will have difficulty with early reading. Comprehension deficits manifest themselves later and are not based on an inability to sound out words. Likewise, a single silent reading comprehension test is insufficient to identify those who are slow readers from those who have language-based comprehension problems (Snyder, Caccamise, & Wise, 2005). At the very least, a thorough evaluation must include the following:

- Oral language skills, especially vocabulary and listening comprehension
- Narrative skills from conversational samples
- Standardized assessment of all aspects of comprehension beyond simple recall of text content, including paraphrasing, summarizing, predicting, and inferencing
- Sampling of grade-appropriate reading comprehension

Intervention for Reading Impairment

Evidence-based practice (EBP) suggests that four possible preschool target areas are strongly related to later reading development: alphabet knowledge, print and word knowledge, phonological awareness, and literate language (Justice & Kaderavek, 2004). Alphabet knowledge consists of knowing the features and names of letters in both upper- and lowercase. This differs from print and word knowledge, which is knowledge of how letters form words and the ways that pages (left to right) and books (front to back) are organized. Phonological awareness, as mentioned before, involves awareness of the sound and syllable structure of oral language. Finally, literate language differs from oral language in its use of vocabulary and syntax, such as elaborated noun phrases, to create text. These written conventions differ from those used in speech. Although primary responsibility for prereading instruction falls upon the classroom teacher, the SLP has expertise in some areas in which teachers are unprepared.

Despite programs such as Head Start, a need for intense exposure to literacy in preschool continues to exist, especially for children from CLD backgrounds (Hammer, Miccio, & Wagstaff, 2003). Given that African American preschoolers with more complex syntax and shape-matching skills have better reading skills by third grade, it would be wise to target these areas for instruction (Craig, Connor, & Washington, 2003).

For preschool and kindergarten children with LI, the transition from prereaders to readers can be facilitated by an integrated multitiered intervention approach using both embedded and explicit approaches and targeting the four areas of (1) alphabet knowledge, (2) print and word knowledge, (3) phonological awareness, and (4) literate language, mentioned previously (Justice & Kaderavek, 2004). Children demonstrate widespread gains in a number of emerging literacy skills when both explicit and implicit methods are used (Justice, Chow, Capellini, Flanigan, & Colton, 2003).

Embedded Approaches

In embedded approaches, children's growth is fostered through high-quality daily literacy experiences and interactions with print that are placed within meaningful literacy activities. The goal is to maximize children's use of print through a literacy-rich environment (Towey, Whitcomb, & Bray, 2004). Other elements may include the following:

- Morning message board with words to count and segment and sounds to blend into words, or for finding words that begin with a selected sound or rhyme
- In-school breakfast and lunch menus with printed words and picture
- Matching games throughout the day using sounds and rhyming
- Recipes with words and pictures
- Music, finger play, and rhyming
- Identifying beginning sounds within themed activities, such as the names of different kinds of trucks, e.g., F-iretruck, M-ixer, D-umptruck, etc.
- Sorting tasks by rhyming

Embedding might include labels on items in the classroom, increased availability of children's books, and shared story reading with adults. These approaches may be more effective than more explicit models in increasing children's positive orientation to reading.

Individual book sharing accompanied by targeted questions can improve both literal and inferential language skills among Head Start preschoolers with LI (van Kleeck, Vander Woude, & Hammett, 2006). Examples of questions and prompts for correct answers are presented in Table 13.3. Book sharing accompanied by dialogue is an excellent activity for promoting oral language, including syntax, semantics, and language comprehension (van Kleeck, 2003).

Sustained and intensive preschool, kindergarten, and first- and second-grade intervention can reduce reading difficulties among at-risk children (Justice, 2006b). As little as a 15- to 20-minute daily block of dedicated literacy time in preschool may be sufficient to forestall reading difficulties for many children (Kame'enui, Simmons, & Coyne, 2000). This increases to 30 to 45 minutes in kindergarten and 90 minutes by first grade.

Book Sharing. The least restrictive environment is often considered to be the home, and as a therapeutic approach, home-based intervention has considerable social validity. Programs such as home book sharing have reported positive results (Justice, Skibbe, McGinty, Piasta, & Petrill, 2011). Success is not ensured for all families, however, and SLPs must carefully examine their methods and the values and expectations of each family.

Shared storybooks can promote development of oral language and emergent literacy skills in young children (Ezell & Justice, 2005). Books are a stable source of linguistic forms and content that can be used as a part of language intervention. Adults can use a variety of strategies, such as open-ended questions, repetition, modeling, expansion, and cloze techniques, to facilitate the child's participation and learning. Used appropriately, shared book reading has been shown to increase vocabulary and overall language and literacy development (Justice & Kaderavek, 2004; Justice, Meier, & Walpole, 2005).

Intervention techniques should not only be effective, but they must also be accomplished with minimal disruption to family routines. While we may expect families to participate in their

TABLE 13.3 Literal and Inferential Questions and Prompts for Use in Guided Reading

Question	Feedback/Prompt
Level I (Literal) What's that?	*Correct:* Repeat correct answer and "Yes, it's a X." *Incorrect:* Build a bridge to the correct answer. "Yes, it's a kind of Y called a . . ." *No response:* Prompt with the beginning sound or syllable, and if still no answer, tell the child and provide more information.
Level II (Literal) What's the bunny doing?	*Correct:* Repeat correct answer and "Yes, he's X-ing (*running, jumping,* etc.)." *Incorrect:* Build a bridge to the correct answer. "Yes, that's the bunny and he's . . ." *No response:* Prompt with the beginning sound or syllable, and if still no answer, tell the child and provide more information.
Level III (Inferential) How do you think the bunny feels when he finds all his friends are hiding?	*Correct:* Repeat correct answer and "Yes, I think he feels X because Y. Do you ever feel X? *Incorrect:* "I think he feels X because . . ." After child gives reason add "Yes, the bunny feels X because (repeat child's reason)." *No response:* "Bunny feels . . ." If no response, "Bunny feels X because Y. Do you ever feel X?"
Level IV (Inferential) What do you think the bunny will do next to find his friends?	*Correct:* "I think so too. The bunny wants to X so he can Z. Shall we keep reading and see?" *Incorrect:* "I think he's going to do X so he can . . ." After correct response, "Yes, I think so, too. He's going to X so he can Y." *No response:* "Bunny wants to Y, so he's going to X."

Source: Information from van Kleeck, Vander Woude, & Hammett (2006).

child's intervention and become agents of change, it is too much to expect that most parents will be able to carry through with very structured training programs that place an undue burden on the family.

Parents from CLD backgrounds who are participating in family literacy programs based on European American practices may encounter programs that do not approximate their patterns of interaction with their children. This could jeopardize success with their children. An SLP would need to exercise caution when attempting to get parents to change their interactive style. Disregarding differences between a program's inherent interaction practices and those of families can result in poor intervention outcomes and limited parent participation (Janes & Kermani, 2001; Kummerer et al., 2007). Culturally relevant intervention programs are essential.

Book sharing is one of a series of pre-reading suggestions for children with ASD. Frequent and repeated shared book reading may increase oral language and attention and decrease echolalia, stereotypic behaviors, and verbal outbursts (Bellon, Ogletree, & Harn, 2000; Koppenhaver & Erickson, 2003; Wolfberg, 1999). Books should contain simple pictures, predictable stories with clear cause-and-effect relationships or goal-directed behavior, events that can be related to everyday experiences, and elements that can easily be contextualized with manipulative props, such as puppets or action figures (Bellon et al., 2000).

Explicit Approaches

In contrast, explicit approaches include direct instruction of discrete skills. Some skill areas, such as phonological awareness, may be best suited to an explicit approach. Ideally, explicit instruction would be provided in the classroom, in small groups, and individually.

TABLE 13.4 Programs for Written Language Intervention

• *Linguistic Remedies* (Wise, Rogan, & Sessions, 2009) provides insightful ideas for applying **language** research to literacy instruction that is individually tailored to a professional's own cases.
• *Lovett Empower Reading*, developed and validated by Maureen Lovett, provides lessons for teaching strategies for accurate and efficient decoding and application of this knowledge to independent reading for meaning, information, and pleasure. Some spelling and reading comprehension activities are included. Other programs focus on both word and syntactic processing and awareness.
• *The Nelson Writing Lab* (Nelson, Bahr, & Van Meter, 2004) offers many effective treatment strategies for both writing and reading, which integrate use of technology and were validated for students with oral as well as written **language** disabilities.
• *Retrieval, Automaticity, Vocabulary, and Engagement with **Language**, and Orthography (RAVE-O)*, developed and validated by Maryanne Wolf and colleagues, provides explicit instruction in phonology, orthography, and morphology with a focus on improving word retrieval and building vocabulary as well.
• *SPELL-2: Spelling Performance Evaluation for **Language** & Literacy* (Masterson, Apel, & Wasowicz, 2006) and *SPELL—Links to Reading and Writing* (Wasowicz, Apel, Masterson, & Whitney, 2004) provide a comprehensive, user-friendly approach to linking assessment and instructional treatment with a focus on phonology, orthography, and morphology.
• *The Wilson Reading System*[6] incorporates multisensory teaching techniques with explicit instruction in phonology, orthography, and morphology.

The classroom teacher is primarily responsible for embedded learning and for explicit whole-class instruction. Through collaboration, intervention team membership, and classroom activities, the SLP can support the classroom teacher while fostering children's growth in literacy.

Children with a specific reading learning disorder need specialized instruction to develop their phonological, orthographic, and morphological awareness and their ability to coordinate this knowledge in word decoding and spelling (Berninger, Raskind, Richards, Abbott, & Stock, 2008; Berninger & Wolf, 2009a, 2009b). Those with SLI, LD, or other written LIs need specialized instruction in word retrieval to overcome their difficulty in applying executive functions to long-term memory search, and in syntactic awareness and text inferencing (Cain & Oakhill, 2007; Silliman & Scott, 2009). Table 13.4 presents evidence-based programs to treat written LI.

By age 3, most children in the majority culture are familiar with books, can recognize their favorite books, and have the rudiments of **print awareness**, such as knowing the direction in which reading proceeds across a page and through a book, being interested in print, and recognizing some letters (Snow et al., 1999). Print awareness includes these skills plus later-developing ones, such as knowing that words are discrete units, being able to identify letters, and using literacy terminology, such as *letter*, *word*, and *sentence*.

Print awareness can be increased among preschool children with print-focused reading activities that emphasize word concepts and alphabetic knowledge (Justice & Ezell, 2002). Print-focus prompts are presented in Table 13.5.

Parents can be taught to use print-based reading strategies that enhance their children's print-referenced behaviors (Justice & Ezell, 2000). Print-focused prompts are easy to teach, and parents have been successful with only minimal training. For example, a parent can easily point to words as she or he reads to a child. As a result, the child learns about print through the behavior of the parent. Print referencing has been shown to facilitate development of word concepts and alphabet knowledge as well as print concepts (Ezell, Justice, & Parsons, 2000; Justice & Ezell, 2002)

Interestingly, language difficulties of young children with SLI are not sufficient to account for their poor print knowledge. Instead, the quality of home literacy experiences seems to play an important role in fostering their print knowledge (McGinty & Justice, 2009). These findings would suggest a strong home literacy component to any intervention with young children with SLI.

TABLE 13.5 Print-Focus Prompts

Strategies	Examples	
Print-Focus Strategies		
Nonverbal	Point to print in text or to print in illustrations	
	Follow print with finger while reading	
Verbal		
Print Conventions	Ask questions:	Do you read this way or this way?
		And this one says?
		Where would you read if you were telling this story?
	Comment:	We start here and turn the pages this way.
		That one tells you what the boy says.
	Requests:	Show me how to hold a book to read.
		Can you show me where it says "Help"?
Word Concepts	Ask questions:	Where is the last word on the page?
		Is "cat" a word?
	Comment:	This word says "cow."
		This says "hungry" and this says "caterpillar." We put them together to make "hungry caterpillar."
	Request:	Show me the first word.
		You point to the words and I'll read.
Alphabet knowledge	Asks questions:	Do you know this letter? What does it say?
		What's the first letter in "bear"?
	Comment:	That's a B. It makes the /b/ sound.
		Where's Spot? Bet we can find her. Spot begins with S, just like your name, Susan.
	Request:	Show me where the P is.

Source: Adapted from Justice & Ezell (2002, 2004).

Curriculum supplements such as *Read It Again!* (RIA; Justice, McGinty, Beckman, & Kilday, 2006) offer downloadable materials (http://myreaditagain.com) for use with fifteen commercially available children's books and are an alternative to high-cost language and literacy curricula, which often require ongoing intensive professional development. RIA offers sixty large-group lessons over a thirty-week period, making it a viable means of enhancing the language and literacy instruction within preschool classrooms and increasing children's grammar and vocabulary and literacy skills, such as rhyming, alliteration, and print awareness (Justice, McGinty, Cabell, Kilday, Knighton, & Huffman, 2010).

For emergent readers who fail to achieve adequate reading, intervention is different from that addressed with prereaders and includes phonemic awareness, phonics, fluency, vocabulary, and reading comprehension. As in prereading difficulties, some of these areas are best addressed by an SLP.

Reading intervention might begin with a two-stage intervention model (van Kleeck, 1995). In stage one, meaning foundation, the reader scaffolds the reading for a child by placing the text in context and asking questions to guide comprehension. The child learns that print contains the meaning and gains phonological awareness and letter knowledge. In stage two, form foundation, phonological awareness, and alphabetic knowledge are emphasized. Phonological training would include syllables and subsyllabic units, such as initial phonemes, or *onsets*, and *rimes*, or the remaining part of the word. Rhyming and alliteration activities also would be used. Training in alphabetic knowledge would include learning uppercase letters, followed by lowercase, copying shapes and letters, sound-letter correspondence, and knowledge of meaning found in books read to the child by others. Four

TABLE 13.6 Levels of Abstraction

Level	Intervention Strategies
I: Matching Perception	Name and label characters, objects, and actions Find characters or objects named Direct adult's attention to a character, object, or action
II: Selection Analysis/ Integration of Perception	Describe characteristics, parts, or personal qualities of characters or objects Describe scenes and actions Recall previous information from text
III: Reorder/Infer	Summarize two or more events or actions in the text Describe similarities or differences in characters, actions, or events in text
IV: Reasoning	Predict what will happen next in text Consider causes for actions or events in text Explain actions or events in task Describe emotions of characters in text and possible influence on behavior

Source: Information from van Kleeck (1995) and others.

levels of abstraction of meaning are presented in Table 13.6. The first two require concrete skills, such as naming and describing, while the latter two require children to make inferences and to reason.

Each child brings a sense of self to the therapeutic situation. In part, this self-concept has grown out of his or her interactions with family and immediate community members. An SLP's failure to recognize and include these dimensions of an individual's social identity can negatively impact intervention (Demmert, McCardle, & Leos, 2006).

Providing culturally responsive intervention is extremely important for children with CLD backgrounds. SLPs can integrate culturally based stories into shared storybook intervention (Inglebret, Jones, & Pavel, 2008).

Responding to children from CLD backgrounds means much more than simply having pictures of black children in the materials being used. Even books translated from another language may have been unintentionally altered to reflect a Eurocentric perspective. Being culturally responsive may involve the SLP's collaborating with people in the community.

Although materials for use with children from CLD backgrounds may already exist, not all stories accurately reflect a culture's norms or values. Again, it is best to consult with members of the ethnic community before using such materials.

Later reading intervention might target both linguistic and metalinguistic skills including recognition of key words, use of all parts of the text such as the glossary and the index, and application of general learning strategies, such as graphic organizers.

Intervention for Phonological Awareness

SLPs have distinct and extensive knowledge related to PA and can play a critical role on educational teams (Cunningham, Perry, Stanovich, & Stanovich, 2004; Moats & Foorman, 2003; Spencer, Schuele, Guillot, & Lee, 2007). Thus, SLPs can contribute to their school teams' efforts to enhance children's PA acquisition in several ways (Schuele & Boudreau, 2008):

- Boost other team members' knowledge by contributing their expertise.
- Provide a unique perspective in assessment decisions.
- Collaborate with classroom teachers and reading specialists to enhance PA instruction within the general education curriculum.
- Provide small-group PA intervention to struggling students.

While classroom instruction focuses on children's achievement of specific curricular outcomes, SLP intervention focuses on the individual learning needs of children who have not achieved these desired classroom goals. I would suggest that you read the excellent article by Schuele and Boudreau (2008) for a more in-depth discussion of PA and EBP than we can have in a text.

Teaching PA is akin to teaching problem-solving and can be accomplished through the SLP's repeated modeling with multiple examples and guided practice by the child (Wanzek, Dickson, Bursuck, & White, 2000). The SLP provides a framework for accomplishing the task. This might take the following form (Schuele & Boudreau, 2008):

- SLP introduces a word, comments on a sound or syllable, as in "The first sound in the *time* is /t/."
- SLP repeats the process and has child repeat the sound or syllable.
- SLP asks the child a question, as in "What's the first sound in *time*?"

While this is a bare-bones example, it can be spruced up with some fun and silliness, such as "Is the first sound in *time* a (cough)?" Through this step-by-step process, the child learns the task as well as the correct answer. Using words in the child's environment or favorite book makes the entire process more functional.

Ideally, each step in teaching supports subsequent steps. For example, there is data to suggest that segmenting a word into phonemes may be easier if the child has used the word in rhyming and matching initial sounds. Previous exposure to the word may provide the child with practice analyzing the characteristics of the word even though the child has never been asked to segment the word's component sounds (Metsala, 1999).

Intervention for phoneme awareness can be effective with preschool children, even those with speech impairments related to sound production (Gillon, 2005). Developmental intervention for phoneme awareness can include the following:

- Phoneme awareness and identification
- Letter identification
- Encoding and decoding print

Phoneme awareness teaching activities can be placed within play activities and can include (Gillon, 2005) the following:

- Phoneme detection (*Find the word that starts with . . . Does . . . begin with . . . ?*)
- Phoneme categorization (*Find all the toys that begin with . . .*)
- Initial phoneme matching (*Ball begins with /b/. Find the one that begins the same as ball. Book. Doll.*)
- Phoneme isolation (*What sound does pony start with?*)

Letter-name and letter-sound intervention can begin with recognition of letters that vary widely in their appearance and accompanying sound. Within words, it's best to begin with the letter in the initial position. Picture cards should contain the word written under the picture, so children can begin to match sound and letter.

Whenever possible, phonological awareness should be taught within meaningful text experiences. In this way, the emergent nature of both literacy and phonological awareness can be used. Environmental signs, such as *stop, women,* and *Main Street,* can be used to enhance training.

Within rhyming, the SLP can use a variety of tasks that vary in the amount of support provided to the child (Adams, Foorman, Lundberg, & Beeler, 1998; Anthony, Lonigan, Driscoll, Phillips, & Burgess, 2003). The child can be asked if two words rhyme, choose one of three words that does not rhyme, match rhyming words, or generate his or her own rhymes (Schuele & Boudreau, 2008).

Rhymes may be more easily recognized by children when articulation of the final sounds are visible, as in labial sounds. Rhyming words that end in consonants (*stop*) seems to be easier than words that end in vowel sounds (*stay*).

Segmenting and blending are based on broader PA skills. It would seem to make sense to target lower level skills, such as rhyming, to the extent that they facilitate development of more complex PA skills, such as segmenting and blending. SLPs and teachers should work to ensure that each child has a sufficient foundation in PA to enable him or her to benefit from general education decoding instruction (Schuele & Dayton, 2000). At the very least, this involves (Schuele & Boudreau, 2008)

- the ability to consistently and independently segment and blend CV, VC, and CVC words.
- an emerging ability to segment and blend words with consonant clusters or blends (CCVC, CVCC).

Once blending and segmenting is established, the SLP can provide a link between PA skills and classroom decoding and spelling instruction by providing practice that facilitates the application of phonemic awareness knowledge to spelling and decoding words (Blachman, Ball, Black, & Tangel, 2000).

Teaching segmentation is easiest for children if the SLP begins with larger units, such as words, and proceeds to smaller units, such as syllables and then phonemes. Within words, however, shorter words with fewer syllables and single consonants are easier than multisyllabic words with blended consonants.

When progressing to multisyllabic words, obvious units, such as syllables in compound words, as in *football* or *cupcake*, are easier than compound words, such as *telephone*, in which the units are not readily identifiable (Schuele & Dayton, 2000). When segmenting words or separating them into their constituent sounds,

- consonants are easier to segment than vowels.
- initial sounds are easier to segment than final sounds.
- syllable final /r/ is particularly difficult.
- continuing phonemes, such as /s/ and /ʃ/, seem to be easier to analyze than stop phonemes, such as /p/ and /t/. It's possible to elongate continuing sounds to make them more salient for children.
- shorter words, such as CV, are easier to segment than longer words, such as CVC.
- initial sounds are easier to segment than final sounds.
- single consonants, as in CV words, are easier to segment than blended consonants, as in CCV.
- blended consonants may be easier to segment if the phonemes are produced in different locations, as in the /st/ in *stop*, than if they are produced in the same location, as in /mp/ in *stamp*.
- segmenting words with blends, such as *bring*, may be easier when the child has had practice segmenting a subunit of that word, such as *ring* (Blachman et al., 2000).

Letter representations can be physically manipulated to add another element to training.

Printed letters can be used to support phoneme learning, especially if letters are used in the classroom. Again, a functional approach tries to incorporate use contexts, such as the classroom, as much as possible. Letters give additional input, are a potential memory aid, and are functional for generalization to reading. For children with deficits in working memory, letters can offer a compensatory visual aid. It is important for the SLP to remember that intervention is for phonological awareness not reading per se. It is very tempting to try to teach reading, but that is not the job of an SLP.

Letter-sound knowledge can be viewed as consisting of recognition, or pointing to a letter or letters when a sound or consonant blend is presented; recall, or saying a sound or sounds when a letter or consonant blend is presented; and reproduction, or writing a letter or consonant blend when the sound or sounds are heard. In general, recognition is easier than recall, which in turn is easier than reproduction (Dodd & Carr, 2003).

Multisensory approaches are also helpful and can make the training interesting. For example, during auditory training children can respond to target sounds by dropping objects into cans, stacking toys, playing hopscotch, or taking turns in any number of child games. Although typically developing children seem to benefit more than children with SLI from computer-supported phonological awareness intervention, the method still holds promise as one aspect of a comprehensive intervention plan (Segers & Verhoeven, 2004).

Vowels offer a particular problem because of the number and inconsistent spelling in English. An SLP can begin with short vowels because they are the nucleus of the longest syllables, called closed syllables. Closed syllables have rimes that end in at least one consonant and may have a maximum of six phonemes in the word, as in *scrimp*. Children can be taught common rimes such as *-ent, -ide, -old,* and *-ick.*

Long vowels can be introduced later, first in the VCe form, in which the "e" is silent, as in *home*; followed by the open syllable with no consonant in the coda, as in *tray* or *she*. Appearing in short syllables or syllables with unusual spellings, long vowels can be taught as intervention assumes more of a reading focus. The inconsistent spelling of long vowels can be seen in *day, weigh,* and *raise.*

Training of the phoneme–grapheme relationship should be approached cautiously following the outline above. Some sound–letter relationships, presented in Table 13.7, are particularly difficult.

Intervention for Morphological Awareness

Reading and spelling accuracy can be improved through instruction in morphological awareness together with other forms of linguistic awareness, including knowledge of phonology, orthography, syntax, and semantics (Kirk & Gillon, 2009). For example, morphological awareness intervention has resulted in improved reading and spelling performance for late elementary school students (Berninger, Nagy, et al., 2003; Butyniec-Thomas & Woloshyn, 1997).

Intervention focuses on increasing awareness of the morphological structure of words, with particular attention to the orthographic rules that apply when suffixes are added to the base word. For

TABLE 13.7 Difficult Phoneme–Grapheme Relationships

Phoneme	Example	Explanation
/r/-controlled vowels	Thr*ough*, tr*ue*, cr*ew*	Inconsistent spelling
diphthongs	Fl*y*, he*igh*t, r*igh*t	Inconsistent spelling
/ɛ/	So*fa*, tel*e*phone	Stress and spelling interact
/Λ/	F*u*n, w*o*n, *o*ne	Multiple spellings
Grapheme	**Example**	**Explanation**
-nk	Tha*nk*s, ri*nk*	Two phonemes /ηk/
x	Ta*x*i, ma*x*imum	Two sounds /ks/
u	t*u*ne, f*u*n	Two pronunciations /U/ and /Λ/
Plural -s	Dog*s*, cat*s*, kiss*es*	Multiple pronunciations
Past -ed	Walk*ed*, jogg*ed*, collid*ed*	Multiple pronunciations
-pt	Ke*pt*, sle*pt*	Final blend has short stop

Source: Information from Hambly & Riddle (2002).

example, the "y" in *happy* and *crazy* changes to an "i" before the *–ly* marker in *happily* and *crazily*. Intervention tasks might include (Kirk & Gillon, 2009)

- segmenting words into syllables and morphemes.
- combining affixes and base words (e.g., comparing the agentive *-er* suffix and the comparative *-er* suffix, as in *healer* vs. *bigger*, helps children understand that suffixes are more than just graphemes, and that they alter the meaning of a word in predictable ways).
- generating new words for each morpheme in a given word.
- identifying base words and common affixes, such as *un-, non-, dis-, -er, -est, -ing, -y, -ed, -iest, -ier, -ly, -ish, -en,* and *–ened*.
- identifying orthographic changes to the base word when a suffix is added (e.g., consonant doubling, as in *shopping*; e-drop, as in *riding*), and *y →i*, as in *funniest*.
- Recognizing semantic relationships between morphologically complex words.

Phonological opacity—the transparent or opaque nature of morphological derivations—affects both reading speed and accuracy. In transparency relationships, a base word does not change when a morphological affix is added, as in *active-actively*. In opaque relationships, the base word changes, as in *piano-pianist*. The more opaque the relationship, the more difficult the word is to read. An SLP can help older students by "morphing" words into parts and helping children to hear the sound changes while appreciating the spelling consistencies, as in *sign-signature*. A fun activity is "Comes From," which employs underlying semantic relationships (Green, 2004). In this activity, the SLP poses questions such as "Does *mother* come from *moth*?"

Intervention for Comprehension

Comprehension relies on many different aspects of processing. When we read, our knowledge and experience blend with the information on the page to form a mental representation of the meaning. An active reader makes inferences from the text and past knowledge and experience that bridge these gaps. An SLP or teacher attempts to facilitate this process through instruction, questions, visual and verbal cues, explanations, and comments (Crowe, 2003). By providing contextually supported intervention, such as establishing the content and setting the scene prior to reading, establishing relationships, and discussing unfamiliar vocabulary and concepts, an SLP or teacher assists students in constructing meaning from print. Using a conversational style, the adult provides cues and feedback as oral group reading occurs. It's important that questions used by adults reflect the level of comprehension targeted and not simply ask all students to recount facts from the page. The strategy should be accompanied by more direct vocabulary instruction, especially for words related to specific curricular topics, such as ecology or geometry (Ehren, 2006).

The effect of different adult strategies is dependent upon when they are used. For example, while semantic strategies prior to reading reduce reading miscues or errors, graphophonemic strategies are more effective during reading (Kouri, Selle, & Riley, 2006). Semantic strategies consist of giving a definition or synonym for key words. In contrast, graphophonemic strategies include encouraging a child to "sound out" a word, calling a child's attention to phonetic regularities, or asking a child to identify initial or final sounds or consonant blends.

Comprehension can be enhanced by inferential thinking that goes beyond the text and helps children integrate their world knowledge with the information on the page. This may consist of dialogue between the teacher and students to help students construct meaning as they read, not just at the conclusion of the story. The teacher can provide background information or encourage students to use their own knowledge sources.

Periodically during reading, students can summarize the story and/or select the main idea or ideas. Finally, they can contemplate alternatives, explain motives, personalize the story and, predict what will happen next in the story based on the information to this point.

Ideally, students will internalize comprehension strategies and use them as they read actively. Three types of strategies are goal-specific strategies, monitoring and repair, and packaging (Ehren, 2005, 2006). Goal-specifc strategies include the following:

- Using context to analyze word meaning
- Activating prior knowledge
- Rereading difficult passages
- Self-questioning to help frame key ideas
- Analyzing text structures to determine type of reading
- Visualizing content
- Paraphrasing in one's own words
- Summarizing

These strategies are used in tandem with the monitoring and repair strategies, in which a reader decides if a reading passage makes sense and, if not, what repairs need to be made so that it does. On the basis of these answers, a reader decides which of the goal-specific strategies to continue, discontinue, or modify. Finally, packaging strategies organize the entire process, planning what to do and how to do it through the other two types of strategies. It's this active aspect of reading that truly constitutes self-regulated reading. Let's take a look at the goal-specific strategies in more detail.

When we analyze children's eye movements while reading, we begin to understand that their eyes are bounding ahead and back, trying to check the accuracy of words within the surrounding meaning. Children are sense-makers, and when they read, they are trying to make sense of the words on the page. In similar fashion they can be taught to use this information to determine word meaning (Owens & Kim, 2007). They can also be helped to use dictionaries and glossaries, to analyze words into roots, and to use sentence structure to acquire word meaning.

Activation of prior knowledge improves comprehension, especially for children with LD. As a student reads, he or she gathers information that is kept current and used to interpret following passages. Once students can successfully access this knowledge, they can be helped to use it to predict subsequent information from the text. In addition, children can be helped in applying past learning and experience to the comprehension task.

Good readers recognize when they have not comprehended a written passage and therefore reread it. Poor readers may not realize that they have missed key points. Several of the strategies presented here will help students with LI recognize what they don't know. When this is highlighted for them, a teacher or SLP can guide them to reread portions of the text.

Self-questioning is a strategy that encourages a reader to be active and to make inferences that the author hopefully intended the reader to make. Students should be encouraged to ask questions about the structure, such as when and where a narrative occurred, and about specific content, such as why a character acted a certain way.

Text structure provides information that assists readers in determining overall organization and important points. Students can be instructed in the use of text structure to assist comprehension, modeling, and guided and independent practice, including "think alouds" to evaluate one's progress. Explorations to be made by a reader include

- the type of text, expository or narrative.
- visual cues that aid in figuring out the organization, such as headings, introductory paragraphs, and topic sentences.
- overall organization.
- the most important ideas.
- devices that signal how ideas are connected.

By helping children with LI visualize the content, written material, especially narration, comes alive. Imagery can be taught as a strategy for increasing comprehension.

Paraphrasing and summarizing can occur at various points in reading, such as the end of a paragraph or a passage. Good readers do this automatically as they read. Paraphrasing demonstrates a child's comprehension by forcing a child to focus on the meaning and to replace content words and/or syntactic structure with equivalent forms. In order to paraphrase and summarize, students with LI may need to be helped in identifying the main idea in what they read.

Identifying the Main Idea

Children with LI often cannot find the main idea or organizing frame even in simple texts. This task is fundamental to success in comprehension and academic success.

Structure of narrative and expository texts differs greatly and affects comprehension and memory. Readers or listeners go through a process of deleting, generalizing, and integrating the propositions of a text until they reach a macrostructure that summarizes the propositions presented. This process is dependent on underlying cognitive classification skills and world knowledge. Text often is evaluated for its "goodness-of-fit" to the reader's expectations.

Informational understanding develops as the readers progressively revise their expectations until they approximate the meaning of the author. Organizational clues supplied by the author enable the reader to interpret the passage and determine the main ideas.

Several textual features signal important information, including graphic features, such as italics, boldface, and type size; syntactic features, such as word order; semantic features, such as summaries and introductions; and schematic features, such as text structure. Of course, it is easiest to determine the overall organization if the topic is stated explicitly in the first sentence.

Good readers are sensitive to the text organization. They "discover" the organizing structure. Many children with LI have difficulty comprehending and producing narratives because they fail to realize the internal organization of the text (Yoshinaga-Itano & Snyder, 1985). These children fail to integrate new information with prior knowledge or fail to use the author's clues. Poor readers use a fragmented organization or impose an unrelated structure.

Intervention might include comprehension strategies, such as predicting, questioning, clarifying, and summarizing; semantic networking; generative tasks in which the child generates a summary sentence; and familiarization with different text structures (Armbuster, Anderson, & Ostertag, 1987; Richgels, McGee, Lomax, & Sheard, 1987; J. Williams, 1988). Summarizing strategies used by older children include deletion of unimportant information, deletion of redundant information, substitution of category names for various category members, and selection or creation of a topic sentence. Direct instruction in these strategies results in the best performance.

Semantic networking or organizing is a method of teaching organization. Helping children organize and reorganize structure during and after reading improves reading comprehension, writing cohesion, retention, and recall.

Ideas are displayed in semantic networks as clusters resembling spiders. Major ideas are circles or other shapes. Lines form related ideas or connect major ideas. Semantic clusters can be taught with a guided study approach that helps the child develop generalizable strategies. Slowly, students adapt and internalize the methods for reading comprehension and for writing.

Organizational patterns are of two types: cluster and episodic. Cluster patterns are for superordination and subordination. In Figure 13.2, the topic, or superordinate aspect, is in the center. Related ideas radiate outward. Episodic organizers representing change move from event to event as in narration. These also can be used for problem-solution and cause-effect diagrams.

Children can begin to use semantic organizers in kindergarten or first grade, drawing pictures for the sequence of events in a narrative. Older children can write events in each cluster, either to aid recall or to structure narratives for telling or retelling. Variations, such as the story map, can help children develop story grammars (Figure 13.2). Similar diagrams, such as the mind map, can be adapted to various purposes, such as a book report, newspaper article, or argument. Likewise, classroom brainstorming can help children realize their prior knowledge by examining all they know about a given topic.

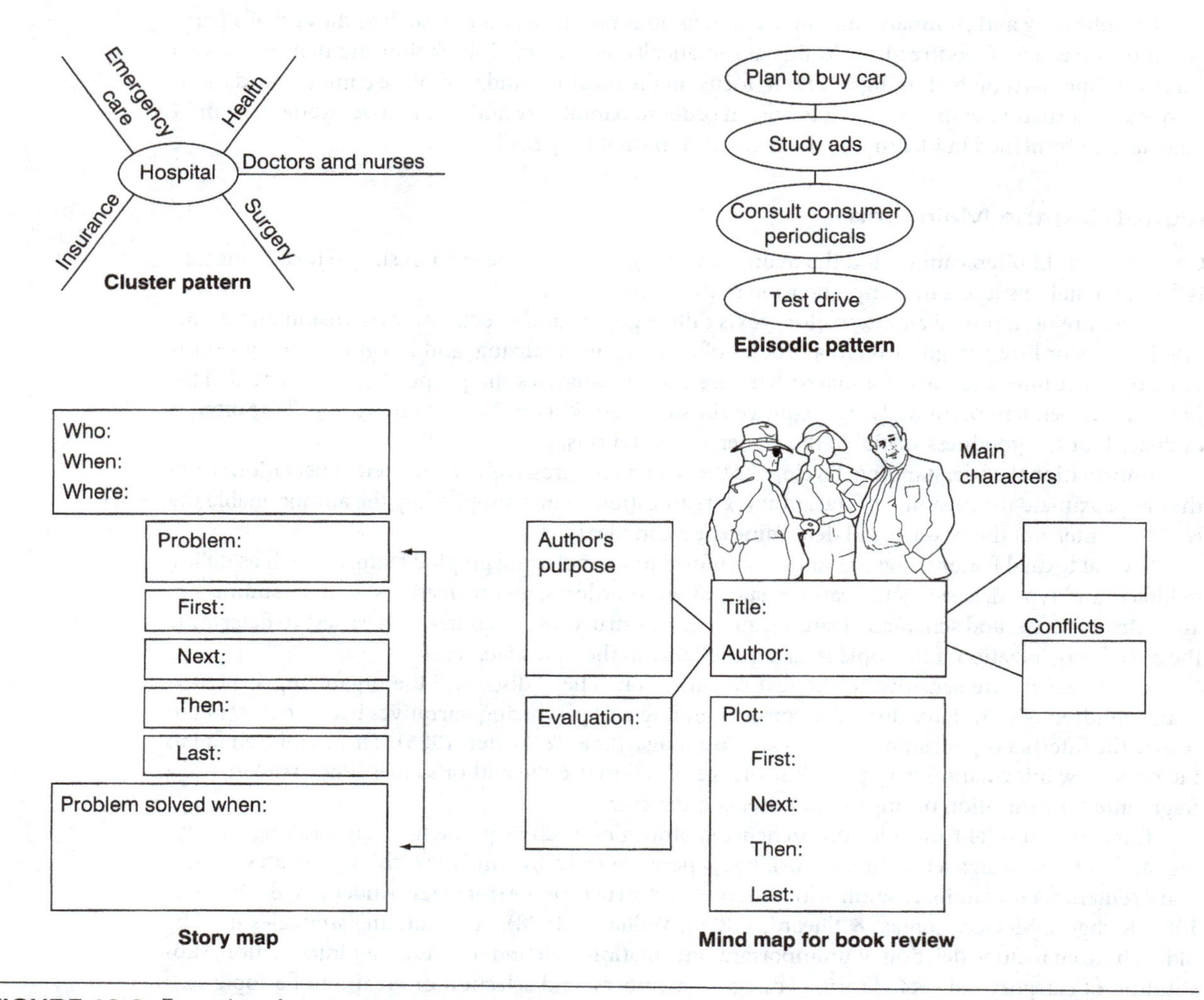

FIGURE 13.2 Examples of semantic networks.

As SLPs, we are interested in language and in helping children make sense of the language they receive and produce. This includes both what they hear and read. Now let's look at writing.

Writing

As with all language modes, writing is a social act. Just like a speaker, the writer must consider the audience. Because the audience is not present when the writing occurs, writing demands more cognitive resources for planning and execution than does speaking. Writing is a complex process that includes the generation of ideas, organization and planning, action based on the plan, revision, monitoring, and self-feedback. More abstract and decontextualized than conversation, writing also requires internal knowledge of the writing form. Forms can be divided into narrative and expository writing.

Expository texts have several forms. The easiest type, especially with familiar content, is sequential or procedurally organized, while others are descriptive with little overall structure. A typical sequential text explains how something is accomplished. Problem-solving, cause-and-effect, and compare-and-contrast genres are the most difficult.

The writing system consists of several processes: text construction, handwriting, spelling, executive function, and memory (Berninger, 2000). Text construction is the process of going from ideas to written texts. This is not the same as actual handwriting and spelling, although all three are correlated. Texts consist of words and sentences that support the ideas of the writer.

Executive function is the self-regulatory aspect of writing. It's the ability to select and sustain attention, organize perception, and flexibly shift perceptual and cognitive setup, as well as control social and affective behavior (Ylvisaker & DeBonis, 2000). Further, executive function includes realistic self-appraisal of strengths and weaknesses and the difficulty of tasks; the ability to set reasonable goals; planning and organizing to achieve each goal; initiating, monitoring, and evaluating your performance in relation to each goal; and revising plans and strategies based on feedback. Intelligence and executive function are not the same thing, although language use and executive function are interdependent.

Young writers must first develop a foundation in text generation and transcription (spelling, handwriting, and punctuation) before they can divert cognitive resources to higher level processes, such as planning and revising. Among upper-level elementary school children, the process of encoding thoughts and ideas into meaningful words, phrases, clauses, and sentences generally limits the planning and revising components of writing seen among older adolescents and adults (Berninger, 2000).

The writing of TD Spanish-speaking early adolescent bilingual English language learners (ELLs) demonstrates similar lexical, syntactic, and discourse sophistication across both languages, indicating that these teens are emerging writers in both Spanish and English (Danzak, 2011). This implies the potential transfer of writing skills across languages.

Memory serves the writer in many ways. Working memory stores ideas as they are worked and reworked by the writer. Short-term memory is used for word recognition while writing. Long-term memory provides content and word knowledge as well as overall format. Automaticity of retrieving letters and words from memory and producing them contributes to the quality of text generation.

Writing Problems

Children with oral language impairments will most likely have writing impairments too. For many children with LI, writing difficulties do not decrease with age, and the gap widens between their writing abilities and those of children developing typically. The content and organization of their writing suffer as more of their cognitive capacity is used for the lower-level mechanics of writing, such as spelling.

Children with LD have difficulties with all aspects of the writing process (Troia, Graham, & Harris, 1999; Vallecorsa & Garriss, 1990; Wong, 2000). Because, they have little knowledge of the writing process and find it frustrating, children with LLD fail to plan, make few substantive revisions, and write very little on a given task. Cognitive capacity is expended on low-order mechanics. Spelling often follows a maladaptive pattern in which words that can be spelled are substituted for those that cannot. In the process, meaning suffers.

In narrative writing as in storytelling, children with LI lack mature internalized story schemes. As noted in Chapter 8, the oral narratives of children with LI are often shorter with fewer episodes, contain fewer details, and often fail to consider the needs of the listener. Listeners are only rarely given cause and effect or character motivation. The oral and written narratives of children with LI have similar characteristics.

In general, children with LI exhibit reduced written productivity as measured by total number of words, total number of utterances, or total number of ideas (Puranik, Lombardino, & Altmann, 2007; Scott & Windsor, 2000). Similarly, these same children exhibit deficits in writing *complexity* as measured by average length of T-units, number of different words, and percentage of complex sentences (Fey, Catts, Proctor-Williams, Tomblin, & Zhang, 2004; Mackie & Dockrell, 2004; Nelson & Van Meter, 2003; Puranik et al., 2007; Scott & Windsor, 2000). Finally, children with LI exhibit reduced *accuracy* as measured by number of spelling or mechanical errors and number of syntax errors (Altmann, Lombardino, & Puranik, 2008; Mackie & Dockrell, 2004; Nelson & Van Meter, 2003; Puranik et al., 2007).

Deficits in Executive Function

When executive function is impaired, communication abilities are diminished, especially in socially demanding or complex linguistic tasks, such as writing. Executive function is especially important for the pragmatic aspects of communication, memory and retrieval, strategic thinking, perspective taking, and generalization.

Executive function impairment is most evident in children with TBI. The high frequency of frontal lobe injury makes executive function particularly vulnerable for these children. Children with ADHD have been described as inattentive and impulsive, disorganized, unable to inhibit behavior, and ineffective learners, characteristics of those with impaired executive function.

When children with LD write, they follow a "retrieve-write" strategy in which they write whatever comes to mind, each sentence stimulating the next, with little thought to planning. The result is that they produce and elaborate very little. Revisions are ineffective and can be characterized by seeming indifference to the audience, inept detection of errors, and difficulty executing intended changes (Graham & Harris, 1999).

Deficits in Spelling

Writing and spelling are separate but correlated processes. Children with written-language deficits due to LD, SLI, or other causes may have problems in either or both. In general, children have more difficulty with spelling if handwriting is also a problem (Berninger, Abbott, Rogan, Reed, Abbott, et al., 1998).

Poor spellers view spelling as arbitrary and random. To them, spelling is difficult and ultimately unlearnable. Beyond the obvious difficulties for poor spellers are the parallel deficits seen in reading. Poor spellers have poor word attack or decoding skills.

The misspellings of the poorest older spellers suggest the following patterns of spelling deficits (Moats, 1995):

- Omission of liquids and nasals in rime or noninitial positions, as in *SEF* for *self* and *RET* for *rent*
- Omission in consonant clusters, especially in the syllable- and word-final positions, as in *FAT* for *fast*
- Omission of unstressed vowel, as in *TELFON* for telephone
- Vowel substitutions, as in *TRI* for *try*
- Consonant substitutions that share some articulatory features, as in "t" for "d" or "m" for "n"
- Omission of plural inflections
- Omission or substitution of past tense inflections
- Misspelling of difficult common words, such as *their/there* and *to/too/two*

Many poor spellers demonstrate primitive phonologically based errors even when they have high levels of orthographic knowledge.

Although most TD spellers shift to greater use of analogy (e.g., *pillage* is spelled like *village*) between second and fifth grade, poor spellers continue to rely on visual matching skills and phoneme position rules because of limited knowledge of sound-letter correspondences (Kamhi & Hinton,

2000). In other words, they continue to use the visual approach to learning that characterizes much younger spellers.

Spelling deficits are only rarely caused by poor visual memory. Usually, deficits in spelling represent poor phonological processing and poor knowledge and use of phoneme-grapheme information.

Assessment of Writing

One method of assessing writing in the classroom is through the use of portfolios of children's writing. Portfolios are a collection of meaningful writing selected by a child, SLP, and teacher that contains samples of the child's writing over time, enabling the child to demonstrate progress. The wide variety helps to increase the validity of the sample. Allowing children to contribute fosters self-growth and monitoring. In addition, selection of teacher and SLP choices fosters collaboration. Guidelines for portfolio use in an initial evaluation are as follows (Manning Kratcoski, 1998):

- Careful determination of the items to be included for variety over time
- Analysis appropriate for the different types of writing and the goals of the assessment
- Appropriate persons contributing items

Items to be included in a portfolio may include SLP observation notes, work samples, and first drafts of writing samples, such as journal or learning log entries, and projects/papers, final drafts of the same, and peer and teacher evaluations.

Executive function is best assessed within overall writing assessment or through dynamic assessment techniques mentioned in Chapter 4. There is a risk in separating the various functions and considering them separately from functional communication tasks (Fey, 1986).

Data Collection

Samples should be written in ink to allow the SLP to note revisions. The teacher or SLP should inform children that edits are fine and encourage them to do their best. It's helpful to allow children to plan and to write drafts. Paper can be provided for notes and plans and should be collected along with the finished product. These can be added to the portfolio mentioned previously. Whenever possible, the SLP can observe the writing process for evidence of planning and organizing, drafting, writing, revising, and editing.

There is little consensus in the professional literature on the best way to collect a written language sample (Hudson, Lane, & Mercer, 2005). Writing samples have been gathered using a variety of methods. While adolescents acquire greater skill with expository writing, it seems appropriate to use narrative writing, such as spontaneous stories of story retelling from a book or video, with younger children. In addition to reflecting the demands of the curriculum, including comprehending read-aloud material, holding key concepts in memory, and reformulating the information, a narrative retelling format gives the SLP some control of the stimulus input and a more reliable gauge of the accuracy of information recalled and the propositions and inferences made (Puranik, Lombardino, & Altmann, 2008). Although constraints of memory load in text-retelling tasks exist for some children with LI, elementary school transcription skills seem to have a greater impact than memory skills (Graham, Berninger, Abbott, Abbott, & Whitaker, 1997).

Personal written narratives can be elicited using a format found on many states' fourth-grade writing examination (Puranik, Lombardino, & Altmann, 2008). This generally takes the following form:

> Think about your favorite thing to do.... Maybe you like to.... Write a story about a fun time that you had doing your favorite thing. Give enough details to show the reader what happened and why it was fun. (Massachusetts Department of Education, 2006)

Of course, this information may need to be simplified for children with LI.

Expository texts can be elicited by a number of procedures. For example, sequential/procedural texts can be elicited by asking the child, "Tell me how you make _____." With the cause-and-effect genre, the SLP might say, "Tell me what might happen if _____." Problem-solving genres can be encouraged with "How would you _____?" It is important to pose familiar and unfamiliar themes. Key words, such as *describe, compare, contrast, cause,* and *solve* can cue the child for the type desired.

Added information can be obtained if children read their paper aloud while being audiotaped. This procedure aids the SLP in interpreting garbled or poorly spelled words.

Data Analysis

Writing can be analyzed on several levels, including textual, linguistic, and orthographic (spelling). At a textual level, the SLP can note compositional length, an indication of the amount of effort; quality, a holistic rating on the nature of the task; and discourse structure, the way in which text is related to the global topic or comments support the topic (Berninger, 2000).

The child's writing can be photocopied for mark-up and analysis. Of interest are the total number of words, clauses, and T-units. The use of T-units can help to avoid long run-on sentences but does not reflect "grammatical accuracy," so further internal analysis must be performed (N. Nelson & Van Meter, 2002). These are outlined in Chapter 8. Writing conventions, such as capitalization and punctuation, plus the use of sentences and paragraphs, should be noted. Spelling can be analyzed as explained below.

By adolescence, the expository writing of typically developing children has made several strides. Changes found in persuasive writing include increases in essay length, mean length of utterance measured in words, relative clause production, and use of literate words (Nippold, Ward-Lonergan, & Fanning, 2005). Literate words include adverbial conjuncts, discussed earlier (*however, finally, in conclusion, personally*), abstract nouns (*kindness, loyalty, benefits, pleasure*), and metalinguistic and metacognitive verbs (*think, remember, reflect, agree, persuade, confess*). The greater flexibility of older writers is seen in presentation of greater numbers of reasons and acknowledgment of diverse perspectives and differing opinions. Average values are presented in Table 13.8. Individual variation is

TABLE 13.8 Parameters of Persuasive Writing by Age

	Age 11	Age 17	Age 24
MLU-W (Mean length of utterance in words)	11.3	13.9	15.9
Range	5.5–19.3	8.9–23.8	11.1–27
Below 1 SD	5.5–8.3	8.9–11.9	11.1–14.6
Total words	146.9	188.5	262.9
Range	33–297	86–321	146–481
Below 1 SD	33–88	86–139	146–215
Word types as percentage of total words			
Adverbial conjuncts	0.3%	0.77%	0.83%
Range	0–3.9%	0–2.8%	0–2.5%
Abstract nouns	2.7%	5.7%	7.8%
Range	0–6.3%	1.8–17.3%	3.7–16.4%
Metaverbs	1.3%	1.9%	2%
Range	0–3.7%	0–5.9%	0–4.6%
Total utterances	13.6	14.7	17.3
Range	4–30	5–33	7–37
Below 1 SD	4–9.8	5–10.6	7–12.7
Relative clauses as percentage of total utterances	11.7%	16.7%	20.8%
Total reasons	6.8	7.9	12.7

Source: Information taken from Nippold, Mansfield, & Billow (2007).

great, and there is much overlap. It's important to recognize that these values will vary by task and represent a 20-minute writing sample based on a presentation of three diverse points of view and the instructions to state one's own perspective supported by several good reasons for the opinion. Readers are urged to consult the original research for data collection methods.

Spelling Assessment

Although it may seem straightforward, spelling deficits are very complex and can be difficult to describe. Collection should be of sufficient quantity to allow for a broad-based analysis of error types.

Data Collection. Spelling deficits should be assessed through both dictation and connected writing (Masterson & Apel, 2000). In dictation, either within standardized testing or from word inventories, the SLP or teacher reads words while the child writes them. Standardized tests include the Test of Written Language (Hammill & Larson, 1996), Test of Written Spelling (Larson & Hammill, 1994), and the Wide Range Achievement Test–3 (Wilkinson, 1995).

Word inventories, either preselected—such as those found in Bear, Invernizzi, Templeton, and Johnston (2000)—or SLP-designed, should be developmental in nature and include several phoneme-grapheme variations, including, but not limited to, single consonants in various positions in words, consonant blends, morphological inflections, diphthongs, digraphs or two letters for one phoneme such as "ch" and "sh," and complex morphologic derivations as in *omit-omission*. The choice of words will vary with the age and functioning level of the child. The number of words must be sufficient to identify patterns of functioning. Using 50 to 100 words is probably adequate, although more is desirable (Masterson & Apel, 2000).

Single-word spelling may be of little real value because decontextualized spelling does not measure a child's ability in a real communicative context. More functional connected writing can be generated in response to pictures or narratives or provided portfolios. In a variation, the child can write an original sentence or narrative using representative words taken from word lists.

Testing tasks that require a child to select correctly spelled words may seen like a good assessment tool but may be of little actual value (Ehri, 2000). These tasks occur infrequently in the real world of the child and thus are not functional for either assessment or intervention.

Data Analysis. Descriptive analysis should focus on orthographic patterns evident in the child's spelling (Bear et al., 2000). While individual errors are significant, error patterns are important for intervention. Of interest are the most frequent and the lowest level patterns.

The SLP tries to determine the type of error reflected in the child's spelling of each incorrect word. It's helpful to analyze base words (*teach*), inflected words (*teaches*), and derived words (*teacher*) separately to see if errors are related to any specific word form. Spelling is the result of segmenting a word into phonemic elements and selecting the appropriate graphemes. In analyzing the spelling sample, the SLP should note consonant blends by location within the syllable and word and by the presence of other phonemes. The SLP should seek phonemic (EKWAT for *equate*), morphologic (omits morphologic markers), or semantic (confuses similar sounding words, as in *there, their,* and *they're*) explanations for error patterns (Bourassa & Treiman, 2001).

Phonological processing and spelling are related for elementary school children, less so for older students who use multiple spelling strategies. If the child uses an incorrect letter, the error most likely represents a problem in phonological awareness. Inserted or deleted letters may represent a speech perception problem.

In addition, the SLP should look at each error to determine the child's orthographic system knowledge. This includes letter selection and position constraints. For example, "ts" is an acceptable blend but is constrained by position and is not acceptable at the beginning of a word, with the exception of the Russian "tsar" and the Japanese "tsunami." Such knowledge addresses the question *Could this be a word?* Has the child's error violated acceptable English spelling or would the resultant word be an acceptable one?

Intervention for Writing Impairment

Intervention for writing may involve both general training and more specific techniques for narrative and expository forms. Generalization is enhanced if intervention is functional, curriculum-based, and within authentic writing projects.

Executive function can be targeted within the writing process using a goal-plan-do-review format. (Ylvisaker, Szekeres, & Feeney, 1998). Although there is little an SLP can do to alleviate the root causes of TBI, ADHD, or other impairments relative to executive function, he or she can provide external support to enable children with these impairments to experience some level of success (Ylvisaker & DeBonis, 2000). This should not be interpreted to mean that the SLP acts as the child's executive function. In that situation, little changes for the child. SLPs give children the tools to facilitate their lives. SLPs change behaviors and processes. In the end, we cannot live our client's lives for them.

Intervention can begin by allowing children to select their own topics. This increases motivation and shifts the focus to ideas. Mechanics will come later. Topic selection works well with small groups of children and the sharing process often generates more ideas.

In the planning phase, the SLP and child can brainstorm ideas for inclusion in the writing (Troia, Graham, & Harris, 1999). Drawings and ideational maps or spider diagrams can help. For narratives, children might draw a few simple pictures and organize them in the appropriate order. Computer programs, such as *The Amazing Writing Machine* (Broderbund, 1999) and *The Ultimate Writing and Creativity Center* (The Learning Company), can also be helpful. It is also useful for the child to focus on the potential audience. The SLP can ask questions such as the following (Graham & Harris, 1999):

Who will read this paper?

What do the readers know?

What do the readers need to know?

Why are you writing?

The SLP and child may prefer to use computers as an assistive technology for writing (MacArthur, 2000). Software, such as *Inspiration* (Inspirations Software, 1997), can aid text generation, and the result is easily modifiable by the child or teacher. Although the technology itself is unlikely to improve writing, it does remove the handwriting difficulties for some children. Typing can also detract from text development, and computer use can result in new burdens for working memory. Having said this, we should note that children with LD who receive training in executive function along with word processing make greater gains in the quality of their writing than children instructed only in executive function. Word processing experience alone, however, does not improve overall quality.

A word about spellcheckers and grammar checkers seems in order. Neither are foolproof, as I'm sure you know. Spellcheckers will be discussed in the following section on spelling. Grammar checkers miss many errors, especially if there are multiple spelling errors, and can easily confuse the writer who is left to figure out just what the error is.

Word-prediction programs, such as *Co:Writer* (D. Johnston, 1998), *Write Away* 2000 (Information Services, 1989), and *Clicker 5* (2005), are helpful, but mostly for spelling (MacArthur, 2000; Ylvisaker & DeBonis, 2000). Most have speech synthesis too. Inputs vary from spelling only to spelling plus grammar. It's important that the word-prediction program's vocabulary match the writing task of the child (MacArthur, 1999). For example, *Co:Writer* incorporates the word frequency and topic of the writer. *Write Away 2000* allows the child or teacher to add vocabulary, and content-specific prompts can be added to expand the vocabulary. In contrast, *Clicker Plus* allows the child or teacher to download specific words.

Finally, speech recognition software allows children to compose by dictation, resulting in longer and higher quality papers by children with LD. Children must be instructed to speak clearly in order to improve speech recognition and to dictate punctuation and formatting. Speech-recognition software cannot overcome oral language difficulties, although these can be moderated with the additional use of grammar checkers.

Narrative Writing

Narrative writing may require explicit instruction in story structure as outlined in Chapter 11. Story maps using pictures or story frames may be necessary initially but should be faded gradually as the child assumes more responsibility for the narrative. Story frames are written starters for each main-story grammar element. The child completes the sentence and continues with that portion of the narrative. Cards or checklists can also be used to remind the child of story grammar elements.

During the writing process, the SLP can use story guides, prompts, and acronyms to aid the child. Story guides are questions that help a student construct the narrative, while prompts are story beginning and ending phrases. Acronyms, such as SPACE for setting, problem, action, and consequent events, can also act as prompts for guiding writing. Children can be encouraged to write more with verbal prompts such as "Tell me more" or "What happened next?"

Feelings and motivations found in mature narratives are often missing from the stories of children with LI. These elements can be targeted with pictures and questions such as "How do you think she felt?" (Roth, 2000).

Expository Writing

Procedures for intervention with expository writing include collaborative planning; individual, independent writing; conferencing with the teacher/SLP and peers; individual, independent revising; and final editing (Wong, 2000). Whatever the expository genre involved, collaborative planning is important, including planning, writing, and revising. In the first step, the child should think aloud and solicit opinions. This is an opportunity for the child to hear alternative views and to reconcile these with his or her own.

For opinion papers, the child first needs to pick a topic. These might come from a prepared list, from the child, or from topics discussed in class. Once the topic is selected and discussed in small groups, with a peer, and/or with the SLP, the SLP can give the child a planning sheet to help organize her or his thoughts. It might include two columns: *What I believe* and *What someone else believes* (Wong, 2000). After the child has completed the sheet, either with help or working alone, the SLP can help the child form dyads of opposing views. This is a great time for verbal repartee, challenging, and helping the child clarify his or her views and prepare for independent writing.

Writing, although independent, can be fostered through the use of a prompt card containing key words for each major section of the paper. Table 13.9 presents a sample prompt card. After the child has completed the paper, he or she conferences with peers for feedback while the SLP mediates. The child revises the paper based on feedback.

At each stage in the process, the child should record progress on a checklist. In addition to providing a model for the writing process, the checklist can motivate the child as she or he finishes each step.

For compare-and-contrast writing, the planning process can be similar. Again, the topic—which entities are to be compared—can come from prepared lists, the child, or the curriculum. Through brainstorming, the child and SLP try to answer the question "How can we compare them?" SLPs should be prepared for some comparisons that are very "original," especially from children who have perceptual deficits and may view the world quite differently from adults.

TABLE 13.9 Sample Prompt Card for Opinion Writing

Section of Paper	Examples
Introduction	In my opinion . . . I believe . . . From my point of view . . . I agree with . . . I disagree with . . . Supporting words: first, second, finally, for example, most important is . . . , consider, think about, remember
Counter Opinion	Although . . . However, . . . On the other hand, . . . To the contrary, . . . Even though . . .
Conclusion	In conclusion . . . After considering both sides, . . . To summarize, . . .

Source: Information from Wong, Butler, Ficzere, & Kuperis (1996).

Again, the child can be helped with writing prompts, such as the following (Ylsivaker & DeBonis, 2000):

In this essay, I'm going to compare and contrast. . .
I have chosen two (any number) features: . . .
In conclusion, . . .

As mentioned previously, peer, teacher, and SLP review and feedback can help the child revise.

Intervention for Spelling

The SLP is not the "spelling teacher." It is as inappropriate for the SLP to teach this week's spelling list as it is to teach this week's vocabulary. Rather the SLP's role is to help children learn to spell.

Much of our previous discussion of phonological awareness intervention is also applicable here. The benefits to spelling of early phonological awareness training are well documented. In addition to spelling better by mid-elementary school than children who did not receive preschool phonological awareness training, children who did receive such training are more likely to employ morphological awareness—knowledge of root words and affixes—when spelling (Kirk & Gillon, 2007).

Words selected for intervention should be individualized for each child and reflect both the curriculum and the child's desires. Spelling intervention should be integrated into real writing and reading within the classroom. It is best if intervention can occur when the child is actually writing and he or she can be reminded of alphabetic and orthographic principles (Scott, 2000). Words misspelled in class can be analyzed by the SLP. Spelling strategies can be discussed with the child using these words.

Spelling can be taught within teaching of general executive function in which the child is taught to proofread, correct, and edit. Peer editing is also effective (Graham, 1999).

Prompted spelling is helping a child identify the sounds in the word, such as the length of the vowel, and the orthographic pattern. With bound morphemes, the SLP might ask the child to recall what happens when the morpheme is added to certain words with long and short vowels, as in *roping* and *ripping*.

If needed, spelling intervention should begin with alphabetic principles, connecting sounds and letters. Targeted words can be taught as explained below but expanded into onset-rime training to facilitate overall spelling ability.

Children with LD benefit from multisensory input such as pictures, objects, or actions (Graham, 1999). Several multisensory study techniques have been proposed. For example, the child (1) says the word; (2) writes it while saying it again; (3) checks spelling; and, (4) if correct, traces it while saying it again; then finally, (5) writes the word and checks the spelling. In a variation, the child pronounces the word carefully. Letters are pronounced in sequence, then recalled. The child then writes the word, checks, and if incorrect, respells and checks again.

In the 8-Step Method (Berninger, Abbott, et al., 1998), first, the SLP sweeps his or her finger over the word and pronounces it out loud. Next, to call attention to the phoneme-grapheme correspondence, the SLP says the word again emphasizing sounds that correspond to colored letter groupings. For example, /b/-/i/-/d/ for "b"-"ea"-"d." On the third pass, the child names the letters as the SLP points to each in sequence. The child then closes his or her eyes and visualizes the word. In step five, while his or her eyes are closed, the child spells the word out loud. Following this step, the child writes the word, then compares it to the sample. In the final step, the SLP reinforces the child's correct spelling. If the child's spelling is incorrect, the SLP points out the difference between the sample and the child's attempt and repeats the previous steps.

Word analysis and sorting tasks can be used to strengthen the alphabetic principle (Scott, 2000). Patterns to be taught should be identified from the child's misspellings. Minimum pairs that differ on the bases of these processes can be used to demonstrate the lexical consequences of misspelling (Masterson & Crede, 1999). The SLP should use known and unknown words to facilitate generalization.

Sorting tasks will differ based on the spelling level of the child (Scott, 2000). Sorting may be of various patterns:

- Morphological (*magic, magical, magically, magician*)
- Phonological (e.g., words that were phonologically identical except for the length of the vowel, as in *-ke* and *-ck* in *bake, back*)
- Orthographic (e.g., length of the vowel or consistent orthographic shape despite phonological variation as in the three variants of *–ed* in *walked, jogged*, and *glided*)
- Syntactic (e.g., by word class as noun, verb, or adjective and learning how these categories interact with various suffixes)
- Semantic (e.g., *to, too, two*)

At the letter-name level of development, words can be sorted or grouped by sounds and location, as in initial consonants or initial digraphs (two letters = one sound, "sh" = /ʃ/). Minimal pairs might contrast short vowels, long and short vowels, single consonants and blends, and one digraph with another. With more mature spellers, the SLP can sort by orthographic patterns, such as vowel patterns, rimes, and homophones. In later stages, words can be grouped by syllable juncture principles and meaning, including inflectional suffixes and simple prefixes and derivational suffixes, consonant doubling with open and closed syllables, compound words, changing final "y" to "i," and word roots. Minimal pairs may contrast variants of inflectional suffixes, such as "-s" and "-es," and base words with derivational suffixes, as in *teach/teacher*.

Computers are helpful and encourage editing, although spellcheckers are not foolproof and the child may learn little. In general, spellcheckers miss words in which the misspelling has inadvertently produced another word. Suggested spellings may also confound the child with poor word attack skills. In addition, suggested spellings may be far afield if the original word has multiple misspellings. Spellcheckers help only about 37 percent of the time for children with LD, a lower percentage than found among children developing typically (MacArthur, Graham, Haynes, & DeLaPaz, 1996).

On the other hand, word-prediction programs reduce spelling errors of children with LI by over half, although the user must get the initial letters correct for the program to work effectively.

If children with LI are taught to spell phonetically when unsure of the correct spelling, spell-checkers generate more correct suggestions. Proofing and editing on a hard copy also seem to increase the number of correctly spelled words. Internet searches can foster spelling learning because correct spelling is needed to complete searches successfully.

Spelling intervention is more meaningful if it occurs within authentic writing exercises, such as curriculum-based writing. Within these activities, children can be taught to ask themselves if they can identify word part or initial or final sounds. They can try to identify similarly sounding words or identify locations where the word has appeared. These can be checked for the correct spelling. When all else fails, the student should try to find the word in the dictionary. This may be facilitated by use of a personal or class dictionary or dictionaries produced for different classroom topics. Computer spellcheckers may also be helpful.

Conclusion

And so, we reach the end of this text. I hope that I have challenged your thinking along the way and that you'll use this book as a reference. Even in the area of literacy, functional communication is important. Using real reading and writing samples. Training for the kinds of reading and writing that the child is encountering in the classroom. And we have come full circle. Intervention in the classroom is about as close as an SLP in the schools can get to the actual use environment of the child. Other aspects of the model that we have discussed may also be present. For example, parents may be involved in their children's training. Cues and consequences should still be as natural as possible. Literacy being as functional as possible is especially important. Remember. . . .

> *Decontextualized training routinely fails at the level of generalization* . . . (Ylvisaker & DeBonis, 2000, p. 43)

Appendix A

Considerations for CLD Children

Most regional and ethnic dialects differ only slightly from the standard or are used by a limited number of individuals. Three ethnic dialects, however, represent rather large segments of the U.S. population and have some very important differences with (MAE) Majority American English. These dialects are African American English, Latino English, and Asian English. African American English is used primarily by working-class African Americans in the urban northern United States and rural African Americans in the South. Not every African American uses African American English, and not everyone who uses it is African American.

Latino English and Asian English are probably misnomers. Latino English, as used here, is a composite of the English used by many speakers who are bilingual Spanish-English and learned English as a second language. Individual variations represent the age of learning and level of mastery, the Spanish dialect used, socioeconomic status, and where the person lives in the United States. Asian English is also a composite, but of bilingual speakers of Asian languages who learned English as a second language. As such, Asian English probably does not exist except to simplify our discussion. Asians speak many languages, and each has a different effect on the learning of English. In addition to the original language learned, other individual differences may reflect the same factors as those of Latino English. Each dialect is discussed in some detail. Where possible, information has been reduced to tables to aid presentation. Each dialect is compared with Majority American English, an idealized norm uninfluenced by the dialectal differences each person possesses.

African American English

African American English reflects the complex racial and economic history of the United States and the migration of African Americans from the rural South to the urban North after World War II. Regional differences exist to some degree. The major variations between (MAE) Majority American English and African American English in phonology, syntax, and morphology are presented in Tables A.1 and A.2.

Latino English

Speakers who are bilingual may move back and forth between both languages in a process called *code switching*. The amount of code switching depends on the speaker's mastery of the two languages and on the audience being addressed. Of course, a great deal of code switching makes the speaker's English incomprehensible to the listener who is monolingual American English.

Most characteristics of Latino English reflect interference points, or points where the two languages differ, thus making learning somewhat more difficult. For example, the speaker of Latino

TABLE A.1 Phonemic Contrasts Between African American English and Majority American English (MAE)

MAE Phonemes	Position in Word		
	Initial	**Medial**	**Final***
/p/		Unaspirated /p/	Unaspirated /p/
/n/			Reliance on preceding nasalized vowel
/w/	Omitted in specific words (*I 'as, too!*)		
/b/		Unreleased /b/	Unreleased /b/
/g/		Unreleased /g/	Unreleased /g/
/k/		Unaspirated /k/	Unaspirated /k/
/d/	Omitted in specific words (*I 'on't know*)	Unreleased /d/	Unreleased /d/
/ŋ/		/n/	/n/
/t/		Unaspirated /t/	Unaspirated /t/
/l/		Omitted before labial consonants (*help-hep*)	"uh" following a vowel (*Bill-Biuh*)
/r/		Omitted or /ə/	Omitted or prolonged vowel or glide
/θ/	Unaspirated /t/ or /f/	Unaspirated /t/ or /f/ between vowels	Unaspirated /t/ or /f/ (*bath-baf*)
/v/	Sometimes /b/	/b/ before /m/ and /n/	Sometimes /b/
/ð/	/d/	/d/ or /v/ between vowels	/d/, /v/, /f/
/z/		Omitted or replaced by /d/ before nasal sound (*wasn't-wud'n*)	

Blends

/str/ becomes /skr/
/ʃr/ becomes /str/
/θr/ becomes /θ/
/pr/ becomes /p/
/br/ becomes /b/
/kr/ becomes /k/
/gr/ becomes /g/

Final Consonant Clusters (second consonant omitted when these clusters occur at the end of a word)

/sk/	/nd/	/sp/
/ft/	/ld/	/dʒd/
/st/	/sd/	/nt/

*Note weakening of final consonants.

TABLE A.2 Grammatical Contrasts Between African American English and Majority American English (MAE)

African American English Grammatical Structure	MAE Grammatical Structure
Possessive -'s	
Nonobligatory where word position expresses possession. Get *mother* coat. It be mother*'s*.	Obligatory regardless of position. Get mother*'s* coat. It's mother*'s*.
Plural -s	
Nonobligatory with numerical quantifier. He got ten *dollar*. Look at the cat*s*.	Obligatory regardless of numerical quantifier. He has ten dollar*s*. Look at the cat*s*.
Regular past -ed	
Nonobligatory; reduced as consonant cluster. Yesterday, I *walk* to school.	Obligatory. Yesterday, I walk*ed* to school.
Irregular past	
Case by case, some verbs inflected, others not. I *see* him last week.	All irregular verbs inflected. I *saw* him last week.
Regular present tense third-person singular -s	
Nonobligatory. She *eat* too much.	Obligatory. She eat*s* too much.
Irregular present tense third-person singular -s	
Nonobligatory. He *do* my job.	Obligatory. He *does* my job.
Indefinite *an*	
Use of indefinite *a*. He ride in a airplane.	Use of *an* before nouns beginning with a vowel. He rode in *an* airplane.
Pronouns	
Pronominal apposition: pronoun immediately follows noun. Momma *she* mad. She ...	Pronoun used elsewhere in sentence or in other sentence; not in apposition. Momma is mad. *She* ...
Future tense	
More frequent use of *be going to* (gonna). I *be going to* dance tonight. I *gonna* dance tonight.	More frequent use of *will*. I *will* dance tonight. I *am going to* dance tonight.
Omit *will* preceding *be*. I *be* home later.	Obligatory use of *will*. I *will* (I'll) *be* home later.
Negation	
Triple negative. *Nobody don't never* like me.	Absence of triple negative. *No* one ever likes me.
Use of *ain't*. I *ain't* going.	*Ain't* is unacceptable form. I*'m not* going.
Modals	
Double modals for such forms as *might, could,* and *should*. I *might could* go.	Single modal use. I *might be able to* go.

(*Continued*)

TABLE A.2 *(Continued)*

African American English Grammatical Structure	MAE Grammatical Structure
Questions	
Same form for direct and indirect. What *it is?* Do you know what *it is?*	Different forms for direct and indirect. What *is it?* Do you know what *it is?*
Relative pronouns	
Nonobligatory in most cases. He the one stole it. It the one you like.	Nonobligatory with *that* only. He's the one *who* stole it. It's the one (that) you like.
Conditional if	
Use of *do* for conditional *if.* I ask *did* she go.	Use of *if.* I asked *if* she went.
Perfect construction	
Been used for action in the distant past. He *been* gone.	*Been* not used. He left a long time ago.
Copula	
Nonobligatory when contractible. He sick.	Obligatory in contractible and uncontractible forms. He's sick.
Habitual or general state	
Marked with uninflected *be.* She *be* workin'.	Nonuse of *be;* verb inflected. She's *working* now.

English may continue to use the Spanish possessive form in which the owner is preceded by the entity owned, as in "the dress of Mary." The major variations between MAE and Latino English in phonology, syntax, and morphology are presented in Tables A.3 and A.4.

Asian English

Chinese culture and language have for centuries influenced all other Asian cultures and languages. Other cultures, such as that of the Indian subcontinents, have influenced nearby Asian neighbors. Colonial occupation, especially by the French in Indochina, also has influenced the culture and language of the affected region.

The most widely used languages—Chinese, Filipino, Japanese, Khmer, Korean, Laotian, and Vietnamese—represent only a portion of the languages of the area. Each language contains many dialects and has distinct linguistic features. It is therefore impossible to speak of an Asian English dialect. Instead, I shall attempt to describe the major overall differences between Asian English and MAE. These major or differences in phonology, syntax, and morphology are listed in Tables A.5 and A.6.

TABLE A.3 Phonemic Contrasts Between Latino English and Majority American English (MAE)

	Position in Word		
MAE Phonemes	**Initial**	**Medial**	**Final***
/p/	Unaspirated /p/		Omitted or weakened
/m/			Omitted
/w/	/hu/		Omitted
/b/			Omitted, distorted, or /p/
/g/			Omitted, distorted, or /k/
/k/	Unaspirated or /g/		Omitted, distorted, or /g/
/f/			Omitted
/d/		Dentalized	Omitted, distorted, or /t/
/ŋ/	/n/	/d/	/n/ (*sing-sin*)
/j/	/d*/		
/t/			Omitted
/ʃ/	/tʃ/	/s/, /tʃ/	/tʃ/ (*wish-which*)
/tʃ/	/ʃ/ (*chair-share*)	/ʃ/	/ʃ/ (*watch-wash*)
/r/	Distorted	Distorted	Distorted
/dʒ/	/d/	/j/	/ʃ/
/θ/	/t/, /s/ (*thin-tin, sin*)	Omitted	/ʃ/, /t/, /s/
/v/	/b/ (*vat-bat*)	/b/	Distorted
/z/	/s/ (*zip-sip*)	/s/ (*razor-racer*)	/s/
/ð/	/d/ (*then-den*)	/d/, /θ/, /v/ (*lather-ladder*)	/d/
Blends /skw/ becomes /eskw/* /sl/ becomes /esl/* /st/ becomes /est/*			
Vowels /I/ becomes /i/ (*bit-beet*)			

*Separates cluster into two syllables.

TABLE A.4 Grammatical Contrasts Between Latino English and Majority American English (MAE)

Latino English Grammatical Structure	MAE Grammatical Structure
Possessive -'s	
Use post-noun modifier. This is the homework *of my brother.*	Post-noun modifier used only rarely. This is my brother*'s* homework.
Article used with body parts. I cut *the* finger.	Possessive pronoun used with body parts. I cut *my* finger.
Plural -s	
Nonobligatory. The *girl* are playing. The *sheep* are playing.	Obligatory, excluding exceptions. The *girls* are playing. The *sheep* are playing.
Regular past -ed	
Nonobligatory, especially when understood. I *talk* to her yesterday.	Obligatory. I *talked* to her yesterday.
Regular third-person singular present tense -s	
Nonobligatory. She *eat* too much.	Obligatory. She *eats* too much.
Articles	
Often omitted. I am going to store. I am going to school.	Usually obligatory. I am going to *the* store. I am going to school.
Subject pronouns	
Omitted when subject has been identified in the previous sentence. Father is happy. Bought a new car.	Obligatory. Father is happy. *He* bought a new car.
Future tense	
Use *go + to.* I *go to* dance.	Use *be + going to.* I *am going to* the dance.
Negation	
Use *no* before the verb. She *no* eat candy.	Use *not* (preceded by auxiliary verb where appropriate). She does *not* eat candy.
Question	
Intonation: no noun-verb inversion. *Maria is* going?	Noun-verb inversion usually. *Is Maria* going?
Copula	
Occasional use of *have.* I *have* ten years.	Use of *be.* I *am* ten years old.
Negative imperatives	
No used for *don't.* *No* throw stones.	*Don't* used. *Don't* throw stones.
Do insertion	
Nonobligatory in questions. You like ice cream?	Obligatory when no auxiliary verb. *Do* you like ice cream?
Comparatives	
More frequent use of longer form (*more*). He is *more* tall.	More frequent use of shorter *-er.* He is tall*er.*

TABLE A.5 Phonemic Contrasts Between Asian English and Majority American English (MAE)

	Position in Word		
MAE Phonemes	**Initial**	**Medial**	**Final**
/p/	/b/****	/b/****	Omission
/s/	Distortion*	Distortion*	Omission
/z/	/s/**	/s/**	Omission
/t/	Distortion*	Distortion*	Omission
/tʃ/	/ʃ/****	/ʃ/****	Omission
/ʃ/	/s/**	/s/**	Omission
/r/, /l/	Confusion***	Confusion***	Omission
/θ/	/s/	/s/	Omission
/dʒ/	/d/ or /z/***	/d/ or /z/***	Omission
/v/	/f/***	/f/***	Omission
	/w/**	/w/**	Omission
/ð/	/z/*	/z/*	Omission
	/d/***	/d/***	Omission

Blends
Addition of /ə/ between consonants***
Omission of final consonant clusters****

Vowels
Shortening or lengthening of vowels (seat-sit, it-eat*)
Difficulty with /I/, /ɔ/ and /æ/, and substitution of /e/ for /æ/**
Difficulty with /I/, /æ/, /ɔ/, and /ə/****

*Mandarin dialect of Chinese only
**Cantonese dialect of Chinese only
***Mandarin, Cantonese, and Japanese
****Vietnamese only

TABLE A.6 Grammatical Contrasts Between Asian English and Majority American English

Asian English Grammatical Structure	Majority American English Grammatical Structure
Plural -*s*	
Not used with numerical adjective: *three cat*	Used regardless of numerical adjective: *three cats*
Used with irregular plural: *the sheeps*	Not used with irregular plural: *the sheep*
Auxiliaries *to be* and *to do*	
Omission: *I going home. She not want eat.*	Obligatory and inflected in the present progressive form: *I am going home. She does not want to eat.*
Uninflected: *I is going. She do not want eat.*	

(*Continued*)

TABLE A.6 (*Continued*)

Asian English Grammatical Structure	Majority American English Grammatical Structure
Verb *have*	
Omission: *You been here.* Uninflected: *He have one.*	Obligatory and inflected: *You have been here.* *He has one.*
Regular past *-ed*	
Omission: *He talk yesterday.* Overgeneralization: *I eated yesterday.* Double-marking: *She didn't ate.*	Obligatory, nonovergeneralization, and single-marking: *He talked yesterday. I ate yesterday. She didn't eat.*
Interrogative	
Nonreversal: *You're late?* Omitted auxiliary: *You like ice cream?*	Reversal and obligatory auxiliary: *Are you late?* *Do you like ice cream?*
Perfect marker	
Omission: *I have write letter.*	Obligatory: *I have written a letter.*
Verb-noun agreement	
Nonagreement: *He go to school. You goes to school.*	Agreement: *He goes to school. You go to school.*
Article	
Omission: *Please give gift.* Overgeneralization: *She go the school.*	Obligatory with certain nouns: *Please give the gift.* *She went to school.*
Preposition	
Misuse: *I am in home.* Omission: *He go bus.*	Obligatory specific use: *I am at home.* *He goes by bus.*
Pronoun	
Subjective/objective confusion: *Him go quickly.* Possessive confusion: *It him book.*	Subjective/objective distinction: *He gave it to her.* Possessive distinction: *It's his book.*
Demonstrative	
Confusion: *I like those horse.*	Singular/plural distinction: *I like that horse.*
Conjunction	
Omission: *You I go together.*	Obligatory use between last two items in a series: *You and I are going together. Mary, John, and Carol went.*
Negation	
Double-marking: *I didn't see nobody.* Simplified form: *He no come.*	Single obligatory marking: *I didn't see anybody.* *He didn't come.*
Word order	
Adjective following noun (Vietnamese): *clothes new.*	Most noun modifiers precede noun: *new clothes.*
Possessive following noun (Vietnamese): *dress her.*	Possessive precedes noun: *her dress.*
Omission of object with transitive verb: *I want.*	Use of direct object with most transitive verbs: *I want it.*

Appendix B

Language Analysis Methods

Assigning Structural Stage/Complex Sentence Development

In Assigning Structural Stage, Miller (J. Miller, 1981) proposes a three-tiered analysis that includes MLU, percentage correct of Brown's 14 morphemes, and sentence analysis. These three measures enable the SLP to determine the stage of development based on Brown's work (Brown, 1973) and to describe the forms used.

Analysis begins by collecting a language sample. The SLP collects 50 to 100 utterances or 15 minutes of conversation, whichever is larger, from the child for analysis. First, the SLP calculates MLU to determine the stage of development and the approximate language age of the child. MLU calculation is discussed in Chapter 7.

After determining MLU, the SLP decides on the analysis method to follow. He or she may choose Assigning Structural Stage and/or Complex Sentence Development. If the MLU of the child is below 3.0, the SLP uses only Assigning Structural Stage. If the child's MLU is above 4.5, the SLP uses only Complex Sentence Development. For MLUs of 3.0 to 4.5, the SLP uses both procedures.

In Assigning Structural Stage, the SLP calculates the percentage correct for Brown's 14 morphemes. A minimum number of occurrences or possibilities of occurrence are needed before the SLP can decide on consistency or inconsistency of use or nonuse. The child should attempt a morpheme at least four times before a percentage correct figure is calculated.

The percentage correct value is determined by dividing the number of correct appearances by the total number of obligatory contexts. After calculating the percentage correct, the SLP again can attempt to describe the child's stage of language development.

Next, the SLP analyzes each utterance within four possible categories of noun phrase, verb phrase, and negative and interrogative development. Utterances are divided into noun and verb phrases where applicable, and each phrase is assigned to the stage of development that best describes its structures. Negative or interrogative utterances are further assigned to stages representing their level of development.

The SLP should be familiar with the information Miller (1981) presents for each stage of development. Some of this information is presented in Table 7.25, although Miller presents a great deal more. The analysis process is demonstrated here by using some of the information in Table 7.25. Consider the child's utterance, "Want a big doggie." The noun phrase a *big doggie* has been expanded by the addition of an article and an adjective to the noun. This noun phrase occurs in the object position of the sentence. Expansion of the noun phrase only in the object position is an example of Brown's Stage II (see intrasentence column of Table 7.25). Therefore, this sentence represents noun phrase development characteristic of Stage II. The verb phrase is unelaborated, and no subject is present. This represents Brown's Stage I development.

Complex Sentence Development is used similarly, but different samples and categories are used for analysis. Analysis is based on a 15-minute sample of the child's communication, rather than on 50 utterances. For children with MLUs between 3.0 and 4.5, these samples can overlap. Five aspects of complex sentences are noted: percentage of both conjoined and embedded sentences within the sample, type of embedding, conjoining, conjunctions, and the number of different conjunctions. At each stage, development is described by the forms exhibited by 50 to 90 percent and by greater than 90 percent of the children.

Limited data from Complex Sentence Development are incorporated into Table 7.25. By post-Stage V, 90 percent of children should be using *and* within a 15-minute sample. To complete a full analysis, the SLP should consult Complex Sentence Development (J. Miller, 1981).

Each sentence is analyzed by using Assigning Structural Stage and/or Complex Sentence Development, and the data are summarized. Most likely, the child will exhibit language forms in each stage of development. Now, the SLP must use his or her skill.

Even mature language users occasionally use language forms that are characteristic of less mature learning. Adults use many one-word utterances everyday. These forms are not the most characteristic forms, however, and the SLP must gather a summary of overall language form to determine most accurately the user's abilities. It is the same with the child with language impairment. The SLP determines those behaviors that are most characteristic of the child. These might be behaviors at a particular stage that the child uses most frequently or behaviors that represent the highest attainment level. The SLP must make this determination.

All data from the two analysis methods—Assigning Structural Stage and Complex Sentence Development—are combined to place the child's language form within a stage or stages of development and to describe the child's language form. The child functioning well below age expectancy may need intervention.

Developmental Sentence Scoring

Developmental Sentence Scoring, the process discussed in *Developmental Sentence Analysis* (L. Lee, 1974), is one of the most widely used and popular methods for assessing children's syntactic and morphological development. Even so, DSS requires considerable study by the SLP to score language samples correctly. Although the instructions are explicit and straightforward, they require a thorough understanding of English syntax and morphology. Because the scale does not evaluate many aspects of children's language, it should be only one aspect of an evaluation battery.

In the following section I discuss the primary aspects of DSS and its most common problems. This survey cannot take the place of a thorough reading of DSS procedures and actual practice with the instrument.

To rate a sample of child language, the SLP collects 50 different consecutive *sentences*. No speaker uses full sentences all the time. Therefore, utterances that do not qualify as sentences simply are omitted, and the remainder is collected until 50 consecutive sentences are amassed. DSS analysis should not be undertaken if fewer than 50 percent of the child's utterances are sentences.

Because the sample should include 50 different consecutive sentences, repeated sentences are discarded unless some change occurs. Run-on sentences of several independent clauses joined by *and* are segmented so that no more than two independent clauses are joined. For example, the following run-on should be divided as noted:

> [We went to the zoo, and I saw monkeys,] [(and) we had a picnic, and I ate a hot dog,] [(and) I fed pigeons, and we came home on the bus.]

The *and* at the beginning of each sentence ("[*and*] we had . . . , *and*] I fed . . .") would not be scored. A sentence may have more than one *and* if the word does not link clauses, but rather is used for compound subjects, verbs, or objects, for example:

> Jorge, Maria, *and* Shanisa were throwing *and* kicking beach balls *and* soccer balls.

TABLE B.1 Language Sample Analysis Using Developmental Sentence Scoring

Developmental sentence scoring form

Name:
D.O.B.:
D.O.K.:
C.A.:
Score

Score:	Indefinite Pronouns	Personal Pronouns	Main verbs	Secondary Verbs	Negatives	Conjunctons	Interrogative Reverses	Wh-Questions	Sentence-Point	Total
I don't know what I like.		*1,1,6*	*4,1*		*4*				*1*	*18*
What you like?		*1*	*1*				*2*			*4*
I don't know.		*1*	*4*		*4*				*1*	*10*
He bes happy.		*2*	*inc*							*2*
I want to go home.		*1*	*1*	*2*					*1*	*5*
What's that?			*1*				*1*	*2*	*1*	*5*
I can't go now.		*1*	*4*		*4*				*1*	*10*

Sentences that begin with a conjunction, such as "Because I falled down," are included in the sample, but the conjunction itself should not be scored because it does not link clauses.

Each sentence is rated on the basis of eight grammatical categories and assigned a score of 1 to 8 points in the applicable categories. Each structure demonstrated in the sentence is scored each time it occurs. For example, sentence 1 in Table B.1, "I don't know what I like," contains the word *I* twice. Therefore, the word receives a score of 1 twice under personal pronouns, in addition to other points.

Sentences that would be acceptable mature forms are given an additional point called a *sentence point*. The sentence point should only be awarded when the sentence is syntactically and semantically correct by mature standards. The following would not receive a sentence point:

Carol and me went to the store.

Nobody didn't go.

I got six pencils in my desk.

In Table B.1, sentence 2, "What you like?" receives a score of 4; it does not receive a sentence point because it is not an acceptable mature sentence. Sentence 3, "I don't know," does receive the sentence point.

Attempt markers and incomplete markers may be awarded for structures. An *attempt marker*—a line or hyphen in place of a score—is awarded when a structure is attempted but incorrect. Naturally, as in sentence 4, "He bes happy," the sentence cannot receive a sentence point. Surface structures that are conversationally appropriate but incomplete receive the incomplete marker *inc* in place of a score. If the structure is conversationally acceptable, it receives a sentence point. For example, in the following exchange, the child's response would receive an incomplete for the main verb, but would receive a sentence point.

SLP: Who let the guinea pig out?

Child: I didn't. (I didn't [let him out].)

Attempt and incomplete markers are difficult to use and confusing for those not familiar with DSS. They do not affect the score and are meant to aid the SLP in deciding where to begin intervention. This decision can be made on the basis of other data.

The point value of each sentence is totaled and added to the value for every other sentence. This overall total is divided by the number of sentences (usually 50) to yield a score. The SLP must remember that this value is a DSS score, not an MLU. The two values are very different.

The SLP then applies the DSS score to a table of ages and scores to compare the child's performance with that of other children at that age. According to the instructions, children whose scores place them below the 10th percentile should be considered for therapy.

The most common problems encountered with DSS are associated with determination of grammatical units and with scoring (Lively, 1984). Readers can refer to Lively (1984) and Hughes, Fey, and Long (1992) for a more thorough discussion.

Modification for CLD Children

The nature of the DSS makes it an inappropriate tool to use for assessing the language abilities of children with CLD backgrounds. Some advances have been made in this area. Black English Sentence Scoring (BESS) is a promising attempt to maintain the DSS format while measuring African American English usage.

Summary

DSS is a good quantitative measure, although no data are available on the relationship of DSS scores to the type and extent of a child's LI (Hughes et al., 1992). Even when matched with peers on the basis of MLU, children with LI tend to have more difficulty with the main verb and pronoun categories and may have difficulty with secondary verbs, negatives, and conjunctions. DSS has shown great resiliency and has been modified for speakers of Black English, expanded to 6- to 10-year-olds, and converted to a computerized version. Although DSS scoring has been computerized in a variant of SALT transcription called Computerized Profiling (Long, Fey, & Channell, 2000), reliability comparisons with hand-scored DSS suggest further refinement of the program may still be needed (Channell, 2003).

Systematic Analysis of Language Transcripts

Systematic Analysis of Language Transcripts (SALT for Windows, Version 6.1) (J. Miller & Chapman, 2003) is one of the most promising computer analysis methods available. Based on Assigning Structural Stage/Complex Sentence Development (J. Miller, 1981), SALT is designed for use with the IBM PCs and Macintosh computers. Within limits, SALT analyzes morphemic, syntactic, and semantic aspects of a language sample.

Although it's difficult to describe computer-aided language sampling and analysis (CLSA) without having the computer in front of us, I'll give a short explanation and suggest that you check out the fine tutorial by Hammett Price, Hendricks, and Cook (2010) and go online to work through the tutorials at the Systematic Analysis of Language Transcripts (SALT) website (www.saltsoftware.com/originaltraining).

CLA can be conceptualized as a four-step process (Hammett Price et al., 2010):

- Eliciting and recording the language sample
- Transcribing the language sample
- Analyzing and interpreting the results of the language sample
- Using the results to plan treatment and monitor response to treatment

Because we have describe elicitation previously in Chapter 6, we won't discuss this step in the present context. Needless to say, you'll need a computer with a sound card and adequate memory; an external microphone; audio recording software, such as Audacity (http://audacity.sourceforge.net); materials for eliciting the sample; software with which to transcribe the sample, such as Transcriber (http://sourceforge.net/projects/trans); and SALT software (Miller & Iglesias, 2006).

Transcribing a Language Sample

The key to using the SALT analysis program is accurate transcription. SALT transcripts are marked with a "C" to indicate the child's utterances and "E" for the examiner's if the transcriber choses to record these also. Each utterance should end with a punctuation mark. Depending on the type of analysis sought, the SLP next segments the child utterances into communication units (C-units), modified communication units, or phonological units (P-units), which are described in the SALT online manual. Finally, the SLP needs to mark the duration of the sample by indicating *0.00* at the beginning and the ending time in minutes and seconds, such as *8.34*, at the end.

Pauses, repetitions, and revisions are placed in parentheses as in *We (saw saw) saw (a) (um) a big horsie*. In addition, long pauses may be marked for duration in seconds, as in *We (saw saw) saw (a) (um)* :03 *a big horsie*.

Once the child's utterances have been transcribed, the SLP is ready to analyze specific features of the child's language. These features must be marked accurately and reliably within the transcript in order for the SALT program to analyze the sample accurately. SALT software includes training samples that demonstrate how to apply the transcription conventions, which can be applied either during the initial transcription process or as a revision. For maximun productivity, the SLP should mark four language features:

- Unintelligible words
- Omissions
- Bound morphemes
- Word and utterance errors

By marking unintelligible words, the SLP excludes these from the analysis. Unintelligible words are marked with an X, unintelligible segments with XX, and whole utterances with XXX.

Omissions are marked with an asterisk. Partial words are followed by an asterisk, as in *We wa* wa* want some candy*. In contrast, omitted bound morphemes and words are included by preceded by an asterisk, as in *Three dog/*s* and *We went *to school* respectively.

Bound morphemes are marked as follows:

- Plurals marked with *s* (bike/s, boy/s)
- Possessives marked with *z* (Suzy/z)
- Past tense (want/ed, play/ed)
- Third person singular (does = do/3s, eats = eat/3s)
- Verb inflections (go/ing, jump/ing)
- Negative contractions (do/n't, can/'t)
- Contractible verb forms (I/'m, we/'re, he/'s)

Each bound morpheme is separated from the root word by a forward slash (/) followed by the encoded morpheme.

Finally, word and utterance errors are followed by EW or EU respectively within brackets, as in *We was* [EW:were] *going too*. Error utterances are simply followed by the [EU] without any attempt to correct as in word errors [EW:were].

Analyzing and Interpreting the Results of the Language Sample

In order to analyze a child's language sample, the SLP opens the SALT program and follows the instructions for creating a new transcript file. This includes generating the header identification information needed by the program, such as the child's name and age. Next, the SLP copies the child's sample from the text file and pastes it into this new transcript file. From the "check" pull-down menu, the SLP can check the file in for any errors that should be corrected prior to analysis. Now, we're ready to go!

By asking the program to generate the standard analyses, the SLP will receive data on the number of intelligible utterances in the sample, elapsed time, words spoken per minute, MLU, number of different word roots, number of mazes, duration of pauses, numbers of omitted words and morphemes, and word and utterance errors. To obtain a standard analyses, the SLP simply chooses the "database" pull-down menu in the SALT program and selects "standard analyses." The window that follows asks the SLP to choose the database from which to draw the comparison sample—either conversation or narrative—whether an age-matched or grade-matched sample is desired, and whether the comparison should be based on the entire transcript or matched on number of words or utterances. Once these choices have been made, SALT will identify the available samples to use for comparison, and the SLP must select which set to use. It's probably best to find a balance that allows a comparison using as many utterances as in the sample while comparing to 25 or more peers if possible (Hammett Price et al., 2010). After the database comparison sample has been chosen, another SALT window will ask the SLP to choose the analyses and the standard deviation desired. AT least initially, it is best to choose "standard measures" and a 1-*SD* interval, which are the default settings (Hammett Price et al., 2010). The output provides data for the standard measures mentioned previously, including the child's score on each measure, the mean score for the children in the database, and how the target child's score compares to that mean in standard deviation units. After gaining familiarity with the standard measures, the SLP can request additional analyses on the sample or produce lists of utterances from the sample that contain a target feature.

Nothing in the SALT analysis or any other CLSA method relieves an SLP of the responsibility of applying her or his professional knowledge of both language development and disorders to interpretation of the results. Interpreting SALT output also requires that the SLP look for both areas of strength and areas of weakness in the child's performance. Although SALT will mark measures with asterisks, revealing discrepancies between the child's performance and that of children in the comparison sample, the SLP must use his or her clinical judgment to interpret the meaning of those discrepancies.

Planning Treatment Goals and Monitoring Response to Treatment

After interpreting SALT data that reveal specific patterns of disordered language performance, the SLP must decide which areas to target for intervention. SALT data can be used to establish a baseline for each goal and to measure mastery.

To assess a child's response to treatment, the SLP can measure the child's progress using tasks similar to the ones used for the original language sampling. This can be accomplished by comparing the child's current sample to the original one either overall or for the specific language feature targeted in intervention. SALT offers a way to compare two samples produced by the same child. By choosing "Link" from the pull-down menu, the SLP can link two samples of the child from the database.

Conclusion

SALT is a very promising and versatile analysis method that is easy for the SLP to use after becoming familiar with entering the transcript into the computer. As with other computer analysis methods, however, it is not the great panacea. At present, most results are a calculation of those features signaled by the SLP when he or she enters the data. Thus, special care is required to ensure that features are signaled accurately.

Appendix

C

Selected English Morphological Prefixes and Suffixes

TABLE C.1 Prefixes and Suffixes

Derivational		*Inflectional*
Prefixes	**Suffixes**	
a- (in, on, into, in a manner)	-able (ability, tendency, likelihood)	-ed (past)
bi- (twice, two)	-al (pertaining to, like, action, process)	-ing (at present)
de- (negative, descent, reversal)	-ance (action, state)	-s (plural)
ex- (out of, from, thoroughly)	-ation (denoting action in a noun)	-s (third person marker)
inter- (reciprocal between, together)	-en (used to form verbs from adjectives)	-'s (possession)
mis- (ill, negative, wrong)	-ence (action, state)	
out- (extra, beyond, not)	-er (used as an agentive ending)	
over- (over)	-est (superlative)	
post- (behind, after)	-ful (full, tending)	
pre- (to, before)	-ible (ability, tendency, likelihood)	
pro- (in favor of)	-ish (belonging to)	
re- (again, backward motion)	-ism (doctrine, state, practice)	
semi- (half)	-ist (one who does something)	
super- (superior)	-ity (used for abstract nouns)	
trans- (across, beyond)	-ive (tendency or connection)	
tri- (three)	-ize (action, policy)	
un- (not, reversal)	-less (without)	
under- (under)	-ly (used to form adverbs)	
	-ment (action, product, means, state)	
	-ness (quality, state)	
	-or (used as an agentive ending)	
	-ous (full of, having, like)	
	-y (inclined to)	

Appendix D

Indirect Elicitation Techniques

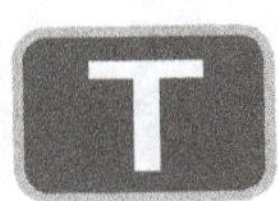

There is an infinite variety of indirect elicitation techniques, although we tend to rely on two old favorites:

Tell me what you see.
Tell me in a whole sentence.

Here are a few conversational techniques that came to mind one day. The list is not exhaustive, merely illustrative.

TABLE D.1 Indirect Elicitation Techniques

Technique	Target	Example
The emperor's new clothes	Negative statements	CLINICIAN: Oh, Shirley, what beautiful yellow boots!
		CHILD: I'm not wearing boots!
Pass it on	Requests for information	CLINICIAN: John, do you know where Linda's project is?
		CHILD: No.
		CLINICIAN: Oh, see if she knows?
		CHILD: Linda, where's your project?
Violating routines ("Silly rabbit")	Imperatives, directives	CLINICIAN: Here's your sandwich.
		CHILD: Nothing in it.
		CLINICIAN: Oh, you must like different sandwiches than I do. What do you want?
		CHILD: Peanut butter.
		CLINICIAN: How do I do it? (There's your opener)
Nonblabbermouth	Requests for information	CLINICIAN: (Place interesting object in front of child) "Boy, is this neat."
		CHILD: What is it?
		CLINICIAN: A flibbideejibbit. (Now STOP. Don't give any more info)
		CHILD: What's it do?

(Continued)

TABLE D.1 (*Continued*)

Technique	Target	Example
What I have	Request for action	CLINICIAN: Oh, I can't wait to show you what I have in this bag. It's really neat. (Wait child out)
Guess what I did	Request for information, past tense verbs	CLINICIAN: Guess what I did yesterday in the park. CHILD: Jogged? Picked flowers? Had a picnic?
Mumble	Contingent query	At height of an interesting story or punchline of a joke, clinician should mumble so that child does not receive message. If needed, increase pressure by asking questions on what was just said.
Ask someone else	Request for information	CLINICIAN: What do you need? CHILD: Sugar. CLINICIAN: I don't know where it is. Why don't you ask Sally where the sugar is?
Rule giving	Requests for objects	CLINICIAN: I have the athletic equipment for recess. If you need some, just ask me. CHILD: I want jump rope.
Request for assistance	Initiating conversation	CLINICIAN: John, can you ask Keith to help me?
Modeling with meaningful intent	I want _____	CLINICIAN: We have lots of colored paper for our project. Now let's see who needs some. I want a green one. (Take one and wait) CHILD: I want blue.
"Screw up" #1	Locatives, prepositions	CLINICIAN: Can you help me dress this doll? (Place shoe on doll's head) How's that? CHILD: No. The shoe goes *on* the doll's foot. CLINICIAN: But now the foot's all gone. CHILD: No. It's *in* the shoe.
"Screw up" #2	Negative statements	CLINICIAN: Here's your snack. (Give child a pencil) CHILD: That's not a snack.
Requests for topic	Statements	CLINICIAN: Now let's talk about your birthday party. (Not shared information)
Expansion of child utterance into desired form	Infinitives	CHILD: I want paste crayon. CLINICIAN: You want crayon to *sing with?* CHILD: No, to color. CLINICIAN: What? CHILD: I want crayon to color.

Appendix

E

Intervention Activities and Language Targets

FIGURE E.1 Activities and Targets

Activities	Nouns	Plurals	Verb tensing	Adjectives/descriptive words	Adverbs	Pronouns	Articles and/or demonstrations	Prepositions/spatial terms	Requests for objects	Requests for assistance	Requests for information	Negatives	Interrogatives	Following directions	Giving directions	Sequencing	Turn taking	Topic introduction and maintenance	Categorization	Register	Presupposition	Conversational repair	Variety of pragmatic features	Auditory processing and memory	Word association	Vocabulary
Barrier tasks														X	X	X					X			X		
Body tracing	X		X	X				X		X				X	X	X										X
Colorforms			X	X			X	X																		
*Cooking			X	X					X	X	X		X	X	X				X							X
Describing pictures that others cannot see	X	X		X			X														X					
Dolls, clothing, and furniture	X	X		X				X												X						X
Dressing	X	X							X					X	X											
Dress-up			X	X		X	X	X												X			X			
Explaining "how-to"				X	X			X				X			X	X		X			X	X				
Farm or zoo play	X	X		X								X							X							X
Guiding others through an activity														X	X	X		X			X					
Treasure hunt—"You're getting warmer"								X						X	X						X					
Interviewing											X		X				X	X		X		X				
"I see something that's ..."				X				X			X		X												X	
Jeopardy											X	X	X												X	
Kitchen play				X					X	X							X	X					X			X

*Making things	X		X	X	X	X	X	X	X	X	X	X		X	X	X	X									X
Map following								X		X	X	X	X	X	X											
Mime														X		X		X			X					
My "ME" book				X	X	X												X								
Music and action songs														X	X	X										
Nature or science activity				X					X	X	X		X	X	X	X	X		X						X	X
Obstacle course			X	X				X		X			X	X	X	X										
Planning an activity			X	X	X	X	X	X										X			X					X
Planting seeds			X	X				X						X	X											X
Playhouse			X			X	X	X												X			X			
Playing teacher												X			X			X		X	X	X	X			
Pretend shopping	X	X								X	X	X	X				X	X	X				X			X
Puppet show																X				X			X			
Putting objects in order				X				X											X						X	
"Safety Town" (Safety curriculum for preschool and kindergarten)					X	X		X		X	X			X	X					X			X			X
Simon Says														X	X	X									X	
Simulated restaurant									X		X		X				X		X	X	X		X			X
Sorting clothing	X	X							X					X					X							
Storytelling (true or make-believe)			X			X	X									X		X				X		X		
Telephone play						X	X				X	X	X				X	X		X	X	X	X	X		
TV commercials				X														X		X	X	X	X			
"Twenty questions" variations				X							X	X	X													
Washing dishes	X	X		X					X	X				X	X											
"What am I?"				X	X	X	X	X			X	X	X					X				X				
"What did you do ...?"			X		X	X	X	X			X		X					X				X				

See third page of table (p. 418)

(Continued)

FIGURE E.1 *(Continued)*

Possible cooking activities: Be sure to check for possible allergies or sensitivities to nuts and milk before using these items.

1. Cookies, cupcakes, muffins
2. Cornbread and butter
3. Edible honeybees—Mix 1/2 cup peanut butter, 1 T. plus 1/3 cup honey, 2 T. sesame seeds, and 2 T. toasted wheat germ. Roll into balls. Make stripes on the bee by dipping a toothpick in cocoa powder and pressing into ball. Use slivered almonds for wings.
4. English muffin pizzas
5. Fruit salad—Use a few vegetables just to confuse the issue and to elicit some language.
6. Ice cream sundaes
7. Instant pudding
8. Milkshakes—Lots of variations here, such as vanilla, chocolate, and banana (use real ones in the blender).
9. Peanut butter and jelly sandwiches.
10. Peanut butter balls—Mix 1/2 cup honey, 1/2 cup peanut butter, 1 cup dry milk, and 1 cup oatmeal. Roll into balls. Refrigerate.
11. Peanut butter "face" sandwiches—Make faces on the bread with a peanut butter base using raisins (eyes), peanut (nose), chocolate chips (mouth), and carrot slivers or coconut (hair).
12. Picnic lunch
13. Popcorn and popcorn balls

**Things to make:

1. Cereal box instrument—Use a strong cereal box with a circular hole cut in the face similar to the hole in a guitar. Stretch various size rubber bands around the box and tack them into wooden blocks that act as bridges.
2. Costumes from grocery bags—Cut eye holes or a hole for face. Cut arm holes if desired. Decorate bag. Slip over child.
3. Cowgirl and cowboy outfits from grocery bags—Bags can easily be cut to resemble vests and yokes. Be sure to fringe them. Add a bandanna and you have the outfit.
4. Decorate a shoebox "room" with scraps of wallpaper.
5. Food sculptures—Use shredded coconut or lettuce, raisins, peanuts, M&Ms, hot cinnamon candies, cheese strips, fruit halves, celery and carrot sticks, olives, marshmallows, gum drops, and toothpicks.
6. Holiday cards
7. Kites
8. Paper bag puppets
9. Paper butterflies
10. Paper flowers
11. Playdough—Mix 2 cups flour, 1 cup water, 1 T. salad oil, 1 cup salt, and food coloring.
12. Potato and sponge prints
13. Sachets—Cloves and crumbled bay leaves and cinnamon sticks in square of cloth. Pull ends of cloth together and tie with a ribbon.
14. Snowmen and snowwomen—Use styrofoam balls, pipecleaners, cloves, and toothpicks.
15. Stained glass windows—Cut out a cardboard mold. Tape aluminum foil over one side of the cut-out sections. Place this side down. Fill the holes with Elmer's glue. Swirl in food coloring. Allow to dry thoroughly. Peel foil. Hang in sunny window..

Note: A variety of language features can be elicited within these activities by using the indirect elicitation techniques in Appendix D and the nonlinguistic strategies in Chapter 10.

Appendix

F

Use of Children's Literature in Preschool Classrooms

Books and Their Uses in Intervention

Targets

Auditory Skills

Auditory Awareness

Rhyming

Aardema, *Bring the rain to Kapiti Plain* (M)
Ahlberg, *Each peach pear plum*
Alborough, *Where's my teddy?*
Anholt & Anholt, *Here come the babies*
Bang, *Ten, nine, eight* (M)
Deming, *Who is tapping at my window?*
deRegniers, *Going for a walk*
Jonas, *This old man*
Kandoian, *Molly's seasons*
Lear, *The owl and the pussycat*
Lotz, *Snowsong shistling*
Lyon, *Together*
Martin, *Brown bear, brown bear, what do you see?*
Martin, *The happy hippopotami*
Martin, *Polar bear, polar bear, what do you hear?*
Patron, *Dark cloud, strong breeze*
Philpot, *Amazing Anthony Ant*
Polushkin, *Mother, mother, I want another*
Seuss, *Hop on pop*
Stickland & Stickland, *Dinosaur roar!*
Wood, *The napping house*

Auditory Memory

Bennett & Cooke, *One cow moo moo*
Hayes, *The grumpalump*
Hutchins, *Don't forget the bacon*
Hutchins, *The surprise party*

Numeroff, *If you give a mouse a cookie*	Auditory and visual memory
Numeroff, *If you give a moose a muffin*	Auditory and visual memory
Neitzel, *The jacket I wear in the snow*	
Offen, *The sheep made a leap*	Following directions
Smalls-Hector, *Jonathan and his mommy* (M)	Following directions

Auditory Attending and Other Skills

Brown, *The noise book*	Discrimination
Calmenson, *It begins with an A*	Attending and synthesis
Carle, *The very hungry caterpillar*	Sequencing, auditory memory
deRegniers, *It does not say meow*	Auditory attending and processing

Word Play

Barrett, *Animals should definitely not act like people*
Calmenson, *It begins with an A*
Carle, *The secret birthday message*
Hutchins, *Don't forget the bacon*

Syntax and Morphology

Verb Tensing

Present Progressive

Allen, *A lion in the night*
Barton, *Harry is a scaredy-cat*
Brown, *The runaway bunny*
Burningham, *Jangle, twang*
DePaola, *Pancakes for breakfast*
Ets, *In the forest*
Gelman, *I went to the zoo*
Hutchins, *The very worst monster*
Keats, *Over in the meadow*
Keats, *Peter's chair*
Krauss, *Bears*
Krauss, *The carrot seed*
Lear, *The owl and the pussycat*
Martin, *Brown bear, brown bear, what do you see?*
Martin, *Polar bear, polar bear, what do you hear?*
Martin & Archambault, *Here are my hands*
Mayer, *There's an alligator under my bed*
Noll, *Jiggle, wiggle, prance*
Peppe, *Odd one out*
Rockwell, *First comes spring*
Rockwell & Rockwell, *At the beach*
Sendak, *Alligators all around*
Van Laan, *Possum come a-knockin'*
Wood, *The napping house*

Future Tense

Allen, *A lion in the night*
Zolotow, *Do you know what I'll do?*

Past Tense

Aardema, *Bring the rain to Kapiti Plain* (M)
Arnold, *Green Wilma*
Arnold, *The simple people*
Baker, *The third-story cat*
Charlip, *Fortunately*
Chorao, *Kate's box*
Cole, *Monster manners*
DePaola, *Charlie needs a cloak*
DePaola, *The knight and the dragon*
Ehlert, *Redlead, yellow leaf*
Ets, *Play with me*
Everitt, *Frida the wondercat*
Ginsburg, *Good morning, chick*
Hayes, *The grumpalump*
Hutchins, *Goodnight owl*
Hutchins, *Rosie's walk*
Keats, *Over in the meadow*
Keats, *Peter's chair*
Kent, *There's no such thing as a dragon*
Knowlton, *Why cowboys sleep with their boots on*
Krauss, *The carrot seed*
Lear, *The owl and the pussycat*
London, *Froggy gets dressed*
London, *Let's go, froggy!*
Mayer, *Just me and my little sister*
Mayer, *There's an alligator under my bed*
Peppe, *Odd one out*
Ruschak, *One hot day*
Scieszka, *The true story of the 3 little pigs*
Tojhurst, *Somebody and the three Blairs*
Wells, *Noisy Nora*

Noun-verb Agreement

Barton, *Airplanes*
Barton, *Airport*
Barton, *Boats*
Brown, *Goodnight moon*
Lewin, *Jafta's mother* (M)
Sendak, *Alligators all around*

Prepositions

Ahlberg, *Each peach pear plum*
Appelt, *Elephants aloft*
Baker, *The third-story cat*
Banchek, *Snake in, snake out*
Brown, *The runaway bunny*
Brown, *A dark dark tale*
Carle, *The secret birthday message*
Chorao, *Kate's box*

Hill, *Spot's birthday party*
Hutchins, *Rosie's walk*
Krauss, *Bears*
Lillie, *Everything has a place*
London, *Let's go, froggy!*
Mayer, *There's an alligator under my bed*
Noll, *Jiggle, wiggle, prance*
Westcott, *The lady with the alligator purse*
Wheeler, *Marmalade's yellow leaf*

Pronouns

Brown, *Arthur's nose*
Brown, *The runaway bunny*
Chorao, *Kate's box*
Mayer, *Just my friend and me*
Mayer, *Just me and my little sister*
Roffey, *Look, there's my hat*

Adjectives/Descriptor words

Asch, *The last puppy* (first/last)
Asch, *Little fish, big fish* (big/little)
Baker, *Hide and snake*
Baker, *White rabbit's coloring book*
Brown, *A dark dark tale*
Collington, *The midnight circus*
Davol, *Black, white, just right* (M)
Day, *Good dog, Carl*
Day, *Carl goes to daycare*
Day, *Carl goes shopping*
Day, *Carl's afternoon in the park*
deRegniers, *It does not say meow*
Geisert, *Oink, oink*
Gill, *The spring hat*
Glassman, *The wizard next door*
Graham, *Full moon soup or the fall of the Hotel Splendide*
Guarino, *Is your mama a llama?*
Guarino, *Tu mama es una llama?*
Hoban, *Is it rough, is it smooth, is it shiny?*
Hoban, *Exactly the opposite*
Hoban, *Is it larger? Is it smaller?*
Hudson & Ford, *Bright eyes, brown skin* (M)
Hutchins, *The very worst monster*
Jonas, *Reflections*
Jonas, *The 13th clue*
Jonas, *The trek*
Jonas, *Where can it be*
Kandoian, *Molly's seasons*
Keats, *Peter's chair*
Lester, *It wasn't my fault*
Martin, *Brown bear, brown bear, what do you see?*
Martin, *When dinosaurs go visiting*
Marzollo & Pinkney, *Pretend you're a cat*

Reiss, *Colors*
Rockwell, *Big wheels*
Viorst, *My mama says*
Wood, *The napping house*

Possessive -'s

Brown, *Arthur's nose*
Chorao, *Kate's box*
Gibbons, *The season of the Arnold's apple tree*
Keats, *Peter's chair*
Kraus, *Whose mouse are you?*
Yabuuchi, *Whose footprints?*

Plurals (Regular -s & irregular)

Brown, *Goodnight moon*
Ehlert, *Redlead, yellow leaf*
Ets, *In the forest*
Gibbons, *The season of the Arnold's apple tree*
Hoban, *Is it larger? Is it smaller?*
Kandoian, *Molly's seasons*
Keats, *Over in the meadow*
Lionni, *A color of his own*
Lukesova, *Julian in the autumn woods*

Third person singular -s

Gibbons, *The season of the Arnold's apple tree*
LeSaux, *Daddy shaves*
Lester, *Clive eats alligators*
Loomis, *In the diner*
Tafuri, *This is the farmer*

Verbs

LeSaux, *Daddy shaves*
Lester, *Clive eats alligators*
Loomis, *In the diner*
Lyon, *Together*
Martin, *When dinosaurs go visiting*
Marzollo & Pinkney, *Pretend you're a cat*
Mayer, *Just my friend and me*
Numeroff, *Dogs don't wear sneakers*
Offen, *The sheep made a leap*
Shaw, *Sheep in a shop*
Shaw, *Sheep on a ship*
Shaw, *Sheep out to eat*
Smalls-Hector, *Jonathan and his mommy* (M)
Westcott, *The lady with the alligator purse*
Zolotow, *Do you know what I'll do?*

Negative and/or Interrogative Sentences

Burningham, *Mr. Gumpy's outing*
Kraus, *Whose mouse are you?*
Numeroff, *Dogs don't wear sneakers*

Use to Elicit SVO sentences

Burningham, *Skip, trip*
Burningham, *Sniff, shout*

Comparative

Hoban, *Is it larger? Is it smaller?*

Superlative

Ruschak, *One hot day*

***But* Clauses**

Scott & Coalson, *Hi*

***And then* Clauses**

Wolf, *And then what?*

***When* Clauses**

Schecter, *When will the snow trees grow?*

***Because* clauses**

Porter-Gaylord, *I love my daddy because*
Zukman & Edelman, *It's a good thing*

Relative clauses

Wood, *Silly Sally*

Pragmatics

Cole, *Monster manners*
Corey, *Everyone takes turns*
Meddaugh, *Martha speaks*

Describing

Graham, *Full moon soup or the fall of the Hotel Splendide*
Lester, *It wasn't my fault*
Marzollo & Wick, *I spy*
Mayer, *Ah-choo* (No words)
Mayer, *A boy, a dog, a frog and a friend* (No words)
Mayer, *Frog goes to dinner* (No words)
Mayer, *Frog on his own* (No words)
Mayer, *Hiccup* (No words)
Mayer, *The great cat chase* (No words)
McCully, *Picnic* (No words)
McNaughton, *Guess who just moved in next door*
McPhail, *Emma's pet*
Novak, *Elmer Blunt's open house*
O'Malley, *Bruno, you're late forschool* (No words)
Raskin, *Nothing ever happens on my block*
Raschka, *Yo! Yes?*
Rathman, *Good night, gorilla*
Roe, *All I am*
Russo, *The great treasure hunt*
Schories, *Mouse around* (No words)

Spier, *Dreams* (No words)
Turkle, *Deep in the forest* (No words)

Discussion

Porter-Gaylord, *I love my daddy because*
Roe, *All I am*
Small, *Imogene's antlers (What if...)*
Zukman & Edelman, *It's a good thing*

Imagining

Barrett, *Cloudy with a chance of meatballs (If...then)*
Small, *Imogene's antlers*
Spier, *Dreams* (No words)

Noticing the "Ridiculous"

Slepian & Seidler, *The hungry thing returns*

Question/Answer

Charles, *What am I?*
Graham, *Full moon soup or the fall of the Hotel Splendide*
Marzollo & Pinkney, *Pretend you're a cat*
Raschka, *Yo! Yes?*

Semantics

Vocabulary

Barton, *Airplanes*
Barton, *Airport*
Barton, *Boats*
Burningham, *Skip, trip*
Burningham, *Sniff, shout*
Carle, *The secret birthday message*
DePaola, *Charlie needs a cloak*
DePaola, *Pancakes for breakfast*
King, *Gus is gone*
King, *Lucy is lost*
Krauss, *Bears*
Marzollo & Wick, *I spy*
Marzollo & Wick, *I spy mystery*
Noll, *Jiggle, wiggle, prance*
Peppe, *Odd one out*
Reiss, *Colors*
Rockwell, *Big wheels*
Rockwell, *My kitchen*
Rockwell, *Things that go*
Rockwell, *Things to play with*
Rockwell & Rockwell, *At the beach*
Viorst, *Alexander and the terrible, horrible, no good, very bad day*
Yabuuchi, *Whose footprints?*

Antonyms

Butterworth & Inkpen, *Nice or nasty: A book of opposites*

Hoban, *Is it rough, is it smooth, is it shiny?*
Hoban, *Exactly the opposite*
Wildsmith, *What the moon saw*

Categories

Barton, *Airplanes*
Barton, *Airport*
Barton, *Boats*
Martin, *Brown bear, brown bear, what do you see?*
Martin, *Polar bear, polar bear, what do you hear?*
Rockwell, *Big wheels*
Rockwell, *My kitchen*
Viorst, *Alexander and the terrible, horrible, no good, very bad day*
Yabuuchi, *Whose footprints?*
Zolotow, *Some things go together*

Word Associations

Zolotow, *Some things go together*

Verbal absurdities

Allard, *The Stupids die*
Allard, *The Stupids have a ball*
Allard, *The Stupids step out*
Barrett, *Animals should definitely not act like people*
Gwynne, *A chocolate moose for dinner*
Gwynne, *A king who rained*
Johnson, *Never babysit the hippopotamuses*

Synonyms

Wood, *The napping house*

Figurative Language

Barrett, *Cloudy with a chance of meatballs*
Gwynne, *A chocolate moose for dinner*
Gwynne, *A king who rained*
Lewin, *Jafta*
Mccauley, *Why the chicken crossed the road*
Numeroff, *If you give a mouse a cookie*
Numeroff, *If you give a moose a muffin*

Speech Sounds

Plosives

Aardema, *Bring the rain to Kapiti Plain* (M)

Initial /b/

Anholt & Anholt, *Here come the babies*
Dunrea, *Deep down underground*
Kent, *There's no such thing as a dragon*

Initial /s/

Arnold, *The simple people*
Barrett, *Cloudy with a chance of meatballs*

Carle, *A house for hermit crab*
Carle, *The very quiet cricket*
Dunrea, *Deep down underground*
Johnson, *The girl who wore snakes* (M)
Kennedy & Hague, *The teddy bears' picnic*
Kraus, *Milton the early riser*
Lewin, *Jafta's mother* (M)
Wood, *Silly Sally*
Zolotow, *Someday*

Initial /k/

Barton, *Harry is a scaredy-cat*
Knowlton, *Why cowboys sleep with their boots on*
Oxenbury, *The car trip*
Sendak, *Pierre*
Viorst, *My mama says*

/s/ blends

Barton, *Harry is a scaredy-cat* (Initial /sk/)
Borden, *Caps, hats, socks, and mittens* (Final /ts, ps/)
Keats, *The snowy day* (Initial /sn/)
Rockwell, *The first snowfall* (Initial /st/)
Rosen & Oxenbury, *We're going on a bear hunt* (Initial /sk/)

Final /ts, ps/ blends

Borden, *Caps, hats, socks, and mittens*

Initial /r/

Brown, *Big red barn*
Dunrea, *Deep down underground*
Capucilli, *Inside a barn in the country*
Carle, *A house for hermit crab*
Carle, *The very busy spider*
Ehlert, *Planting a rainbow*
Stinson, *Red is best*

/v/

Carle, *The very busy spider*

Final /k/

Carlson, *I like me*
DePaola, *Pancakes for breakfast*
Waddell & Oxenbury, *Father Duck*

Initial /k/ blends

Carle, *The very quiet cricket*
Jonas, *Where can it be*

Initial /l/

Carlson, *I like me*
Christelow, *Five little monkeys jumping on the bed*
Hale, *Mary had a little lamb*
Kraus, *Leo the late bloomer*
Shaw, *It looked like spilt milk*
Wood, *Quick as a cricket*

Initial /g/

Dunrea, *Deep down underground*
Galdone, *The three billy goats gruff*
Gantos, *Greedy greeny*
Jonas, *Where can it be*

Initial /h/

McCarthy, *Happy hiding hippos*

Initial /p/

Johnson, *Never babysit the hippopotamuses*
Teague, *Pigsty*

Final /p/

Seuss, *Hop on pop*
Shaw, *Sheep in a shop*
Shaw, *Sheep on a ship*
Shaw, *Sheep out to eat*

Publications to Assist in Classroom Use of Books

Charner, K. (1993). *The giant encyclopedia of theme activities.* Mt. Rainier, MD: Gryphon House.

Gebers, J. (1998). *Books are for talking, too! A sourcebook for using children's literature in speech and language remediation.* Tucson, AZ: Communication Skill Builders.

Jett-Simpson, M. (Ed.). (1989). *Adventures with books: A booklist for pre-K-grade 6.* Urbana, IL: National Council of Teachers of English.

Lockhart, B. (1992). *Read to me, Talk with me (Revised): Language activities based on children's favorite literature.* Tucson, AZ: Communication Skill Builders.

Raines, S.C., & Canady, R.J. (1989). *Story s-t-r-e-t-c-h-e-r-s: Activities to expand children's favorite books.* Mt. Rainier, MD: Gryphon House.

Raines, S.C., & Smith, B.S. (2011). *Story s-t-r-e-t-c-h-e-r-s for the primary grades: Activities to expand children's books,* Silver Spring, MD: Gryphon House.

Trelease, J. (1989). *The new read-aloud handbook.* New York: Penguin.

Glossary

AAC system An integrated group of components used by an individual to enhance communication.

ADHD Characterized by overactivity and an inability to attend for more than short periods of time. Although related to LD, the disorder does not manifest itself in severe perceptual and learning difficulties.

Aided AAC A form of augmentative and alternative communication that incorporates the use of communication devices in addition to the user's body.

Arena assessment A diagnostic assessment in which a common sample of the child's behavior is collected and recorded as parents and professionals observe the entire process and contribute their expertise.

Asperger's syndrome A mild form of pervasive development disorder in which the child exhibits LI and some autistic-like characteristics without the extreme "aloneness" found in many children with ASD.

Assessment The ongoing process, using of multiple tools and methods, of identifying a child's unique needs; the family's priorities, concerns, and resources; and the nature and extent of the EI services needed by both. Typically, assessments focus not on what is *wrong* with a child but on identifying what can be done to help.

Assistive technology (AT) An essential part of early intervention, consisting of adaptations and devices for children and families that enable children to function more independently.

At-risk A broad category of children served by early intervention programs in which there is the potential for both biological and environmental factors to interfere with a child's ability to interact in a typical way with the environment and to develop typically.

Augmentative and alternative communication (AAC) A form of AT and an intervention approach that uses other-than-speech means to complement or supplement an individual's communication abilities and may include a combination of existing speech or vocalizations, gestures, manual signs, communication boards, and speech-output communication devices.

Coaching A process of observing, demonstrating, and providing individualistic feedback to caregivers that can result in the acquisition and use of the skills necessary to provide effective intervention.

Code switching The shifting from one language to another within and/or across different utterances.

Collaborative teaching An educational method that combines consultation, team teaching, direct individual intervention, and side-by-side teaching in which the teacher and speech-language pathologist share the same goals for individual children.

Communication boards Non-electronic aided communication using visual-graphics symbols, such as photographs, line drawings, symbols, or printed words, which are selected by pointing.

Communication event An entire conversation and/or the topic or topics included therein.

Conditional use Using a behavior--sometimes an unacceptable one—that best matches a particular context and may be reinforced intentionally or unintentionally.

Conjunction A word that joins together sentences, clauses, phrases, or words.

Construct validity Accuracy with which or extent to which a measure describes or measures some trait or construct.

Content validity Faithfulness with which a sample or measure represents some attribute or behavior.

Contrast training Training method that teaches a child to discriminate between structures and situations that obligate use of the feature being trained and those features that do not.

Criterion validity Effectiveness or accuracy with which a measure predicts success.

Culture A shared framework of meanings within which a population shapes its way of life. Culture is what one needs to know or believe to function in a manner acceptable to a particular group. It includes, but is not limited to, history and the explanation of natural phenomena; societal roles; rules for interactions, decorum, and discipline; family structure; education; religious beliefs; standards of health, illness, hygiene, appearance, and dress; diet; perceptions of time and space; definitions of work and play; artistical and musical values; life expectations; and aspirations; and communication and language use.

C-unit Nonclausal response to a question in which ellipsis or one main clause plus any attached or embedded subordinate clause or nonclausal structure (T-unit) is evident.

Deafness A profound hearing loss of 90 dB or greater.

Deixis Process of using the speaker's perspective as a reference.

Developmental disabilities (DD) A severe, chronic disability of an individual 5 years of age or older that is attributable to mental or physical impairment or a combination of impairments; manifested before the age 22 years; likely to continue indefinitely; result in substantial functional limitations in three or more areas of life activity; and reflects the individual's need for a combination and sequence of special, interdisciplinary, or generic services, individualized supports, or other forms of assistance that are of lifelong or of extended duration.

Dynamic assessment Assessment tasks suggested for children with limited English proficiency (LEP) that emphasize ability to communicate and learn language rather than ability to use grammar. Typical tasks are narration, conversation, or teach-test paradigms.

Dyslexia A reading disorder, characterized by word recognition and/or reading comprehension abilities two years below the expected level but not due to any known emotional, environmental, intellectual, perceptual, or obvious neurological problem.

Early communication intervention (ECI) An intervention approach primarily focused on a young child's speech, language and/or feeding difficulties.

Early intervention (EI) An educational approach for young children, who have or are at risk of developing a handicapping condition or other special need that may affect their development, providing both remediation and prevention services focused on both child and family.

Echolalia Immediate or delayed whole or partial repetition of previous utterances of others with the same intonational pattern.

Ellipsis Omission of known or shared information in subsequent utterances in which it would be redundant.

Established risk A broad category of children served by early intervention programs, in which there is a strong relationship between the condition and development difficulties.

Evaluation Defined in Part H of the IDEA and conducted to determine a child's eligibility for services. Traditionally, evaluations are structured and formal and rely on the use of standardized instruments.

Evidence-based practice (EBP) Clinical practice based on scientific evidence, clinical experience, and client needs.

Fetal alcohol spectrum disorder (FASD) A continuum of permanent birth defects caused by materinal consumption of alcohol during pregancy that includes, but is not limited to, fetal alcohol syndrome (FAS).

Figure-ground perception Perceptual ability to isolate a stimulus against a background.

Functional language intervention A client-based, communication-first assessment and intervention method that employs language as it is actually used as the vehicle for change.

Hyperactivity A motor difficulty of overactivity often associated with learning disabilities and accompanied by attention problems.

Hyperlexia A variety of Pervasive Developmental Disorder characterized by spontaneous early reading ability and an intense preoccupation with letters and words but little real reading comprehension.

Incidental teaching A naturalistic child-directed intervention strategy used during unstructured activities.

Inclusive schooling An educational philosophy that proposes one integrated educational system—versus the two-tiered system, with regular and special education—based on each classroom becoming a supportive environment for all its members.

Individualized Family Service Plan (IFSP) An intervention plan that addresses both child and family needs that impact the child's development and includes the child and family's current status and the recommended service delivery.

Interdisciplinary team An intervention group consisting of professionals and parents in which a child is assessed by different disciplines independently and the team presents the family with a cohesive report.

Interference The influence of one language on the learning and use of another.

Interjudge reliability The probability of two judges scoring a child's performance on a test in the same manner.

Interlanguage A combination of the rules of two languages plus ad hoc rules from either or both languages.

Internal consistency Degree of relationship among items and the overall test.

Jargon Meaningless combination of words and sounds with the international pattern of speech.

Language impairment A heterogeneous group of developmental and/or acquired disorders and/or delays principally characterized by deficits and/or immaturities in the use of spoken or written language for comprehension and/or production purposes that may involve the form, content, and/or function of language in any combination.

Legal blindness A visual acuity of 20/200 or less in the better eye with the best possible correction as compared to 20/20 for typical vision.

Lexical competition An instantaneous process of comprehension consisting of all the words predicted by our brains from the phonemes we hear and the possible words that will make sense.

Maze Language segments that disrupt, confuse, and slow conversational movements. Mazes may consist of silent pauses, fillers, repetitions, and revisions.

Morbidity Illness or disability.

Multidisciplinary team A group of professionals in which members evaluate a child and determine his/her needs independently with little coordination.

Normed test A standardized test that has been given to a sample of individuals that supposedly represents all individuals for whom the test was designed. Scores are used to determine the typical performance expected for the entire population from whom the sample was drawn.

Orthographic awareness An individual's attention to an active and conscious thought and mindful consideration or orthographic knowledge, such as the regularities of print, that plays an important role in literacy acquisition.

Orthographic knowledge The information stored in our memory that tells us how to represent spoken language in a written form.

Parallel sentence construction A form of priming in which an SLP provides a model of a type of utterance to which a child is expected to provide a similar type of sentence.

PDD-NOS Pervasive Developmental Disorder–Not Otherwise Specified is mild form of PDD lacking the extreme characteristics of ASD.

Perseveration Repetition of the same behavior with a seeming inability to shift to another behavior or to stop.

Phonics Sound-letter correspondence used as the basis for most reading instruction.

Phonological awareness Literacy knowledge of the sounds and the sound and syllable structure of words. Better phonological awareness is related to better reading and spelling skills are to better phonological production.

Presupposition The speaker's assumption about the knowledge level of the listener, or what the listener knows and needs to know.

Preterm Delivery prior to 37 weeks of gestation.

Priming When the utterance of one person influences the structure, vocabulary selection, or sounds used by a second speaker.

Print awareness Literacy knowledge that includes knowing the direction in which reading proceeds across a page and through a book, being interested in print, recognizing letters, knowing that words are discrete units, and using literacy terminology, such as *letter*, *work*, and *sentence*.

Prognosis Estimate of the rate and extent of recovery from illness or injury.

Referential communication Speaker selects and verbally identifies attributes of an entity, thereby enabling the listener to identify the entity accurately.

Reliability Repeatability of a measure, based on the accuracy or precision with which a sample, at one time, represents performance based on either a different but similar sample or the same sample at a different time.

Response to intervention (RTI) A multitiered, problem-solving approach to education that addresses the learning difficulties of all children not just those with LI or other special needs conditions, incorporating both prevention and intervention.

Scanning An indirect method of accessing an AAC device, computer, or a voice-output device in which an individual activates a switch and makes a succession of choices that leads to the desired input.

Semantic networking A method of improving reading comprehension, writing cohesion, retention, and recall by teaching organization of information around a central theme or sequence.

Sensory integration Interpretation and synthesis of information received from two or more senses, such as hearing and vision.

Social disinhibition Inability to inhibit "acting out" behaviors often seen with traumatic brain injury.

Standardized test Test in which items are presented, cued, and consequated in a prescribed manner.

Story grammar Organizational pattern of narratives.

Strategy-based intervention model Training that teaches the child information-processing and problem-solving strategies.

Structural priming When a sentence produced by one speaker influences the structure of the sentences of a second speaker.

Systems model Intervention that targets the child's interactive systems or contexts.

Topic The subject matter about which the speaker is either providing or requesting information.

Transdisciplinary team A group of parents and facilitators from multiple disciplines who share responsibility for assessing, planning, and implementing intervention for a child, while at the same time contributing their own unique expertise and producing an integrated service plan through consensus or collaboration.

Total blindness A complete lack of form and visual light perception.

T-units (minimal terminal units) A main clause plus any attached or embedded subordinate clause or nonclausal structure.

Type-token ratio (TTR) Ratio of the number of different words to the total number of words, used as a measure of vocabulary and word retrieval.

Unaided AAC A from of augmentative and alternative communication that does not require any equipment and relies on the user's body to relay messages.

Validity Effectiveness of a test in representing, describing, or predicting an attribute. A test's ability to assess what it purports to measure.

Working memory Memory in which information is kept active while processed.

References

Adams, C. (2002). Practitioner review: The assessment of language pragmatics. *Journal of Child Psychology and Psychiatry, 43,* 973–987.

Adams, M., Foorman, B., Lundberg, I., & Beeler, T. (1998). *Phonemic awareness in young children: A classroom curriculum.* Baltimore: Paul H. Brookes.

Ad-hoc Committee on Service Delivery in Schools. (1993). American Speech-Language-Hearing Association (ASHA). Rockville, MD: ASHA.

Alderete, A., Frey, S., McDaniel, N., Romero, J., Westby, C., & Roman, R. (2004, November). *Developing vocabulary in school.* Paper presented at the American Speech-Language-Hearing Association Annual Convention, Philadelphia.

Allen, J. B., & Mason, J. M. (1989). *Risk makers, risk takers, risk breakers: Reducing the risks for young literacy learners.* Portsmouth, NH: Heinemann.

Allen, K., Feenaughty, L., Filippini, E., Johnson, M., Kanuck, A. Kroecker, J., Loccisano, S., Lyle, K., Nieto, J., Wind, K., Young, S., & Owens, R. E. (In press). Noun phrase elaboration in children's language samples. *Journal of Communication Disorders.*

Alloway, T. (2007). *The Automated Working Memory Assessment.* London: Pearson Assessment.

Alloway, T., & Archibald, L. (2008). Working memory and learning in children with developmental-coordination disorder and specific language impairment. *Journal of Learning Disabilities, 41,* 251–262.

Alloway, T. P., Gathercole, S. E., Kirkwood, H., & Elliott, J. (2009). The cognitive and behavioural characteristics of children with low working memory. *Child Development, 80,* 606–621.

Alt, M., Plante, E., & Creusere, M. (2004). Semantic features in fast-mapping: Performance of preschoolers with specific language impairment versus preschoolers with normal language. *Journal of Speech, Language, and Hearing Research,* 47, 407–420.

Altmann, L., Lombardino, L. J., & Puranik, C. (2008). Sentence production in students with dyslexia. *International Journal of Language & Communication Disorders, 43(1),* 55–76.

American Association on Intellectual and Developmental Disability. (2008). The AAIDD definition. Accessed August 11, 2008, from www.aamr.org/Policies/faq_intellectual_disability.shtml

American College of Obstetricians and Gynecologists. (2002, September). Perinatal care at the threshold viability. *ACOG Practice Bulletin,* 38.

American Psychiatric Association. (2000). *Diagnostic and statistical manual of mental disorders* (4th ed., revised). Washington, DC: Author.

American Speech-Language-Hearing Association. (2004a). Admission/discharge criteria in speech-language pathology. *ASHA Supplement, 24,* 65–70.

American Speech-Language-Hearing Association. (2005). *Roles and responsibilities of speech-language pathologists in service delivery for persons with mental retardation and developmental disabilities: Position statement.* Rockville, MD: Author.

American Speech-Language-Hearing Association. (2008a). *Core knowledge and skills in early intervention speech-language pathology practice.* Retrieved from www.asha.org/policy on March 15, 2012

American Speech-Language-Hearing Association. (2008b). *Roles and responsibilities of speech-language pathologists in early intervention: Guidelines.* Retrieved from www.asha.org/policy on March 15, 2012

American Speech-Language-Hearing Association. (2008c). *Roles and responsibilities of speech-language pathologists in early intervention: Position statement.* Retrieved from www.asha.org/policy on March 15, 2012

American Speech-Language-Hearing Association. (2008d). *Roles and responsibilities of speech-language pathologists in early intervention: Technical report.* Retrieved from www.asha.org/policy on March 15, 2012

American Speech-Language-Hearing Association. (2009). *Demographic profile of ASHA members providing bilingual and Spanish-language services.* Retrieved from www.asha.org/uploaded/Files/Demographic-Profile-Bilingual-Spanish-Service-Members.pd#search=%22bilingual%22 on March 15, 2012

American Speech-Language-Hearing Association. (2010). *2010 Schools survey report: SLP caseload characteristics.* Retrieved from www.asha.org/uploadedFiles/Schools10Caseload.pdf on March 15, 2012

Anderson, D., Lord, C., & Heinz, S. J. (2005, May). *Growth in language abilities among children with ASD and other developmental disabilities.* Poster presented at the International Meeting for Autism Research, Boston, MA.

Angelo, D. H. (2000). Impact of augmentative and alternative communication devices on families. *Augmentative and Alternative Communication* 16, 37–47.

Anthony, J., & Lonigan, C. (2004). The nature of phonological awareness: Converging evidence from four studies of preschool and early grade school children. *Journal of Educational Psychology*, 96, 43–55.

Anthony, J., Lonigan, C., Driscoll, K., Phillips, B., & Burgess, S. (2003). Phonological sensitivity: A quasi-parallel progression of word structure units and cognitive operation. *Reading Research Quarterly, 38*, 470–487.

Apel, K. (2010). Kindergarten children's initial spoken and written word learning in a storybook context. *Scientific Studies in Reading, 14*(5), 440–463.

Apel, K. (2011). What is orthographic knowledge? *Language, Speech, and Hearing Services in Schools, 42*, 592–603.

Apel, K., & Lawrence, J. (2011). Contributions of morphological awareness skills to word-level reading and spelling in first-grade children with and without speech sound disorder. *Journal of Speech, Language, and Hearing Research, 54*, 1312–1327.

Apel, K., & Thomas-Tate, S. (2009). Morphological awareness skills of fourth-grade African American students. *Language, Speech, and Hearing Services in Schools, 40*, 312–324.

Applebee, A. N. (1978). *The child's concept of story.* Chicago: University of Chicago Press.

Applequist, K. L., & Bailey, D. B. (2000). Navajo caregivers' perceptions of early intervention services. *Journal of Early Intervention. 23*, 47–61.

Archibald, L. M., & Gathercole, S. E. (2006a). Non-word repetition: A comparison of tests. *Journal of Speech, Language, and Hearing Research, 49*, 970–983.

Archibald, L. M., & Gathercole, S. E. (2006b). Visuospatial immediate memory in specific language impairment. *Journal of Speech, Language, and Hearing Research, 49*, 265–277.

Archibald, L. M., & Gathercole, S. E. (2006c). Short-term and working memory in specific language impairment. *International Journal of Language and Communication Disorders, 41(6)*, 675–693.

Archibald, L. M., & Gathercole, S. (2007). The complexities of complex memory span: Storage and processing deficits in specific language impairment. *Journal of Memory and Language, 57*, 177–194.

Archibald, L. M., & Joanisse, M. (2009). On the sensitivity and specificity of nonword repetition and sentence recall to language and memory impairments in children. *Journal of Speech, Language, and Hearing Research, 52*, 899–914.

Armbuster, B. B., Anderson, T. H., & Ostertag, J. (1987). Does text structure/summarization instruction facilitate learning from expository text? *Reading Research Quarterly, 22*, 331–346.

Atchison, B. J. (2007). Sensory modulation disorders among childrne with a history of trauma: A frame of reference for speech-language pathologists. *Language, Speech, and Hearing Services in Schools, 38*, 109–116.

August, D., Snow, C., Carlo, M., Proctor, C. P., Rolla de San Francisco, A., Duursma, E., & Szuber, A. (2006). Literacy development in elementary school second-language learners. *Topics in Language Disorders, 26*, 351–364.

Baddeley, A. D. (2000). The episodic buffer: New component of working memory? *Trends in Cognitive Sciences, 4*, 417–423.

Baddeley, A. D. (2003). Working memory and language: An overview. *Journal of Communication Disorders, 36*, 189–208.

Bailey, D. B. (2004). Assessing family resources, priorities, and concerns. In M. McLean, M. Wolery, & D. Bailey (Eds.), *Assessing infants and preschoolers with special needs* (3rd ed., pp. 172–203). Upper Saddle River, NJ: Pearson Merrill Prentice Hall.

Barras, C., Geoffrois, E., Wu, Z., & Liberman, M. (1998-2008). Transcriber (Version 1.5) [Computer software]. Amsterdam, The Netherlands: DGA.

Barrow, I. M., Holbert, D., & Rastatter, M. P. (2000). Effect of color on developmental picture vocabulary naming of 4-, 6-, and 8-year-old children. *American Journal of Speech-Language Pathology, 9*, 310–318.

Bashir, A. S., & Hook, P. E. (2009). Fluency: A key link between word identification and comprehension. *Language, Speech, and Hearing Services in Schools, 40*, 196–200.

Battle, D. E. (2002). Language development and disorders in culturally and linguistically diverse children. In D. Bernstein & E. Tiegerman-Farber (Eds.), *Language and communication disorders in children* (pp. 354–386). Boston: Allyn and Bacon.

Bauer, S. (1995a). Autism and the pervasive developmental disorders: Part I. *Pediatrics in Review, 16*(4), 130–136.

Bauer, S. (1995b). Autism and the pervasive developmental disorders: Part II. *Pediatrics in Review, 16*(5), 168–176.

Bayliss, D., Jarrold, C., Baddeley, A., Gunn, D., & Leigh, E. (2005). Mapping the developmental constraints on working memory span performance. *Developmental Psychology, 41*, 579–597.

Bear, D., Invernizzi, M., Templeton, S., & Johnston, F. (2000). *Words their way: Word study for phonics, vocabulary, and spelling instruction* (2nd ed.). Upper Saddle River, NJ: Prentice Hall.

Beck, A. R., & Dennis, M. (1997). Speech-language pathologists and teachers' perceptions of classroom-based interventions. *Language, Speech, and Hearing Services in Schools, 28*, 146–153.

Beckett, C., Bredenkamp, D., Castle, C., Groothues, C., O'Connor, T. G., & Rutter, M., & the English and Romanian Adoptees Study Team. (2002). Behavior patterns associated with institutional deprivation: A study of children adopted from Romania. *Developmental and Behavioral Pediatrics, 23*, 297–303.

Bedore, L. M., & Leonard, L. B. (2000). The effects of inflectional variation on fast mapping of verbs in English and Spanish. *Journal of Speech, Language, and Hearing Research, 43*, 21–33.

Bedore, L. M., & Leonard, L. B. (2001) Grammatical morphology deficits in Spanish-speaking children with specific language, *Journal of Speech, Language, and Hearing Research*, 44, 905–924.

Bedore, L. M., Peria, E. D., Garcia, M., & Cortez, C. (2005). Conceptual versus monolingual scoring: When does it make a difference? *Language, Speech, and Hearing Services in Schools*, 36, 188–200.

Bellon, M., Ogletree, B., & Harn, W. (2000). Repeated storybook reading as a language intervention for children with autism: A case study on the application of scaffolding. *Focus on Autism and Other Developmental Disabilities*, 15(1), 52–58.

Bencini, G. M., & Valian, V. V. (2008). Abstract sentence representations in 3-year-olds: Evidence from language production and comprehension. *Journal of Memory and Language, 59*, 97–113.

Bergman, R. L., Piacentini, J., & McCracken, J. (2002). Prevalence and description of selective mutidm in a school-based sample. *Journal of the American Academy of Child and Adolescent Psychiatry, 41*, 938–946.

Berman, R. A., & Verhoven, L. (2002). Cross-linguistic perspectives on the development of text-production abilities: Speech and writing. *Written Language and Literacy, 5(1)*, 1–43.

Bernheimer, L., & Weismer, T. (2007). "Let me tell you what I do all day. . .": The family story at the center of interventon research and practice. *Infants and Young Children, 20(3)*, 192–201.

Berninger, V. W. (2000). Development of language by hand and its connections to language by ear, mouth, and eye. *Topics in Language Disorders*, 20, 65–84.

Berninger, V. W. (2007a). *PAL II Reading and Writing Diagnostic Test Battery.* San Antonio, TX: The Psychological Corporation.

Berninger, V. W. (2007b). *PAL II user guides* (2nd version). San Antonio, TX: The Psychological Corporation/Pearson.

Berninger, V. W. (2008). Defining and differentiating dyslexia, dysgraphia, and language learning disability within a working memory model. In E.Silliman & M. Mody (Eds.), *Langugae impairment and reding disability–Interactions among brain, behavior, and experience* (pp, 103–134). New York: Guilford Press.

Berninger, V. W., Abbott, R., Rogan, L., Reed, L., Abbott, S., Brooks, A., Vaughan, K., & Graham, S. (1998). Teaching spelling to children with specific learning disabilities: The mind's ear and eye beats the computer and pencil. *Learning Disability Quarterly*, 21, 106–122.

Berninger, V. W., Abbott, R. D., Swanson, H. L., Lovitt, D., Trivedi, P., Lin, S-J., Gould, L., Youngstrom, M., Shimada, S., & Amtmann, D. (2010). Relationship of word- and sentence-level working memory to reading and writing in second, fourth, and sixth grade. *Language, Speech, and Hearing Services in Schools, 41*, 179–193.

Berninger, V. W., Nagy, W. E., Carlisle, J., Thomson, J., Hoffer, D., Abbott, S., et al. (2003). Effective treatment for children wirh dyslexia in grades 4-6: Behavioral and brain evidence. In B. R. Foorman (Ed.), *Preventing and remediating reading difficulties: Bringing science to scale* (pp. 381–417). Baltimore: York Press.

Berninger, V. W., Raskind, W., Richards, T., Abbott, R., & Stock, P. (2008). A multidisciplinary approach to understanding development dyslexia within working-memory architecture: Genotypes, phenotypes, brain, and instruction. *Development Neuropsychology*, 33, 707–744.

Berninger, V. W., Winn, W. D., Stock, P., Abbott, R. D., Eschen, K., Shi-Ju, L., Garcia, N., & Nagy, W. (2008). Tier 3 specialized writing instruction for students with dyslexia. *Reading and Writing*, 21, 95–129.

Berninger, V. W., & Wolf, B. (2009a). *Helping students with dyslexia dysgraphia make connections: Differential instruction lesson plans in reading and writing.* Baltimore, MD: Paul H. Brookes.

Berninger, V. W., & Wolf, B. (2009b). *Teaching students with dyslexia and dysgraphia: Lessons from teaching and science.* Baltimore, MD: Paul H. Brookes.

Bernstein Ratner, N. (2006). Evidence-based practice. An examination of its ramifications for the practice of speech-language pathology. *Language, Speech, and Hearing Services in Schools, 37*, 257–267.

Beukelman, D. R., & Mirenda, P. (2005). *Augmentative and alternative communication: Supporting children and adults with complex communication needs* (3rd ed.). Baltimore: Paul H. Brookes.

Bialystok, E., Craik, F., & Luk, G. (2008a). Cognitive control and lexical access in younger and older bilinguals. *Journal of Experimental Psychology: Learning, Memory, and Cognition, 34*, 859–873.

Bialystok, E., Craik, F. I. M., & Luk, G. (2008b). Lexical access in bilinguals: Effects of vocabulary size and executive control. *Journal of Neurolinguistics, 21*, 522–538.

Bialystok, E., Luk, G., Peets, K., & Yang, S. (2010). Receptive vocabulary differences in monolingual and bilingual children. *Bilingualism; Language and Cognition, 13*, 525–531.

Bibby, P., Eikeseth, S., Martin, N., Mudford, O., & Reeves, D. (2001). Progress and outcomes for children with autism receiving parent-managed intensive interventions. *Research in Developmental Disabilities, 22*, 425–447.

Biemiller, A. (2001). Teaching vocabulary: Early, direct, and sequential. *American Educator, 25*, 24–28.

Binger, C., & Light, J. C. (2006). Demographics of preschoolers who require augmentative and alternative communication. *Language Speech and Hearing Services in Schools, 37*, 200–208.

Bishop, D. V. (1985) Automated LARSP [Computer program]. Manchester, England: University of Manchester.

Bishop, D. V. (2003). *Children's Communication Checklist — 2.* London, England: The Psychological Corporation.

Bishop, D. V. (2006). *Children's Communication Checklist—2 U.S. Edition.* New York: The Psychological Corporation.

Bishop, D. V., Adams, C., & Rosen, S. (2006). Resistance of grammatical impairment to computerized comprehension training in children with specific and non-specific language impairments. *International Journal of Language and Communication Disorders, 41, 19–40.*

Bishop, D. V., & Baird, G. (2001). Parent and teacher report of pragmatic aspects of communication: Use of the Children's Communication Checklist in a clinical setting. *Developmental Medicine and Child Neurology, 43,* 809–818.

Bishop, D. V., & Donlan, C. (2005). The role of syntax in encoding and recall of pictorial narratives: Evidence from specific language impairment. *British Journal of Developmental Psychology, 23,* 25–46.

Bishop, D. V., North, T., & Donlan, C. (1995). Genetic basis of specific language impairment: Evidence from a twin study. *Developmental Medicine and Child Neurology, 37,* 56–71.

Bishop, D. V., Price, T. S., Dale, P. S., & Plomin, R. (2003). Outcomes of early language delay: II. Etiology of transient and persistent language difficulties. *Journal of Speech, Language, and Hearing Research, 46,* 561–575.

Blachman, B. (1984). Relationship of rapid naming ability and language analysis skills in kindergarten and first grade reading achievement. *Reading Research Quarterly, 13,* 223–253.

Blachman, B., Ball, E., Black, R., & Tangel, D. (2000). *Road to the code: A phonological awareness program for young children.* Baltimore: Paul. H. Brookes.

Blackstone, S. W., & Hunt-Berg, M. (2003) *Social networks: An assessment and intervention planning inventory for individuals with complex communication needs and their communication partners.* Monterey, CA: Augmentative Communication.

Bliss, L. S., McCabe, A., & Mahecha, N. R. (2001). Analyses of narratives from Spanish-speaking children. *Contemporary Issues in Communication Science and Disorders, 28,* 133–139.

Bock, J. K., & Griffin, Z. M. (2000). The persistence of structural priming: Transient activation or implicit learning? *Journal of Experimental Psychology: General, 129,* 177–192.

Bock, K., Dell, G., Chang, F., & Onishi, K. (2007). Persistent structural priming from language comprehension to language production. *Cognition, 104,* 437–458.

Boland, A. M., Haden, C. A., & Ornstein, P. A. (2003). Boosting children's memory by training mothers in the use of an elaborative conversational style as an event unfolds. *Journal of Cognition and Development, 4(1),* 39–65.

Bono, M. A., Daley, T., & Sigman, M. (2004). Relations among joint attention, amount of intervention and language gain in autism. *Journal of Autism and Developmental Disorders, 34,* 495–505.

Bono, M. A., & Sigman, M. (2004). Relations among joint attention, amount of intervention and language gain in autism. *Journal of Autism and Developmental Disorders, 34,* 495–505.

Bopp, K. D., Mirenda, P., & Zumbo, B. D. (2009). Behavior predictors of language development over 2 years in children with autism spectrum disorders. *Journal of Speech, Language, and Hearing Research, 52,* 1106–1120.

Botting, N, & Conti-Ramsden, G. (2003). Autism, primary pragmatic difficulties, and specific language impairment: Can we distinguish them using psycholinguistic markers? *Developmental Medicine and Child Neurology, 45,* 515–524.

Boudreau, D. M. (2005). Use of a parent questionnaire in emergent and early literacy assessment of preschool children, *Language, Speech, and Hearing Services in Schools, 36,* 33–47.

Boudreau, D. M. (2007). Narrative abilities in children with language impairment. In R. Paul (Ed.), *Language disorders from a developmental perspective: Essays in honor of Robin S. Chapman* (pp. 331–356). Mahwah, NJ: Erlbaum.

Boudreau, D. M., & Costanza-Smith, A. (2011). Assessment and treatment of working memory deficits in school-age children: The role of the speech-language pathologist. *Language, Speech, and Hearing Services in Schools, 42,* 152–166.

Boudreau, D. M., & Hedberg, N. L. (1999). A comparison of early literacy skills in children with specific language impairment and their typically developing peers. *American Journal of Speech-Language Pathology, 8,* 249–260.

Boudreau, D. M., & Larsen, J. (2004, November). *Strategies for teaching narrative abilities to schoolaged children.* Paper presented at the American Speech-Language-Hearing Association Annual Convention, Philadelphia.

Bourassa, D. C., & Treiman, R. (2001). Spelling development and disability: The importance of linguistic factors. *Language, Speech, and Hearing Services in Schools, 32(3),* 172–181.

Bowers, L., Huisingh, R., LoGiudice, C., & Orman, J. (2004a). *Word Test 2: Adolescent.* East Moline, IL: LinguaSystems.

Bowers, L., Huisingh, R., LoGiudice, C., & Orman, J. (2004b). *Word Test 2: Elementary.* East Moline, IL: LinguaSystems.

Boyce, N., & Larson, V. L. (1983). *Adolescents' communication: Development and disorders.* Eau Claire, WI: Thinking Publications.

Bracken, B. (1988). Rate and sequence of positive and negative poles in basic concept acquisition. *Language, Speech, and Hearing Services in Schools*, 19, 410–417.

Brackenbury, T., & Fey, M. E. (2003). Quick incidental verb learning in 4-year-olds: Identification and generalization. *Journal of Speech, Language, and Hearing Research, 46,* 313–327.

Brackenbury, T., & Pye, C. (2005). Semantic deficits in children with language impairments: Issues for clinical assessment. *Language, Speech, and Hearing Services in Schools*, 36, 5–16.

Bradshaw, M. L., Hoffman, P. R., & Norris, J. A. (1998). Efficacy of expansion and cloze procedures in the development of interpretations by preschool children exhibiting delayed language and development. *Language, Speech, and Hearing Services in Schools, 29,* 85–95.

Brady, N. C. (2000). Improved comprehension of object names following voice output communication aid use: Two case studies. *Augmentative and Alternative Communication, 16,* 197–204.

Braillion, A., & DuBois, G. (2005). [Letter to the editor]. *The Lancet, 365,* 1387.

Braten, I., & Stromso, H. (2003). A longitudinal think-aloud study of spontaneous strategic processing during the reading of multiple expository texts. *Reading and Writing: An Interdisciplinary Journal, 16,* 195–218.

Brinton, B., & Fujiki, M. (1989). *Conversational management with language-impaired children: Pragmatic assessment and intervention.* Rockville, MD: Aspen.

Brinton, B., Robinson, L. A., & Fujiki, M. (2004). Description of a program for social language intervention: "If you can have a conversation, you can have a relationship." *Language, Speech, and Hearing Services in Schools,* 35, 283–290.

Brinton, B., Spackman, M. P., Fujiki, M., & Ricks, J. (2007). What should Chris say? The ability of children with specific language imapirment to recognize the need to dissemble emotions in social situations. *Journal of Speech, Language, and Hearing Research, 50,* 798–811.

Brocki, K. C., Randall, K. D., Bohlin, G., & Kerns, K. A. (2008). Working memory in school-aged children with attention-deficit/hyperactivity disorder combined type: Are deficits modality specific and are they independent of impaired inhibitory control? *Journal of Clinical and Experimental Neuropsychology, 30,* 749–759.

Bromberger, P., & Permanente, K. (2004). Premies. University of Michigan Health Services. Updated November 30, 2004. Accessed September 16, 2008, from www.med.umich.edu/1libr/pa/pa_premie_hhg.htm

Brown, R. (1973). *A first language: The early stages.* Cambridge, MA: Harvard University Press.

Bull, R., & Scerif, G. (2001). Executive functioning as a predictor of children's mathematics ability: Shifting, inhibition, and working memory. *Developmental Neuropsychology, 19,* 273–293.

Burgess, S., & Turkstra, L. S. (2010). Quality of communication life in adolescents with high-functioning autism and Asperger syndrome: A feasibility study. *Language, Speech, and Hearing Services in Schools, 41,* 474–487.

Buschbacher, P. W., & Fox, L. (2003). Understanding and intervening with the challenging behavior of young children with autism spectrum disorder. *Language, Speech, and Hearing Services in Schools, 34,* 217–227.

Buttrill, J., Niizawa, J., Biemer, C., Takahashi, C., & Hearn, S. (1989). Serving the language learning disabled adolescent: A strategies-based model. *Language, Speech, and Hearing Services in Schools, 20,* 185–204.

Butyniec-Thomas, J., & Woloshyn, V. E. (1997). The effects of explicit-strategy and whole-language instruction on students' spelling ability. *Journal of Experimental Education, 65,* 293–302.

Buysse, V., & Wesley, P. (2006). *Consultation in early childhood settings.* Baltimore: Paul. H. Brookes.

Cabell S. Q., Justice, L. M., Piasta, S. B., Curenton, S. M., Wiggins, A., Turnbull, K. P., & Petscher, Y. (2011). The impact of teacher responsivity education on preschoolers' language and literacy skills. *American Journal of Speech-Language Pathology,* 20, 315–330.

Cabell, S. Q., Justice, L. M., Zucker, T. A., & Kilday, C. R. (2009). Validity of teacher report for assessing the emergent literacy skills of at-risk preschoolers. *Language, Speech, and Hearing Services in Schools, 40,* 161–173.

Caesar, L. G., & Kohler, P. D. (2007). The state of school-based bilingual assessment: Actual practice versus recommended guidelines. *Language, Speech, and Hearing Services in Schools, 38,* 190–200.

Cain, K., & Oakhill, J. (Eds.). (2007). *Children's comprehension problems in oral and written language. A cognitive perspective.* New York: Guilford Press.

Cain, K., Oakhill, J. V., & Bryant, P. E. (2001). Children's reading comprehension ability: Concurrent prediction by working memory, verbal ability, and component skills. *Journal of Educational Psychology, 96,* 31–42.

Calfee, R., Norman, K., & Wilson, K. (1999). *Interactive Reading Assessment Systems—Revised.* Accessed August 16, 2008, from http://cehs.unl.edu/wordworks/docs/IRAS.pdf

Calvert, M. B., & Murray, S. L. (1985). Environmental Communication Profile: An assessment procedure. In C. S. Simon (Ed.), *Communication skills and classroom success: Assessment of language-learning disabled students* (pp. 135-165). Austin, TX: Pro-Ed.

Campbell, P. H., Milbourne, S. A., Dugan, L. M., & Wilcox, M. J. (2006). A review of evidence on practices for teaching young children to use assistive technology devices. *Topics in Early Childhood Special Education, 26,* 3–14.

Cannizzaro, M. S., & Coelho, C. A. (2002). Treatment of story grammar following traumatic brain injury: A pilot study. *Brain Injury, 16,* 1065–1073.

Cardenas-Hagan, E., Carlson, C. D., & Pollard-Durodola, S. D. (2007). The cross-linguistic transfer of early literacy skills: The role of initial L, and L2 skills and language instruction. *Language, Speech, and Hearing Services in Schools,* 3, 249–259.

Carrow, E. (1979). *Carrow Elicited Language Inventory.* McAllen, TX: DLM and Teaching Resources.

Carrow-Woolfolk, E. (1999). *Test of Auditory Comprension of Language* (3rd ed.). Austin, TX: Pro-Ed.

Catts, H. W. (1997). The early identification of language-based reading disabilities. *Language, Speech, and Hearing Services in Schools, 28,* 86–89.

Catts, H. W., Adlof, S. M., & Ellis Weismer, S. (2006). Language deficits in poor comprehenders: A case for the simple view of reading. *Journal of Speech, Language, and Hearing Research, 49,* 278–293.

Catts, H. W., Fey, M. E. Tomblin, J. B., & Zhang, X. (2002). A longitudinal investigation of reading outcomes in children with language impairments. *Journal of Speech, Language, and Hearing Research, 45,* 1142–1157.

Catts, H. W., Hogan, T. P., & Adlof, S. M. (2005). Developmental changes in reading and reading disabilities. In H. W. Catts & A. Kamhi (Eds.), *The connections between language and reading disabilities* (pp. 25-40). Mahwah, NJ: Erlbaum.

Catts, H. W., Hogan, T. P., & Fey, M. E. (2003). Subgrouping poor readers on the basis of individual differences in reading-related abilities. *Journal of Learning Disabilities, 36(2),* 151–164.

Centers for Disease Control and Prevention. (2007). Morbidity and mortality weekly report. *MMWR Surveillance Summaries, 56,* 1–40.

Chakrabarti, S., & Fombonne, E. (2001). Pervasive developmental disorders in preschool children. *Journal of the American Medical Association, 285,* 3093–3099.

Champion, T. B., Hyter, Y. D., McCabe, A., & Bland-Stewart, L. M. (2003). A matter of vocabulary: Performances of low-income African American Head Start children on the Peabody Picture Vocabulary Test—III. *Communication Disorders Quarterly, 24(3),* 121–127.

Chaney, C. (1992). Language development, metalinguistic skills, and print awareness in 3-year-old children. *Applied Psycholinguistics, 13,* 485–514.

Chang, F., Early, D., & Winton, P. (2005). Early childhood teacher preparation in special education at 2- and 4-year institutions of higher education. *Journal of Early Intervention,* 27, 110–124.

Channell, R. W. (2003). Automated Developmental Sentence Scoring using computerized profiling software. *American Journal of Speech-Language Pathology, 12,* 369–375.

Chao, P., Bryan, T., Burstein, K., & Cevriye, E. (2006). Family-centered intervention for young children at-risk for language and behavior problems. *Early Childhood Education Journal, 34,* 147–153.

Chapman, R. S. (1981). Exploring children's communicative intents. In J. Miller (Ed.), *Assessing language production in children* (pp. 22-25). Baltimore: University Park Press.

Chapman, R. S., Sindberg, H., Bridge, C., Gigstead, K., & Hasketh, L. (2006). Effect of memory support and elicited production on fast mapping of new words by adolescents with Down syndrome. *Journal of Speech, Language, and Hearing Research, 49,* 3–15.

Charman, T. R., Baron-Cohen, S., Swettenham, J., Baird, G., Drew, A., & Cox, A. (2003). Predicting language outcome in infants with autism and pervasive developmental disorder. *International Journal of Language and Communication Disorders, 38,* 265–285.

Choudhury, N., & Benasich, A. A. (2003). A family aggregation study: The influence of family history and other risk factors on language development. *Journal of Speech, Language, and Hearing Research, 46,* 261–272.

Cirrin, F. M., Schooling, T. L., Nelson, N. W., Diehl, S. F., Flynn, P. F., Staskowski, M., Torrey, T. Z., & Adamczyk, D. F. (2010). Evidence-based systematic review: Effects of different service delivery models on communication outcomes for elementary school-age children. *Language, Speech, and Hearing Services in Schools, 41,* 233–264.

Clay, M. M. (1979). *The early detection of reading difficulties: A diagnostic survey with recovery procedures.* Exeter, NH: Heinemann.

Cochrane, R. (1983). Language and the atmosphere of delight. In H. Winitz (Ed.), *Treating language disorders: For clinicians by clinicians* (pp. 143–162). Baltimore University Park Press.

Coggins, T. (1991). Bringing context back into assessment. *Topics in Language Disorders, 11*(4), 43–54.

Coggins, T., Olswang, L., Carmichael Olson, H., & Timler, G. (2003). On becoming socially competent communicators: The challenge for children with fetal alcohol exposure. *International Review of Research in Mental Retardation. 27,* 121–150.

Cohen, W., Hodson, A., O'Hare, A., Boyle, J., Durrani, T., McCartney, E., & Watson, J. (2005). Effects of computer-based intervention through acoustically modified speech (Fast ForWord) in severe mixed receptive-expressive language impairment: Outcomes from a randomized controlled trial. *Journal of Speech, Language, and Hearing Research, 48,* 715–729.

Colozzo, P., Garcia, R., Megan, C., Gillam, R., & Johnson, J (2006, June). *Narrative assessment in SLI: Exploring interactions between content and form.* Poster session presented at the annual meeting of the Symposium, on Research in Child Language Disorders, Madison, WI.

Condouris, K., Meyer, E., & Tager-Flusberg, H.(2003). The relationship between standardized measures of language and measures of spontaneous speech in children with autism. *American Journal of Speech-Language Pathology, 12,* 349–358.

Conti-Ramsden, G., & Botting, N. (2004). Social difficulties and victimization in children with SLI at 11 years of age. *Journal of Speech, Language, and Hearing Research, 47,* 145–161.

Conti-Ramsden, G., Botting, N., & Durkin, K. (2008). Parental perspectives during the transition to adulthood of adolescents with a history of Specific Language Impairment (SLI). *Journal of Speech, Language, and Hearing Research, 51,* 84–96.

Conti-Ramsden, G., & Durkin, K. (2007). Phonological short-term memory, language and literacy: Developmental relationships in early adolescence in young people with SLI. *Journal of Child Psychology and Psychiatry, 48,* 147–156.

Conti-Ramsden, G., & Durkin, K. (2008). Language and independence in adolescents with and without a history of Specific Language Impairment (SLI). *Journal of Speech, Language, and Hearing Research, 51,* 70–83.

Conti-Ramsden, G., Durkin, K., & Simkin, Z. (2010). Language and social factors in the use of cell phone technology by adolescents with and without Specific Language Impairment (SLI). *Journal of Speech, Language, and Hearing Research, 53,* 196–208.

Conti-Ramsden, G., Simkin, Z., & Pickles, A. (2006). Estimating familial loading in SLI: A comparison of direct assessment versus personal interview. *Journal of Speech, Language, and Hearing Research, 49,* 88–101.

Corriveau, K., Posquine, E., & Goswami, U. (2007). Basic auditory processing skills and specific language impairment: A new look at an old hypothesis. *Journal of Speech, Language, and Hearing Research, 50,* 647–666.

Cowan, N., Nugent, L., Elliott, E., Ponomarev, I., & Saults, S. (2005). The role of attention in the development of short-term memory: Age differences in the verbal span of apprehension. *Child Development, 70,* 1082–1097.

Craig, H. K., Connor, C. M., & Washington, J. A. (2003). Early positive predictors of later reading comprehension for African American students: A preliminary investigation. *Language, Speech, and Hearing Services in Schools, 34,* 31–43.

Craig, H. K., & Washington, J. A. (2002). Oral language expectations for African American preschoolers and kindergarteners. *American Journal of Speech-Language Pathology,* 11, 59–70.

Craig, H. K., Washington, J. A., & Thompson-Porter, C. (1998). Average C-unit lengths in the discourse of African American children from low-income urban homes. *Journal of Speech, Language, and Hearing Research,* 41, 433–444.

Craig, H. R., Zhang, L., Hensel, S. L., & Quinn, E. J. (2009). African American English-speaking students: An examination of the relationship between dialect shifting and reading outcomes. *Journal of Speech, Language, and Hearing Research, 52,* 839–855.

Crais, E. R. & Roberts, J. (1991). Decision making in assessment and early intervention planning. *Language, Speech, and Hearing Services in Schools, 22,* 19–30.

Crais, E. R., & Roberts, J. (2004). Assessing communication skills. In M. McLean, M. Wolery, & D. Bailey (Eds.), *Assessing infants and preschoolers with special needs* (3rd ed., pp. 345–411). Upper Saddle River, NJ: Pearson/Merrill/Prentice Hall.

Creaghead, N. A. (1992). Classroom interactional analysis/script analysis. *Best Practices in School Speech Language Pathology, 2,* 65–72.

Cress, C. J. (2003). Responding to a common early AAC question: "Will my child talk?" *Perspectives on Augmentative and Alternative Communication, 12,* 10–11.

Cress, C. J., & Marvin, C. A. (2003). Common questions about AAC services in early intervention. *Augmentative and Alternative Communication, 19,* 254–272.

Crowe, L. K. (2003). Comparison of two reading feedback strategies in improving the oral and written language performance of children with language learning disabilities. *American Journal of Speech-Language Pathology, 12,* 16–27.

Crowhurst, M., & Piche, G. L. (1979). Audience and mode of discourse effects on syntactic complexity in writing at two grade levels. *Research in the Teaching of English, 13,* 101–109.

Crumrine, L., & Lonegan, H. (1998). *Pre-Literacy Skills Screening.* Chicago: Applied Symbolix.

Crystal, D. (1982). *Profiling linguistic disability.* London, UK: Edward Arnold.

Crystal, D., Fletcher, P., & Garman, R. (1976). *The grammatical analysis of language disability.* New York: Elsevier.

Cunningham, A., Perry, K., Stanovich, K., & Stanovich, P. (2004). Disciplinary knowledge of K-3 teachers and their knowledge calibration in the domain of early literacy. *Annals of Dyslexia, 54,* 139–167.

Cunningham, M., & Cox, E. O. (2003, February). Hearing assessment in infants and children: Recommendations beyond neonatal screening. *Pediatrics, 111*(2), 436–440.

Curenton, S., & Justice, L. (2004). African American and Caucasian preschoolers' use of decontextualized language: Literate language features in oral narratives. *Language, Speech, and Hearing Services in Schools, 35,* 240–253.

Dale, P. S., Price, T. S., Bishop, D. V. M., & Plomin, R. (2003). Outcomes of early language delay: I. Predicating persistent and transient language difficulties at 3 and 4 years. *Journal of Speech, Language, and Hearing Research, 46,* 544–560.

Damico, J. S. (1991a). Clinical Discourse Analysis: A functional language assessment technique. In C. S. Simon (Ed.), *Communication skills and classroom success: Assessment and therapy methodologies for language and learning disabled students* (pp. 125–150). Eau Claire, WI: Thinking Publications.

Damico, J. S. (1992). Systematic observation of communication interaction. *Best Practices in School Speech-Language Pathology, 2,* 133–144.

Damico, J. S., & Oller, J. (1985). *Spotting language problems* San Diego: Los Amigos Research Associates.

Danahy Ebert, K., & Kohnert, K. (2011). Sustained attention in children with primary language impairment: A meta-analysis. *Journal of Speech, Language, and Hearing Research, 54,* 1372–1384.

Danzak, R. L. (2011). The integration of lexical, syntactic, and discourse features in bilingual adolescents' writing: An exploratory approach. *Language, Speech, and Hearing Services in Schools, 42,* 491–505.

Davis, J. W., & Bauman, K. J. (2008). *School enrollment in the United States: 2006.* Washington, DC: U.S. Bureau of the Census.

Deevy, P., Wisman Weil, L., Leonard, L. B., & Goffman, L. (2010). Extending use of the NRT to preschool-age children with and without Specific Language Impairment.

Language, Speech, and Hearing Services in Schools, 41, 277–288.

DeKroon, D. M. A., Kyte, C. S., & Johnson, C. J. (2002). Partner influences on the social pretend play of children with language impairments. *Language, Speech, and Hearing Services in Schools, 33,* 253–267.

Demmert, W. G., McCardle, P., & Leos, K. (2006). Conclusions and commentary. *Journal of American Indian Education, 45 (2),* 77–88.

Dempsey, L., Jacques, J., Skarakis-Doyle, E., & Lee, C. (2002, November). *The relationship between preschoolers' comprehension monitoring ability and their knowledge of truth conditions.* Paper presented at the annual convention of the American Speech-Language-Hearing Association, Atlanta, GA.

Denham, S. A., & Burton, R. (1996). Social-emotional intervention for at-risk 4-year-olds. *Journal of School Psychology, 34,* 223–245.

Dennis, M., Lazenby, A. L., & Lockyer, L. (2001). Inferential language in high-functioning children with autism. *Journal of Autism and Developmental Disorders,* 31(1), 47–54.

de Rivera, C, Girolametto, L., Greenberg, J., & Weitzman, E. (2005). Children's responses to educators' questions in day care play groups. *American Journal of Speech-Language Pathology, 14,* 14–26.

DeThorne, L. S., Petrill, S. A., Hart, S. A., Channell, R. W., Campbell, R. J., Deater-Deckard, K., Thompson, L. A., & Vandenbergh, D. J. (2008). Genetic effects on children's conversational language use. *Journal of Speech, Language, and Hearing Research, 51,* 423–435.

de Valenzuela, J. S., Copeland, S. R., Qi, C. H., & Park, M. (2006). Examining educational equity: Revisiting the disproportionate representation of minority students in special education. *Exceptional Children, 72,* 425–441.

deVilliers, J. G. (2004). Cultural and linguistic fairness in the assessment of semantics. *Seminars in Speech and Language, 25,* 73–90.

Dickinson, D. K., & DeTemple, J. (1998). Putting parents in the picture: Maternal reports of preschoolers' literacy as a predictor of early reading. *Early Childhood Research Quarterly, 13,* 241–261.

Dickinson, D. K., & Tabors, P. O. (2001). *Beginning literacy with language: Young children learning at home and school.* Baltimore: Paul H. Brookes.

Dickinson, D. K., Darrow, C. L., & Tinubu, T. A. (2008). Patterns of teacher-child conversations in Head Start classrooms: Implications for an empirically grounded approach to professional development. *Early Education and Development, 19,* 396–429.

Diehl, S. F., Ford, C., & Federico, J. (2005). The communication journey of a fully included child with an autism spectrum disorder. *Topics in Language Disorders, 25*(4), 375–387.

Dinnebeil, L. A., Pretti-Frontczak, K., & Mclnemey, W. (2009). A consultative itinerant approach to service delivery: Considerations for the early childhood community. *Language, Speech, and Hearing Services in Schools, 40,* 435–445.

Dodd, B., & Carr, A. (2003). Young children's letter-sound knowledge. *Language, Speech, and Hearing Services in Schools, 34,* 128–137.

Dollaghan, C. A. (2004). Evidence-based practice in communication disorders: What do we know and when do we know it? *Journal of Communication Disorders, 37,* 391–400.

Dollaghan, C. A., & Campbell, T. (1998). Nonword repetition and child language impairment. *Journal of Speech, Language, and Hearing Research, 41,* 1136–1146.

Dore, J. (1974). A pragmatic description of early language development. *Journal of Psycholinguistic Research, 3,* 343–350.

Dore, J. (1986). The development of conversational competence. In R. Schiefelbusch (Ed.), *Language competence: Assessment and intervention* (pp. 3–60). San Diego: College-Hill.

Douglas, J. M. (2010). Relation of executive functioning to pragmatic outcome following severe traumatic brain injury. *Journal of Speech, Language, and Hearing Research, 53,* 365–382.

Drager, K. D., Light, J. C, Carlson, R., D'Silva, K., Larsson, B., Pitkin, L., & Stopper, G. (2004). Learning of dynamic display AAC technologies by typically developing 3-year-olds: Effect of different layouts and menu approaches. *Journal of Speech, Language, and Hearing Research, 47,* 1133–1148.

Drager, K. D., Light, J. C, Curran Speltz, J., Fallon, K. A., & Jeffries, L. Z. (2003). The performance of typically developing 2 ½-year-olds on dynamic display AAC technologies with different system layouts and language organizations. *Journal of Speech, Language, and Hearing Research, 46,* 298–312.

Duchan, J. F. (1997). A situated pragmatics approach for supporting children with severe communication disorders. *Topics in Language Disorders, 17*(2), 1–18.

Duchan, J. F., & Weitzner-Lin, B. (1987). Nurturant-naturalistic intervenion for language-impaired children: Implications for planning lessons and tracking progress. *Asha, 29*(7), 45–49.

Dunn, L. M., & Dunn, D. M. (2007). *Peabody Picture Vocabulary Test* (PPVT) (4th ed.). Boston Pearson.

Dunst, C. J. (2002). Family-centered practices: Birth through high school. *Journal of Special Education, 36,* 139–147.

Dunst, C. J., Hamby, D., Trivette, C. M., Raab, M., & Bruder, M. B. (2000). Everyday family and community life and children's naturally occurring learning opportunities. *Journal of Early Intervention, 23(3),* 151–164.

Dunst, C. J., & Trivette, C. M. (2009a). Let's be PALS: An evidence-based approach to professional development. *Infants and Young Children, 22,* 164–176.

Ebbels, S. (2007). Teaching grammar to school-aged children with specific language impairment using shape coding. *Child Language Teaching and Therapy, 23,* 67–93.

Edmonston, N. K., & Thane, N. L. (1990, April). Children's concept comprehension: *Acquisition, assessment, intervention*. Paper presented at the Annual Convention of the New York State Speech-Language-Hearing Association, Kiamesha Lake.

Ehren, B. J. (2000). Maintaining a therapeutic focus and sharing responsibility for student success: Keys to in-classroom speech-language services. *Language, Speech, and Hearing Services in Schools, 31*, 219–229.

Ehren, B. J. (2005). Looking for evidence-based practice in reading comprehension instruction. *Topics in Language Disorders, 25*, 310–321.

Ehren, B. J. (2006). Partnerships to support reading comprehension for students with language impairment. *Topics in Language Disorders, 26*, 42–54.

Ehri, L. C. (2000). Learning to read and learning to spell: Two sides of a coin. *Topics in Language Disorders, 20(3)*, 19–36.

Eigsti, L., & Cicchetti, D. (2004). The impact of child maltreatment on the expressive syntax at 60 months. *Developmental Science, 7*, 88–102.

Eisenberg, S. L. (2005). When comprehension is not enough: Assessing infinitival complements through elicitation. *American Journal of Speech-Language Pathology, 14*, 92–106.

Eisenberg, S. L., McGovern Fersko, T., & Lundgren, C. (2001). The use of MLU for identifying language impairment in preschool children: A review. *American Journal of Speech-Language Pathology, 10*, 323–342.

Ellis Weismer, S., & Evans, J. L. (2002). The role of processing limitations in early identification of specific language impairment. *Topics in Language Disorders, 22*(3), 15–29.

Ellis Weismer, S., & Hesketh, L. J. (1998). The impact of emphatic stress on novel word learning by children with specific language impairment. *Journal of Speech, Language, and Hearing Research, 41*, 1444–1458.

Ellis Weismer, S., Plante, E., Jones, M., & Tomblin, J. B. (2005). A functional magnetic resonance imaging investigation of verbal working memory in adolescents with specific language impairment. *Journal of Speech, Language, and Hearing Research, 48*, 405–425.

Ellis Weismer, S., Tomblin, J. B., Zhang, X., Buckwalter, P., Chynoweth, J. G., & Jones, M. (2000). Non-word repetition performance in school-age children with and without language impairment. *Journal of Speech, Language, and Hearing Research, 43*, 865–878.

Ertmer, D. J., Strong, L. M., & Sadagopan, N. (2003). Beginning to communicate after cochlear implantation: Oral language development in a young child. *Journal of Speech, Language, and Hearing Research, 46*, 328–340.

Ervin, M. (2001, June 26). SLI—What we know and why it matters. *ASHA Leader*.

Ervin-Tripp, S. (1977). Wait for me roller skate. In S. Ervin-Tripp & C. Mitchell-Kerner (Eds.), *Child discourse* (pp. 165–188). New York: Academic Press.

Evans, J. L., & Craig, H. K. (1992). Language sample collection and analysis. Interview compared to freeplay assessment contexts. *Journal of Speech and Hearing Research, 35*, 343–353.

Ezell, H. K., & Justice, L. M. (2005). *Shared storybook reading: Building young children's language and emergent literacy skills*. Baltimore: Paul H. Brookes.

Ezell, H. K., Justice, L. M., & Parsons, D. (2000). Enhancing the emergent literacy skills of preschoolers with communication disorders: A pilot investigation. *Child Language Teaching and Therapy, 16*, 121–160.

Fallon, K. A., & Katz, L. A. (2011). Providing written language services in the schools: The time is now. *Language, Speech, and Hearing Services in Schools, 42*, 3–17.

Fallon, K. A., Light, J. C., & Kramer Paige, T. (2001). Enhancing vocabulary selection for preschoolers who require augmentative and alternative communication (AAC). *American Journal of Speech-Language Pathology, 10*, 81–94.

Feldman, H. M., Dollaghan, C. A., Campbell, T.R, Colborn, D. K., Janosky, J., Kurs-Lasky, M., Rockette, H. E., Dale, P. S., & Paradise, J. L. (2003). Parent-reported language skills in relation to otitis media during the first 3 years of life. *Journal of Speech, Language, and Hearing Research, 46*, 273–287.

Fenson, L., Marchman, V. A., Thai, D., Dale, P., Reznick, J. S., & Bates, E. (2007). *The MacArthur-Bates Communicative Development Inventories: User's guide and technical manual* (2nd ed.). Baltimore, MD: Paul H. Brookes.

Fey, M. E. (1986). *Language intervention with young children*. San Diego: College-Hill.

Fey, M. E., Catts, H., Proctor-Williams, K., Tomblin, B., & Zhang, X. (2004). Oral and written story composition skills of children with language impairment. *Journal of Speech, Language, and Hearing Research, 47*, 1301–1318.

Fey, M. E., Finestack, L. H., Gajewski, B. J., Popescu, M., & Lewine, J. D. (2010). A preliminary evaluation of Fast ForWord-Language as an adjuvant treatment in language intervention. *Journal of Speech, Language, and Hearing Research, 53*, 430–449.

Fey, M. E., & Frome Loeb, D. (2002). An evaluation of the facilitative effects of inverted yes-no questions on the acquisition of auxiliary verbs. *Journal of Speech, Language, and Hearing Research, 45*, 160–174.

Fey, M. E., Long, S. H., & Finestack, L. H. (2003). Ten principles of grammar facilitation for children with specific language impairments. *American Journal of Speech-Language Pathology, 12*, 3–15.

Fiestas, C. E., & Pefia, E. D. (2004). Narrative discourse in bilingual children: Language and task effects. *Language, Speech, and Hearing Services in Schools, 35*, 155–168.

Filipek, P., Accordo, P., Baranek, G., Cook, E., Dawson, G., Gordon, B., Gravel, J., Johnson, C , Kallen, R., Levy, S., Minshew, N., Prizant, B., Rapin, I., Rogers, S., Stone, W., Teplin, S., Tuchman, R., 8c Volkmaret, F. (1999). The screening and diagnosis of autism spectrum disorders.

Journal of Autism and Developmental Disorders, 29, 49–58.
Finestack, L. H., & Fey, M. E. (2009). Evaluation of a deductive/procedure to teach grammatical inflections to children with language impairment. *American Journal of Speech-Language Pathology, 18,* 289–302.
Finneran, D. A., Francis, A. L., & Leonard, L. B. (2009). Sustained attention in children with Specific Language Impairment (SLI). *Journal of Speech, Language, and Hearing Research, 52,* 915–929.
Finneran, D. A., Leonard, L. B., & Miller, C. (in press). Speech disruptions in the sentence formulation of school-age children with specific language impairment. *International Journal of Language and Communication Disorders.*
Flax, J. F., Realpe-Bonilla, T., Hirsch, L. S., Brzustowicz, L. M., Bartlett, C. W., & Tallal, P. (2003). Specific language impairment in families: Evidence for co-occurrence with reading impairments. *Journal of Speech, Language, and Hearing Research, 46,* 530–543.
Flenthrope, J. L., & Brady, N. C. (2010). Relationships between early gestures and later language in children with fragile X syndrome. *American Journal of Speech-Language Pathology, 19,* 135–142.
Folger, J., & Chapman, R. (1978). A pragmatic analysis of spontaneous imitations. *Journal of Child Language, 5,* 25–38.
Fombonne, E. (2003a). The prevalence of autism. *Journal of the American Medical Association, 289, 87–89.*
Fombonne, E. (2003b). Epidemiological surveys of autism and other pervasive developmental disorders: An update. *Journal of Autism and Developmental Disorders, 33,* 365–382.
Fontes, L. A. (2002). Child discipline and physical abuse in immigrant Latino families: Reducing violence and misunderstandings. *Journal of Counseling and Development, 80,* 31–40.
Ford, J. A., & Milosky, L. M. (2003). Inferring emotional reactions in social situations: Differences in children with language impairment. *Journal of Speech, Language, and Hearing Research, 46,* 21–30.
Ford, J. A., & Milosky, L. M. (2008). Inference generation during discourse and its relation to social competence: An online investigation of abilities of children with and without language impairment. *Journal of Speech, Language, and Hearing Research, 51,* 367–380.
Foster, W. A., & Miller, M. (2007). Development of the literacy achievement gap: A longitudinal study of kindergarten through third grade. *Language, Speech, and Hearing Services in Schools, 38,* 173–181.
Fried-Oken, M. (1987). Qualitative examination of children's naming skills through test adaptations. *Language, Speech, and Hearing Services in Schools, 18,* 206–216.
Fried-Patti, S. (1999). Specific language impairment: Continuing clinical concerns. *Topics in Language Disorders, 20*(1), 1–13.
Fry, R. (2007). *The changing racial and ethnic composition of U.S. public schools.* Washington, DC: Pew Hispanic Center.
Fujiki, M., Brinton, B., Isaacson, T., & Summers, C. (2001). Social behavior of children with language impairment on the playground. A pilot study. *Language, Speech, and Hearing Services in Schools, 32,* 101–113
Galaburda, A. L. (2005). Neurology of learning disabilities: What will the future bring? The answer comes from the successes of the recent past. *Journal of Learning Disabilities, 28,* 107–109.
Gallagher, A., Frith, U., & Snowling, M. J. (2000). Precursors of literacy delay among children at genetic risk of dyslexia. *Journal of Child Psychology and Psychiatry and Allied Disciplines, 41,* 202–213.
Garcia, S. B., Mendez-Perez, A., & Ortiz, A. A. (2000). Mexican American mothers' beliefs about disabilities: Implications for early childhood intervention. *Remedial and Special Education, 21,* 90–100.
Garnett, K. (1986). Telling tales: Narratives and learning disabled children. *Topics in Lamguage Disorders, 6*(2), 44–56.
Gathercole, S. E. (2006). Nonword repetition and word learning: The nature of the relationship. *Applied Psycholinguistics, 27,* 513–543.
Gathercole, S. E., & Alloway, T. (2006). Short-term and working memory impairments in neurodevelopmental disorders: Diagnosis and remedial support. *Journal of Child Psychology and Psychiatry, 47,* 4–15.
Gathercole, S. E., & Alloway, T. P. (2008). Working memory and classroom learning. In S. K. Thurman & C. A. Fiorello (Eds.), *Applied cognitive research in K–3 classrooms* (pp. 17–40). New York: Routledge/Taylor & Francis Group.
Gathercole, S. E., Alloway, T. P., Willis, C., & Adams, A. (2006). Working memory in children with reading disabilities. *Journal of Experimental Child Psychology, 93,* 265–281.
Gathercole, S. E., & Baddeley, A. D. (1993). Phonological working memory: A critical building block for reading development and vocabulary acquisition. *European Journal of Psychology of Education, 8,* 259–272.
Gathercole, S. E., & Baddeley, A. (1996). *The Children's Test of Nonword Repetition.* London: The Psychological Corporation.
Gathercole, S. E., Lamont, E., & Alloway, T. P. (2004). Working memory in the classroom. In S. J. Pickering & G. D. Phye (Eds.), *Working memory and education* (pp. 219–240). Hillsdale, NJ: Erlbaum.
Gaulin, C., & Campbell, T. (1994). Procedure for assessing verbal working memory in normal school-age children: Some preliminary data. *Perceptual and Motor Skills, 79,* 55–64.
Gavens, N., & Barrouillet, P. (2004). Delays of retention, processing efficiency and attentional resources in working memory span development. *Journal of Memory and Language, 51,* 644–657.

Gazelle, J., & Stockman, I. J. (2003). Children's story retelling under different modality and task conditions: Implications for standardizing language sampling procedures. *American Journal of Speech-Language Pathology, 12,* 61–72.

German, D. J. (1992). Word-finding intervention for children and adolescents. *Topics in Language Disorders, 13*(1), 33–50.

German, D. J. (2000). *Test of Word Finding, second edition (TWF-Z).* Austin, TX: Pro-Ed.

German, D. J., & Newman, R. S. (2004). The impact of lexical factors on children's word-finding errors. *Journal of Speech, Language, and Hearing Research, 47,* 624–636.

Ghaziuddin, M., & Mountain-Kimchi, K. (2004). Defining the intellectual profile of Asperger syndrome: Comparison with high-functioning autism. *Journal of Autism and Developmental Disorders, 34,* 279–284.

Gilchrist, A., Green, J., Cox, A., Burton, D., Rutter, M., & Le Couteur, A. (2001). Development and current functioning in adolescents with Asperger syndrome: A comparative study. *Journal of Child Psychology and Psychiatry and Allied Disciplines, 42,* 227–240.

Gill, C., Klecan-Aker, J., Roberts, T., & Fredenburg, K. (2003). Following directions: Rehearsal and visualization strategies for children with specific language impairment. *Child Language Teaching and Therapy, 19,* 85–103.

Gillam, R. B., & Bedore, L. M. (2000). Language science. In R. B. Gillam, T. P. Marquardt, & F. R. Martin (Eds.), *Communication sciences and disorders: From science to clinical practice* (pp. 385–408). San Diego: Singular.

Gillam, R. B., Frome Loeb, D., Hoffman, L. M., Bohman, T., Champlin, C. A., Thibodeau, L., Widen, J., Brandel, J., & Friel-Patti, S. (2008). The efficacy of Fast ForWord language intervention in school-age children with language impairment: A randomized controlled trial. *Journal of Speech, Language, and Hearing Research, 51* , 97–119.

Gillam, R. B., Hoffman, L. M., Marler, J. A., & Wynn-Dancy, M. L. (2002). Sensitivity to increased task demands: Contributions from data-driven and conceptually driven information processing deficits. *Topics in Language Disorders, 22*(3), 30–48.

Gillam, R. B., & Johnston, J. R. (1985). Development of print awareness in language-disordered preschoolers. *Journal of Speech and Hearing Research, 28,* 521–526.

Gillam, R. B., & Pearson, N. A. (2004). *Test of Narrative Language.* Austin, TX: Pro-Ed.

Gillam, R. B., & van Kleek, A. (1996). Phonological awareness training and short-term working memory: Clinical implications. *Topics in Language Disorders, 17,* 72–81.

Gillam, S. L., & Gillam, R. B. (2006). Making evidence-based decisions about child language intervention in schools. *Language, Speech, and Hearing Services in Schools, 37,* 304–315.

Gillon, G. T. (2005). Facilitating phoneme awareness development in 3- and 4-year-old children with speech impairment. *Language, Speech, and Hearing Services in Schools, 36,* 308–324.

Girolametto, L., & Weitzman, E. (2002). Responsiveness of child care providers in interactions with toddlers and preschoolers. *Language, Speech, and Hearing Services in Schools, 33,* 268–281.

Girolametto, L., Weitzman, E., & Greenberg, J. (2003). Training day care staff to facilitate children's language. *American Journal of Speech-Language Pathology, 12,* 299–311.

Girolametto, L., Wiigs, M., Smyth, R., Weitzman, E., & Pearce, P. S. (2001). Children with a history of expressive vocabulary delay: Outcomes at 5 years of age. *American Journal of Speech-Language Pathology, 10,* 358–369.

Glenberg, A. M., Brown, M., & Levin, J. R. (2007). Enhancing comprehension in small reading groups using a manipulation strategy. *Contemporary Educational Psychology, 32,* 389–399.

Glenberg, A. M., Jaworski, B., & Rischal, M. (2005). *Improving reading improves math.* Unpublished manuscript, University of Wisconsin, Madison.

Glennen, S. L., & Masters, M. G. (2002). Typical and atypical language development in infants and toddlers adopted from Eastern Europe. *American Journal of Speech-Language Pathology, 11,* 417–433.

Goffman, L., & Leonard, J. (2000). Growth of language skills in preschool children with specific language impairment. *American Journal of Speech-Language Pathology, 9,* 151–161.

Goldbart, J., & Marshall, J. (2004). "Pushes and pulls" on the parents of children who use AAC. *Augmentative and Alternative Communication, 20,* 194–208.

Goldenberg, C. (2008). Teaching English language learners what the research does—and does not—say. *American Educator, 32*(2), 8–44.

Goldenberg, R. L., Culhane, J. F., Iams, J. D., & Romero, R. (2008). Epidemiology and causes of preterm birth. *Lancet,* 5(371), 75–84.

Goldstein, B. A. (2006). Clinical implications of research on language development and disorders in bilingual children. *Topics in Language Disorders, 26,* 305–321.

Goldstein, H., English, K., Shafer, K., & Kaczmarek, L. (1997). Interaction among preschoolers with and without disabilities: Effects of across-the-day peer intervention. *Journal of Speech, Language, and Hearing Research, 40,* 33–48.

Goldstein, H., & Strain, P. S. (1988). Peers as communication intervention agents: Some new strategies and research findings. *Topics in Language Disorders, 9*(1), 44–59.

Goldstein, H., Walker, D., & Fey, M. (2005, Nov.). *Comparing strategies for promoting communication of infants and toddlers.* Seminar presented at the Association for Speech and Hearing Conference (ASHA), San Diego, CA.

Gorman, B. K., Fiestas, C. E., Peña, E. D., & Reynolds Clark, M. (2011). Creative and stylistic devices employed by children during a storybook narrative task:

A cross-cultural study. *Language, Speech, and Hearing Services in Schools, 42,* 167–181.

Graham, S. (1999). Handwriting and spelling instruction for students with learning disabilities: A review. *Learning Disability Quarterly, 22,* 78–98.

Graham, S., Berninger, V., Abbott, R., Abbott, P., & Whitaker, D. (1997). Role of mechanics in composing of elementary school students: A new methodological approach. *Journal of Educational Psychology, 89,* 170–182.

Graham, S., & Harris, K. R. (1999). Assessment and intervention in overcoming writing difficulties: An illustration from the self-regulation strategy development model. *Language, Speech, and Hearing Services in Schools, 30,* 255–264.

Granlund, M., Bjorck-Åkesson, E., Wilder, J., & Ylven, R. (2008). AAC interventions for children in a family environment: Implementing evidence in practice. *Augmentative and Alternative Communication, 24,* 207–219.

Gray, S. (2003). Word learning by preschoolers with specific language impairment: What predicts success? *Journal of Speech, Language, and Hearing Research, 46,* 56–67.

Gray, S. (2005). Word learning by preschoolers with specific language impairment: Effect of phonological or semantic cues. *Journal of Speech, Language, and Hearing Research, 48,* 1452–1467.

Gray, S., & Brinkley, S. (2011). Fast mapping and word learning by preschoolers with specific language impairment in a supported learning context: Effect of encoding cues, phonotactic probability, and object familiarity. *Journal of Speech, Language, and Hearing Research, 54,* 870–884.

Green, L. (2004, November). *Morphology and literacy: Implications for students with reading disabilities.* Paper presented at the American Speech-Language-Hearing Annual convention, Philadelphia.

Greenhalgh, K. S., & Strong, C. J. (2001). Literate language features in spoken narratives of children with typical language and children with language impairments. *Language, Speech, and Hearing Services in Schools, 32,* 114–126.

Griffin, T. M., Hemphill, L., Camp, L., & Wolf, D. P. (2004). Oral discourse in the preschool years and later literacy skills. *First Language, 24,* 123–147.

Grigorenko, E. L. (2005). A conservative meta-analysis of linkage and linkage-association studies of developmental dyslexia. *Scientific Studies of Reading, 9,* 285–316.

Grisham-Brown, J. L., Hemmeter, M. L., & Pretti-Frontczak, K. L. (2005). *Blended practices for teaching young children in inclusive settings.* Baltimore: Paul H. Brookes.

Griswold, K. E., Barnhill, G. P., Smith-Myles, B., Hagiwara, T., & Simpson, R. L. (2002). Asperger syndrome and academic achievement. *Focus on Autism and Other Developmental Disabilities,* 77(2), 94–102.

Grossman, R. B., Bemis, R. H., Plesa Skwerer, D., & Tager-Flusberg, H. (2010). Lexical and affective prosody in children with high-functioning autism. *Journal of Speech, Language, and Hearing Research, 53,* 778–793.

Gruenewald, L., & Pollack, S. (1984). *Language interaction in teaching and learning.* Baltimore: University Park Press.

Gullo, F., & Gullo, J. (1984). An ecological language intervention approach with mentally retarded adolescents. *Language, Speech, and Hearing Services in Schools, 15,* 182–191.

Guo, L. Y., Tomblin, J. B., & Samelson, V. (2008). Speech disruptions in the narratives of English-speaking children with Specific Language Impairment. *Journal of Speech, Language, and Hearing Research, 51,* 722–738.

Gutierrez-Clellan, V. F., & Peña, E. D. (2001). Dynamic assessment of diverse children: A tutorial. *Language, Speech, and Hearing Services in Schools, 32,* 212–224.

Gutierrez-Clellan, V. F., & Quinn, R. (1993). Assessing narratives of children from diverse cultural-lingual groups. *Language, Speech, and Hearing Services in Schools, 24,* 2–9.

Gutierrez-Clellen, V. F., Restrepo, M. A., Bedore, L., Peña, E., & Anderson, R. (2000). Language sample analysis in Spanish-speaking children: Methodological considerations. *Language, Speech, and Hearing Services in Schools, 31,* 88–98.

Gutierrez-Clellan, V. F., & Simon-Cereijido, G. (2007). The discriminant accuracy of a grammatical measure of Latino English-speaking children. *Journal of Speech, Language, and Hearing Research, 50,* 968–981.

Hadley, P. A., & Holt, J. (2006). Individual differences in the onset of tense marking: A growth curve analysis. *Journal of Speech, Hearing, and Language Research, 49,* 984–1000.

Hadley, P. A., & Short, H. (2005). The onset of tense marking in children at risk for specific language impairment. *Journal of Speech, Language, and Hearing Research, 48,* 1344–1362.

Halpern, R. (2000). Early childhood intervention for low-income children and families. In J. P. Shonkoff & S. J. Meisels (Eds.), *Handbook of early childhood intervention* (2nd ed., pp. 361–386). Cambridge, England: Cambridge University Press.

Hambly, C., & Riddle, L. (2002, April). *Phonological awareness training for school-age children.* Paper presented at the annual convention of the New York State Speech-Language-Hearing Association, Rochester.

Hamm, B., & Mirenda, P. (2006). Post-school quality of life for individuals with developmental disabilities who use AAC. *Augmentative and Alternative Communication, 22,* 134–146.

Hammer, C. S., Lawrence, F. R., & Miccio, A. W. (2007). Bilingual children's language abilities and early reading outcomes in Head Start and kindergarten. *Language, Speech, and Hearing Services in Schools, 38,* 237–248.

Hammer, C. S., & Miccio, A. W. (2006). Early language and reading development of bilingual preschoolers from low-income families. *Topics in Language Disorders, 26,* 322–337.

Hammer, C. S., Miccio, A. W., & Wagstaff, D. A. (2003). Home literacy experiences and their relationship to bilingual preschoolers' developing English literacy abilities: An initial investigation. *Language, Speech, and Hearing Services in Schools, 34,* 20–30.

Hammer, C. S., Rodriguez, B. L., Lawrence, F. R., & Miccio, A. W. (2007). Puerto Rican mothers' beliefs on home literacy practices. *Language, Speech, and Hearing Services in Schools, 38,* 216–224.

Hammett Price, L., Hendricks, S., & Cook, C. (2010). Incorporating computer-aided language sample analysis into clinical practice. *Language, Speech, and Hearing Services in Schools, 41,* 206–222.

Hammill, D. D., Brown, V. L., Larson, S. C., & Wiederholt, J. L. (2007). *Test of Adolescent and Adult Language* (4th ed.). Austin, TX: Pro-Ed.

Hammill, D. D., & Larson, S. (1996). *Test of Written Language–3.* Austin, TX: Pro-Ed.

Hammill, D. D., & Newcomer, P. (2007). *Test of Language Development—Intermediate* (4th ed.). Austin, TX: Pro-Ed.

Hancock, T. B., & Kaiser, A. P. (2006). Enhanced milieu teaching. In R. J. McCauley & M. E. Fey (Eds.), *Treatment of language disorders in children* (pp. 203–236). Baltimore: Paul H. Brookes.

Hanft, B. E., Miller, L. J., & Lane, S. J. (2000). Towards a consensus in terminology in sensory integration theory and practice: Part I. Taxonomy of neurophysiologic processes. *Sensory Integration Special Interest Section Quarterly, 23,* 1–4.

Hanft, B. E., Rush, D. D., & Shelden, M. L. (2004). *Coaching families and colleagues in early childhood.* Baltimore, MD: Paul H. Brookes.

Harris Wright, H., & Newhoff, M. (2001). Narration abilities of children with language-learning disabilities in response to oral and written stimuli. *American Journal of Speech-Language Pathology, 10,* 308–319.

Hart, K. I., Fujiki, M., Brinton, B., & Hart, C. H. (2004). The relationship between social behavior and severity of language impairment. *Journal of Speech, Language, and Hearing Research, 47,* 647–662.

Hartley, S. L., & Sikora, D. M. (2009). Which DSM-IV-TR criteria best differentiate high-functioning autism spectrum disorder from ADHD and anxiety disorders in older children? *Autism, 13,* 485–509.

Hartsuiker, R. J., Bernolet, S., Schoonbaert, S., Speybroeck, S., & Vanderelst, D. (2008). Syntactic priming persists while the lexical boost decays: Evidence from written and spoken dialogue. *Journal of Memory and Language, 58,* 214–238.

Hashimoto, N., McGregor, K. K., & Graham, A. (2007). Conceptual organization at 6 and 8 years of age: Evidence from the semantic priming of object decisions. *Journal of Speech, Language, and Hearing Research, 50,* 161–176.

Hassink, J. M., & Leonard, L. B. (2010). Within-treatment factors as predictors of outcomes following conversational recasting. *American Journal of Speech-Language Pathology,* 19, 213–224.

Hayiou-Thomas, M. E., Harlaar, N., Dale, P. S., & Plomin, R. (2010). Preschool speech, language skills, and reading at 7, 9, and 10 years: Etiology of the relationship. *Journal of Speech, Language, and Hearing Research, 53,* 311–332.

Hayward, D., Gillam, R. B., & Lien, P. (2007). Retelling a script-based story: Do children with and without language impairments focus on script or story element? *Journal of Speech-Language Pathology, 16,* 235–245.

Health Resources and Services Administration (HRSA). (2005). *Women's Health USA 2005.* Rockville, MD: U.S. Department of Health and Human Services.

Hedberg, N. L., & Stoel-Gammon, C. (1986). Narrative analysis: Clinical procedures. *Topics in Language Disorders, 7,* 58–69.

Heilmann, J. J., Miller, J., Iglesias, A., Fabiano-Smith, L., Nockerts, A., & Digney-Andriacchi, K. (2008). Narrative transcription accuracy and reliability in two languages. *Topics in Language Disorders, 28,* 178–188.

Heilmann, J. J., Miller, J. F., & Nockerts, A. (2010). Using language sample databases. *Language, Speech, and Hearing Services in Schools, 41,* 84–95.

Heilmann, J. J., Miller, J. F., Nockerts, A., & Dunaway, C. (2010). Properties of the narrative scoring scheme using narrative retells in young school-age children. *American Journal of Speech-Language Pathology, 19,* 154–166.

Heilmann, J. J., Nockerts, A., & Miller, J. F. (2010). Language sampling: Does the length of the transcript matter? *Language, Speech, and Hearing Services in Schools, 41,* 393–404.

Hemphill, L., Uccelli, P., Winner, K., Chang, C., & Bellinger, D. (2002). Narrative discourse in young children with histories of early corrective heart surgery. *Journal of Speech, Language, and Hearing Research, 45,* 318–331.

Henry, J., Sloane, M., & Black-Pond, C. (2007). Neurobiology and neurodevelopmental impact of childhood traumatic stress and prenatal alcohol exposure. *Language, Speech, and Hearing Services in Schools, 38,* 99–108.

Henry, M. (1990). *Words.* Los Gatos, CA: Lex.

Hernandez, D. J. (2004). *Demographic change and the life circumstances of immigrant families..* Albany: University at Albany, State University of New York Press.

Hickmann, M., & Schneider, P. (2000). Cohesion and coherence anomalies and their effects on children's referent introduction in narrative retell. In M. Perkins & S. Howard (Eds.), *New directions in language development and disorders* (pp. 251–260). New York: Plenum.

Hixson, P. K. (1983). DSS Computer Program [Computer program]. Omaha, NE: Computer Language Analysis.

Hoffman, L. M., & Gillam, R. B. (2004). Verbal and spatial information processing constraints in children with specific language impairment. *Journal of Speech, Language, and Hearing Research, 47,* 114–125.

Hood, J., & Rankin, P. M. (2005). How do specific memory disorders present in the school classroom? *Pediatric Rehabilitation, 8,* 272–282.

Hooper, S. J., Roberts, J. E., Zeisel, S. A., & Poe, M. (2003). Core language predictors of behavioral functioning in early elementary school children: Concurrent and longitudinal findings. *Behavioral Disorders, 29(1),* 10–21.

Horohov, J. E., & Oetting, J. B. (2004). Effects of input manipulations on the word learning abilities of children with and without specific language impairment. *Applied Psycholinguistics, 25,* 43–65.

Horton-Ikard, R., & Weismer, S. E. (2007). A preliminary examination of vocabulary and word learning in African American toddlers from middle and low socioeconomic status homes. *American Journal of Speech-Language Pathology, 16(4),* 381–392.

Horwitz, S. M., Irwin, J. R., Briggs-Gowan, M. J., Heenan, J. M. B., Mendoza, J., & Carter, A. S. (2003). Language delay in a community cohort of young children. *Journal of the American Academy of Child & Adolescent Psychiatry, 42,* 932–940.

Howlin, P., Goode, S., Hurton, J., & Rutter, M. (2004). Adult outcome for children with autism. *Journal of Child Psychology and Psychiatry, 45,* 212–229.

Howlin, P., Mawhood, L., & Rutter, M. (2000). Autism and developmental receptive language disorder—A follow-up comparison in early adult life: Social, behavioral, and psychiatric outcomes. *Journal of Child Psychology and Psychiatry, 41,* 561–578.

Hubbs-Tait, L., Culp, A. M., Huey, E., Culp, R., Starost, H., & Hare, C. (2002). Relation of Head Start attendance to children's cognitive and social outcomes: Moderation by family risk. *Early Childhood Research Quarterly, 17,* 539–558.

Hudson, R., Lane, H., & Mercer, C. (2005). Writing prompts: The role of various priming conditions on the compositional fluency of developing writers. *Reading and Writing: An Interdisciplinary Journal, 18,* 473–495.

Hugdahl, K., Gundersen, H., Brekke, C., Thomsen, T., Rimol, L. M., Ersland, L., & Niemi, J. (2004). fMRI brain activation in a Finnish family with specific language impairment compared with a normal control group. *Journal of Speech, Language, and Hearing Research, 47,* 162–172.

Hughes, D., Fey, M., & Long, S. (1992). Developmental sentence scoring: Still useful after all these years. *Topics in Language Disorders, 12(2),* 1–12.

Humphries, T., Cardy, J. O., Worling, D. E., & Peets, K. (2004). Narrative comprehension and retelling abilities of children with nonverbal learning disabilities. *Brain and Cognition, 56,* 77–88.

Hustad, K. C., Morehouse, T. B., & Gutmann, M. (2002). AAC strategies for enhancing the usefulness of natural speech in children with severe intelligibility challenges. In J. Reichle, D. Beukelman, & J. Light (Eds.), *Implementing an augmentative communication system: Exemplary strategies for beginning communicators* (pp. 433–452). Baltimore:. Paul H. Brookes.

Hutson-Nechkash, P. (1990). *Storybuilding: A guide to structuring oral narratives.* Eau Claire, WI: Thinking Publications.

Hutson-Nechkash, P. (2001). *Narrative tool box: Blueprints for storytelling.* Eau Claire, WI: Thinking Publications.

Hwa-Froelich, D. A., & Westby, C. E. (2003). Frameworks of education: Perspectives of Southeast Asian parents and Head Start staff. *Language, Speech, and Hearing Services in Schools, 34,* 299–319.

Hyter, Y. D., Atchinson, B., & Blashill, M. (2006). *A model of supporting children at risk: The School Intervention Program (SIP).* Unpublished manuscript.

Individuals with Disabilities Education Improvement Act of 2004, P. L. 108–446, 118 Stat. 2647 (2004).

Inglebret, E., Jones, C., & Pavel, D. M. (2008). Integrating American Indian/Alaska Native culture into shared storybook intervention. *Language, Speech, and Hearing Services in Schools, 39,* 521–527.

lrwin, J., Carter, A., & Briggs-Gowan, M. (2002). The social-emotional development of latetalking toddlers. *Journal of the American Academy of Child & Adolescent Psychiatry, 41,* 1324–1332.

Isaacs, G. J. (1996). Persistence of non-standard dialect in school-age children. *Journal of Speech and Hearing Research, 39,* 434–441.

Isaki, E., Spauiding, T. J., & Plante, E. (2008). Contributions of language and memory demands to verbal memory performance in language-learning disabilities. *Journal of Communication Disorders, 41,* 512–530.

Iverson, J. M., & Braddock, B. A. (2011). Gesture and motor skill in relation to language in children with language impairment. *Journal of Speech, Language, and Hearing Research, 54,* 72–86.

Ivy, LJ., & Masterson, J. J. (2011). A comparison of oral and written English styles in African American students at different stages of writing development. *Language, Speech, and Hearing Services in Schools, 42,* 31–40.

Jackson, S., Pretti-Frontczak, K., Harjusola-Webb, S., Grisham-Brown, J., & Romani, J. M. (2009). Response to Intervention: Implications for early childhood .professionals. *Language, Speech, and Hearing Services in Schools,* 40, 424–434.

Jackson, S. C., & Roberts, J. E. (2001). Complex syntax production of African American preschoolers. *Journal of Speech, Language, and Hearing Research, 44,* 1083–1096.

Jacobson, P. F., & Schwartz, R. G. (2005). English past tense use in bilingual children with language impairment. *American Journal of Speech-Language Pathology, 14,* 313–323.

Jacobson, S., & Jacobson, J. (2000). Teratogenic insult and neurobehavioral function in infancy and childhood. In C. Nelson (Ed.), *Minnesota Symposia on Child Psychology* (pp. 61–112). Hillsdale, NJ: Erlbaum.

Jacoby, G. P., Lee, L., & Kummer, A. W. (2002). The number of individual treatment units necessary to facilitate functional communication improvements in the speech and language of young children. *American Journal of Speech-Language Pathology, 11,* 370–380.

Janes, H., & Kermani, H. (2001). Caregivers' story reading to young children in family literacy programs: Pleasure or punishment? *Journal of Adolescent & Adult Literacy, 44,* 458–466.

Jankovic, J. (2001). Tourette's syndrome. *The New England Journal of Medicine, 345,* 1184–1192.

Jarrold, C., Baddeley, A. D., & Phillips, C. E. (2002). Verbal short-term memory in Down syndrome: A problem of memory, audition, or speech? *Journal of Speech, Language, and Hearing Research, 45,* 531–544.

Jaycox, L. H., Zoellner, L., & Foa, E. B. (2002). Cognitive-behavior therapy for PTSD in rape survivors. *Journal of Clinical Psychology, 58,* 891–906.

Jerome, A. C., Fujiki, M., Brinton, B., & James, S. L. (2002). Self-esteem in children with specific language impairment. *Journal of Speech, Language, and Hearing Research, 45,* 700–714.

Johnson, D. E. (2000). Medical and developmental sequelae of early childhood institutionalization in Eastern European adoptees. In C. A. Nelson (Ed.), *The Minnesota Symposia on Child Psychology: The effects of early adversity on neurobiological development, 31,* (pp. 113-162). Mahwah, NJ: Erlbaum.

Johnston, J. R., & Kamhi, A. (1984). The same can be less: Syntactic and semantic aspects of the utterances of language impaired children. *Merrill-Palmer Quarterly, 30,* 65–86.

Johnston, J. R., & Wong, M. Y. A. (2002). Cultural differences in beliefs and practices concerning talk to children. *Journal of Speech, Language, and Hearing Research, 45,* 916–926.

Johnston, S. S., Reichle, J., & Evans, J. (2004). Supporting augmentative and alternative communication use by beginning communicators with severe disabilities. *American Journal of Speech Language Pathology, 13,* 20–30.

Jones Moyle, M., Ellis Weismer, S., Evans, J. L., & Lindstrom, M. J. (2007). Longitudinal relationships between lexical and grammatical development in typical and late-talking children. *Journal of Speech, Language, and Hearing Research, 50,* 508–528.

Juel, C. (1988). Learning to read and write: A longitudinal study of 54 children from first through fourth grades. *Journal of Educational Psychology, 80,* 437–447.

Justice, L. M. (2006). Evidence-based practice, response to intervention, and the prevention of reading difficulties. *Language, Speech, and Hearing Services in Schools, 37,* 284–297.

Justice, L. M., Bowles, R. P., Kaderavek, J. N., Ukrainetz, T. A., Eisenberg, S. L., & Gillam, R. B. (2006). The index of narrative microstructure: A clinical tool for analyzing school-age children's narrative performances. *American Journal of Speech-Language Pathology, 15,* 177–191.

Justice, L. M., Chow, S., Capellini, C., Flanigan, K., & Colton, S. (2003). Emergent literacy intervention for vulnerable preschoolers: Relative effects of two approaches. *American Journal of Speech-Language Pathology, 12,* 320–332.

Justice, L. M., & Ezell, H. K. (2000). Enhancing children's print and word awareness through home-based parent intervention. *American Journal of Speech-Language Pathology, 9,* 257–269.

Justice, L. M., & Ezell, H. K. (2002). Use of storybook reading to increase print awareness in at-risk children. *American Journal of Speech-Language Pathology, 11,* 17–29.

Justice, L. M., & Ezell, H. K. (2004). Print referencing: An emergent literacy enhancement strategy and its clinical applications. *Language, Speech, and Hearing Services in Schools, 35,* 185–193.

Justice, L. M., Invernizzi, M. A., & Meier, J. D. (2002). Designing and implementing an early literacy screening protocol: Suggestions for the speech-language pathologist. *Language, Speech, and Hearing Services in Schools, 33,* 84–101.

Justice, L. M., & Kaderavek, J. (2004). Embedded-explicit emergent literacy intervention I: Background and description of approach. *Language, Speech, and Hearing Services in Schools, 35,* 201–211.

Justice, L. M., Mashburn, A., Hamre, B., & Pianta, R. C. (2008). Quality of language instruction in preschool classrooms serving at-risk pupils. *Early Childhood Research Quarterly, 23,* 51–68.

Justice, L. M., Mashburn, A., Pence, K. L., & Wiggins, A. (2008). Experimental evaluation of a preschool language curriculum: Influence on children's expressive language skills. *Journal of Speech, Language, and Hearing Research, 51,* 983–1001.

Justice, L. M., McGinty, A. S., Beckman, A. R., & Kilday, C. R. (2006). *Read It Again! Language and literacy supplement for preschool programs.* Charlottesville, VA: Preschool Language and Literacy Lab, Center for Advanced Study of Teaching and Learning, University of Virginia.

Justice, L. M., McGinty, A. S., Cabell, S. Q., Kilday, C. R., Knighton, K., & Huffman, G. (2010). Literacy curriculum supplement for preschoolers who are academically at risk: A feasibility study. *Language, Speech, and Hearing Services in Schools, 41,* 161–178.

Justice, L. M., Meier, J., & Walpole, S. (2005). Learning new words from storybooks: An efficacy study with at-risk kindergartners. *Language, Speech, and Hearing Services in, Schools, 36, 17–33* .

Justice, L. M., & Schuele, C. M. (2004). Phonological awareness: Description, assessment, and intervention. In J. Bernthal & N. Bankson (Eds.), *Articulation and phonological disorders* (5th ed., pp. 376–405). Boston: Allyn & Bacon.

Justice, L. M., Skibbe, L. E., McGinty, A. S., Piasta, S. B., & Petrill, S. (2011). Feasibility, efficacy, and social validity of home-based storybook reading itervention for children with language impairment. *Journal of Speech, Language, and Hearing Research, 54,* 523–538.

Kaderavek, J. N., & Sulzby, E. (1998, November). *Low versus high orientation towards literacy in children.* Paper presented at the annual convention of the American Speech-Language-Hearing Association, San Antonio, TX.

Kaderavek, J. N., & Sulzby, E. (2000). Narrative production by children with and without specific language impairment: Oral narratives and emergent readings. *Journal of Speech, Language, and Hearing Research, 43,* 34–49.

Kaiser, A. P., Hancock, T., & Neitfield, J. P. (2000). The effects of parent-implemented enhanced milieu teaching on social communication of children who have autism [Special issue]. *Journal of Early Education and Development, 4,* 423–446.

Kame'enui, E. J., Simmons, D. C., & Coyne, M. D. (2000). Schools as host environments: Towards a schoolwide reading improvement model. *Annals of dyslexia, 50,* 33–51.

Kamhi, A. G., & Hinton, L. N. (2000). Explaining individual differences in spelling ability. *Topics in Language Disorders, 20*(3), 37.

Kamhi, A. G., & Johnston, J. (1992). Semantic assessment: Determining propositional complexity. *Best Practices in School Speech-Language Pathology, 2,* 99–107.

Kapantzoglou, M., Restrepo, M. A., & Thompson, M. S. (2012). Dynamic assessment of word learning skills: Identifying language impairment in bilingual children. *Language, Speech, and Hearing Services in Schools, 43,* 81–96.

Kapp, S. A., McDonald, T. P., & Diamond, K. L. (2001). The path to adoption for children of color. *Child Abuse and Neglect, 21,* 215–229.

Kashinath, S., Woods, J., & Goldstein, H. (2006). Enhancing generalized teaching strategy use in daily routines by parents of children with autism. *Journal of Speech, Language, and Hearing Research, 49,* 466–485.

Katzir, T., Kim, Y., Wolf, M., O'Brien, B., Kennedy, B., Lovett, M., & Morris, R. (2006). Reading fluency: The whole is more than the parts. *Annals of Dyslexia, 56,* 51–82.

Kay-Raining Bird, E., Cleave, P. L., White, D., Pike, H., & Helmkay, A. (2008). Written and oral narratives of children and adolescents with Down syndrome. *Journal of Speech, Language, and Hearing Research, 51,* 436–450.

Kemp, N., Lieven, E., & Tomasello, M. (2005). Young children's knowledge of the "determiner" and "adjective" categories. *Journal of Speech, Language, and Hearing Research, 48,* 592–609.

Kemper, A. R., & Downs, S. M. (2000, May). A cost-effectiveness analysis of newborn hearing screening strategies. *Archives of Pediatric and Adolescent Medicine, 154*(5), 484–488.

Kent-Walsh, J., & Light, J. (2003). *Communication partner training in AAC: A literature review.* Paper presented at the Pennsylvania Speech-Language-Hearing Association annual convention, Harrisburg, PA.

Ketelaars, M. P., Alphonsus Hermans, T. S. L., Cuperus, J., Jansonius, K., & Verhoeven, L. (2011). Semantic abilities in children with pragmatic language impairment: The case of picture naming skills. *Journal of Speech, Language, and Hearing Research, 54,* 87–98.

Kibby, M., Marks, W., Morgan, S., & Long, C. (2004). Specific impairment in developmental reading disabilities: A working memory approach. *Journal of Learning Disabilities, 37,* 349–363.

Kirk, C., & & Gillon, G. T. (2007). Longitudinal effects of phonological awareness intervention on morphological awareness in children with speech impairment. *Language, Speech and Hearing Services in Schools, 38,* 342–352.

Kirk, C., & Gillon, G. T. (2009). Integrated morphological awareness intervention as a tool for improving literacy *Language Speech, and Hearing Services in Schools, 40,* 341–351.

Kjelgaard, M. M., & Tager-Flusberg, H. (2001). An investigation of language impairment in autism: Implications for genetic subgroups. *Language and Cognitive Processes, 16,* 287–308.

Klee, T. (1992). Developmental and diagnostic characteristics of quantitative measures of children's language production. *Topics in Language Disorders, 12*(2), 28–41.

Klee, T., Carson, D. K., Gavin, W. J., Hall, L., Kent, A., & Reece, S. (1998). Concurrent and predictive validity of an early language screening program. *Journal of Speech, Language, and Hearing Research, 41,* 627–641.

Klee, T., Schaffer, M., Mays, S., Membrino, I., & Mougey, K. (1989). A comparison of the age-MLU relationship in normal and specifically language impaired preschool children. *Journal of Speech and Hearing Disorders, 54,* 226–233.

Klein, H. B., Moses, N., & Jean-Baptiste, R. (2010). Influence of context on the production of complex sentences by typically developing children. *Language, Speech, and Hearing Services in Schools, 41,* 289–302.

Kline, A., & Volkmar, F. R. (2000). Treatment and intervention guidelines for individuals with Asperger's syndrome. In A. Kline, F. R. Volkmar, & S. S. Sparrow (Eds.), *Asperger's syndrome* (pp. 340–366). New York: Guilford.

Klingberg, T., Fernell, W., Oelson, P., Johnson, M., Gustafsson, P., Dahltrom, K., & ... Westerberg, H. (2005). Computerized training of working memory in children with. ADHD: A randomized, controlled trial. *Journal of the American Academy of Child and Adolescent Psychiatry, 44,* 177–186.

Klingner, J. K., Vaughn, S., & Boardman, A. (2007). *Teaching reading comprehension to students with learning difficulties.* New York: Guilford.

Knoche, L., Peterson, C. A., Edwards, C. P., & Jeon, H. (2006). Child care for children with and without disabilities:

The provider, observer, and parent perspectives. *Early Childhood Research Quarterly, 21,* 93–109.

Kohnert, K. J. (2008). *Language disorders in bilingual children and adults.* San Diego, CA: Plural.

Kohnert, K. J., & Bates, E. (2002). Balancing bilinguals II: Lexical comprehension and cognitive processing in children learning Spanish and English. *Journal of Speech, Language, and Hearing Research, 45,* 347–359.

Kohnert, K., Kennedy, M. R. T., Glaze, L., Kan, P. F., & Carney, E. (2003). Breadth and depth of diversity in Minnesota: Challenges to clinical competency. *American Journal of Speech-Language Pathology, 12,* 259–272. doi: 10.1044/1058-0360(2003/072).

Kohnert, K. J., Yim, D., Nett, K., Kan, P. F., & Duran, L. (2005). Intervention with linguistically diverse preschool children: A focus on developing home languages. *Language, Speech, and Hearing Services in Schools, 36,* 251–263.

Konopka, A., & Bock, K. (2005, March). *Helping syntax out: How, much do words do?* Paper presented at the CUNY Conference on Human Sentence Processing, Tucson, AZ.

Koppenhaver, D., & Erickson, K. (2003). Natural emergent literacy supports for preschoolers with autism and severe communication impairments. *Topics in Language Disorders, 23(4),* 283–292.

Koramoa, J., Lynch, M. A., & Kinnair, D. (2002). A continuum of childrearing: Responding to traditional practices. *Child Abuse Review, 11,* 415–421.

Kouri, T. A. (2005). Lexical training through modeling and elicitation procedures with late talkers who have specific language impairment and developmental delays. *Journal of Speech, Language, and Hearing Research, 48,* 157–171.

Kouri, T. A., Selle, C. A., & Riley, S. A. (2006). Comparison of meaning and graphophonemic feedback strategies for guided reading instruction of children with language delays. *American Journal of Speech-Language Pathology, 15,* 236–246.

Kovarsky, D., & Duchan, J. (1997). The interactional dimensions of language therapy. *Language, Speech, and Hearing Services in Schools, 28,* 297–307.

Krantz, L. R., & Leonard, L. B. (2007). The effect of temporal adverbials on past tense production by children with specific language impairment. *Journal of Speech, Language, and Hearing Research, 50,* 137–148.

Krashen, S., & Brown, C. L. (2005). The ameliorating effects of high socioeconomic status: A secondary analysis. *Bilingual Research Journal, 29,* 185–196.

Kristensen, H. (2000). Selective mutism and comorbidity wih developmental disorder/delay, anxiety disorder, and elimination disorder. *Journal of the American Academy of Child and Adolescent Psychiatry, 39,* 249–256.

Kummerer, S. E., Lopez-Reyna, N. A., & Hughes, M. T. (2007). Mexican immigrant mothers' perceptions of their children's communication disabilities, emergent literacy development, and speech-language therapy program. *American Journal of Speech-Language Pathology, 16,* 271–282.

Lahey, M. (1988). *Language disorders and language development.* New York: Macmillan.

Laing Gillam, S., Fargo, J. D., & St. Clair Robertson, K. (2009). Comprehension of expository text: Insights gained from think-aloud data. *American Journal of Speech-Language Pathology, 18,* 82–94.

Landa, R. (2000). Social language use in Asperger syndrome and high-functioning autism. In A.Klin, F. Volkmar, & S. Sparrow (Eds.), *Asperger syndrome* (pp. 125-158). New York: Guilford Press.

Lane, S. J. (2002). Sensory modulation. In A. Bundy, S. Lane, & E. Murray (Eds.), *Sensory integration: Theory and practice* (pp. 101–122). Philadelphia: F. A. Davis.

Langdon, H. W., & Cheng, L. L. (2002). *Collaborating with interpreters and translators: A guide for communication disorders professionals.* Eau Claire, WI: Thinking Publications.

La Paro, K. M., Justice, L., Skibbe, L. E., & Planta, R. C. (2004). Relations among maternal, child, and demographic factors and the persistence of preschool language impairment. *American Journal of Speech-Language Pathology, 13,* 291–303.

Larroque, B., Ancel, P. Y., Marret, S., Marchand, L., Andre, M., Arnaud, C., Pierrat, V., Roze, J. C., Messer, J., Thiriez, G., Burguet, A., Picaud, J. C., Breart, G., & Kaminski, M. (2008). Neurodevelopmental disabilities and special care of 5-year-old children born before 33 weeks of gestation (the EPIPAGE study): A longitudinal cohort study. *Lancet,* 371(9615), 813–820.

Larson, S., & Hammill, D. (1994). *Test of Written Spelling–3.* Austin, TX: Pro-Ed.

Larson, V. L., & McKinley, N. L. (1987). *Communication assessment and intervention strategies for adolescents.* Eau Claire, WI: Thinking Publications.

Larson, V. L., & McKinley, N. L. (2003). *Communication solutions for older students: Assessment and intervention.* Eau Claire, WI: Thinking Publications.

Law, J. (2004). The implications of different approaches to evaluating intervention: Evidence from the study of language delay/disorders. *Folia phoniatrica et logopaedica,* 56, 199–219.

Law, J., Garrett, Z., & Nye, C. (2004). The efficacy of treatment for children with developmental speech and language delay/disorder. A meta-analysis. *Journal of Speech, Language, and Hearing Research, 47,* 924–943.

Law, J., Rush, R., Schoon, I., & Parsons, S. (2009). Modeling developmental language difficulties from school entry into adulthood: Literacy, mental health, and employment outcomes. *Journal of Speech, Language, and Hearing Research, 52,* 1401–1416.

Lee, L. (1974). *Developmental sentence analysis.* Evanston, IL: Northwestern University Press.

Lehto, J., Juujarvi, P., Kooistra, L., & Pulkkinen, L. (2003). Dimensions of executive functioning: Evidence from children. *British Journal of Developmental Psychology, 21,* 59–80.

Leonard, L. B. (2009). Is expressive language disorder an accurate diagnostic category? *American Journal of Speech-Language Pathology, 18,* 115–123.

Leonard, L. B. (2011). The primacy of priming in grammatical learning and intervention: A tutorial. *Journal of Speech, Language, and Hearing Research, 54,* 608–621.

Leonard, L. B., Camarata, S. M., Brown, B., & Camarata, M. N. (2004). Tense and agreement in the speech of children with specific language impairment: Patterns of generalization through intervention. *Journal of Speech, Language, and Hearing Research, 47,* 1363–1379.

Leonard, L. B., Camarata, S. M., Pawlowska, M., Brown, B., & Camarata, M. N. (2006). Tense and agreement morphemes in the speech of children with specific language impairment during intervention: Phase 2. *Journal of Speech, Language, and Hearing Research, 49,* 749–770.

Leonard, L. B., Deevy, P., Kurtz, R., Krantz Chorev, L., Owen, A., Polite, E., Elam, D., & Finneran, D. (2007). Lexical aspect and the use of verb morphology by children with specific language impairment. *Journal of Speech, Language, and Hearing Research, 50,* 759–777.

Leonard, L. B., Ellis Weismer, S., Miller, C., Francis, D., Tomblin, J. B., & Kail, R. (2007). Speed of processing, working memory, and language impairment in children. *Journal of Speech, Language, and Hearing Research, 50,* 408–428.

Leonard, M. A., Milich, R., & Lorch, E. P. (2011). Pragmatic language use in mediating the relation between hyperactivity and inattention and social skills poblems. *Journal of Speech, Language, and Hearing Research, 54* , 567–579.

Leonard, L. B., Miller, C. A., Deevy, P., Rauf, L., Gerber, E., & Charest, M. (2002). Production operations and the use of nonfinite verbs by children with specific language impairment. *Journal of Speech, Language, and Hearing Research, 45,* 744–758.

Leonard, L. B., Miller, C. A., Grela, B., Holland, A. L., Gerber, E., & Petucci, M. (2000). Production operations contribute to the grammatical morpheme limitations of children with specific language impairment. *Journal of Memory and Language, 43,* 362–378.

Leslie, L., & Caldwell, J. (2000). *Qualitative Reading Inventory-III.* New York: Longman.

Lewis, B. A., Freebairn, L., & Taylor, H. G. (2000). Follow-up of children with early expressive phonology disorders. *Journal of Learning Disabilities, 25,* 586–597.

Lewis, B. A., Freebairn, L., & Taylor, H. G. (2002). Correlates of spelling abilities in children with early speech sound disorders. *Reading and Writing: An Interdisciplinary Journal, 15,* 389–407.

Lidz, C. S., & Peña, E. D. (1996). Dynamic assessment: The model, its relevance as a nonbiased approach, and its application to Latino American preschool children. *Language, Speech, and Hearing Services in Schools, 27,* 367–372.

Light, J. C., & Drager, K. D. (2002). Improving the design of augmentative and alternative technologies for young children. *Assistive Technology, 14,* 17–32.

Light, J. C., & Drager, K. D. (2005). *Maximizing language development with young children who require AAC.* Paper presented at the annual convention of the American Speech-Language-Hearing Association, San Diego.

Light, J. C., & Drager, K. D. (2007). AAC technologies for young children with complex communication needs: State of the science and future research directions. *Augmentative and Alternative Communication, 23,* 204–216.

Light, J. C., Drager, K., & Nemser, J. (2004). Enhancing the appeal of AAC technologies for young children: Lessons from the toy manufacturers. *Augmentative and Alternative Communication, 20,* 137–149.

Light, J., Page, R., Curran, J., & Pitkin, L. (2007). Children's ideas for the design of AAC assistive technologies for young children with complex communication needs . *Augmentative and Alternative Communication,* 23, 274–287.

Light, J. C., Parsons, A., & Drager, K. D. (2002). "There's more to life than cookies": Developing interactions for social closeness with beginning communicators who use AAC. In J. Reichle, D. Beukelman, & J. Light (Eds.), *Exemplary practices for beginning communicators: Implications for AAC* (pp. 187–218). Baltimore: Paul H. Brookes.

Liiva, C. A., & Cleave, P. L. (2005). Roles of initiation and responsiveness in access and participation for children with specific language impairment. *Journal of Speech, Language, and Hearing Research, 48,* 868–883.

Lindamood, C., & Lindamood, R. (2004). *Lindamood Auditory Conceptualization Test* (3rd ed.). Austin, TX: Pro-Ed.

Linderholm, T., Everson, M. G., van den Broek, P., Mischinski, M., Crittenden, A., & Samuels, J. (2000). Effects of causal text revisions on more and less skilled readers: Comprehension of easy and difficult text. *Cognition and Instruction, 18,* 525–556.

Lindsey, D. (2003). *The welfare of children* (2nd ed.). New York: Oxford University Press.

Liss, M., Harel, B., Fein, D., Allen, D., Dunn, M., Feinstein, C., et al. (2001). Predictors and correlates of adaptive functioning in children with developmental disorders. *Journal of Autism and Developmental Disorders, 31,* 219–230.

Lively, M. (1984). Developmental sentence scoring: Common scoring errors. *Language, Speech, and Hearing Services in Schools, 15,* 154–168.

Lohmann, H., & Tomasello, M. (2003). The role of language in the development of false belief understanding: A training study. *Child Development, 74,* 1130–1144.

Lomax, R. G., & McGee, L. M. (1987). Young children's concepts about print and reading: Toward a model of word acquisition. *Reading Research Quarterly, 22,* 237–256.

Long, S. H. (2001). About time: A comparison of computerized and manual procedures for grammatical and phonological analysis. *Clinical Linguistics & Phonetics, 15*(5), 399–426.

Long, S. H., & Channell, R. W. (2001). Accuracy of four language analysis procedures performed automatically. *American Journal of Speech-Language Pathology, 10,* 180–188.

Long, S. H., & Fey, M. E. (1988). Computerized Profiling Version 6.1 (Apple II series) [Computer program]. Ithaca, NY: Ithaca College.

Long, S. H., & Fey, M. E. (1989). Computerized Profiling Version 6.2 (Macintosh and MS-DOS series) [Computer program]. Ithaca, NY: Ithaca College.

Long, S. H., Fey, M. E., & Channell, R. W. (1998). Computerized Profiling (Version 9.0 MSDOS) [Computer software], Cleveland, OH., Case Western Reserve University.

Long, S. H., Fey, M. E., & Channell, R. W. (2000). Computerized Profiling (Version 9.2.7, MS-DOS) [Computer software]. Cleveland, OH: Department of Communication Sciences, Case Western Reserve University.

Lonigan, C. J., Burgess, S. R., Anthony, J. S., & Barker, T. A. (1998). Development of phonological sensitivity in 2- to 5-year-old children. *Journal of Educational Psychology, 90,* 294–311.

Loomes, C., Rasmussen, C., Pei, J., Manji, S., & Andrew, G. (2008). The effect of rehearsal training on working memory span of children with fetal alcohol spectrum disorder. *Research in Developmental Disabilities, 29,* 113–124.

Loosli, S., Buschkuehl, M., Perrig, W., & Jaeggi, S. (2008, July). *Working memory training enhances reading in 9-11 year old healthy children.* Poster presented at the Jean Piaget Archives 18th Advanced Course, Geneva, Switzerland.

Lord, C., Risi, S., & Pickles, A. (2004). Trajectory of language development in autistic spectrum disorders. In M. L. Rice & S. F. Warren (Eds.), *Developmental language disorders: From phenotypes to etiologies* (pp. 1–38). Mahwah, NJ: Erlbaum.

Losh, M., & Capps, L. (2003). Narrative ability in high-functioning children with autism or Asperger's syndrome. *Journal of Autism and Developmental Disorders, 33,* 239–251.

Lowe, E., Slater, A., Wefley, J., & Hardie, D.(2002). *A status report on hunger and homelessness in America's cities 2002: A 25-city survey.* Washington, DC: U.S. Conference of Mayors.

Luckasson, R., Borthwick-Duffy, S., Buntinx, W. H., Coulter, D. L., Craig, E. M., Reeve, A., Schalock, R. L., Snell, M. E., Spitalnik, D. M., Spreat, S., & Tasse, M. J. (2002). *Mental retardation: Definition, classification, and systems of supports, 10th Edition.* Washington, DC: American Association on Mental Retardation.

Lugo-Neris, M. J., Wood Jackson, C., & Goldstein, H. (2010). Facilitating vocabulary acquisition of young English language learners. *Language, Speech, and Hearing Services in Schools, 41,* 314–327.

Lund, N. J., & Duchan, J. F. (1993). *Assessing children's language in naturalistic contexts.* Englewood Cliffs, NJ: Prentice-Hall.

Lund, S., & Light, J. (2006). Long term outcomes for individuals who use augmentative and alternative communication: Part I—What is a good outcome? *Augmentative and Alternative Communication, 22,* 284–299.

Lynch, E. W., & Hanson, M. J. (Eds.) (2004). *Developing cross-cultural competence: A guide for working with young children and their families.* (3rd ed.) Baltimore: Paul H. Brookes.

Lyon, G. R., Shaywitz, S. E., & Shaywitz, B. A. (2003). A definition of dyslexia. *Annals of Dyslexia,* 53, 1–14.

Lyytinen, P., Poikkeus, A., Laakso, M., Eklund, K., & Lyytinen, H. (2001). Language development and symbolic play in children with and without familial risk of dyslexia. *Journal of Speech, Language, and Hearing Research, 44,* 873–885.

MacArthur, C. A. (1999). Word processing with speech synthesis and word prediction: Effects on the dialogue journal writing of students with learning disabilities. *Learning Disability Quarterly, 21,* 1–16.

MacArthur, C. A. (2000). New tools for writing: Assistive technology for students with writing difficulties. *Topics in Language Disorders, 20*(4), 85–104.

MacArthur, C. A., Graham, S., Haynes, J. A., & DeLaPaz, S. (1996). Spelling checkers and students with learning disabilities: Performance comparisons and impact on spelling. *Journal of Special Education, 30,* 35–57.

Mackie, C., & Dockrell, J. (2004). The nature of written language deficits in children with SLI. *Journal of Speech, Language, and Hearing Research, 47,* 1469–1483.

Maclean, M., Bryant, P., & Bradley, L. (1987). Rhymes, nursery rhymes, and reading in early childhood. *Merrill-Palmer Quarterly, 33,* 255–282.

MacWhinney, B. (2000a). *The CHILDES project: Tools for analyzing talk* (3rd ed.). Mahwah, NJ: Erlbaum.

MacWhinney, B. (2000b). CLAN [Computer software]. Pittsburgh, PA: Carnegie Mellon University.

Magill, J. (1986). *The nature of social deficits of children with autism.* Unpublished doctoral dissertation, University of Alberta, Edmonton.

Mainela-Arnold, E., & Evans, J. (2005). Beyond capacity limitations: Determinants of wordrecall performance on verbal working memory span tasks in children with SLI. *Journal of Speech, Language, and Hearing Research, 48,* 897–909.

Mainela-Arnold, E., Evans, J. J., & Alibali, M. W. (2006). Understanding conservation delays in children with specific language impairment: Task representations revealed in speech and gesture. *Journal of Speech, Language, and Hearing Research, 49,* 1267–1279.

Mainela-Arnold, E., Evans, J. L., & Coady, J. A. (2008). Lexical representations in children with SLI: Evidence from a frequency-manipulated gating task. *Journal of speech, Language, and Hearing Research, 51,* 381–393.

Mainela-Arnold, E., Evans, J. L., & Coady, LA. (2010). Explaining lexical-semantic deficits in Specific Language Impairment: The role of phonological similarity, phonological working memory, and lexical competition. *Journal of Speech, Language, and Hearing Research, 53,* 1742–1756.

Manhardt, J., & Rescorla, L. (2002). Oral narrative skills of late talkers at ages 8 and 9. *Applied Psycholinguistics, 23,* 1–21.

Mann, V., & Singson, M. (2003). Linking morphological knowledge to English decoding ability: Large effects of little suffixes. In E. Assink & D. Sandra (Eds.), *Reading complex words: Cross-language studies* (pp. 1–25). Dordrecht, the Netherlands: Kulwer.

Manning Kratcoski, A. (1998). Guidelines for using portfolios in assessment and evaluation. *Language, Speech, and Hearing Services in Schools, 29,* 3–10.

March of Dimes. (2007). Premature birth. Updated February 2007. Accessed Sept 15, 2008, from www.marchofdimes.com/prematurity/21326_115 7. asp

Maridaki-Kassotaki, K. (2002). The relation between phonological memory skills and reading ability in Greek-speaking children: Can training of phonological memory contribute to reading development? *European Journal of Psychology of Education, 1 7,* 63–73.

Markowitz, J., Carlson, E., Frey, W., Riley, J., Shimshak, A., Heinzen, H., et al. (2006). *Preschoolers' characteristics, services, and results: Wave 1 overview report from the Pre-Elementary Education Longitudinal Study (PEELS).* Available from www.peels.org

Marsh, H. W., Cairns, L., Relich, J., Barnes, J., & Debus, R. L. (1984). The relationship between dimensions of self-attribution and dimensions of self-concept. *Journal of Educational Psychology, 76,* 3–32.

Martin, J. A. et al. (2006, September 29). Births: Final data for 2004. *National Vital Statistics Reports, 55*(1).

Marton, K., Kelmenson, L., & Pinkhasova, M. (2007). Inhibition control and working memory capacity in children with SLI. *Psychologia, 50,* 110–121.

Marton, K., & Schwartz, R. G. (2002). Working memory capacity and language processes in children with specific language impairment. *Journal of Speech, Language, and Hearing Research, 45,* 1138–1153.

Massachusetts Department of Education. (2006). *Massachusetts Comprehensive Assessment System.* Retrieved July 23, 2007, from the Massachusetts Department of Education Web site: www.doe.mass.edu/mcas

Masterson, J. J., & Apel, K. (2000). Spelling assessment: Charting a path to optimal intervention. *Topics in Language Disorders, 20*(3), 50–65.

Masterson, J. J., Apel, K., & Wasowicz, J. (2006). SPELL-2: *Spelling Performance Evaluation for Language & Literacy.* Evanston, IL: Learning By Design.

Masterson, J. J., & Crede, L. A. (1999). Learning to spell: Implications for assessment and intervention. *Language, Speech, and Hearing Services in Schools, 30,* 243–354.

Masterson, J. J., & Perrey, C. D. (1999). Training analogical reasoning skills in children with language disorders. *American Journal of Speech-Language Pathology, 8,* 53–61.

Mattes, L. J. (1995). *Spanish Language Assessment Procedures: A Communication Skills Inventory* (3rd ed.). Oceanside, CA: Academic Communication Associates.

Mawhood, L., Howlin, P., & Rutter, M. (2000). Autism and developmental receptive language disorder—A comparative follow-up in early adult life. I: Cognitive and language outcomes. *Journal of Child Psychology and Psychiatry and Allied Disciplines, 41,* 547–559.

Mayer, M. (1969). *Frog, where are you?* New York: Dial Books.

Mayer, M., & Mayer, M. (1975). *One frog too many.* New York: Penguin Putnam.

McCabe, A., & Bliss, L. S. (2004–2005). Narratives from Spanish-speaking children with impaired and typical language development. *Imagination, Cognition and Personality, 24,* 331–346.

McCabe, A., Bliss, L., Barra, G., & Bennett, M. (2008). Comparison of personal versus fictional narratives of children with language impairment. *American Journal of Speech-Language Pathology, 17,* 194–206.

McCabe, A., & Rollins, P. R. (1994). Assessment of preschool narrative skills. *American Journal of Speech Language Pathology, 3*(1), 45–56.

McCardle, P., Scarborough, H. S., & Catts, H. W. (2001). Predicting, explaining, and preventing children's reading difficulties. *Learning Disabilities Research & Practice, 16(4),* 230–239.

McCathren, R. B., Yoder, P. J., & Warren, S. F. (2000). Testing predictive validity of the Communication Composite of the Communication and Symbolic Behavior Scales. *Journal of Early Intervention, 23,* 36–46.

McCauley, R. J. (1996). Familiar strangers: Criterion-referenced measures in communication disorders. *Language, Speech, and Hearing Services in Schools, 27,* 122–131.

McCormack, J., Harrison, L. J., McLeod, S., & McAllister, L. (2011). A nationally representative study of the association between communication impairment at 4–5 years and children's life activities at 7–9 years. *Journal of Speech, Language, and Hearing Research, 54,* 1328–1348.

McDuffie, A., & Yoder, P. (2010). Types of parent verbal responsiveness that predict language in young children with Autism Spectrum Disorder. *Journal of Speech, Language, and Hearing Research, 53,* 1026–1039.

McDuffie, A., Yoder, P., & Stone, W. (2005). Prelinguistic predictors of vocabulary in young children with autism spectrum disorders. *Journal of Speech, Language, and Hearing Research, 48,* 1080–1097.

McGinty, A. S., & Justice, L. M. (2009). Predictors of print knowledge in children with Specific Language Impairment: Experiential and developmental factors. *Journal of Speech, Language, and Hearing Research, 52,* 81–97.

McGregor, K. K. (2000). The development and enhancement of narrative skills in a preschool classroom: Towards a solution to clinician-client mismatch. *American Journal of Speech-Language Pathology, 9,* 55–71.

McGregor, K. K., Newman, R. M., Reilly, R. M., & Capone, N. C. (2002). Semantic representation and naming in children with specific language impairment. *Journal of Speech, Language, and Hearing Research, 45*, 998–1014.

McLeod, S., & Harrison, L. J. (2009). Epidemiology of speech and language impairment in a nationally representative sample of 4- to 5-year-old children. *Journal of Speech, Language, and Hearing Research, 52*, 1213–1229.

Meilijson, S. R., Kasher, A., & Elizur, A. (2004). Language performance in chronic schizophrenia: A pragmatic approach. *Journal of Speech, Language, and Hearing Research, 47*, 695–713.

Mental Health Research Association. (2007). Childhood schizophrenia. Retrieved July 20, 2007, from www.narsad.org/dc/childhood_disorders/schizophrenia.html

Mentis, M., & Lundgren, K. (1995). Effects of prenatal exposure to cocaine and associated risk factors on language development. *Journal of Speech and Hearing Research, 38*, 1303–1318.

Metsala, J. (1999). Young children's phonological awareness and nonword repetition as a function of vocabulary development. *Journal of Educational Psychology, 91*, 3–19.

Miles, S., & Chapman, R. S. (2002). Narrative content as described by individuals with Down syndrome and typically developing children. *Journal of Speech, Language, and Hearing Research, 45*, 175–189.

Miles, S., Chapman, R., & Sindberg, H. (2006). Sampling context affects MLU in the language of adolescents with Down syndrome. *Journal of Speech, Language, and Hearing Research, 49*, 325–337.

Millar, D. C., Light, J. C., & Schlosser, R. W. (2000). The impact of AAC on natural speech development: A meta-analysis. In *Proceedings of the 9th Biennial Conference of the International Society for Augmentative and Alternative Communication* (pp. 740–741). Washington, DC: ISAAC.

Millar, D. C., Light, J. C., & Schlosser, R. W. (2006). The impact of augmentative and alternative communication intervention on the speech production of individuals with developmental disabilities: A research review. *Journal of Speech, Language, and Hearing Research, 49*, 248–264.

Miller, C. A., & Deevy, P. (2006). Structural priming in children with and without specific language impairment. *Clinical Linguistics & Phonetics, 20*, 387–399.

Miller, C. A., Kail, R., Leonard, L. B., & Tomblin, J. B. (2001). Speed of processing in children with specific language impairment. *Journal of Speech, Language, and Hearing Research, 44*, 416–433.

Miller, C. A., Leonard, L. B., Kail, R. V., Zhang, X., Tomblin, J. B., & Francis, D. J. (2006). Response time in 14-year-olds with language impairment. *Journal of Speech, Language, and Hearing Research, 49*, 712–728.

Miller, J. F. (1981). *Assessing language production in children: Experimental procedures*. Baltimore: University Park Press.

Miller, J. F., & Chapman R. S. (2003). SALT for Windows, Version 6.1 [Computer program]. Muscoda, WI: SALT Software, LLC.

Miller, J. F., Freiberg, C., Rolland, M., & Reeves, M. A. (1992). Implementing computerized language sample analysis in the public school. *Topics in Language Disorders, 12*(2), 69–82.

Miller, J. F., & Iglesias, A. (2006). Systematic Analysis of Language Transcripts (SALT), English & Spanish (Version 9) [Computer software]. Madison, WI: Language Analysis Lab, University of Wisconsin—Madison.

Miller, L. (1999a). *Two friends*. New York: Smart Alternatives.

Miller, L. (1999b). *Bird and his ring*. New York: Smart Alternatives.

Miller, L., & Hendric, N. (2000). Health of children adopted from China. *Pediatrics, 105* (6). Available at www.pediatrics.org/cgi/content/full/105/6/e76

Minear, M., & Shah, P. (2006). Sources of working memory deficits in children and possibilities for remediation. In S. E. Pickering & G. D. Phye (Eds.), *Working memory and education* (pp. 273–297). Mahwah, NJ: Erlbaum.

Miolo, G., Chapman, R. S., & Sindberg, H. A. (2005). Sentence comprehension in children with Down syndrome and typically developing children: Role of sentence voice, visual context, and auditory-verbal short-term memory. *Journal of Speech, Language, and Hearing Research, 48*, 172–188.

Mirenda, P., Smith, V., Fawcett, S., & Johnston, J. (2003, November). *Language and communication intervention outcomes for young children with autism*. Paper presented at the American Speech-Language-Hearing Association Annual Meeting.

Mirrett, P. L., Roberts, J. E., & Price, J. (2003). Early intervention practices and communication intervention strategies for young males with fragile X syndrome. *Language, Speech, and Hearing Services in Schools, 34*, 320–331.

Moats, L. (1995). *Spelling development, disability, and instruction*. Baltimore, MD: York.

Moats, L., & Foorman, B. (2003). Measuring teacher's content knowledge of language and reading. *Annals of Dyslexia, 53*, 23–45.

Montgomery, J. W. (2000a). Relation of working memory to off-line and real-time sentence processing in children with specific language impairment. *Applied Psycholinguistics, 21*, 117–148.

Montgomery, J. W. (2002b). Understanding the language difficulties of children with specific language impairments: Does verbal working memory matter? *American Journal of Speech-Language Pathology, 11*, 77–91.

Montgomery, J. W. (2005). Effects of input rate and age on the real-time language processing of children with specific language impairment. *International Journal of Language and Communication Disorders, 40*, 171–188.

Montgomery, J. W. (2008). Role of auditory attention in the real-time sentence processing of children with specific language impairment: A preliminary investigation. *International Journal of Language and Communication Disorders, 43*, 499–527.

Montgomery, J. W., & Evans, J. (2009). Complex sentence comprehension and working memory in children with specific language impairment. *Journal of Speech, Language, and Hearing Research, 52,* 269–288.

Montgomery, J. W., Evans, J. L., & Gillam, R. B. (2009). Relation of auditory attention and complex sentence comprehension in children with specific language impairment: A preliminary study. *Applied Psycholinguistics, 30,* 123–151.

Montgomery, J. W., Magimairaj, B. M., & Finney, M. C. (2010). Working memory and Specific Language Impairment: An update on the relation and perspectives on assessment and treatment. *American Journal of Speech-Language Pathology, 19,* 78–94.

Montgomery, J. W., Polunenko, A., & Marinellie, S. A. (2009). Role of working memory in children's understanding of spoken narrative: A preliminary investigation. *Applied Psycholinguistics, 30,* 485–509.

Montgomery, J. W., & Windsor, J. (2007). Examining the language performances of children with and without specific language impairment: Contributions of phonological short-term memory and processing speed. *Journal of Speech, Language, and Hearing Research, 50,* 778–797.

Moore, S. M. & Perez-Mendez, C. (2006). Working with linguistically diverse families in early intervention: Misconceptions and missed opportunties. *Seminars in Speech and Language, 27,* 187–198.

Moran, C., & Gillon, G. (2005). Inference comprehension of adolescents with traumatic brain injury: A working memory hypothesis. *Brain Injury, 19,* 743–751.

Mordecai, D. R., Palin, M. W., & Palmer, C. B. (1985). Lingquest 1 [Computer program]. Columbus, OH: Macmillan.

Mosse, E. K., & Jarrold, C. (2011). Evidence for preserved novel word learning in Down syndrome suggests multiple routes to vocabulary acquisition. *Journal of Speech, Language, and Hearing Research, 54* , 1137–1152.

Mundy, P., Block, J., Delgado, C., Pomaes, Y., Van Hecke, A. V., & Parlade, M. V. (2007). Individual differences and the development of joint attention in infancy. *Child Development, 78,* 938–954.

Muñoz, M. L., Gillam, R. B., Peña, E. D., & Gulley-Faehnle, A. (2003). Measures of language development in fictional narratives of Latino children. *Language, Speech, and Hearing Services in Schools, 34,* 332–342.

Murray, D. S., Ruble, L. A., Willis, H., & Molloy, C. A. (2009). Parent and teacher report of social skills in children with Autism Spectrum Disorders. *Language, Speech, and Hearing Services in Schools, 40,* 109–115.

Nail-Chiwetula, B. J., & Bernstein Ratner, N. (2006). Information literacy for speech-language pathologists: A key to evidence-based practice. *Language, Speech, and Hearing Services in Schools, 37,* 157–167.

Naremore, R. C. (2001, April). *Narrative frameworks and early literacy.* Seminar presentation by Rochester Hearing and Speech Center and Nazareth College, Rochester, NY.

Nash, M., & Donaldson, M. L. (2005). Word learning in children with vocabulary deficits. *Journal of Speech, Language, and Hearing Research, 48,* 439–458.

Nathan, L., Stackhouse, J., Goulandris, N., & Snowling, M. J. (2004). The development of early literacy skills among children with speech difficulties: A test of the "critical age hypothesis." *Journal of Speech, Language, and Hearing Research, 47,* 377–391.

Nation, K., Clarke, P., Marshall, C. M., & Durand, M. (2004). Hidden language impairments in children: Parallels between poor reading comprehension and Specific Language Impairment. *Journal of Speech, Language, and Hearing Research, 47,* 199–211.

Nation, K., & Frazier Norbury, C. (2005). Why reading comprehension fails. *Topics in Language Disorders, 25,* 21–32.

National Institute of Child Health and Human Development (NICHD) Early Child Care Research Network. (2005). Pathways to reading: The role of oral language in the transition to reading. *Developmental Psychology, 41* (2), 428–442.

National Joint Committee on Learning Disabilities. (1991). Learning disabilities: Issues on definition (A position paper). *Asha, 33,* (Suppl. 5), 18–20.

Neisworth, J. T., & Bagnato, S. J. (2004). The mismeasure of young children. *Infants & Young Children, 17*(3), 198–212.

Nelson, D. L., & Zhang, N. (2000). The ties that bind what is known to the recall of what is new. *Psychonomic Bulletin & Review, 7* , 604–617.

Nelson, N. W. (1992). Targets of curriculum-based language assessment. *Best Practices in School Speech-Language Pathology, 2,* 73–86.

Nelson, N. W. (1994). Curriculum-based language assessment and intervention across grades. In G. P. Wallach & K. G. Butler (Eds.), *Language learning disabilities in school-age children and adolescents* (pp. 104–131). Boston: Allyn & Bacon.

Nelson, N. W., Bahr, C., & Van Meter, A. (2004). *The Writing Lab approach to language instruction and intervention.* Baltimore, MD: Paul H. Brookes.

Nelson, N. W., & Van Meter, A. M. (2002). Assessing curriculum-based reading and writing samples. *Topics in Language Disorders, 22*(2), 35–59.

Nelson, N. W., & Van Meter, A. (2003, June). *Measuring written language abilities and change through the elementary years* . Poster session presented at the annual meeting of the Symposium for Research in Child Language Disorders, Madison, WI.

Newman, R. S., & German, D. J. (2002). Effects of lexical factors on lexical access among typical language-learning children and children with word-finding difficulties. *Language and Speech, 45,* 285–317.

Nicholas, J. G., & Geers, A. E. (2007, August). Will they catch up? The role of age at cochlear implantation in the spoken language development of children with severe to profound hearing loss. *Journal of Speech, Language, Hearing Research, 50*, 1048–1062.

Nickisch, A., & von Kries, R. (2009). Short-term memory (STM) constraints in children with Specific Language Impairment (SLI): Are there differences between receptive and expressive SLI? *Journal of Speech Language, and Hearing Research, 52*, 578–595.

Nicolson, R., Lenane, M., Singaracharlu, S., Malaspina, D., Giedd, J. N., Hamburger, S. D., Gochman, P., Bedwell, J., Thaker, G. K., Fernandez, T., Wudarsky, M., Hommer, D. W., & Rapoport, J. L. (2000). Premorbid speech and language impairments in childhood-onset schizophrenia: Association with risk factors. *American Journal of Psychiatry, 157*, 794–800.

Nippold, M. A. (2000). Language development during the adolescent years: Aspects of pragmatics, syntax, and semantics. *Topics in Language Disorders, 20*(2), 15–28.

Nippold, M. A. (2004). Research on later language development: International perspectives. In R. A. Berman (Ed.), *Language development across childhood and adolescence: Volume 3. Trends in language acquisition research* (pp. 1–8). Amsterdam, The Netherlands: John Benjamins.

Nippold, M. A. (2007). *Later language development: School-age children, adolescents, and young adults* (3rd ed.). Austin, TX: Pro-Ed.

Nippold, M. A. (2011). Language intervention in the classroom: What it looks like. *Language, Speech, and Hearing Services in Schools, 42*, 393–394.

Nippold, M. A., Hesketh, L. J., Duthie, J. K., & Mansfield, T. C. (2005). Conversational versus expository discourse: A study of syntactic development in children, adolescents, and adults. *Journal of Speech, Language, and Hearing Research, 48* (5), 1048–1064.

Nippold, M. A., Mansfield, T. C., & Billow, J. L. (2007). Peer conflict explanations in children, adolescents, and adults: Examining the development of complex syntax. *American Journal of Speech-Language Pathology, 16*, 179–186.

Nippold, M. A., Mansfield, T. C., Billow, J. L., & Tomblin, J. B. (2008). Expository discourse in adolescents with language impairments: Examining syntactic development. *American Journal of Speech-Language Pathology, 17*, 356–366.

Nippold, M. A., & Sun, L. Knowledge of morphologically complex words: A developmental study of older children and young adolescents. *Language, Speech, and Hearing Services in Schools, 39*, 365–373.

Nippold, M. A., Ward-Lonergan, J., & Fanning, J. L. (2005). Persuasive writing in children, adolescents, and adults: A study of syntactic, semantic, and pragmatic development. *Language, Speech, and Hearing Services in Schools, 36*, 125–138.

Norbury, C. F., & Bishop, D. V. (2003). Narrative skills of children with communication impairments. *International Journal of Language and Communication Disorders, 38*, 287–313.

Norris, J. A., & Hoffman, P. R. (1990b). Language intervention within naturalistic environments. *Language, Speech, and Hearing Services in Schools, 21*, 72–84.

Odom, S. L. (2000). What do we know and where do we go from here? *Topics in Early Childhood Special Education, 20*, 20–27.

Oetting, J. B., Cleveland, L. H., & Cope, R. F. (2008). Empirically derived combinations of tools and clinical cutoffs: An illustrative case with a sample of culturally/linguistically diverse children. *Language, Speech, and Hearing Services in Schools, 39*, 44–53.

Oller, J. W. (2003, September 1). Specific language impairment. Accessed on May 22, 2012, from www.speechpathology.com/ask-the-experts/twins-and-language-development-overview-904

Olswang, L. B., Coggins, T. E., & Timler, G. R. (2001) Outcome measures of school-age children with social communication. *Topics in Language Disorders, 22*(1), 50–73.

Olswang, L. B., Svensson, L., & Astley, S. (2010). Observation of classroom social communication: Do children with Fetal Alcohol Spectrum Disorders spend their time differently than their typically developing peers? *Journal of Speech, Language, and Hearing Research*, 53, 1687–1703.

Olswang, L. B., Svensson, L., Coggins, T. E., Beilinson, J., & Donaldson, A. L. (2006). Reliability issues and solutions for coding social communication performance in classroom settings. *Journal of Speech, Language, and Hearing Research, 49*, 1058–1071.

O'Neil-Pirozzi, T. M. (2003). Language functioning of residents in family homeless shelters. *American Journal of Speech-Language Pathology, 12*, 229–242.

O'Neil-Pirozzi, T. M. (2009). Feasibility and benefit of parent participation in a program emphasizing preschool child language development while homeless. *American Journal of Speech-Language Pathology, 18*, 252–263.

O'Shaughnessy, T. E., & Swanson, H. L. (2000). A comparison of two reading interventions for children with reading disabilities. *Journal of Learning Disabilities, 33*, 257–277.

Owen, A. J. (2010). Factors affecting accuracy of past tense production in children with Specific Language Impairment and their typically developing peers: The influence of verb transitivity, clause location, and sentence type. *Journal of Speech, Language, and Hearing Research, 53*, 993–1014.

Owens, R. (1978). *Speech acts in the early language of non-delayed and retarded children: A taxonomy and distributional study.* Unpublished doctoral dissertation, Ohio State University, Columbus.

Owens, R. E. (2012). *Language development: An introduction* (8th ed.). Boston: Pearson.

Owens, R. E., & Kim, K. (2007, November). *Holistic reading and semantic investigation intervention with struggling readers.* Paper presented at Annual Convention of the American Speech-Language-Hearing Association, Boston.

Paez, M., & Rinaldi, C. (2006). Predicting English word reading skills for Spanish-speaking students in first grade. *Topics in Language Disorders, 26,* 338–350.

Paradis, J. (2005). Grammatical morphology in children learning English as a second language: Implications of similarities with specific language impairment. *Language, Speech, and Hearing Services in Schools, 36,* 172–187.

Paradis, J. (2007). Bilingual children with specific language impairment: Theoretical and applied issues. *Applied Psycholinguistics, 28,* 551–564.

Paradis, J., Crago, M., Genesee, F., & Rice, M. (2003). French-English bilingual children with specific language impairment: How do they compare with their monolingual peers? *Journal of Speech, Language, and Hearing Research, 46,* 1–15. doi: 10.1044/1092-4388(2003/009).

Parente, R., & Hermann, D. (1996). Retraining memory strategies. *Topics in Language Disorders, 17(1),* 45–57.

Patterson, J. L. (2000). Observed and reported expressive vocabulary and word combinations in bilingual toddlers. *Journal of Speech, Language, and Hearing Research, 43,* 121–128.

Patton Terry, N., McDonald Connor, C., Thomas-Tate, S., & Love, M. (2010). Examining relationships among dialect variation, literacy skills, and school context in first grade. *Journal of Speech, Language and Hearing Research, 53,* 126–145.

Paul, R. (1996). Clinical implications of the natural history of slow expressive language development. *American Journal of Speech-Language Pathology, 5*(2), 5–22.

Paul-Brown, D., & Caperton, C. J. (2001). Inclusive practices for preschool-age children with specific language impairment. In M. J. Guralnick (Ed.), *Early childhood inclusion: Focus on change* (pp. 433–463). Baltimore: Paul H. Brookes.

Pearce, W., McCormack, P., & James, D. (2003). Exploring the boundaries of SLI: Findings from morphosyntactic and story grammar analyses. *Clinical Linguistics & Phonetics, 17,* 325–334.

Peets, K. F. (2009). The effects of context on the classroom discourse skills of children with language impairment. *Language, Speech, and Hearing Services in Schools, 40,* 5–16.

Peña, E. D. (2002, April). *Solving the problems of biased speech and language assessment with bilingual children.* Paper presented at the Annual Convention of the New York State Speech-Language-Hearing Association, Rochester.

Peña, E. D., Gillam, R. B., Bedore, L. M., & Bohman, T. M. (2011). Risk for poor performance on a language screening measure for bilingual preschoolers and kindergarteners. *American Journal of Speech-Language Pathology, 20,* 302–314.

Peña, E. D., Iglesias, A., & Lidz, C. S. (2001). Reducing test bias through dynamic assessment of children's word learning ability. *American Journal of Speech-Language Pathology, 10,* 138–154.

Pence, K. L., Justice, L. M., & Wiggins, A. K. (2008). Preschool teachers' fidelity in implementing a comprehensive language-rich curriculum. *Language, Speech, and Hearing Services in Schools, 39,* 329–341.

Perzsolt, F., Ohletz, A., Gardner, D., Ruatti, H., Meier, H., Schlotz-Gorton, N., & Schrott, L. (2003). Evidence-based decision making: The 6-step approach. *American College of Physicians Journal Club, 139(3),* 1–6.

Petersen, D. B., Laing Gillam, S., Spencer, T., & Gillam, R. B. (2010). The effects of literate narrative intervention on children with neurologically based language impairments: An early stage study. *Journal of Speech, Language, and Hearing Research, 53,* 961–981.

Petersen, E. A. (2003). A practical guide to early childhood curriculum: Linking thematic, emergent, and skill-based planning to children's outcomes (2nd ed.). Boston: Allyn & Bacon.

Pham, G., Kohnert, K., & Mann, D. (2011). Addressing clinician-client mismatch: A preliminary intervention study with a bilingual Vietnamese-English preschooler. *Language, Speech, and Hearing Services in Schools, 42,* 408–422.

Phelps-Terasaki, D., & Phelps-Gunn, T. (1992). *Test of Pragmatic Language.* East Moline, IL: Linguisystems.

Philofsky, A., Hepburn, S. L., Hayes, A., Hagerman, R., & Rogers, S. J. (2004). Language and cognitive functioning and autism symptoms in young children with fragile X syndrome. *American Journal on Mental Retardation, 109,* 208–218.

Pianta, R., Howes, C., Burchinal, M., Bryant, D., Clifford, R., Early, D., & Barbarin, O. (2005). Features of pre-kindergarten programs, classrooms, and teachers: Do they predict observed classroom quality and child-teacher interactions? *Applied Developmental Science, 9,* 144–159.

Pickering, M. J., & Ferreira, V. S. (2008). Structural priming: A critical review. *Psychological Bulletin, 134,* 427–459.

Pickering, S., & Gathercole, S. (2001). *Working Memory Test Battery for Children.* London: Harcourt Assessment.

P.L. 106-402. (2000), *The Developmental Disabilities Assistance and Bill of Rights Act.*

Pokorni, J. L., Worthington, C. K., & Jamison, P. J. (2004). Phonological awareness intervention: Comparison of Fast For Word, Earobics, and LiPS. *Journal of Educational Research, 97,* 147–157.

Prelock, P. A., Beatson, J., Bitner, B., Broder, C., & Ducker, A. (2003). Interdisciplinary assessment of young children with autism spectrum disorder. *Language, Speech, and Hearing Services in Schools, 34,* 194–202.

Prelock, P. A., Miller, B. L., & Reed, N. L. (1995). Collaborative partnerships in a language in the classroom program. *Language, Speech, and Hearing Services in Schools, 26,* 286–292.

Prendeville, J., & Ross-Allen, J. (2002). The transition process in the early years: Enhancing speech-language pathologists' perspective. *Language, Speech, and Hearing Services in Schools, 33,* 130–136.

Preschool Curriculum Evaluation Research Consortium. (2008). *Effects of preschool curriculum programs on school readiness* (NCER 2008-2009). Washington DC: National Center for Education Research, Institute of Education Sciences, U.S. Department of Education. Retrieved from http://ncer.ed.gov.

Preterm Birth: Causes, Consequences, and Prevention, (2006). *Institute of Medicine.* Updated July 2006. Accessed September 16, 2008, from www.iom.edu/Object.File/Master/35/975/pretermbirth.pdf

Pretti-Frontczak, K. L., & Bricker, D. D. (2004). *An activity-based approach to early intervention* (3rd ed.). Baltimore: Paul H. Brookes.

Price, J. R., Roberts, J. E., Hennon, E. A., Berni, M. C., Anderson, K. L., & Sideris, J. (2008). Syntactic complexity during conversation of boys with Fragile X syndrome and Down syndrome. *Journal of Speech, Language, and Hearing Research, 51,* 3–15.

Proctor-Williams, K., Fey, M. E., & Frome Loeb, D. (2001). Parental recasts and production of copulas and articles by children with specific language impairment and typical language. *American Journal of Speech-Language Pathology, 10,* 155–168.

Pruitt, S. L., & Oetting, J. B. (2009). Past tense marking by African American English–speaking children reared in poverty. *Journal of Speech, Language, and Hearing Research, 52,* 2–15.

Pruitt, S. L., Oetting, J. B., & Hegarty, M. (2011). Passive participle marking by African American English-speaking children reared in poverty. *Journal of Speech, Language, and Hearing Research, 54,* 598–607.

Prutting, C. A. (1983). Scientific inquiry and communicative disorders: An emerging paradigm across six decades. In T. Gallagher & C. Prutting (Eds.), *Pragmatic assessment and intervention issues in language* (pp. 247–267). San Diego: College-Hill.

Prutting, C. A., & Kirchner, D. M. (1983). Applied pragmatics. In T. M. Gallagher & C. A. Prutting (Eds.), *Pragmatic assessment and intervention issues in language* (pp. 29–64). Austin, TX: Pro-Ed.

Prutting, C. A., & Kirchner, D. M. (1987). A clinical appraisal of the pragmatic aspects of language. *Journal of Speech and Hearing Disorders, 52,* 105–119.

Pry, R., Petersen, A., & Baghdadli, A. (2005). The relationship between expressive language level and psychological development in children with autism 5 years of age. *Autism: The International Journal of Research and Practice, 9,* 179–189.

Puranik, C. S., Lombardino, L. J., & Altmann, L. J. (2007). Writing through retellings: An exploratory study of language impaired and dyslexic populations. *Reading and Writing: An Interdisciplinary Journal, 20,* 251–272.

Pye, C. (1987). Pye Analysis of Language (PAL) [Computer program]. Lawrence: University of Kansas.

Qi, C. H., & Kaiser, A. P. (2004). Problem behaviors of low-income children with language delays: An observational study. *Journal of Speech, Language, and Hearing Research, 47,* 595–609.

Qi, C. H., Kaiser, A. P., Milan, S. E., Yzquierdo, Z., & Hancock, T. B. (2003). The performance of low-income African American children on the Preschool Language Scale–3. *Journal of Speech, Language, and Hearing Research, 46,* 576–590.

Qi, C. H., Kaiser, A. P., Milan, S. E., & Hancock, T. B. (2006). Language performance of low-income African American and European American preschool children on the Peabody Picture Vocabulary Test—III. *Language, Speech, and Hearing Services in Schools, 37,* 5–16.

Quail, M., Williams, C., & Leitao, S. (2009). Verbal working memory in specific language impairment: The effect of providing visual support. *International Journal of Speech-Language Pathology, 11,* 220–233.

Raab, M., & Dunst, C. (2007). *Influence of child interests on variations in child behavior and functioning.* (Winterberry Research Syntheses, Vol. 1, No. 21). Asheville, NC: Winterberry Press.

Rankin, P. M., & Hood, J. (2005). Designing clinical interventions for children with specific memory disorders. *Pediatric Rehabilitation, 8,* 283–297.

Redmond, S. M. (2002). The use of rating scales with children who have language impairments. *American Journal of Speech-Language Pathology, 11,* 124–138.

Redmond, S. M., & Rice, M. L. (2001). Detection of irregular verb violations by children with and without SLI. *Journal of Speech, Language, and Hearing Research, 44,* 655–669.

Redmond, S. M., & Rice, M. L. (2002). Stability of behavioral ratings of children with SLI. *Journal of Speech, Language, and Hearing Research, 45,* 190–201.

Reed, V. A., & Spicer, L. (2003). The relative importance of selected communication skills for adolescents' interactions with their teachers: High school teachers' opinions. *Language, Speech, and Hearing Services in Schools, 34,* 343–357.

Reichle, J., Beukelman, D., & Light, J. (2002). *Implementing an augmentative communication system: exemplary strategies for beginning communicators.* Baltimore, MD: Paul H. Brookes.

Reichle, J., Dropik, P. L., Alden-Anderson, E., & Haley, T. (2008). Teaching a young child with autism to request assistance conditionally: A preliminary study. *American Journal of Speech-Language Pathology, 17,* 231–240.

Reichle, J., & McComas, J. (2004). Conditional use of a request for assistance. *Disability and Rehabilitation, 26,* 1255–1262.

Reid, D. K., Hresko, W. P., & Hammill, D. D. (2001). *Test of Early Reading Ability.* Austin, TX: Pro-Ed.

Reilly, J., Losh, M., Bellugi, U., & Wulfeck, B. (2004). Frog, Where are you? Narratives in children with specific language impairment, early focal brain injury and Williams syndrome. *Brain & Language, 88,* 229–247.

Rescorla, L. A. (2005). Age 13 language and reading outcomes in late talking toddlers. *Journal of Speech, Language, and Hearing Research, 48*, 459–473.

Rescorla, L. A. (2009). Age 17 language and reading outcomes in late-talking toddlers: Support for a dimensional perspective on language delay. *Journal of Speech, Language, and Hearing Research, 52* , 16–30.

Rescorla, L., & Roberts, J. (2002). Nominal versus verbal morpheme use in late talkers at ages 3 and 4. *Journal of Speech, Language, and Hearing Research, 45*, 1219–1231.

Rescorla, L. A., Ross, G. S., & McClure, S. (2007). Language delay and behavioral/emotional problems in toddlers: Findings from two developmental clinics. *Journal of Speech, Language, and Hearing Research, 50*, 1063–1078.

Restrepo, M. A. (1998). Identifiers of predominantly Spanish-speaking children with language impairment. *Journal of Speech, Language, and Hearing Research, 41*, 1398–1411.

Restrepo, M. A., Castilla, A. P., Schwanenflugel, P. J., Neuharth-Pritchett, S., Hamilton, C. E., & Arboleda, A. (2010). Supplemental oral language program in sentence length, complexity, and grammaticality in Spanish-speaking children attending English-only preschools. *Language, Speech, and Hearing Services in Schools, 41*, 3–13.

Restrepo, M. A., & Kruth, K. (2000). Grammatical characteristics of a Spanish–English bilingual child with specific language impairment. *Communication Disorders Quarterly, 21*, 66–76. doi: 10.1177/152574010002100201.

Rhyner, P. M., Kelly, D. J., Brantley, A. L., & Krueger, D. M. (1999). Screening low-income African American children using the BLT–2S and the SPELT–P. *American Journal of Speech-Language Pathology, 8* (1) , 44–52.

Riccio, C. A., Cash, D. L., & Cohen, M. J. (2007). Learning and memory performance of children with specific language impairment (SLI). *Applied Neuropsychology, 14*, 255–261.

Rice, M. L., Ash, A., Betz, S., Francois, J., Kepler, A., Klager, E., & Smolik, F. (2004). *Transcription and coding manual for analysis of language samples: Kansas Language Transcript Database*. Lawrence: University of Kansas.

Rice, M. L., Cleave, P. L., & Oetting, J. B. (2000). The use of syntactic cues in lexical acquisition by children with SLI. *Journal of Speech, Language, and Hearing Research, 43*, 582–594.

Rice, M. L., Hoffman, L., & Wexler, K. (2009). Judgments of omitted BE and DO in questions as extended finiteness clinical markers of Specific Language Impairment (SLI) to 15 years: A study of growth and asymptote. *Journal of Speech, Language, and Hearing Research*, 52, 1417–1433.

Rice, M. L., Redmont, S. M., & Hoffman, L. (2006). Mean length of utterance in children with specific language impairment and in younger control children shows concurrent validity and stable and parallel growth trajectories. *Journal of Speech, Language, and Hearing Research, 49*, 793–808.

Rice, M. L., Smolik, F., Perpich, D., Thompson, T., Rytting, N., & Blossom, M. (2010). Mean length of utterance levels in 6-month intervals for children 3 to 9 years with and without language impairments. *Journal of Speech, Language, and Hearing Research, 53*, 333–349.

Rice, M. L., Snell, M. A., & Hadley, P. A. (1990). The Social Interactive Coding System (SICS): An online, clinically relevant descriptive tool. *Language, Speech, and Hearing Services in Schools, 21*, 2–14.

Rice, M. L., Tomblin, J. B., Hoffman, L., Richman, W. A., & Marquis, J. (2004). Grammatical tense deficits in children with SLI and nonspecific language impairment: Relationships with nonverbal IQ over time. *Journal of Speech, Language, and Hearing Research, 47*, 816–834.

Riches, N. G., Tomasello, M., & Conti-Ramsden, G. (2005). Verb learning in children with SLI: Frequency and spacing effects. *Journal of Speech, Language, and Hearing Research, 48*, 1397–1411.

Richgels, D., McGee, D., Lomax, R., & Sheard, C. (1987). Awareness of four text structures: Effects on recall of expository text. *Reading Research Quarterly, 22*, 177–196.

Richman, D. M., Wacker, D. P., & Winborn, L. (2001). Response efficiency during functional communication training: Effects of effort and response allocation. *Journal of Applied Behavior Analysis, 34*, 73–36.

Rispoli, M., & Hadley, P. (2001). The leading-edge: The significance of sentence disruption in the development of grammar. *Journal of Speech, Language, and Hearing Research, 44*, 1131–1143.

Roberts, J. E., Long, S. H., Malkin, C., Barnes, E., Skinner, M., Hennon, E. A., & Anderson, K. (2005). A comparison of phonological skills with fragile X syndrome and Down syndrome. *Journal of Speech, Language, and Hearing Research, 48*, 980–995.

Roberts, J. E., Martin, G. E., Maskowitz, L., Harris, A. A., Foreman, J., & Nelson, L. (2007). Discourse skills of boys with fragile X syndrome in comparison to boys with Down syndrome. *Journal of Speech, Language, and Hearing Research, 50*, 475–492.

Roberts, J. E., Mirrett, P., & Burchinal, M. (2001). Receptive and expressive communication development in young males with fragile X syndrome. *American Journal of Mental Retardation, 106*, 216–231.

Roberts, M. Y., & Kaiser, A. P. (2011). The effectiveness of parent-implemented language interventions: A meta-analysis. *American Journal of Speech-Language Pathology, 20*, 180–199.

Roberts, M. Y., Kaiser, A. P., & Wright, C. (2010). *Parent training: Specific strategies beyond "Try this at home."* Paper presented at the annual convention of the American Speech-Language-Hearing Association, Philadelphia.

Robertson, C., & Salter, W. (1997). *Phonological Awareness Test (PAT)*. East Moline, IL: Linguisystems.

Rodekohr, R., & Haynes, W. O. (2001). Differentiating dialect from disorder: A comparison of two processing tasks and a standardized language test. *Journal of Communication Disorders, 34,* 255–272.

Rodriguez, B. L., Hines, R., & Montiel, M. (2009). Mexican American mothers of low and middle socioeconomic status: Communication behaviors and interactive strategies during shared book reading. *Language, Speech and Hearing Services in Schools, 40,* 271–282.

Rodriguez, B. L., & Olswang, L. B. (2003). Mexican-American and Anglo-American mothers' beliefs and values about child rearing, education, and language impairment. *American Journal of Speech-Language Pathology, 12,* 452–462.

Rollins, P. R., McCabe, A., & Bliss, L. (2000). Culturally sensitive assessment of narrative in children. *Seminars in Speech and Language, 21,* 223–234.

Rolstad, K., Mahoney, K., & Glass, G. V. (2005). The big picture: A meta-analysis of program effectiveness research on English language learners. *Educational Policy, 19,* 572–594. doi: 10.1177/0895904805278067.

Romski, M. A., & Sevcik, R. A. (2005). Augmentative communication and early intervention: Myths and realities. *Infants and Young Children, 18,* 174–185.

Romski, M. A., Sevcik, R. A., Cheslock, M. B., & Hyatt, A. (2002). Enhancing communication competence in beginning communicators: Identifying a continuum of AAC language intervention strategies. In J. Reichle, D. Beukelman, & J. Light (Eds.), *Implementing an augmentative communication system: Exemplary strategies for beginning communicators* (pp. 1–23). Baltimore, MD: Paul H. Brookes.

Romski, M. A., Sevcik, R. A., & Forrest, S. (2001). Assistive technology and augmentative communication in early childhood inclusion. In M. J. Guralnick (Ed.), *Early childhood inclusion: Focus on change* (pp. 465–479). Baltimore: Paul H. Brookes.

Romski, M. A., Sevcik, R. A., Adamson, L. B., Smith, A., Cheslock, M., & Bakeman, R. (2001). Parent perceptions of the language development of toddlers with developmental delays before and after participation in parent-coached language interventions. *American Journal of Speech-Language Pathology, 20,* 111–118.

Roper, N., & Dunst, C. J. (2003). Communication intervention in natural environments. *Infants & Young Children, 16,* 215–225.

Ross, B., & Cress, C. J. (2006). Comparison of standardized assessments for cognitive and receptive communication skills in young children with complex communication needs. *Augmentative and Alternative Communication, 22,* 100–111.

Rossetti, L. M. (2001). *Communication intervention: Birth to three* (2nd ed.). Albany, NY: Singular.

Roth, F. P. (1986). Oral narrative abilities of learning-disabled students. *Topics in Language Disorders, 7*(1), 1–30.

Roth, F. P. (2000). Narrative writing: Development and teaching with children with writing difficulties. *Topics in Language Disorders, 20*(4), 15–28.

Rouse, C. E., & Krueger, A. B. (2004). Putting computerized instruction to the test: A randomized evaluation of a "scientifically based" reading program. *Economics of Education Review, 23,* 323–338.

Rowland, C., & Schweigert, P. D. (2000). Tangible symbols, tangible outcomes. *Augmentative and Alternative Communication, 16,* 61–78.

Rubin, E., & Lennon, L. (2004). Challenges in social communication in Asperger's syndrome and high-functioning autism. *Topics in Language Disorders, 24,* 271–285.

Rubin, K. H., Burgess, K. B., & Coplan, R. J. (2002). Social withdrawal and shyness. In P. K. Smith & C. H. Hart (Eds.), *Blackwell handbook of childhood social development* (pp. 329–352). Malden, MA: Blackwell.

Rutter, M. L., Kreppner, J. M., & O'Connor, T. G. (2001). Specificity and heterogeneity in children's responses to profound institutional privation. *British Journal of Psychiatry, 179* (2), 97–103.

Rvachew, S., Ohberg, A., Grawburg, M., & Heyding, J. (2003). Phonological awareness and phonemic perception in 4-year-old children with delayed expressive phonological skills. *American Journal of Speech-Language Pathology, 12,* 463–471.

Salameh, E., Håkansson, G., & Nettelbladt, U. (2004). Developmental perspectives on bilingual Swedish-Arabic children with and without language impairment: A longitudinal study. *International Journal of Language and Communication Disorders, 39,* 65–91. doi:10.1080/13682820310001595628.

Salas-Provance, M. B., Erickson, J. G., & Reed, J. (2002). Disabilities as viewed by four generations of one Hispanic family. *American Journal of Speech-Language Pathology, 11,* 151–162.

Samuel, A. (2001). Knowing a word affects the fundamental perception of the sounds within it. *Psychological Science, 12,* 348–351.

Sandall, S. R., McLean, M., & Smith, B. (2001). *DEC recommended practices in early intervention/early childhood special education.* Longmont, CO: Sopris West.

Savage, C., Lieven, E., Theakston, A., & Tomasello, M. (2003). Testing the abstractness of children's linguistic representations: Lexical and structural priming of syntactic constructions in young children. *Developmental Science, 6,* 557–567.

Sawyer, D. (1987). *Test of Awareness of Language Segments.* Rockville, MD: Aspen.

Sawyer, D. J. (2006). Dyslexia: A generation of inquiry. *Topics in Language Disorders, 26,* 95–109.

Scally, C. (2001). Visual design: Implications for developing dynamic display systems. *Perspectives on Augmentative and Alternative Communication, 10*(4), 16–19.

Scarborough, H. S. (1990). Index of productive syntax. *Applied Linguistics, 11,* 1–22.

Scarborough, H. S. (2001). Connecting early language and literacy to later reading (dis)abilities: Evidence, theory, and practice. In S. B. Neuman & D. K. Dickinson (Eds.),

Handbook of early literacy research (pp. 97–110). New York: Guilford.

Scarborough, H. S., Wyckoff, J., & Davidson, R. (1986). A reconsideration of the relationship between age and mean utterance length. *Journal of Speech and Hearing Research, 29*, 394–399.

Scheffner Hammer, C., Farkas, G., & Maczuga, S. (2010). The language and literacy development of Head Start children: A study using the family and child experiences survey database. *Language, Speech, and Hearing Services in Schools, 41*, 70–83.

Schlosser, R. W., & Lee, D. L. (2000). Promoting generalization and maintenance in augmentative and alternative communication: A meta-analysis of 20 years of effectiveness research. *Augmentative and Alternative Communication, 16*, 208–226.

Schneider, P. (2008, June). *Referent introduction in stories by children and adults.* Poster presented at the triennial meeting of the International Association for the Study of Child Language, Edinburgh, Scotland.

Schneider, P., & Dubé, R. (2005). Story presentation effects on children's retell content. *American Journal of Speech-Language Pathology, 14*, 52–60.

Schneider, P., Dubé, R. V., & Hayward, D. (2009). *The Edmonton Narrative Norms Instrument.* Available from www.rehabmed.ualberta.ca/spa/enni

Schneider, P., & Hayward, D. (2010). Who does what to whom: Introduction of referents in children's storytelling from pictures. *Language, Speech, and Hearing Services in Schools, 41*, 459–473.

Schore, A. N. (2001). The effects of early relational trauma on right brain development, affect regulation, and infant mental health. *Infant Mental Health Journal, 22*, 201–269.

Schuele, C. M. (2001). Socioeconomic influences on children's language acquisition. *Journal of Speech-Language Pathology and Audiology, 25*(2), 77–88.

Schuele, C. M., & Boudreau, D. (2008). Phonological awareness intervention: Beyond the basics. *Language, Speech, and Hearing Services in Schools, 39*, 3–20.

Schuele, C. M., & Dayton, N. D. (2000). *Intensive Phonological Awareness Program.* Nashville, TN: Authors.

Scientific Learning Corporation. (1998). *Fast ForWord Language* [Computer software]. Berkley, CA: Author.

Scientific Learning Corporation. (2009). *Scientific learning products.* Retrieved from www.scilearn.com/products/index.php?source=Google&adgroup=ffw39-22-8

Scott, C. M. (2000). Principles and methods of spelling instruction: Applications for poor spellers. *Topics in Language Disorders, 20*(3), 66–82.

Scott, C. M., & Erwin, D. L. (1992). Descriptive assessment of writing: Process and products. *Best Practices in School Speech-Language Pathology, 2*, 87–98.

Scott, C. M., Nippold, M. A., Norris, J. A., & Johnson, C. J. (1992, November) *School-age children and adolescents: Establishing language norms.* Paper presented at the Annual Convention of the American Speech-Language-Hearing Association, San Antonio, TX.

Scott, C. M., & Windsor, J. (2000). General language performance measures in spoken and written discourse produced by school-age children with and without language learning disabilities. *Journal of Speech, Language, and Hearing Research, 43*, 324–339.

Segebart DeThorne, L., Hart, S. A., Petrill, S. A., Deater-Deckard, K., Thompson, L. A., Schatschneider, C., & Dunn Davison, M. (2006). Children's history of speech-language difficulties: Genetic influences and association with reading-related measures. *Journal of Speech, Language, and Hearing Research, 49*, 1280–1293.

Segebart DeThorne, L., Petrill, S. A., Schatschneider, C., & Cutting, L. (2010). Conversational language use as a predictor of early reading development: Language history as a moderating variable. *Journal of Speech, Language, and Hearing Research, 53*, 209–223.

Segebert DeThorne, L., & Watkins, R. V. (2001). Listeners' perceptions of language use in children. *Language, Speech, and Hearing Services in Schools, 32*, 142–148.

Segers, E., & Verhoeven, L. (2004). Computer-supported phonological awareness intervention for kindergarten children with specific language impairment. *Language, Speech, and Hearing Services in Schools, 35*, 229–239.

Seigneuric, A., Ehrlich, J., Oakhill, J. V., & Yuill, N. M. (2000). Working memory resources and children's reading comprehension. *Reading and Writing: An Interdisciplinary Journal, 13*, 81–103.

Selber Beilinson, J., & Olswang, L. B. (2003). Facilitating peer-group entry in kindergartners with impairments in social communication. *Language, Speech, and Hearing Services in Schools, 34*, 154–166.

Self, T. L., Hale, L. S., & Crumrine, D. (2010). Pharmacotherapy and children with Autism Spectrum Disorder: A tutorial for speech-language pathologists. *Language, Speech, and Hearing Services in Schools, 41*, 367–375.

Semel, E., Wiig, E., & Secord, W. (2003). *Clinical Evaluation of Language Fundamentals, Fourth Edition.* San Antonio, TX: The Psychological Corporation.

Sénéchal, M., LeFevre, J., Smith-Chant, B. L., & Colton, K. V. (2001). On refining theoretical models of emergent literacy: The role of empirical evidence. *Journal of School Psychology, 39*(5), 439–460.

Seung, H., & Chapman, R. (2000). Digit span in individuals with Down syndrome and in typically developing children: Temporal aspects. *Journal of Speech, Language, and Hearing Research, 43*, 609–620.

Seymour, H. N., Roeper, T. W., & deVilliers, J. (2003). *Diagnostic Evaluation of Language Variance (DELV).* San Antonia, TX: Psychological Corporation.

Shane, H. C. (2006). Using visual scene displays to improve communication and communication instruction in persons with Autism Spectrum Disorders. *Perspectives in*

Augmentative and Alternative Communication, 15(1), 8–13.
Shaywitz, S. E., & Shaywitz, B. A. (2003). Neurobiological indices of dyslexia. In H. L. Swanson, K. R. Harris, & S. Graham (Eds.), *Handbook of learning disabilities* (pp. 514–531). New York: Guilford.
Sheng, L., & McGregor, K. A. (2010). Object and action naming in children with Specific Language Impairment. *Journal of Speech, Language, and Hearing Research, 53*, 1704–1719.
Shimpi, P. M., Gámez, P. B., Huttenlocher, J., & Vasilyeva, M. (2007). Syntactic priming in 3-and 4-year-old children: Evidence for abstract representations of transitive and dative forms. *Developmental Psychology, 43*, 1334–1346.
Shipley, K., Maddox, M., & Driver, J. (1991). Children's development of irregular past tense verb forms. *Language, Speech, and Hearing Services in Schools, 22*, 115–122.
Shiro, M. (2003). Genre and evaluation in narrative development. *Journal of Child Language, 30*, 165–195.
Shumway, S., & Wetherby, A. M. (2009). Communicative acts of children with Autism Spectrum Disorders in the second year of life. *Journal of Speech, Language, and Hearing Research, 52*, 1139–1156.
Sigafoos, J., & Drasgow, E. (2001). Conditional use of aided and unaided AAC: A review and clinical case demonstration. *Focus on Autism and Other Developmental Disabilities, 16*, 152–161.
Sigafoos, J., O'Reilly, E., Drasgow, E., & Reichle, J. (2002). Strategies to achieve socially acceptable escape and avoidance. In J. Reichle, D. Beukelman, & J. Light (Eds.), *Exemplary practices for beginning communicators: Implications for AAC* (pp. 157–186). Baltimore: Paul H. Brookes.
Siller, M., & Sigman, M. (2002). The behaviors of parents of children with autism predict the subsequent development of their children's communication. *Journal of Autism and Developmental Disorders, 32*, 77–89.
Silliman, E. R., Bahr, R., Beasman, J., & Wilkinson, L. C. (2000). Scaffolds for learning to read in an inclusion classroom. *Language, Speech, and Hearing Services in Schools, 31*, 265–279.
Silliman, E. R., & Scott, C. (2009). Research-based oral language intervention routes to the academic language of literacy: Finding the right road. In S. Rosenfield & V. Berninger (Eds.), *Implementing evidence-based interventions in school settings* (pp. 107–145). New York: Oxford University Press.
Simon, C. S. (1984). *Evaluating communicative competence: A functional-pragmatic procedure*. Tucson, AZ: Communication Skill Builders.
Simon, C. S. (1989). *Classroom communication screening procedure for early adolescents: A handbook for assessment and intervention*. Tempe, AZ: Communi-Cog Publications.
Skarakis-Doyle, E. (2002). Young children's detection of violations in familiar stories and emerging comprehension monitoring. *Discourse Processes, 33*(2) 175–197.
Skarakis-Doyle, E., & Dempsey, L. (2008). The detection and monitoring of comprehension errors by preschool children with and without language impairment. *Journal of Speech, Language, and Hearing Research, 51*, 1227–1243.
Skarakis-Doyle, E., Dempsey, L., Campbell, W., Lee, C., & Jaques, J. (2005, June). *Constructs underlying emerging comprehension monitoring: A preliminary study.* Poster session presented at the 26th Annual Symposium on Research in Child Language Disorders, Madison, WI.
Skarakis-Doyle, E., Dempsey, L., & Lee, C. (2008). Language comprehension impairment in preschool children. *Language, Speech, and Hearing Services in Schools, 39*, 54–65.
Smith, V., Mirenda, P., & Zaidman-Zait, A. (2007). Predictors of expressive vocabulary growth in children with autism. *Journal of Speech, Language, and Hearing Research, 50*, 149–160.
Smith-Myles, B., Hilgenfeld, T., Barnhill, G., Griswold, D., Hagiwara, T., & Simpson, R. (2002). Analysis of reading skills in individuals with Asperger syndrome. *Focus on Autism and Other Developmental Disabilities, 17*(1), 44–47.
Snow, C. E., Scarborough, H. S., & Burns, M. S. (1999). What speech-language pathologists need to know about early reading. *Topics in Language Disorders, 20*(1), 48–58.
Snowling, M., Bishop, D. V. M., & Stothard, S. E. (2000). Is preschool language impairment a risk factor for dyslexia in adolescence? *Journal of Child Psychology and Psychiatry, 41*, 587–600.
Snyder, L., Caccamise, D., & Wise, B. (2005). The assessment of reading comprehension. *Topics in Language Disorders, 25*, 33–50.
Snyder, L. E., Dabasinskas, C., & O'Connor, E. (2002). An information processing perspective on language impairment in children: Looking at both sides of the coin. *Topics in Language Disorders, 22*(3), 1–14.
Southwood, F., & Russell, A. F. (2004). Comparison of conversation, freeplay, and story generation as methods of language elicitation. *Journal of Speech, Language, and Hearing Research, 47*, 366–376.
Spaulding, T. J. (2010). Investigating mechanisms of suppression in preschool children with Specific Language Impairment. *Journal of Speech, Language, and Hearing Research, 53*, 725–738.
Spaulding, T. J., Plante, E., & Farinella, K. A. (2006), Eligibility criteria for language impairment: Is the low end of normal always appropriate? *Language, Speech, and Hearing Services in Schools, 37*, 61–72.
Spaulding, T. J., Plante, E., & Vance, R. (2008). Sustained selective attention skills of preschool children with specific language impairment: Evidence for separate attentional capacities. *Journal of Speech Language, and Hearing Research, 51*, 16–34.

Spencer, E., Schuele, C. M., Guillot, K., & Lee, M. (2007). *Phonological awareness skill of speech-language pathologists and other educators.* Manuscript submitted for publication.

Spinelli, F., & Terrell, B. (1984). Remediation in context. *Topics in Language Disorders, 5*(1), 29–40.

Stanovich, K. E. (2000). *Progress in understanding reading: Scientific foundations and new frontiers.* New York: Guilford Press.

Stanton-Chapman, T. L., Chapman, D. A., Kaiser, A. P., & Hancock, T. B. (2004). Cumulative risk and low-income children's language development. *Topics in Early Childhood Special Education, 24,* 227–238.

Steffani, S. A. (2007, Spring). Identifying embedded and conjoined complex sentences: Making it simple. *Contemporary Issues in Communication Science and Disorders, 34,* 44–54.

Stein, N., & Glenn, C. (1979). An analysis of story comprehension in elementary school children. In R. Freedle (Ed.), *New directions in discourse processing* (Vol. 2, pp. 53–120). Norwood, NJ: Ablex.

Stevens, C., Fanning, J., Coch, D., Sanders, L., & Neville, H. (2008). Neural mechanisms of selective auditory attention are enhanced by computerized training: Electrophysiological evidence from language-impaired and typically developing children. *Brain Research, 1205,* 55–69.

Stickler, K. R. (1987). *Guide to analysis of language transcripts.* Eau Claire, WI: Thinking Publications.

Stockman, I. J. (2007). Social-political influences on research practices: Examining language acquisition by African American children. In B. Bailey & C. Lucas (Eds.), *Sociolinguistic variation: Theory, method, and applications* (pp. 297–317). Cambridge, England: Cambridge University Press.

Stockman, I. J. (2008). Toward validation of a minimal competence phonetic core for African American children. *Journal of Speech, Language, and Hearing Research, 51,* 1244–1262.

Stockman. I. J. (2010), A review of developmental and applied language research on African American children: From a deficit to difference perspective on dialect differences. *Language, Speech, and Hearing Services in Schools, 41,* 23–38.

Stockman, I. J., Karasinski, L., & Guillory, B. (2008). The use of conversational repairs by African American preschoolers. *Language, Speech, and Hearing Services in Schools, 39,* 461–474.

Stone, W. L., & Yoder, P. J. (2001). Predicting spoken language level in children with autism spectrum disorders. *Autism, 5,* 341–361.

Storkel, H. L. (2001). Learning new words: Phonotactic probability in language development. *Journal of Speech, Language, and Hearing Research, 44,* 1321–1337.

Storkel, H. L. (2004). The emerging lexicon of children with phonological delays: Phonotactic constraints and probability in acquisition. *Journal of Speech, Language, and Hearing Research, 47,* 1194–1212.

Storkel, H. L., & Adlof, S. M. (2009). The effect of semantic set size on word learning by preschool children. *Journal of Speech, Language, and Hearing Research, 52,* 306–320.

Storkel, H. L., & Maekawa, J. (2005). A comparison of homonym and novel word learning: The role of phonotactic probability and word frequency. *Journal of Child Language, 32,* 827–853.

Storkel, H. L., & Morrisette, M. L. (2002). The lexicon and phonology: Interactions in language acquisition. *Language, Speech, and Hearing Services in Schools, 33,* 24–37.

Storkel, H. L., & Rogers, M. A. (2000). The effect of probabilistic phonotactics on lexical acquisition. *Clinical Linguistics & Phonetics, 14,* 407–425.

Streissguth, A., & O'Malley, K. D. (2001). Neuropsychiatric implications and long-term consequences of fetal alcohol spectrum disorders. *Seminars in Clinical Neuropsychiatry, 5,* 177–190.

Strong, C. J., & North, K. H. (1996). *The magic of stories: Literature-based language intervention.* Eau Claire, WI: Thinking Publications.

Sturm, J. M., & Nelson, N. W. (1997). Formal classroom lessons: New perspectives on a familiar discourse event. *Language, Speech, and Hearing Services in Schools, 28,* 255–273.

Sullivan, P. M., & Knutson, J. F. (2000). Maltreatment and disabilities: A population-based epidemiological study. *Child Abuse & Neglect, 24,* 1257–1275.

Sun, L., & Nippold, M. A. (2012). Narrative writing in children and adolescents: Examining the literate lexicon. *Language, Speech, and Hearing Services in Schools, 43,* 2–13.

Sundara, M., Demuth, K., & Kuhl, P. K. (2011). Sentence-position effects on children's perception and production of English third person singular *–s. Journal of Speech, Language, and Hearing Research, 54,* 55–71.

Swanson, H. L., & Beebe-Frankenberger, M. (2004). The relationship between working memory and mathematical problem solving in children at risk and not at risk for math disabilities. *Journal of Educational Psychology, 96,* 471–491.

Tabors, P. O., Roach, K. A., & Snow, C. E. (2001). Home language and literacy environment: Final results. In D. K. Dickinson & P. O. Tabors (Eds.), *Beginning literacy with language: Young children learning at home and school* (pp. 111–138). Baltimore: Paul H. Brookes.

Tabors, P. O., Snow, C. E., & Dickinson, D. K. (2001). Homes and schools together: Supporting language and literacy development. In D. K. Dickinson & P. O. Tabors (Eds.), *Beginning literacy with language* (pp. 313–334). Baltimore: Paul H. Brookes.

Tager-Flusberg, H. (2004). Do autism and specific language impairment represent overlapping language disorders? In M. L. Rice & S. F. Warren (Eds.), *Develop-*

mental language disorders: From phenotypes to etiologies (pp. 31–52). Mahwah, NJ: Erlbaum.

Tager-Flusberg, H., Paul, R., & Lord, C. E. (2005). Language and communication in autism. In F. Volkmar, R. Paul, A. Klin, & D. J. Cohen (Eds.), *Handbook of autism and pervasive developmental disorder: Vol. 1* (3rd ed., pp. 335–364). New York: Wiley.

Tallal, P. (2000). Experimental studies of language learning impairments: From research to remediation. In D. V. M. Bishop & L. B. Leonard (Eds.), *Speech and language impairments in children* (pp. 131–155). Baltimore, MD: Paul H. Brookes.

Thal, D., Jackson-Maldonado, D., & Acosta, D. (2000). Validity of a parent-report measure of vocabulary and grammar for Spanish-speaking toddlers. *Journal of Speech, Language, and Hearing Research, 43*, 1087–1100.

Theodore, R. M., Demuth, K., & Shattuck-Hufnagel, S. (2011). Acoustic evidence for positional and complexity effects on children's production of plural–*s*. *Journal of Speech, Language, and Hearing Research, 54*, 539–548.

Thiemann, K. S., & Goldstein, H. (2004). Effects of peer training and written text cueing on social communication of school-age children with pervasive developmental disorder. *Journal of Speech, Language, and Hearing Research, 47*, 126–144.

Thistle, J. J., & Wilkinson, K. (2009). The effects of color cues on typically developing preschoolers' speed of locating a target line drawing: Implications for augmentative and alternative communication display design. *American Journal of Speech-Language Pathology, 18*, 231–240.

Thomas-Tate, S., Washington, J., Craig, H., & Packard, M. (2006). Performance of African American preschool and kindergarten students on the Expressive Vocabulary Test. *Language, Speech, and Hearing Services in Schools, 37*, 143–149.

Thomas-Tate, S., Washington, J., & Edwards, J. (2004). Standardized assessment of phonological awareness skills in low-income African American first graders. *American Journal of Speech-Language Pathology, 13*, 182–190.

Thordardottir, E. (2008). Language-specific effects of task demands on the manifestation of specific language impairment: A comparison of English and Icelandic. *Journal of Speech, Language, and Hearing Research, 51*, 922–937.

Thorell, L., Lindqvist, S., Nutley, S., Bohlin, G., & Klingberg, T. (2009). Training and transfer effects of executive functions in preschool children. *Developmental Science, 12*, 106–113.

Thorne, J. C. (2004). *The Semantic Elaboration Coding System*. Unpublished training manual, University of Washington, Seattle.

Thorne, J. C., Coggins, T. E., Carmichael Olson, H., & Astley, S. J. (2007). Exploring the utility of narrative analysis is diagnostic decision making: Picture-bound reference, elaboration, and fetal alcohol spectrum disorders. *Journal of Speech, Language, and Hearing Research, 50*, 459–474.

Thorum, A. R. (1986). *Fullerton Language Tests for Adolescents* (2nd ed.). Austin, TX: Pro-Ed.

Thothathiri, M., & Snedeker, J. (2008). Syntactic priming during language comprehension in three- and four-year-old children. *Journal of Memory and Language, 58*, 188–213.

Throneburg, R. N., Calvert, L. K., Sturm, J. M., Paramboukas, A. M., Paul, P. (2000). A comparision of service delivery models: Effects on curricular vocabulary skills in the school setting. *American Journal of Speech-Language Pathology, 9*, 10–20.

Tilstra, J., & McMaster, K. (2007). Productivity, fluency, and grammaticality measures from narratives: Potential indicators of language proficiency? *Communication Disorders Quarterly, 29*, 43–53.

Timler, G. R., Olswang, L., & Coggins, T. (2005). "Do I know what I need to do?" A social communication intervention for children with complex clinical profiles. *Language, Speech, and Hearing Services in Schools, 36*, 73–84.

Timler, G. R., Vogler-Elias, D., & McGill, K. F. (2007). Strategies for promoting generalization of social communication skills in preschoolers and school-aged children. *Topics in Language Disorders, 27*, 167–181.

Tomasello, M. (2003). *Constructing a language: A usage based theory of language acquisition.* Cambridge, MA: Harvard University Press.

Tomblin, J. B., Barker, B. A., Spencer, L. J., Zhang, X., & Gantz, B. J. (2005). The effect of age at cochlear implant initial stimulation on expressive language growth in infants and toddlers. *Journal of Speech, Language, and Hearing Research, 48*, 853–867.

Tomblin, J. B., Mainela-Arnold, E., & Zhang, X. (2007). Procedural learning in adolescents with and without specific language impairment. *Language Learning and Development, 3*, 269–293.

Tomblin, J. B., Zhang, X., Buckwalter, P., & O'Brien, M. (2003). The stability of primary language disorders: Four years after kindergarten diagnosis. *Journal of Speech, Language, and Hearing Research, 46*, 1283–1296.

Tönsing, K. M., & Tesner, H. (1999). Story grammar analysis of pre-schoolers' narratives: An investigation into the influence of task parameters. *The South African Journal of Communication Disorders, 46*, 37–44.

Torgesen, J. K., & Bryant, B. R. (1994). *Test of Phonological Awareness*. Austin, TX: Pro-Ed.

Torgesen, J. K., Rashotte, C. A., & Alexander, A. W. (2001). Principles of fluency instruction in reading: Relationships with established empirical outcomes. In M. Wolf (Ed.), *Dyslexia, fluency and the brain* (pp. 332–355). Timonium, MD: York Press.

Towey, M., Whitcomb, J., & Bray, C. (2004, November). *Print-sound-story-talk: A successful early reading first program.*

Paper presented at the American Speech-Language-Hearing Association Annual Convention, Philadelphia.

Troia, G. A., Graham, S., & Harris, K. R. (1999) Teaching students with learning disabilities to mindfully plan when writing. *Exceptional Children, 65*, 235–252.

Tsatsanis, K. D., Foley, C., & Donehower, C. (2004). Contemporary outcome research and programming guidelines for Asperger's syndrome and high-functioning autism. *Topics in Language Disorders, 24*, 249–259.

Tucker, J., & McGuire, W. (2004). *Epidemiology of preterm birth.* London, UK: BMJ Publishing Group Ltd.

Turkstra, L. S., Ciccia, A., & Seaton, C. (2003). Interactive behaviors in adolescent conversation dyads. *Language, Speech, and Hearing Services in Schools, 34*, 117–127.

Tyack, D., & Gottsleben, R. (1977). *Language sampling, analysis, and training: A handbook for teachers and clinicians.* Palo Alto: Consulting Psychologists Press.

Uccelli, P., & Páez, M. M. (2007). Narrative and vocabulary development of bilingual children from kindergarten to first grade: Developmental changes.

Ukrainetz, T. A., & Gillam, R. B. (2009). The expressive elaboration of imaginative narratives by children with Specific Language Impairment. *Journal of Speech, Language, and Hearing Research, 52*, 883–898.

Ukrainetz, T. A., Justice, L. M., Kaderavek, J. N., Eisenberg, S. L., Gillam, R. B., & Harm, H. M. (2005). The development of expressive elaboration in fictional narratives. *Journal of Speech, Language, and Hearing Research, 48*, 1363–1377.

Ullman, M., & Pierpoint, E. (2005). Specific language impairment is not specific to language: The procedural deficit hypothesis. *Cortex, 41*, 399–433.

U.S. Conference of Mayors. (2003). *A status report on hunger and homelessness in America's cities: 2003.* Washington, DC: Author.

U.S. Department of Education, National Center for Education Statistics. (2006). *The condition of education 2006* (NCES 2006-071), Indicator 2. Available from nces.ed.gov/pubs2006/2006071.pdf.

U.S. Department of Education, Office of English Language Acquisition, Language Enhancement, and Academic Achievement for Limited English Proficient Students. (2008). *The Biennial Report to Congress on the Implementation of the Title III State Formula Grant Program: School Years 2004-06.* Washington, DC: Author.

U.S. Department of Health and Human Services, Administration on Children, Youth and Families. (2007). *Child Maltreatment 2005.* Washington, DC: U.S. Government Printing Office.

U.S. Department of Health and Human Services' Substance Abuse and Mental Health Administration. (2008). *Fetal alcohol spectrum disorders.* Retrieved August 1, 2008, from www.fascenter.samhsa.gov

U.S. Department of State. (2007). *Immigrant visas offered to orphans coming to the U.S.* Retrieved from travel.state.gov/family/adoption/stats/stats_451.html

U.S. Government Accountability Office. (2005). *Report to the Chairman and Ranking Minority Member, Subcommittee on Human Rights and Wellness, Committee on Government Reform, House of Representatives: Special education, children with autism.* (GAO-05-220). Washington, DC: Author.

U.S. National Library of Medicine. (2010, December 15). *Mental retardation.* Accessed January 2, 2011, from U.S. Department of Health and Human Services, National Institutes of Health, www.nlm.nih.gov/medlineplus/ency/article/001523.htm

Vallecorsa, A. L. & Garriss, E. (1990). Story composition skills in middle-grade students with learning disability. *Exceptional Children, 57*, 48–54.

van Kleeck, A. (1995). Emphasizing form and meaning separately in prereading and early reading instruction. *Topics in Language Disorders, 16*(1), 27–49.

van Kleeck, A. (2003). Research on book sharing: Another critical look. In A. van Kleeck, S. A. Stahl, & E. Bauer (Eds.), *On reading to children: Parents and teachers* (pp. 271–320). Hillside, NJ: Erlbaum.

van Kleeck, A., Vander Woude, J. & Hammett, L. (2006). Fostering literal and inferential language skills in Head Start preschoolers with language impairment using scripted-sharing discussions. *American Journal of Speech-Language Pathology, 15*, 89–95.

Vandereet, J., Maes, B., Lembrechts, D., & Zink, I. (2010). Predicting expressive vocabulary acquisition in children with intellectual disabilities: A 2-year longitudinal study. *Journal of Speech, Language, and Hearing Research, 53*, 1673–1686.

Vigil, A., & van Kleeck, A. (1996). Clinical language teaching: Theories and principles to guide our responses when children miss our language targets. In M. Smith & J. Damico (Eds.), *Childhood language disorders* (pp. 64–96). New York: Thieme.

Virtue, S., & Haberman, J., Clancy, Z., Parrish, T., & Beeman, M. (2006). Neural activity of inferences during story comprehension. *Brain Research, 1084*, 104–114.

Virtue, S., & van den Broek, P. (2004). Hemispheric processing of anaphoric inferences: The activation of multiple antecedents. *Brain and Language, 93*, 327–337.

Virtue, S., van den Broek, P., & Linderholm, T. (2006). Hemispheric processing of inferences: The effects of textual constraint and working memory capacity. *Memory & Cognition, 34*, 1341–1355.

Volden, J. (2002). Features leading to judgments of inappropriacy in the language of speakers with autism: A preliminary study. *Journal of Speech-Language Pathology and Audiology, 26*(3), 138–146.

Volden, J. (2004). Conversational repair in speakers with autism spectrum disorder. *International Journal of Language and Communication Disorders, 39*, 171–189.

Volden, J., & Phillips, L. (2010). Measuring pragmatic language in speakers with Autism Spectrum Disorders: Comparing the children's Communication Checklist-2 and the Test of Pragmatic Language. *American Journal of Speech-Language Pathology, 19,* 204–212.

Vygotsky, L. (1978). *Mind in society: The development of higher psychological processes.* Cambridge, MA: Harvard University Press.

Wadman, R., Durkin, K., & Conti-Ramsden, G. (2008). Self-esteem, shyness, and sociability in adolescents with Specific Language Impairment (SLI). *Journal of Speech, Language, and Hearing Research, 51,* 938–952.

Wagner, R. E., Torgesen, J. K., & Rashotte, C. (1999). *Comprehensive Test of Phonological Processing (CTOPP).* Austin, TX: Pro-Ed.

Wahlberg, T., & Magliano, J. P. (2004). The ability of high-functioning individuals with autism to comprehend written discourse. *Discourse Processes, 38*(1), 119–144.

Waite, M. C., Theodoros, D. G., Russell, T. G., & Cahill, L. M. (2010). Internet-based telehealth assessment of language using the CELF-4. *Language, Speech and Hearing Services in Schools, 41,* 445–458.

Walker, D. R., Thompson, A., Zwaigenbaum, L., Goldberg, J., Bryson, S. E., Mahoney, W. J., Strawbridge, C. P., & Szatmarim P. (2004). Specifying PDD-NOS: A comparison of PDD-NOS, Asperger syndrome, and autism. *Journal of the American Academy of Child and Adolescent Psychiatry, 43,* 172–180.

Wallace, G., & Hammill, D. D. (2002). *Comprehensive Receptive and Expressive Vocabulary Test* (2nd ed.). Austin, TX: Pro-Ed.

Wanzek, J., Dickson, S., Bursuck, W., & White, J. (2000). Teaching phonological awareness to students at risk for reading failure: An analysis of four instructional programs. *Learning Disabilities Research & Practice, 15,* 226–239.

Warren, S. F., & Rogers-Warren, A. (1985). Teaching functional language: An introduction. In S. Warren & A. Rogers-Warren (Eds.), *Teaching functional language* (pp. 3–24). Baltimore: University Park Press.

Washington, J. A., Craig, H. K., & Kushmaul, A. J. (1998). Variable use of African American English across two language sampling contexts. *Journal of Speech, Language, and Hearing Research, 41,* 1115–1124.

Wasik, B. A., Bond, M. A., & Hindman, A. (2006). The effects of a language and literacy intervention on Head Start children and teachers. *Journal of Educational Psychology, 98,* 63–74.

Wasowicz, J., Apel, K., Masterson, J. J., & Whitney, A. (2004). *SPELL—Links to Reading and Writing.* Evanston, IL: Learning By Design.

Watson, L. R., & Ozonoff, S. (2000). Pervasive developmental disorders. In T. L. Layton, E. Crais, & L. R. Watson (Eds.), *Handbook of early language impairment in children: Nature* (pp. 109–161). Albany, NY: Delmar.

Watt, N., Wetherby, A., & Shumway, S. (2006). Prelinguistic predictors of language outcome at 3 years of age. *Journal of Speech, Language, and Hearing Research, 49,* 1224–1237.

Way, I., Yelsma, P., Van Meter, A. M., & Black-Pond, C. (2007). Understanding alexithymia and language skills in children: Implications for assessment and intervention. *Language, Speech, and Hearing Services in Schools, 38,* 128–139.

Wayman, K. I., Lynch, E. W., & Hanson, M. J. (1990). Home-based early childhood services: Cultural sensitivity in a family systems approach. *Topics in Early Childhood Special Education, 10*(4), 56–75.

Weiner, F. (1988). Parrot Easy Language Sample Analysis (PELSA) [Computer program]. State College, PA: Parrot Software.

Weinreb, L. F., Buckner, J. C., Williams, V., & Nicholson, J. (2006). A comparison of the health and mental health status of homeless mothers in Worcester, Mass: 1993 and 2003. *American Journal of Public Health, 96,* 1444–1448.

Weitzman, E., & Greenberg, J. (2002). *Learning language and loving it* (2nd ed.). Toronto: The Hanen Center.

Wells, G. (1985). *Language development in the pre-school years.* New York: Cambridge University Press.

Wentzel, M. (2000, November 29). UR first to identify autistic gene. (Rochester, NY) *Democrat and Chronicle,* pp. 1A, 10A.

Westby, C. E. (1984). Development of narrative language abilities. In G. Wallach & K. Butler (Eds.), *Language learning disabilities in school-age children* (pp. 103–127). Baltimore: Williams & Wilkins.

Westby, C. E. (1992). Narrative assessment. *Best Practices in School Speech-Language Pathology, 2,* 53–64.

Westby, C. E. (1997). There's more to passing than knowing the answers. *Language, Speech, and Hearing Services in Schools, 28,* 244–287.

Westby, C. E. (2005). Assessing and facilitating text comprehension problems. In H. Catts & A. Kamhi (Eds.), *Language and reading disabilities* (pp. 157–232). Boston: Allyn & Bacon.

Westby, C. E. (2007). Child maltreatment: A global issue. *Language, Speech, and Hearing Services in Schools, 38,* 140–148.

Westby, C. E., Van Dongen, R., & Maggart, Z. (1989). Assessing narrative competence. *Seminars in Speech and Language, 10,* 63–76.

Westerveld, M. F., & Moran, C. A. (2011). Expository language skills of young school-age children. *Language, Speech, and Hearing Services in Schools, 42,* 182–193.

Wetherby, A. M., & Prizant, B. M. (1993). *Communication and Symbolic Behavior Scales.* Chicago: Riverside.

Wetherby, A. M., Prizant, B. M., & Schuler, A. (2000). Understanding the nature of communication and language impairments. In A. Wetherby & B. Prizant (Eds.), *Autism spectrum disorders: A transactional developmental perspective* (pp. 109–141). Baltimore: Paul H. Brookes.

Wetherby, A. M., & Woods, J. J. (2006). Early social interaction project for children with autism spectrum disorders beginning in the second year of life: A preliminary study. *Topics in Early Childhood Special Education, 26,* 67–82.

Whitehouse, A. J. (2010). Is there a sex ratio difference in the familial aggregation of Specific Language Impairment? A meta-analysis. *Journal of Speech, Language, and Hearing Research, 53,* 1015–1025.

Wiederholt, J. L., & Bryant, B. R. (2001). *Gray Oral Reading Test.* Austin, TX: Pro-Ed.

Wiig, E. H. (1995). Teaching prosocial communication. In D. F. Tibbits (Ed.), *Language intervention: Beyond the primary grades. For clinicians by clinicians.* Austin, TX: Pro-Ed.

Wiig, E. H., & Semel, E. M. (1984). *Language assessment and intervention for the learning disabled* (2nd ed.). New York: Merrill/Macmillan.

Wilcox, M. J., Bacon, C. K., & Greer, D. C. (2005). *Evidence-based early language intervention: Caregiver verbal responsivity training.* Accessed on June 23, 2010, from www.asu.edu/clas/icrp/research/presentations/p1/pdf2.pdf

Wilcox, M. J., & Woods, J. (2011). Participation as a basis for developing early intervention outcomes. *Language, Speech, and Hearing Services in Schools, 42,* 365–378.

Wilkinson, G. S., (1995). *Wide Range of Achievement Test–3.* Wilmington, DE: Jastak Associates.

Williams, J. P. (1988). Identifying main ideas: A basic aspect of reading comprehension. *Topics in Language Disorders, 8(3),* 1–13.

Williams, K. (1997). *Expressive Vocabulary Test.* Circle Pines, MN: American Guidance Service.

Willis, D., & Silovsky, J. (1998). Prevention of violence at the societal level. In P. Trickett & C. Schellenach (Eds.), *Violence against children in the family and the community* (pp. 401–416). Washington, DC: American Psychological Association.

Windsor, J., Kohnert, K., Loxtercamp, A., & Kan, P. (2008). Performance on nonlinguistic visual tasks by children with language impairment. *Applied Psycholinguistics, 29,* 237–268.

Windsor, J., Scott, C. M., & Street, C. K. (2000). Verb and noun morphology in the spoken and written language of children with language learning disabilities. *Journal of Speech, Language, and Hearing Research, 43,* 1322–1336.

Wing, C., Kohnert, K., Pham, G., Cordero, K. N., Ebert, K. D., Kan, P. F., & Blaiser, K. (2007). Culturally consistent treatment for late talkers. *Communication Disorders Quarterly, 29* (1), 20–27.

Wise, B., Rogan, L., & Sessions, L. (2009). Training teachers in evidence-based intervention: The story of linguistic remedies. In S. Rosenfield & V. Berninger (Eds.), *Handbook on implementing evidence based academic interventions* (pp. 443–477). Oxford, England: Oxford University Press.

Wixson, K., Bosky, A., Yochum, M., & Alvermann, D. (1984). An interview for assessing students' perceptions of classroom reading tasks. *The Reading Teacher, 37,* 346–352.

Wolf, M. (2007). *Proust and the squid: The story and science of the reading brain.* New York: HarperCollins Books.

Wolf, M., & Denkla, M. (2005). *Rapid Automatized Naming and Rapid Alternating Stimulus Tests.* Hydesville, CA: Psychological and Educational Publications.

Wolf, M., & Katzir-Cohen, T. (2001). Reading fluency and its intervention. *Scientific Studies of Reading,* 5, 211–239.

Wolfberg, P. (1999). *Play and imagination in children with autism.* New York: Teachers College Press.

Wolter, J. A., & Apel, K. (2010). Initial acquisition of mental graphemic representations in children with language impairment. *Journal of Speech, Language, and Hearing Research, 53,* 179–195.

Wolter, J. A., Wood, A., & D'zatko, K. W. (2009). The influence of morphological awareness on the literacy development of first-grade children. *Language, Speech, and Hearing Services in Schools, 40,* 286–298.

Wong, B. Y. (2000). Writing strategies instruction for expository essays for adolescents with and without learning disabilities. *Topics in Language Disorders, 20(4),* 244.

Wong, B. Y., Butler, D. L., Ficzere, S. A., & Kuperis, S. (1996). Teaching low achievers and students with learning disabilities to plan, write, and revise opinion essays. *Journal of Learning Disabilities, 29(2),* 197–212.

Woodcock, R. W. (1998). *Woodcock Reading Mastery Test–Revised.* Circle Pines, MN: American Guidance Services.

Woods, J. J., & Wetherby, A. M. (2003). Early identification of and intervention for infants and toddlers who are at risk for autism spectrum disorder. *Language, Speech, and Hearing Services in Schools, 34,* 180–193.

Woods, J. J., Wilcox, M. J., Friedman, M., & Murch, T. (2011). Collaborative consultation in natural environments: Strategies to enhance family-centered supports and services. *Language, Speech, and Hearing Services in Schools, 42,* 379–392.

World Health Assembly. (2001). Retrieved from www.who.int/classifications/icf/whaen.pdf

World Health Organization (1981). *The global strategy for health for all by the year 2000.* Geneva, Switzerland: Author.

World Health Organization. (2005). *International statistical classification of diseases and related health problems, Tenth Revision.* Geneva, Switzerland: Author.

World Health Organization. (2010). *Mental retardation: From knowledge to action.* Accessed January 2, 2011 at www.searo.who.int/en/Section1174/Section1199/Section1567/Section1825_8090.htm

Ylvisaker, M., & DeBonis, D. (2000). Executive function impairment in adolescence: TBI and ADHD. *Topics in Language Disorders, 20(2),* 29–57.

Ylvisaker, M., Szekeres, S. F., & Feeney, T. (1998). Cognitive rehabilitation: Executive functions. In M. Ylvisaker (Ed.), *Traumatic brain injury rehabilitation: Children and adolescents* (pp. 221–269). Boston: Butterworth-Heinemann.

Yoder, P. J., & McDuffie, A. (2002). Treatment of primary language disorders in early childhood: Evidence of efficacy.

In P. Accardo, B. Rogers, & A. Capute (Eds.), *Disorders of language development* (pp. 151–177). Baltimore, MD: York Press.

Yoder, P. J., Molfese, D., & Gardner, E. (2011). Initial mean length of utterance predicts the relative efficacy of two grammatical treatments in preschoolers with Specific Language Impairment. *Journal of Speech, Language, and Hearing Research, 54,* 1170–1181.

Yoder, P. J., & Warren, S. F. (2002). Effects of prelinguistic milieu reaching and parent responsivity education on dyads involving children with intellectual disabilities. *Journal of Speech, Language, and Hearing Research, 45,* 1158–1174.

Yoshinaga-Itano, C., & Snyder, L. (1985). Form and meaning in the written language of hearing impaired children. *Volta Review, 87*(5), 75–90.

Young, E., Diehl, J., Morris, D., Hyman, S., & Bennetto, L. (2005). The use of two language tests to identify pragmatic language problems in children with autism spectrum disorders. *Language, Speech, and Hearing Services in Schools, 36,* 62–72.

Zimmerman, I. L., Steiner, V. G., & Pond, R. E. (2002). *Preschool Language Scale, Fourth Edition, Spanish Edition.* San Antonio, TX: Harcourt Assessment.

Zipoli, R. P., & Kennedy, M. (2005). Evidence-based practice among speech-language pathologists: Attitudes, utilization, and barriers. *American Journal of Speech-Language Pathology, 14,* 208–220.

Zwaigenbaum, L., Bryson, S. E., Rogers, T., Roberts, W., Brian, J., & Szatmaxi, P. (2005). Behavioural manifestations of autism in the first year of life. *International Journal of Developmental Neuroscience, 23,* 143–152.

Author Index

Subject Index

D